Neuroscience for Neurosurgeons

Neuroscience for Neurosurgeons

Edited by

Farhana Akter
Harvard University

Nigel Emptage
University of Oxford

Florian Engert
Harvard University

Mitchel S. Berger
University of California–San Francisco

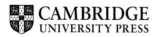
CAMBRIDGE
UNIVERSITY PRESS

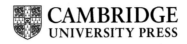

Shaftesbury Road, Cambridge CB2 8EA, United Kingdom

One Liberty Plaza, 20th Floor, New York, NY 10006, USA

477 Williamstown Road, Port Melbourne, VIC 3207, Australia

314–321, 3rd Floor, Plot 3, Splendor Forum, Jasola District Centre, New Delhi – 110025, India

103 Penang Road, #05–06/07, Visioncrest Commercial, Singapore 238467

Cambridge University Press is part of Cambridge University Press & Assessment, a department of the University of Cambridge.

We share the University's mission to contribute to society through the pursuit of education, learning and research at the highest international levels of excellence.

www.cambridge.org
Information on this title: www.cambridge.org/9781108831468

DOI: 10.1017/9781108917339

First published 2024 (version 1, January 2024)

Printed in the United Kingdom by CPI Group Ltd, Croydon CR0 4YY

A catalogue record for this publication is available from the British Library.

Library of Congress Cataloging-in-Publication Data
Names: Akter, Farhana (Surgeon), editor. | Emptage, Nigel, editor. | Engert, Florian, editor. | Berger, Mitchel S., editor.
Title: Neuroscience for neurosurgeons / edited by Farhana Akter, Nigel Emptage, Florian Engert, Mitchel S. Berger.
Description: Cambridge, United Kingdom; New York, NY: Cambridge University Press, 2023. | Includes bibliographical references and index.
Identifiers: LCCN 2023017267 | ISBN 9781108831468 (hardback) | ISBN 9781108917339 (ebook)
Subjects: MESH: Neurosurgical Procedures | Nervous System Diseases – physiopathology | Nervous System – physiology
Classification: LCC RD592.8 | NLM WL 368 | DDC 617.4/8092–dc23/eng/20230703
LC record available at https://lccn.loc.gov/2023017267

ISBN 978-1-108-83146-8 Hardback

....

Every effort has been made in preparing this book to provide accurate and up-to-date information that is in accord with accepted standards and practice at the time of publication. Although case histories are drawn from actual cases, every effort has been made to disguise the identities of the individuals involved. Nevertheless, the authors, editors, and publishers can make no warranties that the information contained herein is totally free from error, not least because clinical standards are constantly changing through research and regulation. The authors, editors, and publishers therefore disclaim all liability for direct or consequential damages resulting from the use of material contained in this book. Readers are strongly advised to pay careful attention to information provided by the manufacturer of any drugs or equipment that they plan to use.

Contents

Contributors

Adib A. Abla
University of California San Francisco, California, USA

Kingsley Abode-Iyamah
Mayo Clinic, Jacksonville, FL, USA

Farhana Akter
Harvard University, Cambridge, MA, USA

Michael Argenziano
Columbia University College of Physicians and Surgeons, New York, NY, USA

Oluwatobi Ariyo
Harvard University, Cambridge, MA, USA

David M. Ashley
Duke University School of Medicine, Durham, NC, USA

Joel S. Beckett
David Geffen UCLA School of Medicine, CA, USA

Joseph S. Bell
UCLA Department of Neurosurgery, Los Angeles, CA, USA

Dhiego Bastos
Brigham and Women's Hospital, Boston, MA, USA

Karol P. Budohoski
University of Utah, Utah, USA

Allison Chang
Harvard University, Cambridge, MA, USA

Megan Chau
Northwestern University, Evanston, IL, USA

Rachel Chau
Harvard University, Cambridge, MA, USA

Pakawat Chongsathidkiet
Duke University Medical Center, Durham, NC, USA

Cecilia Dalle Ore
University of California San Francisco, San Francisco, CA, USA

Gaetano De Biase
Mayo Clinic, Jacksonville, FL, USA

Massimiliano Del Bene
Fondazione IRCCS Istituto Neurologico Carlo Besta, Milan, Italy and European Institute of Oncology IRCCS, Milan, Italy

Francesco DiMeco
Fondazione IRCCS Istituto Neurologico Carlo Besta, Milan, Italy, University of Milan, Milan, Italy, and Johns Hopkins Medical School, Baltimore, MD, USA

Christophe Dupre
Harvard University, Cambridge, MA, USA

Phan Q. Duy
Yale School of Medicine, New Haven, CT, USA

Roberto Eleopra
Fondazione IRCCS Istituto Neurologico Carlo Besta, Milan, Italy

Nigel Emptage
University of Oxford, Oxford, UK

Peter E. Fecci
Duke University Medical Center, Durham, NC, USA and Duke University Center for Brain and Spine Metastasis, Durham, NC, USA

T.J. Florence
David Geffen UCLA School of Medicine, CA, USA

Alexandra J. Golby
Brigham and Women's Hospital, Boston, MA, USA

Matthew M. Grabowski
Cleveland Clinic Neurological Institute, Cleveland, OH, USA

Maya Harary
UCLA Department of Neurosurgery, Los Angeles, CA, USA

Shawn L. Hervey-Jumper
University of California San Francisco, San Francisco, CA, USA

Dominique M. O. Higgins
Columbia University College of Physicians and Surgeons, New York, NY, USA

Langston T. Holly
David Geffen UCLA School of Medicine, CA, USA

Katrina Hon
Harvard University, Cambridge, MA, USA

Shifa Hossain
Harvard University, Cambridge, MA, USA

Jason H. Huang
Baylor Scott and White Health, Medical Center, Temple, TX, USA and Texas A&M University Health Science Center, College of Medicine, Temple, TX, USA

Charlotte J. Huie
University of California San Francisco (UCSF), San Francisco, CA, USA

Andrew S. Jack
University of Alberta, Edmonton, AB, Canada and University of California San Francisco (UCSF), San Francisco, CA, USA

Line Jacques
University of California San Francisco (UCSF), San Francisco, CA, USA

Yike Jin
Johns Hopkins Hospital, Baltimore, MD, USA

Kristopher T. Kahle
Yale School of Medicine, New Haven, CT, USA

Maria Kaltchenko
Harvard University, Cambridge, MA, USA

Jason K. Karimy
Yale School of Medicine, New Haven, CT, USA

Kristin A. Keith
Baylor Scott and White Health, Medical Center, Temple, TX, USA and Texas A&M University Health Science Center, College of Medicine, Temple, TX, USA

Gabriel Kreiman
Harvard Medical School, Boston, MA, USA

Kumaresh Krishnan
Harvard University, Cambridge, MA, USA

Anthony T. Lee
University of California San Francisco, San Francisco, CA, USA

Yingda Li
Westmead Hospital, Sydney, Australia

Ann Liu
Johns Hopkins Hospital, Baltimore, MD, USA

Justin T. Low
Duke University School of Medicine, Durham, NC, USA

Paul McCormick
Columbia University College of Physicians and Surgeons, New York, NY, USA

Ravi Medikonda
Johns Hopkins Hospital, Baltimore, MD, USA

Maxwell D. Melin
UCLA-Caltech Medical Scientist Training Program, Los Angeles, CA, USA

Alaa Montaser
Boston Children's Hospital, Boston, MA, USA

Ziev B. Moses
Rush University Medical Center, Chicago, IL, USA

Zachary T. Miller
Harvard University, Cambridge, MA, USA

Parisa Nikrouz
Maidstone and Tunbridge Wells NHS Trust, Kent, UK

John E. O'Toole
Rush University Medical Center, Chicago, IL, USA

John A. Persing
Yale School of Medicine, New Haven, CT, USA

Nader Pouratian
UT Southwestern Medical Center, Dallas, TX USA

Francesco Prada
Fondazione IRCCS Istituto Neurologico Carlo Besta, Milan, Italy, University of Virginia Health Science Center, Charlottesville, VA, USA, and Focused Ultrasound Foundation, Charlottesville, VA, USA

Xingping Qin
Harvard School of Public Health, Boston, MA, USA

Umar Raza
National University of Medical Sciences (NUMS), Rawalpindi, Pakistan

Benjamin C. Reeves
Yale School of Medicine, New Haven, CT, USA

Charles Reilly
Harvard University, Cambridge, MA, USA

Eric W. Sankey
Duke University Medical Center, Durham, NC, USA

David J. Segar
Brigham and Women's Hospital, Boston, MA, USA

John T. Smetona
Yale School of Medicine, New Haven, CT, USA

Edward R. Smith
Boston Children's Hospital, Boston, MA, USA

Hiro Sparks
UCLA David Geffen School of Medicine, Los Angeles, CA, USA

Ethan S. Srinivasan
Duke University Medical Center, Durham, NC, USA

Jasmine A. Thum
Brigham and Women's Hospital, Boston, MA, USA

Matthew Trawczynski
Rush University Medical Center, Chicago, IL, USA
Vadim Tsvankin
Colorado Brain and Spine Institute, Denver, CO, USA

Vadim Tsvankin
Colorado Brain and Spine Institute, Denver, CO, USA

Pavan S. Upadhyayula
Columbia University College of Physicians and Surgeons, New York, NY, USA

Michael Y. Wang
University of Miami Miller School of Medicine, Miami, FL, USA

Timothy F. Witham
Johns Hopkins Hospital, Baltimore, MD, USA

Ye Wu
Nanjing University of Science and Technology, Nanjing, Jiangsu, China

Will Xiao
Harvard Medical School, Boston, MA, USA

Shun Yao
The First Affiliated Hospital, Sun Yat-sen University, Guangzhou, Guangdong, China

Mengmi Zhang
Harvard Medical School, Boston, MA, USA

Neuroanatomy

Farhana Akter, Charles Reilly, Christophe Dupre, and Shifa Hossain

1.1 Anatomical Planes and Orientation of the Brain

The neuroaxis of humans and other bipedal orthograde animals is different from that of quadruped animals. Example axes include the anteroposterior axis, rostrocaudal axis and the dorsoventral axis (Figure 1.1). The brain is usually visualized in sections cut through three orthogonal planes: sagittal (longitudinal), coronal, and transverse (axial) planes.

1.2 Vascular Supply to the Brain

The brain requires 15–20% of the resting cardiac output and is exquisitely sensitive to oxygen deprivation. Two main pairs of arteries supply blood to the brain: the internal carotid arteries and the vertebral arteries. Within the cranial vault, an anastomotic circle, called the Circle of Willis (Figure 1.3), forms from the terminal branches of these arteries.

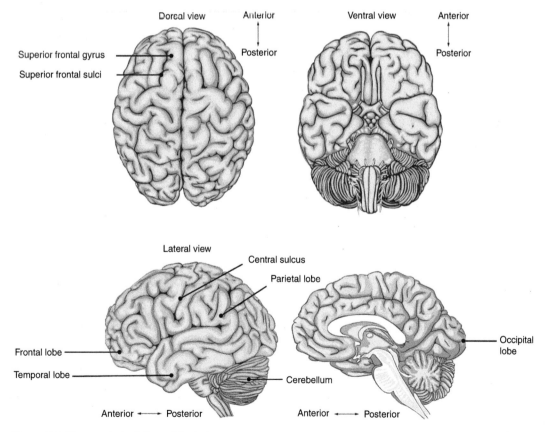

Figure 1.1 Planes and orientations of the brain.

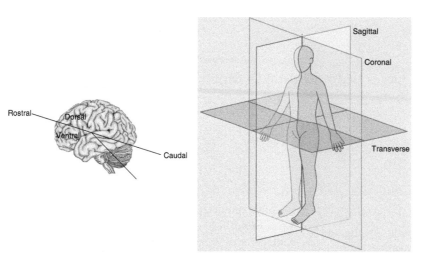

Figure 1.2 Planes and orientations of the body.

The brachiocephalic trunk arises from the aorta and bifurcates into the right common carotid and right subclavian artery. The left common carotid artery and subclavian artery branches off directly from the aortic arch. The common carotid arteries divide at the level of the thyroid cartilage (C4) into external and internal carotid arteries. The carotid sinus, a dilation at the base of the internal carotid artery, is a baroreceptor (stretch receptor) that detects changes in systemic blood pressure. Intimately related to it, is the carotid body, made up of glomus type I chemoreceptor cells and glomus type II supporting cells. The chemoreceptors are primarily sensors of partial pressure of oxygen (PaO_2). The central chemoreceptors in the medulla oblongata are the primary sensors of the partial pressure of carbon dioxide ($PaCO_2$) and pH, however the carotid bodies also play a secondary role.

The external carotid artery divides into the superficial temporal artery and the maxillary artery within the parotid gland and gives rise to six branches (superior thyroid artery, lingual artery, facial artery, ascending pharyngeal artery, occipital artery, and posterior auricular artery). The maxillary artery gives rise to the middle meningeal artery, which passes through the foramen spinosum to enter the cranial cavity.

The internal carotid artery enters the cranial cavity via the carotid canal in the petrous part of the temporal bone, passes through the cavernous sinus and penetrates the dura into the subarachnoid space. Distal to the cavernous sinus, it gives rise to the following branches: ophthalmic artery, posterior communicating artery, anterior choroidal artery, and anterior cerebral artery. It then continues as the middle cerebral artery. The anterior cerebral artery supplies the frontal lobes and medial aspects of the parietal and occipital lobes (Figure 1.4).

The middle cerebral artery is the largest cerebral artery and supplies the somatosensory and motor cortex, basal ganglia, and the cerebral white matter. It can be divided into four main surgical segments, denominated M1 (sphenoidal/horizontal), M2 (insular), M3 (opercular), and M4 (cortical) segments. M1 gives rise to the lenticulostriate perforating end arteries supplying the basal ganglia and internal capsule. Occlusion of these vessels can cause lacunar infarcts, the most common type of ischemic stroke. Hypertensive lipohyalinosis of these vessels can lead to the formation of Charcot-Bouchard aneurysms and these are a principal cause of intracerebral hemorrhage. The cortical branches of MCA arise from all of its segments and supply most of the lateral surface of the brain and include the anterior temporal arteries from M1, lateral frontobasal artery from M2, and parietal branches from M4. The vertebral arteries arise from the subclavian artery and pass though the foramen transversarium in the cervical vertebrae. The vertebral arteries enter the cranium via the foramen magnum and merge to form the basilar artery. Branches of this artery include the anterior and posterior inferior cerebellar arteries supplying the brainstem and the cerebellum alongside the superior cerebellar arteries. The basilar artery bifurcates into the posterior cerebral arteries and supplies the occipital lobes.

1.2.1 Circle of Willis

An anastomotic circle is formed around the optic chiasm between the anterior cerebral arteries (via the anterior

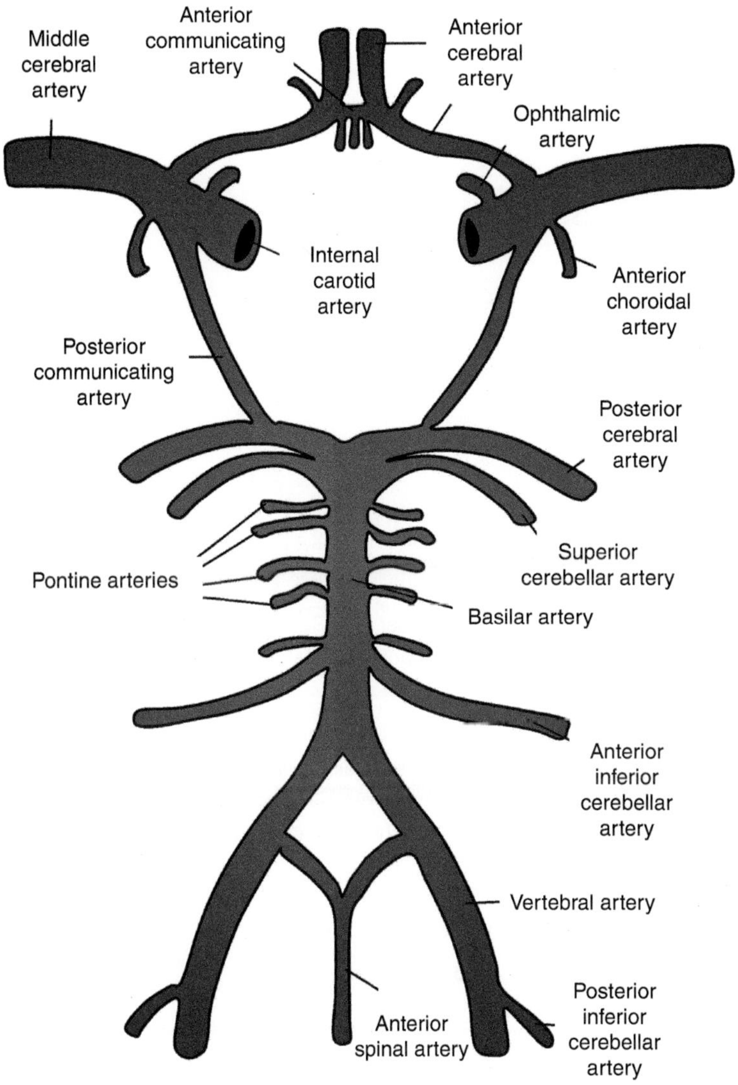

Figure 1.3 Circle of Willis.

Figure 1.3 Circle of Willis.

communicating artery) and the posterior cerebral arteries (via the posterior communicating arteries).

1.2.2 Cerebral Venous Drainage

The superficial system of veins draining the cerebral cortex include the superior cerebral veins, middle cerebral veins, inferior cerebral veins, superior and inferior anastomotic veins. The superficial veins drain into the superior and inferior sagittal sinuses (Figure 1.4).

The deep veins include subependymal veins, the great cerebral vein, and medullary veins. The deep veins drain into the great cerebral vein and then to the straight or transverse sinuses.

The dural venous sinuses are valveless structures found between the periosteal and meningeal layer of the dura mater and drain into the internal jugular vein. The straight, superior, and inferior sagittal sinuses are found in the falx cerebri of the dura mater and converge at the confluence of sinuses. From here the transverse sinus, located bilaterally in the tentorium cerebelli, curves into the sigmoid sinus and then to the internal jugular vein, which exits at the jugular foramen. The great cerebral vein and the inferior sagittal sinus continue as the straight sinus.

The cavernous sinus is clinically relevant due to its vulnerability as a site of infection. It contains the internal

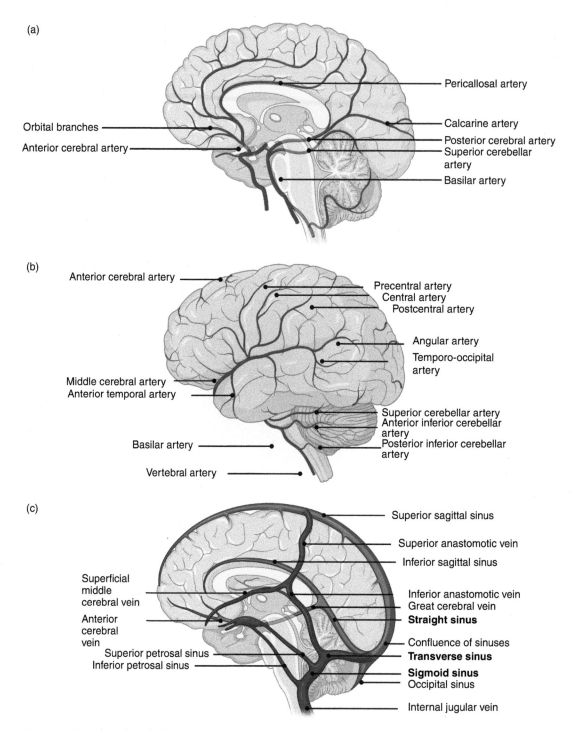

Figure 1.4 Arterial supply to the brain and venous drainage.

carotid artery, abducens nerve, oculomotor nerve, trochlear nerve, and the ophthalmic and maxillary branches of the trigeminal nerve. The sinus is connected to the valveless facial vein via the superior ophthalmic vein, allowing reverse blood flow to the sinus, and is therefore a potential route of intracranial infection. The cavernous sinus also receives venous drainage from the central vein of the retina, the sphenoparietal sinus, the superficial middle cerebral vein, and the pterygoid plexus. These empty into the superior and inferior petrosal sinuses and, ultimately, into the internal jugular vein. The left and right cavernous sinuses are connected in the midline by the anterior and posterior intercavernous sinuses.

1.2.3 Lymphatics of the Brain

It has been a longstanding belief that the vertebrate brain does not contain a classic lymphatic drainage system. Instead, it was thought the brain has a "glymphatic system," a perivascular pathway that allows cerebrospinal fluid (CSF) to recirculate through the brain interstitium along perivascular spaces near the cerebral arteries. This pathway was also thought to be responsible for the clearance of interstitial solutes along perivascular channels near the veins, mediated by astroglial water channels. However, recent findings have provided evidence of a functional lymphatic system in the brain, which acts to transport interstitial fluid (ISF) and

solutes from the parenchyma to the deep cervical lymph nodes. The lymphatic system also helps maintain the water and ion balance of the ISF and allows communication with the immune system. The lymphatic vessels are associated with the superior sagittal and transverse sinus and the dural middle meningeal arteries. It is likely that the lymphatic system works in conjunction with other efflux pathways, such as via the dural arachnoid granulations.

1.3 Bones of the Skull

The skull is a supportive protection for the brain and is formed by intramembranous ossification of cranial and facial bones. The calvarium is the roof of the cranium and is comprised of the frontal, occipital, and parietal bones (Figure 1.5). The base of the cranium is comprised of the ethmoid, occipital, temporal, parietal, frontal, and sphenoid bones. The junction between the latter four bones is known as the pterion and is of clinical relevance because

(a)

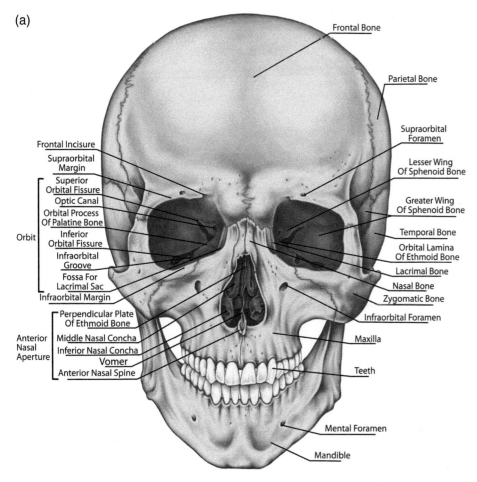

Frontal Bone
Parietal Bone
Supraorbital Foramen
Lesser Wing Of Sphenoid Bone
Greater Wing Of Sphenoid Bone
Temporal Bone
Orbital Lamina Of Ethmoid Bone
Lacrimal Bone
Nasal Bone
Zygomatic Bone
Infraorbital Foramen
Maxilla
Teeth
Mental Foramen
Mandible

Frontal Incisure
Supraorbital Margin
Superior Orbital Fissure
Optic Canal
Orbital Process Of Palatine Bone
Inferior Orbital Fissure
Infraorbital Groove
Fossa For Lacrimal Sac
Infraorbital Margin
Orbit
Perpendicular Plate Of Ethmoid Bone
Middle Nasal Concha
Inferior Nasal Concha
Vomer
Anterior Nasal Spine
Anterior Nasal Aperture

Figure 1.5 The skull and facial skeleton.

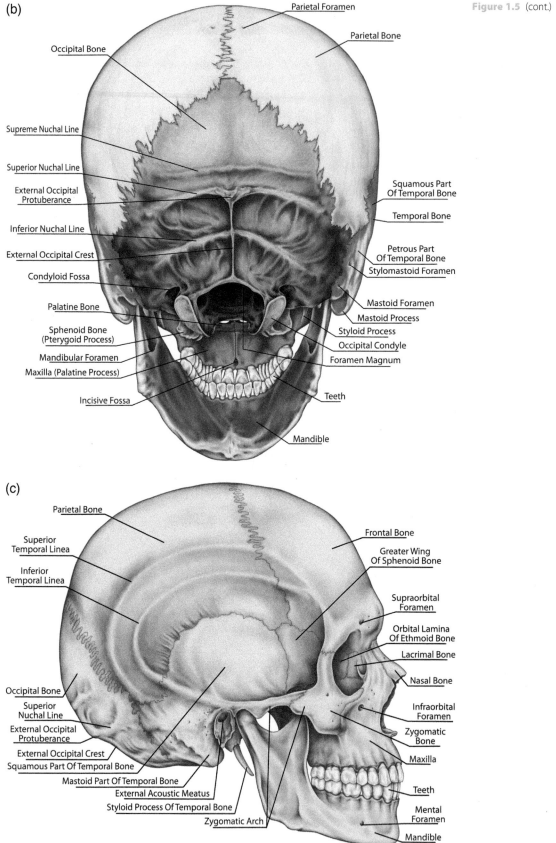

(b)

Parietal Foramen

Parietal Bone

Occipital Bone

Supreme Nuchal Line

Superior Nuchal Line

External Occipital Protuberance

Inferior Nuchal Line

External Occipital Crest

Condyloid Fossa

Palatine Bone

Sphenoid Bone (Pterygoid Process)

Mandibular Foramen

Maxilla (Palatine Process)

Incisive Fossa

Squamous Part Of Temporal Bone

Temporal Bone

Petrous Part Of Temporal Bone

Stylomastoid Foramen

Mastoid Foramen

Mastoid Process

Styloid Process

Occipital Condyle

Foramen Magnum

Teeth

Mandible

(c)

Parietal Bone

Superior Temporal Linea

Inferior Temporal Linea

Frontal Bone

Greater Wing Of Sphenoid Bone

Supraorbital Foramen

Orbital Lamina Of Ethmoid Bone

Lacrimal Bone

Nasal Bone

Occipital Bone

Superior Nuchal Line

External Occipital Protuberance

External Occipital Crest

Squamous Part Of Temporal Bone

Mastoid Part Of Temporal Bone

External Acoustic Meatus

Styloid Process Of Temporal Bone

Zygomatic Arch

Infraorbital Foramen

Zygomatic Bone

Maxilla

Teeth

Mental Foramen

Mandible

Figure 1.5 (cont.)

(d)

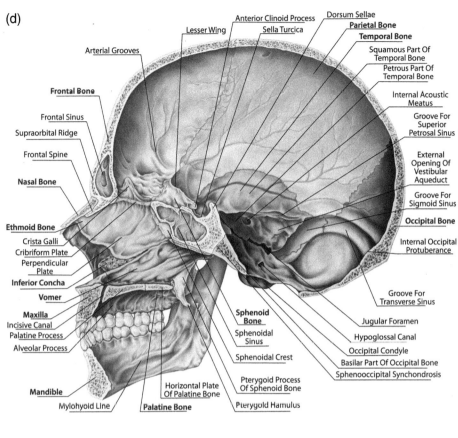

(e)

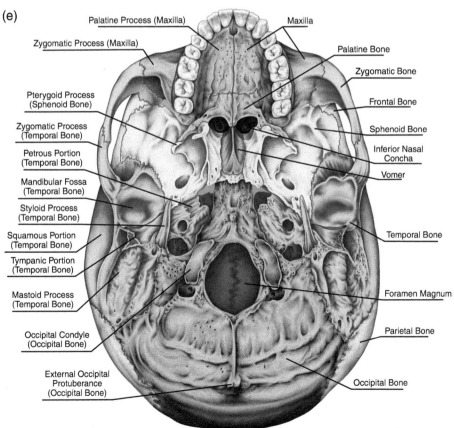

Figure 1.5 (cont.)

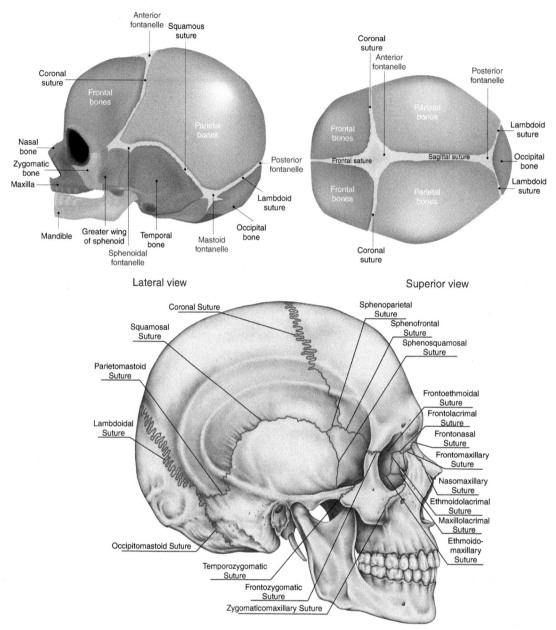

Figure 1.6 Sutures of the brain.

it overlies the middle meningeal artery, which can rupture following fractures to this region, leading to the formation of extradural hematomas.

Cranial fractures may be accompanied by facial bone fractures and should be sought for when assessing the trauma patient. The most common facial fractures include those of the nasal bone, maxilla, mandible, and zygomatic arch. Other areas prone to damage are the sutures, and these include the coronal, sagittal, and lambdoid sutures (Figure 1.6). In neonates, incompletely fused sutures give rise to fontanelles – the frontal fontanelle between the coronal and sagittal sutures and the occipital fontanelle between the sagittal and lambdoid sutures.

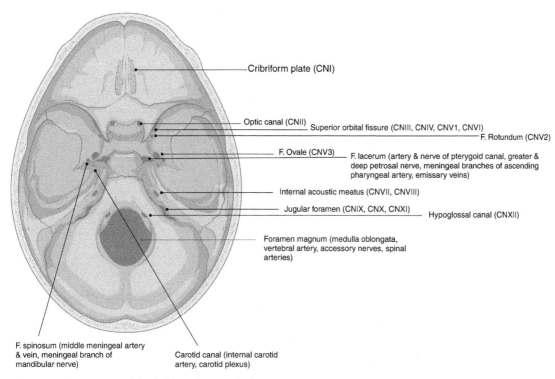

Cribriform plate (CNI)

Optic canal (CNII)
Superior orbital fissure (CNIII, CNIV, CNV1, CNVI)
F. Rotundum (CNV2)

F. Ovale (CNV3)
F. lacerum (artery & nerve of pterygoid canal, greater & deep petrosal nerve, meningeal branches of ascending pharyngeal artery, emissary veins)

Internal acoustic meatus (CNVII, CNVIII)

Jugular foramen (CNIX, CNX, CNXI)
Hypoglossal canal (CNXII)

Foramen magnum (medulla oblongata, vertebral artery, accessory nerves, spinal arteries)

F. spinosum (middle meningeal artery & vein, meningeal branch of mandibular nerve)

Carotid canal (internal carotid artery, carotid plexus)

Figure 1.7 Superior view of the skull base showing the foramina.

1.4 The Cranial Fossae

The cranial cavity is divided into three regions known as fossae. The anterior cranial fossa overlies the nasal and orbital regions and accommodates parts of the frontal lobe. It is made up of the frontal, ethmoid, and sphenoid bones. The frontal crest on the frontal bone and the crista galli of the ethmoid bone are the sites of attachment for a part of the dura mater that divides the cerebral hemispheres, known as the falx cerebri. The cribriform plate supporting the olfactory bulb is lateral to the crista galli, and contains a foramen transmitting the olfactory nerve and two ethmoidal foramina (anterior and posterior, transmitting the anterior and posterior ethmoidal vessels and nerves, respectively). The plate is very thin and can fracture following facial trauma, resulting in CSF rhinorrhea and anosmia.

The anterior fossa is separated from the middle fossa by the lesser wing of the sphenoid bone. The anterior clinoid processes of these bones are the site of attachment for the tentorium cerebelli (dura mater dividing the cerebrum and cerebellum). The middle cranial fossa consists of the sphenoid and temporal bones. Within the central part of the fossa is the sella turcica, a bony prominence which supports the pituitary gland within the hypophysial fossa. The posterior wall of the sella turcica is formed by the dorsal sellae, which separate the middle cranial fossa from the posterior cranial fossa. The lateral parts of the middle cranial fossa are formed by the greater wings of the sphenoid bone and the squamous and petrous parts of the temporal bones and provide structural support to the temporal lobes. Both the sphenoid and temporal bones contain numerous foramina for transmitting vessels and nerves. The posterior cranial fossa is comprised of the occipital bone and the temporal bones and contains the brainstem and cerebellum. The foramina of the skull are most considered in the context of the cranial nerves and are shown in Figure 1.7.

1.5 Layers of the Scalp

The scalp contains several layers, and these include skin, dense connective tissue, epicranial aponeurosis, loose areolar connective tissue, and the periosteum (Figure 1.8). The scalp is supplied by branches of the external carotid artery (superficial temporal, posterior

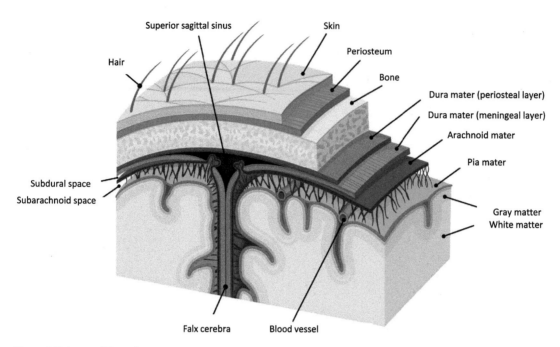

Figure 1.8 Layers of the scalp.

auricular, and occipital arteries) and the ophthalmic artery (supraorbital and supratrochlear arteries). Venous drainage includes a superficial system following the arterial supply (superficial temporal, occipital, posterior auricular, supraorbital, and supratrochlear veins). The temporal region of the skull is drained by the pterygoid venous plexus, which drains into the maxillary vein. The scalp veins connect to the diploic veins of the skull via valveless emissary veins, allowing a connection between the scalp and the dural venous sinuses. The nerves innervating the scalp include the trigeminal nerve branches (supratrochlear, supraorbital, zygomaticotemporal, and auriculotemporal nerves). The cervical nerve branches supplying the scalp include the lesser occipital nerve, the greater occipital nerve, the great auricular nerve, and the third occipital nerve.

1.6 Meninges

The brain and spinal cord are covered with membranous layers called the meninges. From outer to inner these are the dura, arachnoid, and pia mater.

1.6.1 Dura Mater

This layer is found underneath the bones and consists of the outer periosteal layer and the inner meningeal layer

and in between houses the dural venous sinuses. The meningeal layer folds inward to form the dural reflections and forms compartments. These compartments are the falx cerebri, the tentorium cerebelli, the falx cerebelli (separates the cerebellar hemispheres), and the diaphragma sellae (allows the passage of the pituitary stalk). Blood collecting in between the skull and the outer periosteal layer is known as an extradural hematoma and usually occurs due to damage to the middle meningeal artery. A subdural hematoma occurs due to damage of the cerebral veins between the dura and the arachnoid mater.

1.6.2 Arachnoid Mater

The arachnoid mater consists of avascular connective tissue. Below it lies the subarachnoid space containing CSF, which re-enters the circulation via the dural venous sinuses through small projections called arachnoid granulations.

1.6.3 Pia Mater

This is a highly vascularized layer that adheres to the brain surface and follows the contours of the brain into the gyri of the cerebral hemispheres and the folia of the cerebellum. The pia mater and arachnoid mater are joined by connective tissue in the subarachnoid space and together are known as leptomeninges. There are compartments where the two are not in close approximation, resulting in naturally enlarged CSF filled pools called the subarachnoid cisterns.

1.7 Organization of the Sympathetic and Parasympathetic Nervous Systems

The autonomic nervous system is composed of the sympathetic nervous system (SNS) and the parasympathetic nervous system (PNS) and acts to regulate the body's unconscious actions. The SNS stimulates the so-called "fight or flight" response and the PNS is involved in "rest and digest" responses (Box 1.1).

A major anatomical component of the SNS are a pair of nerve fibers that span the skull to coccyx, known as the sympathetic chains. There are two types of neurons involved in sympathetic signal transmission and these are the short preganglionic neurons that originate from T1 to L2–L3, which synapse with postganglionic neurons that extends to the rest of the body. At the synapses, the preganglionic neurons release acetylcholine, which activates the nicotinic acetylcholine receptors in the postganglionic neurons to release norepinephrine, and these subsequently bind to adrenergic receptors in the target tissue leading to sympathetic effects (Figure 1.9). The postganglionic neurons of sweat glands release acetylcholine to activate muscarinic receptors. The chromaffin cells of the adrenal medulla act as a postganglionic neuron and release norepinephrine and epinephrine.

Box 1.1

Organ	Parasympathetic Response	Sympathetic Response
Iris	Miosis and accommodation due to constriction of the sphincter muscles via the short ciliary nerves originating from the Edinger–Westphal nucleus of cranial nerve III	Pupil dilation (adrenergic innervation to the dilator pupillae muscle via the long ciliary nerves, arising from the superior cervical ganglion)
Salivary glands	Increased watery secretion via cranial nerves IX (parotid gland) and chorda tympani of VII (submandibular and sublingual glands) leading to acetylcholine release onto M3 muscarinic receptors	Reduced saliva secretion (innervation via fibers arising from the superior cervical ganglion resulting in norepinephrine release acting on alpha- and beta-adrenergic receptors)
Lacrimal glands	Increased secretion (preganglionic fibers reach the pterygopalatine ganglion via the greater petrosal nerve and the nerve of the pterygoid canal to synapse with postganglionic fibers)	Reduced secretion (innervation via fibers originating in the superior cervical ganglion, which reach the pterygopalatine ganglion via the internal carotid plexus and the deep petrosal nerve)
Heart	Negative chronotopy, inotropy and reduced conduction velocity and coronary artery vasoconstriction via the vagus nerve	Positive chronotropy, inotropy and increased conduction velocity via the cardiac nerves from the lower cervical and upper thoracic ganglia
Lung	Bronchial muscle contraction (vagus nerve)	Bronchial muscle relaxation (thoracic sympathetic ganglia)
Stomach	Increased peristalsis and motility and pyloric sphincter relaxation allowing gastric emptying via the vagus nerve	Reduced gastric motility and peristalsis and pyloric sphincter constriction preventing gastric emptying via the celiac plexus (T5–T12)
Gallbladder	Contraction (vagus nerve)	Relaxation (T7–T9 through the celiac plexus)
Internal urethral sphincter	Relaxation	Constriction
Detrusor muscle of bladder	Contraction (via pelvic splanchnic nerves to allow bladder emptying)	Relaxation (via sympathetic branches from the inferior hypogastric plexus to allow bladder filling)
Penis	Erection (pelvic nerve)	Ejaculation (peristaltic contraction of vas deferens, seminal vesicles, and prostatic smooth muscles via the hypogastric nerve and ejaculation via the pudendal nerve)
Adrenal medulla		Norepinephrine and epinephrine secretion

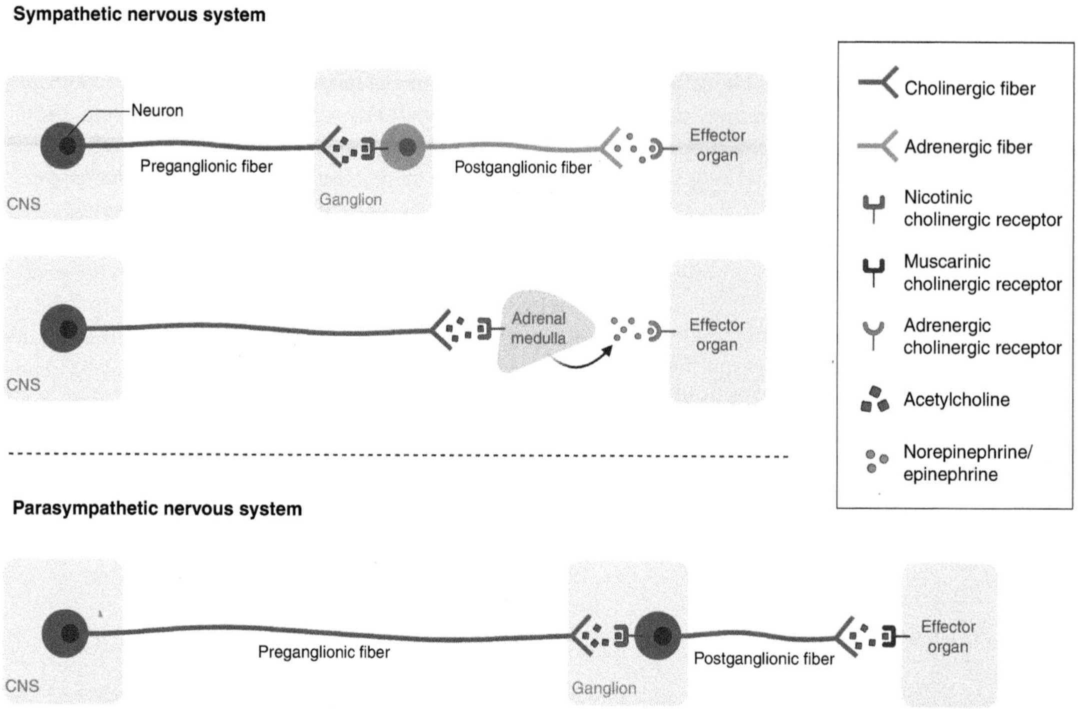

Sympathetic nervous system

Figure 1.9 Sympathetic and parasympathetic fibers. CNS; central nervous system.

Sympathetic nerves arise in the spinal cord in the intermediolateral nucleus of the lateral gray column. Axons leave the spinal cord through the anterior root and pass near the sensory ganglion to enter the anterior rami of spinal nerves. The axons terminate at the paravertebral or prevertebral ganglia. The main prevertebral ganglia (celiac, mesenteric and aorticorenal ganglia) are located anterior to the aorta and vertebral column and receive preganglionic axons via the splanchnic nerves. The paravertebral ganglia are located bilaterally ventrolateral to the vertebral column. There are three paravertebral ganglia and these are the superior cervical ganglion, middle cervical ganglion and inferior cervical ganglion.

1.7.1 Sympathetic Ganglia Supplying the Head and Neck: Cervical Ganglia

There are three cervical ganglia that supply the head and neck (the superior, middle, and inferior cervical ganglia). The superior ganglion is found posterior to the carotid artery and gives rise to a number of postganglionic nerves: the internal and external carotid nerves, the nerve to the pharyngeal plexus, the superior cardiac branch, and the gray rami communicantes. The middle ganglion may be absent, but when present is found anterior to the inferior thyroid artery. Its postganglionic fibers are the gray rami communicantes, the thyroid branches, and the middle cardiac branch. The inferior cervical ganglion is situated anteriorly to the C7 vertebra. Its branches are the gray rami communicantes, branches to the subclavian and vertebral arteries, and the inferior cardiac nerve. Damage to sympathetic fibers en route to the head and neck can lead to Horner's syndrome, a condition presenting with partial ptosis of the upper eyelid, miosis (constricted pupil) and hemi-facial anhidrosis (absence of sweating).

1.7.2 Parasympathetic Ganglia Supplying the Head and Neck

The parasympathetic fibers supplying the head and neck are found in four brainstem nuclei associated with a cranial nerve. They synapse in a peripheral ganglion near the target viscera. There are four parasympathetic ganglia located within the head –ciliary, otic, pterygopalatine, and submandibular. They receive fibers from the oculomotor, facial, and glossopharyngeal nerves (the vagus nerve only innervates structures in the thorax and abdomen).

The ciliary ganglion is located within the bony orbit. Its preganglionic fibers are from the Edinger–Westphal nucleus, associated with the oculomotor nerve. Its postganglionic fibers leave the ganglion via the short ciliary nerves to innervate the sphincter pupillae and the ciliary muscles. Sympathetic nerves from the internal carotid plexus and sensory fibers from the nasocilary nerve pass through the ganglion without synapsing.

The pterygopalatine ganglion is located within the pterygopalatine fossa and is supplied by fibers from the superior salivatory nucleus (associated with the facial nerve). Its postganglionic fibers join branches of the maxillary nerve to supply the lacrimal gland, the nasopharynx, and the palate.

Sympathetic fibers from the internal carotid plexus and sensory branches from the maxillary nerve pass through the pterygopalatine ganglion without synapsing.

The submandibular ganglion is located inferiorly to the lingual nerve and is supplied by fibers from the superior salivatory nucleus. These fibers are carried within a branch of the facial nerve, the chorda tympani. This nerve travels along the lingual branch of the mandibular nerve to reach the ganglion and leaves the ganglion to the submandibular and sublingual glands. Sympathetic fibers from the facial artery plexus pass through the submandibular ganglion. They are thought to innervate glands in the base of the oral cavity.

The otic ganglion is located inferiorly to the foramen ovale within the infratemporal fossa. It is medial to the mandibular branch of the trigeminal nerve. The ganglion is supplied by fibers from the inferior salivatory nucleus (associated with the glossopharyngeal nerve). Parasympathetic fibers travel within the lesser petrosal nerve, a branch of the glossopharyngeal nerve, to reach the otic ganglion. The parasympathetic fibers travel along the auriculotemporal nerve (a branch of the mandibular division of the trigeminal nerve) to provide secretomotor innervation to the parotid gland. Sympathetic fibers from the superior cervical chain pass through the otic ganglion, where they travel with the middle meningeal artery to innervate the parotid gland.

1.8 Structures of the Brain

The nervous system forms during the third week of development. At the cranial end of the neural tube,

three expansions (vesicles) develop: the forebrain (prosencephalon), the midbrain (mesencephalon), and the hindbrain (rhombencephalon). Further division separates the prosencephalon into the diencephalon (thalamus and hypothalamus) and the telencephalon (cerebrum). The mesencephalon consists of the tectum, cerebral aqueduct, tegmentum, and the cerebral peduncles. The rhomboencephalon consists of the pons, the medulla, and the cerebellum. The cavities within the primary brain vesicles are precursors of the ventricular system. The caudal parts of the neural tube form the spinal cord.

1.9 Forebrain

The structures in the forebrain include the cerebral cortex and subcortical structures of the limbic system including the amygdala, hypothalamus, thalamus, hippocampus, basal ganglia, and cingulate gyrus.

1.10 Cerebrum

The largest part of the brain is the cerebrum, containing two hemispheres separated by the falx cerebri of the dura mater. The visible surface of the cerebral hemisphere is a folded sheet of neural tissue called the cerebral cortex, characterized by sulci (depressions) and gyri (elevations). Some of the larger folds include the lateral sulcus (also known as the Sylvian fissure), which separates the temporal lobe from the frontal and parietal lobes, the central sulcus (dividing the frontal and parietal lobes), and the parieto-occipital sulcus, which separates the occipital and parietal lobes (Figure 1.10). The two cerebral hemispheres are connected by a white-matter tract called the corpus callosum. The tissue separating the two hemispheres is called the longitudinal fissure. The septum pellucidum continues from the corpus callosum to the fornix and separates the anterior horns of the lateral ventricles. The calcarine fissure separates the occipital lobe into the inferior lingual gyrus and the superior cuneus.

The cerebrum is made up of gray matter (containing cell bodies and dendrites) and white matter (consisting of glial cells and myelinated axons). The cerebrum can be divided into four lobes. The frontal lobe subserve decision-making and executive control. The parietal lobe is vital for sensory perception and integration. The occipital lobe is the visuospatial processing area of the brain for color, form and motion. The temporal lobe contains cortical areas that process auditory stimuli, encoding of memory and language comprehension.

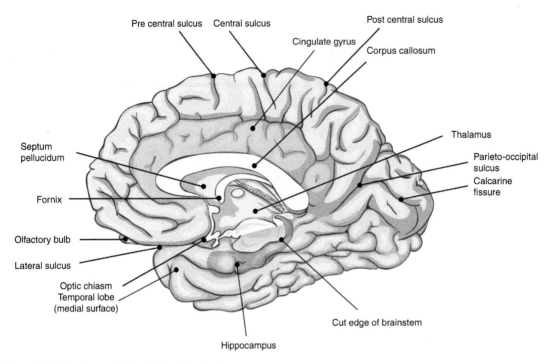

Pre central sulcus Central sulcus

Post central sulcus

Cingulate gyrus

Corpus callosum

Thalamus

Septum
pellucidum

Parieto-occipital
sulcus

Calcarine
fissure

Fornix

Olfactory bulb

Lateral sulcus

Optic chiasm
Temporal lobe
(medial surface)

Cut edge of brainstem

Hippocampus

Figure 1.10 Structures of the brain (medial surface).

1.10.1 Brodmann's Map

The cerebral cortex can also be subdivided into 52 functional regions, numbered by the neuroanatomist Korbinian Brodmann based on cytological structure. The primary motor cortex (Brodmann area 4) is anterior to the central sulcus (Figure 1.10). It contains large neurons called Betz cells, which send axons to the spinal cord and is important for planning and execution of movements. The topographic map of the motor cortex is arranged with an "overrepresentation" of neurons responsible for complex motor behaviors (Figure 1.11). The premotor cortex (Brodmann area 6) also plays a role in planning movement; however, its function is less well understood. The supplementary motor area (Brodmann area 6) contributes to the control of movement. The primary somatosensory cortex (Brodmann areas 3, 2, and 1) is found in the parietal lobe, posterior to the central sulcus. It processes afferent somatosensory input and helps integrate sensory and motor information required for skilled movement. The primary visual cortex (Brodmann area 17) is at the occipital pole. The extra striate cortex is adjacent to the visual cortex and processes specific features of visual information. It can be separated into two streams. The ventral stream is from the primary visual cortex to the temporal lobe and is important for pattern and object recognition. The dorsal stream from the striate cortex into the parietal lobe is responsible for spatial recognition of motion and location. The primary auditory cortex is responsible for recognition of auditory stimuli and is in the lateral temporal lobe. Wernicke's area (Brodmann area 22) is located in the superior temporal gyrus of the dominant cerebral hemi- sphere. It is important for comprehension of written and spoken language, and therefore any damage to this area leads to fluent but nonsensical speech. Broca's area (Brodmann areas 44 and 45) is located in the dominant prefrontal cortex and is involved in language processing and speech production. Lesions in this region lead to expressive aphasia, where the patient retains comprehension but cannot create fluent speech.

1.10.2 Layers of The Cerebral Cortex

The cerebral neocortex is arranged in six layers. The outermost layer is the molecular layer (layer I), containing fibers that run parallel to the cortical surface with very few neurons. Layer II is the outer granular

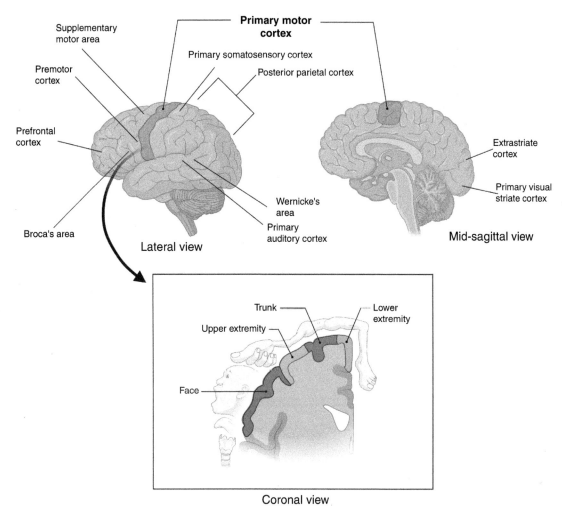

Figure 1.11 Topographic map of the primary motor cortex.

layer, containing small, rounded neurons. Below this is the outer pyramidal layer (layer III), containing pyramidal neurons. Next is the inner granular layer (layer IV), containing spiny stellate and pyramidal cells. It is a major input layer and receives specific sensory inputs from thalamocortical afferent fibers. The primary sensory cortex has a well-developed layer IV, but the output layers are less well developed. Layer IV is well developed in the primary visual cortex and contains the stria of Gennari, a band of myelinated axons that runs parallel to the surface of the cerebral cortex. The inner pyramidal later (layer V) contains many output neurons. The primary motor cortex has a very enlarged layer V containing large Betz cells, which send axons to the contralateral motor nuclei of cranial nerves and to

the lower motor neurons in the ventral horn of the spinal cord. Finally, layer VI is the innermost, multiform layer containing morphologically heterogenous population of neurons and sends efferent fibers to the thalamus.

Certain parts of the cortex are arranged differently: the hippocampus has three layers and the cingulate gyrus has four to five layers.

1.10.3 Vascular Supply

The branches of the anterior, middle, and posterior cerebral arteries are responsible for the blood supply to the cerebrum. The venous drainage of the cerebrum is via cerebral veins that empty into the dural venous sinuses (Figure 1.4).

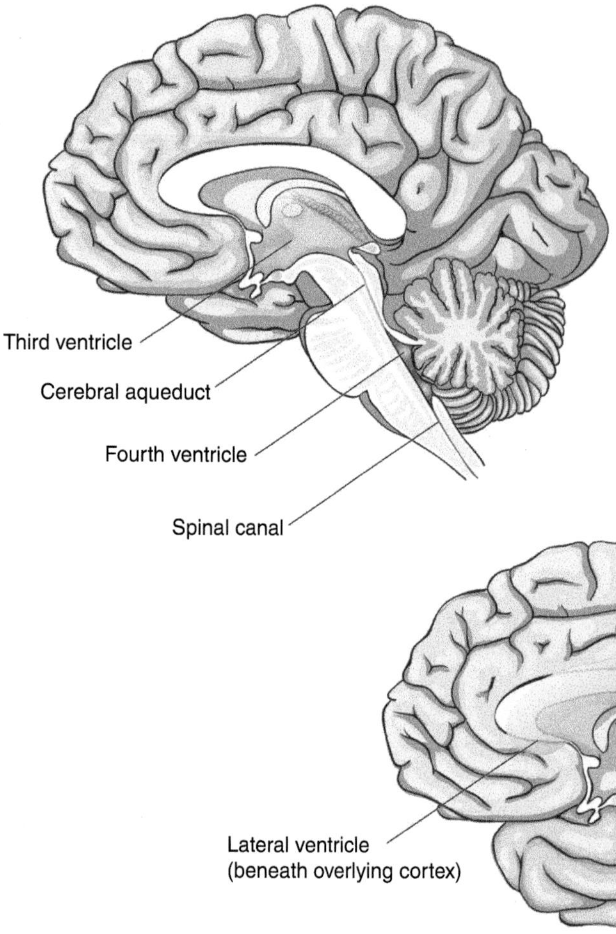

Figure 1.12 The ventricular system

Third ventricle

Cerebral aqueduct

Fourth ventricle

Spinal canal

Lateral ventricle
(beneath overlying cortex)

1.11 Ventricles

The ventricles (Figure 1.12) are lined by ependymal cells, ciliated glial cells, which form the choroid plexus, a structure where CSF is produced (Figure 1.13). This provides hydromechanical protection by acting as a shock absorber and providing buoyancy.

The ventricular system is composed of four connecting cavities derived from the neural tube. The right and left ventricles and the third ventricle are part of the forebrain, while the fourth ventricle is part of the hindbrain.

During development, the fluid-filled cavity of the primary vesicles become the lateral ventricles. They communicate with the third ventricle via the foramen of Monro in the diencephalon. The third ventricle communicates with the fourth ventricle in the hindbrain via the cerebral

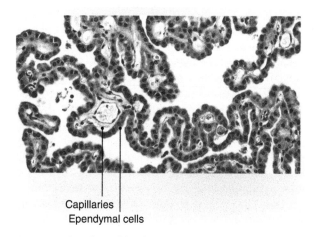

Capillaries
Ependymal cells

Figure 1.13 Histology of the choroid plexus

aqueduct (of Sylvius), which is continuous with the central canal of the spinal cord. The fourth ventricle is also connected to the subarachnoid space by a median aperture (the foramen of Magendie) and two lateral apertures (the foramina of Luschka).

1.12 Higher Association Areas of the Cortex

Higher association areas of the cortex are involved in complex processing of various sensory modalities, cognition and emotion. The prefrontal and limbic association areas are important for regulation of cognition, abstract reasoning, complex emotions and self-awareness. The cingulate and parahippocampal gyri are involved in expression of emotions and formation of memories. The hippocampal formation is important for declarative memory. It contains the Cornu Ammonis (CA) regions, the subiculum, and the dentate gyrus, and is found in the medial temporal lobe in the inferior horn of the lateral ventricle. The amygdala is a subcortical nucleus in the medial temporal lobe and is connected to the orbitofrontal cortex, the hypothalamus, and the nucleus accumbens.

1.13 Limbic System

The limbic system is a part of the brain involved in behavioral and emotional responses. There are several important structures within the limbic system and these include the basal ganglia, thalamus, hypothalamus, hippocampus, amygdala, and the cingulate gyrus.

1.13.1 Basal Ganglia

The basal ganglia are situated at the base of the forebrain and top of the midbrain. They are a group of subcortical nuclei connected to the cerebral cortex, thalamus, and the brainstem. The basal ganglia are responsible for control of voluntary motor movements, procedural learning, cognition, and emotion. They con- sist of several distinct structures (Figure 1.14) and these include the caudate nucleus and putamen (together known as the neostriatum) separated by the internal capsule). The internal capsule is the site of the passage of many fibers including the efferent corticobulbar fibers, corticospinal fibers, efferent corticopontine fibers, and afferent thalamocortical fibers.

The caudate receives inputs from the prefrontal cortex and the putamen receives inputs from the sensorimotor cortex. They send outputs to the external and internal globus pallidus and then to the thalamus and cerebral cortex, forming a subcortical loop. The internal segment projects to the motor areas of the thalamus and the medial nucleus of the thalamus. The external segment projects to the subthalamic nucleus (STN), which also projects to the internal globus pallidus.

The neostriatum also projects to the substantia nigra par compacta (SNPC), which contains dopaminergic neurons and to the pars reticulata, which contains mainly GABAergic neurons and is one of the output nuclei of the basal ganglia to the thalamus (alongside the internal globus pallidus) and plays a vital role in movement execution. The neostriatum is supplied by small branches of the middle and anterior cerebral arteries. The neostriatum and internal capsule are commonly affected in stroke. Damage to the internal capsule leads to contralateral weakness. The most affected region of the internal capsule is the genu, where corticospinal fibers to the head, neck, and part of the upper limb are located.

1.13.1.1 Connections of the Basal Ganglia

The striatum receives input from the cerebral cortex and the SNPC (Figure 1.15). The striatum sends inhibitory connections to the internal and external globus pallidus. The external region therefore disinhibits the STN, which then sends excitatory input to the internal globus pallidus. This sends inhibitory input to the thalamus, leading to inhibition of information flow to the cerebral cortex.

The basal ganglia also project to the medial dorsal nucleus of the thalamus, which then projects to the prefrontal association cortex. This region is involved in higher cortical and executive function.

Parkinson's disease results from degeneration of dopaminergic neurons of the SNPC and excessive inhibition of the thalamus. The SNPC projects to both direct and indirect pathways in the striatum. Due to the presence of two different types of dopamine receptors, the net effect is to excite the direct pathway and inhibit the indirect pathway. However, the loss of the neurons in Parkinson's disease upsets the fine balance of these pathways and reduces excitation of the motor cortex, resulting in poverty of movement.

1.13.2 Thalamus

The thalamus is located in the forebrain and contains nuclei with connections to the cerebral cortex, the hippocampus, the mammillary bodies, and the fornix.

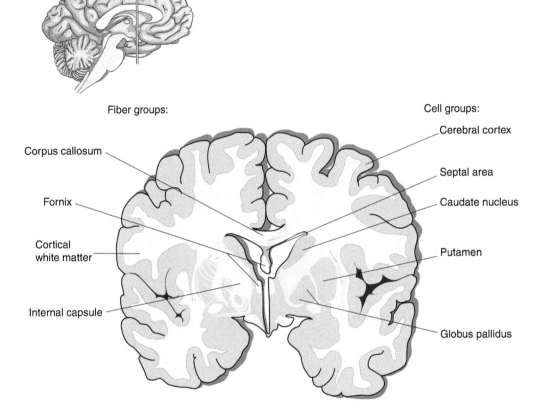

Figure 1.14 Cross-section of the basal ganglia.

Fiber groups:

Cell groups:

Corpus callosum

Fornix

Cortical
white matter

Internal capsule

Cerebral cortex

Septal area

Caudate nucleus

Putamen

Globus pallidus

The thalamus is divided into three major nuclear groups (anterior, medial, and ventral) (Figure 1.16). The ventral group contains ascending somatosensory relays (ventroposterior nuclei) and relays from the cerebellum and basal ganglia (ventrolateral). It also contains the motor association areas (ventro-anterior nuclei). The lateral and medial geniculate nuclei are found posteriorly. The anterior group projects to the cingulate gyrus and receives input from the mammillary bodies of the hypothalamus. The medial nuclei and the pulvinar receive input from the cerebral cortex and form the cortico-thalamo-cortical relays, which project to areas of the association cortex. These are the prefrontal cortex and the temporal–parietal–occipital association cortex, which mainly receive input from the medial nuclei and the pulvinar, respectively.

The thalamus is supplied by the posterior cerebral artery and branches of the posterior communicating artery. The thalamus is involved in learning, episodic memory, regulation of sleep, and wakefulness. Lesions in the anterior thalamus can lead to obstruction of the interventricular foramen of Monro and lesions in the posteriomedial thalamus can obstruct the third ventricle and cerebral aqueduct, leading to the development of hydrocephalus.

1.13.3 Cingulate Gyrus

The cingulate gyrus is situated above the corpus callosum (Figure 1.10). The anterior part relays signals between the right and left hemispheres and is involved in autonomic functions and cognitive processes such as reward behavior, empathy, and emotion. The posterior part becomes continuous with the most medial part of the temporal lobe, the parahippocampal gyrus. The cingulate gyrus is thought to be involved in retrieving episodic memory information. Dysfunction of this gyrus is found in schizophrenia and depression. Deep brain stimulation of the subgenual cortex of the gyrus is used to treat intractable

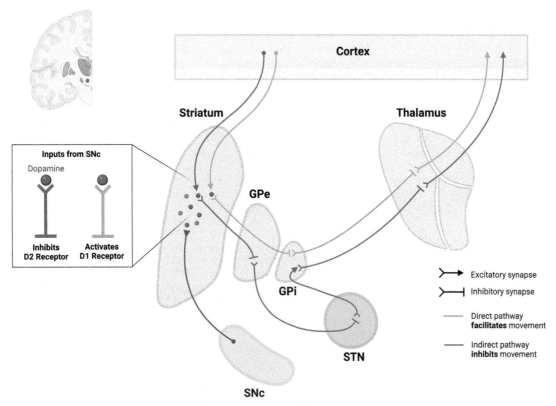

Figure 1.15 Basal ganglia connections.

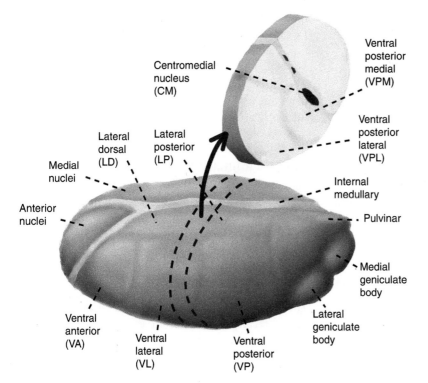

Figure 1.16 Nuclei of the thalamus.

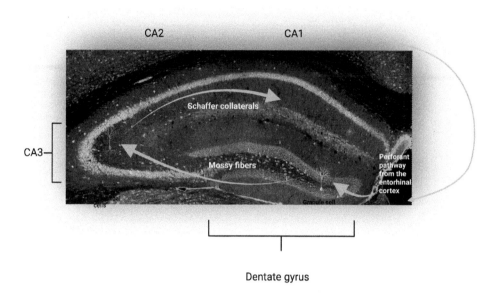

Figure 1.17 Cornu Ammonis axons of the hippocampus.

depression. Output fibers are mainly to the parahippocampal gyrus and are linked by the cingulum, a white-matter tract.

1.13.4 Hippocampus

The hippocampus is a seahorse-shaped structure and the hippocampal formation refers to the hippocampus proper (Cornu Ammonis), the dentate gyrus, and the subiculum. It is found in the temporal lobe, medial to the inferior horn of the lateral ventricle.

The hippocampus has been studied extensively and is used as a model system for electrophysiological studies, particularly for investigating neural plasticity. Damage to the hippocampus is commonly seen in patients with dementia, particularly Alzheimer's disease.

Hippocampal tissue is made up of layers and these include, from outer to inner: an external plexiform layer; a stratum oriens layer containing basal dendrites and basket cells; a pyramidal cell layer containing the primary cells of the hippocampus; a stratum radiatum layer; and the stratum lacunosum-moleculare layers containing the perforate pathway made up of pyramidal cell apical dendrites and afferent fibers from the entorhinal cortex. The external plexiform layer contains the alvear pathway, and this contains pyramidal cell axons through which information from the hippocampus is passed to the inferior horn of the lateral ventricle before reaching the entorhinal cortex. In addition, the hippocampus also contains distinct regions. The shape of the hippocampus has been described as similar to a seahorse or a ram's horn (Cornu Ammonis). The abbreviation CA is used to name the different regions: CA1, CA2, CA3, and CA4 (Figure 1.17).

1.13.4.1 Dentate Gyrus

The dentate gyrus contains granule cells and axons called mossy fibers, which synapse with the pyramidal cells in the CA3 field of the hippocampus. They also contain some pyramidal cells in the polymorphic cell layer.

1.13.4.2 Hippocampal Inputs

The hippocampus receives information from the lateral perforate and medial perforate pathways in the entorhinal cortex (Figure 1.18), the prefrontal cortex, the anterior cingulate gyrus, the pre- mammillary region, and the reticular formation of the brainstem. It also receives input from the thalamus to field CA1 and from the serotonin, norepineph- rine, and dopamine systems. The medial septal nucleus sends cholinergic and γ-aminobutyric acid (GABA)-ergic inputs to the hippocampus.

The largest input and output pathway of the hippocampus is via the fornix, which connects it to other structures including the mammillary bodies of the hypothalamus, prefrontal cortex and the lateral septal area. The entorhinal cortex (part of the parahippocampal gyrus) receives output from the deeper layers of the hippocampus and gives input to the superficial layers.

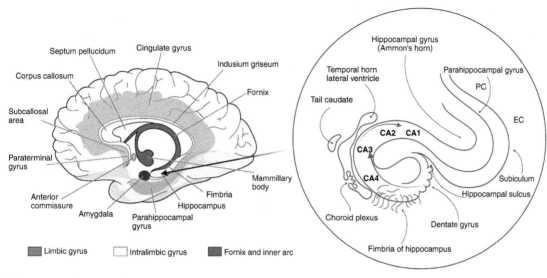

Figure 1.18 Hippocampal connections.

The fornix has two branches: the precommissural and the postcommissural pathways. The former connects to the septal nuclei, preoptic nuclei, ventral striatum, orbital cortex, and anterior cingulate gyrus. The postcommissural branch connects to the anterior nucleus of the thalamus and mammillary bodies of the hypothalamus. In Korsakoff's syndrome, these bodies are damaged and hence patients have trouble learning new memories. The anterior thalamic nuclei connect to the cingulate cortex, which connects back to the entorhinal cortex and creates the Papez circuit, which is involved in learning, memory, and emotion.

1.13.4.3 Hippocampus and Memory

Memory is the ability to acquire, store, and retrieve information and are formed through learning. The process of learning activates engram cells, a population of cells that have undergone cellular changes as a result of learning and when reactivated by the original stimulus leads to memory recall.

1.13.4.3.1 Spatial Memory

The hippocampus is well known to be involved in spatial memory and navigation. Within the hippocampus are found place cells, which contain information regarding the spatial context in which a memory took place in one specific location. These cells cluster in place fields and fire action potentials when an animal passes a certain location. Place-cell responses have been seen in the pyramidal cells of the hippocampus and the granule cells of the dentate gyrus. This is in contrast to the grid cells found

in the entorhinal cortex, which generate a map of firing patterns covering entire regions. The spatial firing sequences appear to be stored in the hippocampus during exploration and can be retrieved at a later time. The dorsal hippocampus is responsible for spatial memory, verbal memory, and learning conceptual information, and there appear to be more place cells in the dorsal region. The ventral hippocampus functions in fear conditioning and affective processes.

1.13.4.3.2 Explicit Versus Implicit Memory

Declarative or explicit memories are available in the consciousness as semantic facts or episodic memories (Figure 1.19). The areas of the brain involved are the hippocampus, the neocortex, and the amygdala. Nondeclarative memories, also known as implicit memories, are memories of skills, and rely on the basal ganglia and cerebellum. Short-term memories (seconds to minutes) are brief memories including working memory and rely heavily on the prefrontal cortex. These memories can be consolidated into long-term memory.

Formation of explicit memory begins with consolidation and storage of encoded information in the hippocampus. Over time, certain memories can be transferred to the neocortex as general knowledge. The amygdala interacts with the hippocampus and neocortex to stabilize a memory and form new memories related to fear.

One of the earlier findings of how the hippocampus impacts memory consolidation came from the study of Henry Molaison, a patient who had a bilateral temporal

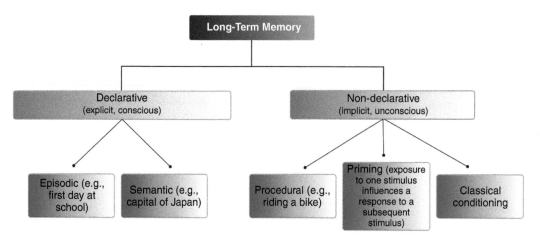

Figure 1.19 Declarative versus non-declarative memory.

lobectomy to treat his epileptic seizures. The surgery led to deficits including an inability to complete tasks that required long-term episodic memory and an inability to create new long-term memories. His spatial orientation was also severely affected. His long-term memory of events many years before the accident was largely intact and his procedural memory and intelligence were unaffected. This showed that the medial temporal lobe containing the hippocampus is important for declarative but not procedural memory consolidation.

Neurophysiological theories of synaptic plasticity based on the cellular models that underpin synaptic plasticity including long-term potentiation (LTP) and long-term depression (LTD) (see Chapter 5 for further details) can be used to explain the neural basis of learning and memory. Donald Hebb was the first to postulate that activation or inactivation of extant synaptic contacts depends on the synchronous impulse activity of pre- and postsynaptic nerve cells.

One of the most fascinating features of the hippocampus is its capacity for plasticity. Action potentials travel down the Schaffer collaterals and stimulate the release of glutamate into the synaptic cleft, which stimulates the α-amino-3-hydroxy-5-methyl-4-isoxazo-lepropionic acid (AMPA) and N-methyl-D-aspartate (NMDA) receptors. Once the AMPA receptors open, sodium travels into the postsynaptic membrane and elicits a membrane depolarization. With a large enough stimulation, a large amount of glutamate will be released, allowing a large membrane depolarization that removes the magnesium block typically seen at the NMDA receptor. This allows both sodium and calcium to enter the postsynaptic membrane. The calcium activates protein kinases and stimulates a cascade of short- and long-term changes. In the short term, there is insertion of AMPA receptors (Figure 1.20), and in the long term there are changes in transcription factors and increased protein translation. This forms the basis of LTP.

On the contrary, LTD is induced by prolonged low-frequency stimulation, which leads to prolonged calcium activation of phosphatase enzymes and an eventual removal of AMPA receptors and pruning of spines.

1.13.4.3.3 Implicit Memory

Implicit memory involves several different brain regions. Classical conditioning involves various sensory and motor systems. Operant conditioning involves the striatum and cerebellum and fear conditioning involves the amygdala.

Classic (Pavlov) conditioning refers to learning that occurs when a neutral stimulus becomes associated with a stimulus that naturally produces a behavior. It was first observed by the Russian physiologist Ivan Pavlov, who exposed dogs to sounds (neutral stimulus) immediately before receiving food (natural stimulus producing behavior). Initially, the dogs began to salivate only when they saw the food; however, later, the dogs learned to associate the sound with the food and began salivating as they heard the sound. The food is the unconditioned stimulus as it naturally leads to a behavior. The conditioned stimulus is the neutral tone, which upon repeated presentation leads to the same behavior as the unconditioned stimulus. Classic conditioning involves enhanced synaptic strength due to presynaptic facilitation, where there is increased release of neurotransmitters from the presynaptic cells under the action of an additional neuron.

Normal synaptic transmission

Induction of long-term potentiation

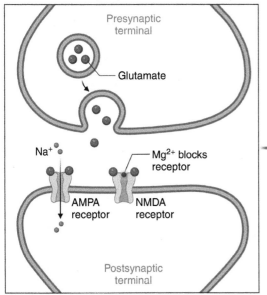

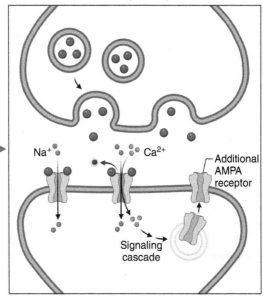

During low-frequency synaptic transmission, Mg^{2+} blocks the NMDA receptor.

High-frequency transmission expels Mg^{2+} from the NMDA receptor, allowing Na$^+$ and Ca^{2+} influx. Ca^{2+} then triggers a signaling cascade, increasing the number of AMPA receptors at the synapse.

Figure 1.20 Long-term potentiation.

Habituation is a type of non-associative learning where a repetitive stimulus leads to a decrement in the response intensity. Sensitization is the increment in response intensity in response to a stimulus. Experiments performed in the sea slug, *Aplysia californica*, by Eric Kandel were crucial in establishing the importance of synaptic changes to learning and memory. It was demonstrated that upon stimulation of the siphon receptors, the motor neuron is activated directly or indirectly through the excitatory interneuron as the gill is withdrawn. However, with repeated stimulation, there is reduced release of synaptic transmitters from the sensory neurons and therefore there is less withdrawal of the gill (habituation). This would typically occur when an animal repeatedly encounters a harmless stimulus. However, when the animal encounters a harmful stimulus, a vigorous response occurs to not only the harmful stimulus but also the harmless stimulus (sensitization). When the head or tail of the *Aplysia* is stimulated by an electric shock, there is activation of the facilitatory interneurons. These synapse with the sensory neurons of the head, and there is increased transmitter release leading to excitation of the excitatory interneurons and the motor neurons to the gill (Figure 1.21). Dishabituation refers to the restoration of a full-strength response that was weakened by habituation.

Operant conditioning, is learning that occurs based on the consequences of behavior (e.g. reinforcement or punishment). This is a voluntary behavioral response and according to the law of effect, the behavior is strengthened or weakened by the learner based on their desired result. The early studies on operant conditioning were performed by Edward Thorndike and B. F. Skinner. The "Skinner box" was designed to study the principles of animal behavior in a controlled environment.

1.13.5 Amygdala

The amygdala is one of two almond-shaped clusters of nuclei found medially within the temporal lobe and is responsible for emotions such as fear and aggression. Emotion is a subjective state and consists of a physical response involving the autonomic motor and endocrine systems. It also requires conscious registration, and this involves both the cerebral cortex and the amygdala. The amygdala is also involved in memory formation, reward processing, and decision making.

1.13.5.1 Inputs

The amygdala receives inputs from the hypothalamus, septal area, and the orbital cortex.

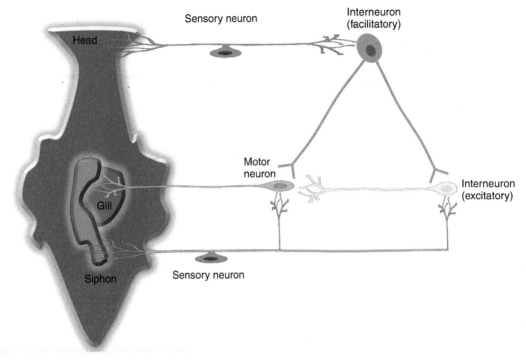

Figure 1.21 *Aplysia californica* experiments performed to demonstrate habituation and sensitization.

1.13.5.2 Outputs

The major outputs of the amygdala include the ventral amygdalofugal pathway, the stria terminalis, the hippocampus, the entorhinal cortex, and the dorsomedial nucleus of the thalamus. The amygdala connects to the hypothalamus via the stria terminalis and the ventral amygdalofugal pathway, the latter of which also connects to the anterior olfactory nucleus, the anterior perforated substance in the forebrain, the piriform cortex, the orbitofrontal cortex, the anterior cingulate cortex, and the ventral striatum. This pathway is particularly important in associative learning and the linking of behavior with reward and punishment. The stria terminalis continues as precommissural and postcommissural branches. The precommissural branch travels to the septal area and the postcommissural branch to the hypothalamus. The stria terminalis also projects to the habenula (involved in reward and aversion processing), which is part of the epithalamus. See section 1.15.

1.13.5.3 Amygdala and Fear Conditioning

The amygdala is involved in Pavlovian fear conditioning, a behavioral paradigm that involves learning to associate stimuli with certain adverse effects. In fear conditioning, an animal associates a neutral conditional stimulus, such as a tone, with an aversive unconditional stimulus, such as an electric foot shock, and responds by freezing even when it is not receiving the aversive stimulus. Fear extinction refers to the reduction in the conditioned fear responses after repeated presentation of the conditioned stimulus without the unconditioned stimulus that had elicited the fear.

1.13.6 Nucleus Accumbens

The nucleus accumbens is part of the striatum. It receives input from the orbitofrontal cortex, the cingulate cortex, and the amygdala and is involved in emotion and motivation.

1.13.7 Prefrontal Cortex

The prefrontal cortex is located in the frontal lobe and is implicated in personality development, decision making, and reasoning. Its role was discovered from the symptoms and signs that Phineas Gage (an American railroad construction worker) developed following an accident that involved a rod being driven into his brain resulting in irreversible damage to his frontal lobe.

The medial part of the prefrontal cortex connects with the amygdala, the hippocampus, and the temporal lobe.

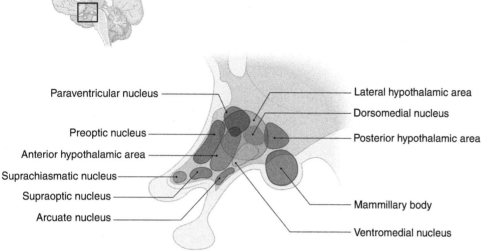

Figure 1.22 Hypothalamic nuclei.

Paraventricular nucleus

Preoptic nucleus

Anterior hypothalamic area

Suprachiasmatic nucleus

Supraoptic nucleus

Arcuate nucleus

Lateral hypothalamic area

Dorsomedial nucleus

Posterior hypothalamic area

Mammillary body

Ventromedial nucleus

The lateral part connects to the basal ganglia, the premotor cortex, the supplemental motor area, the thalamus, and the cingulate cortex. The orbitofrontal region forms connections with the amygdala, the medial part of the thalamus, the hypothalamus, and the basal ganglia.

1.13.8 Olfactory Bulb

The olfactory nerve projects to the olfactory bulb in the forebrain. The bulb is separated from the olfactory epithelium by the cribriform plate. It contains neurons involved in olfaction and receives sensory input from axons of the olfactory receptor neurons in the olfactory epithelium and outputs to the mitral cell axons. It then sends olfactory information to the amygdala, the orbitofrontal cortex, and the hippocampus. It also receives information from the amygdala, the neocortex, the hippocampus, the locus coeruleus, and the substantia nigra.

The bulb is divided into the main and accessory parts. The main bulb connects to the amygdala via the piriform cortex of the primary olfactory cortex. Associative learning between certain odors and behaviors takes place in the amygdala. The accessory bulb forms a parallel pathway.

1.13.9 Hypothalamus

The hypothalamus is bordered by the optic chiasm anteriorly and the mammillary bodies posteriorly. The function of the hypothalamus is to maintain homeostasis. It links the nervous system to the endocrine system via the pituitary gland, which is located below it. It contains four

regional groups of nuclei (Figure 1.22): the preoptic region (which contains the preoptic nucleus), the supraoptic region (which contains suprachiasmatic, supraoptic, paraventricular, and anterior nuclei), the tuberal region (which contains dorsomedial, ventromedial, arcuate, premammillary and lateral tuberal nuclei), and the mammillary region (which contains mammillary and posterior nuclei). The medial preoptic nucleus secretes gonadotropin-releasing hormone (GnRH), which is responsible for the secretion of luteinizing hormone (LH) and follicle-stimulating hormone (FSH) by the pituitary. The paraventricular and supraoptic nuclei both produce the peptide hormones and antidiuretic hormone (ADH). The paraventricular nucleus also releases thyrotropin-releasing hormone (TRH), corticotropin-releasing hormone (CRH), and somatostatin. TRH is responsible for the formation and secretion of the thyroid-stimulating hormone (TSH) in the pituitary gland, which in turn regulates the production of thyroid hormones in the thyroid gland. TRH also stimulates the release of prolactin from the pituitary gland. Corticotropin-releasing hormone activates the release of adrenocorticotropic hormone (ACTH) from the pituitary gland. Somatostatin regulates the endocrine and digestive systems. The anterior nucleus is involved in thermoregulation by stimulating the PNS, and causes hyperthermia if damaged. The suprachiasmatic nucleus regulates the circadian rhythm and pineal gland function. The ventromedial nuclei mediate satiety. The lateral nuclei mediate hunger via orexin neurons. The arcuate nuclei secrete prolactin, growth hormone releasing hormone (GHRH), and GnRH. Dorsomedial nuclei regulate blood pressure and heart rate. The posterior nuclei release vasopressin and are involved in thermoregulation via the SNS. The mammillary nuclei are involved in memory.

1.13.9.1 Hypothalamus and Sleep

Sleep is a reversible state of reduced consciousness that is important for regulation of inflammatory processes, removal of toxins via the glymphatic system, maintenance of a reduced metabolic rate and memory consolidation. Sleep deprivation has negative consequences for the cardiovascular system, endocrine regulation, glucose tolerance and mental health. Sleep can be measured using polysomnography (PSG), which has been used to reveal distinct sleep states. Normally, people transition between nonrapid eye movement (NREM) stages and rapid eye movement (REM) stages and this is regulated by reciprocal inhibition of monoaminergic and cholinergic neurons. There is increased activity of cholinergic neurons and decreased activity of adrenergic and serotonergic neurons during REM sleep and this is reversed in NREM sleep. NREM sleep occurs during the transition from being awake to sleeping and is characterized by light sleeping with slowing of brain waves. Rapid eye movement sleep is characterized by rapid eye movements with faster breathing and increased heart rate and blood pressure.

The sleep cycle is regulated by the circadian rhythm and is controlled by the suprachiasmatic nucleus (SCN) of the hypothalamus. The circadian rhythm is a biological clock maintained in a 24-hour pattern by clock genes such as *Per*, *tim*, and *Cry*. The retina sends inputs to the SCN, which can regulate the circadian rhythm and sleep by releasing a number of hormones such as norepinephrine, and this can stimulate the pineal gland to release melatonin. Activation of the ventrolateral preoptic (VLPO) area is also important in initiating sleep. Wakefulness is regulated by ascending arousal pathways activating the cortical system and uses chemicals such as norepinephrine, serotonin, dopamine, acetylcholine, histamine, and orexin.

1.14 Pituitary Gland

The pituitary gland is functionally and anatomically linked to the hypothalamus (via the infundibulum; Figure 1.23) and is responsible for releasing several hormones. It is located in the sella turcica of the sphenoid bone and is covered by the diaphragma sellae. The gland is divided into the anterior (adenohypophysis) lobe – derived from an outpouching of the roof of the pharynx called Rathke's pouch – and the posterior lobe. The anterior lobe is divided into three parts: Pars anterior (hormone secretion), Pars intermedia, and Pars tuberalis. The posterior (neurohypophysis) lobe releases two hormones (oxytocin and vasopressin) that are initially produced in the hypothalamus.

The anterior pituitary is supplied by the superior hypophyseal artery (a branch of the internal carotid

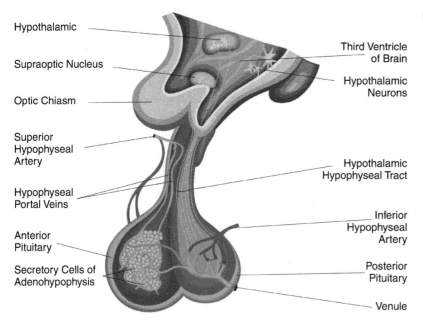

Figure 1.23 The pituitary gland.

Hypothalamic

Supraoptic Nucleus

Optic Chiasm

Superior Hypophyseal Artery

Hypophyseal Portal Veins

Anterior Pituitary

Secretory Cells of Adenohypophysis

Third Ventricle of Brain

Hypothalamic Neurons

Hypothalamic Hypophyseal Tract

Inferior Hypophyseal Artery

Posterior Pituitary

Venule

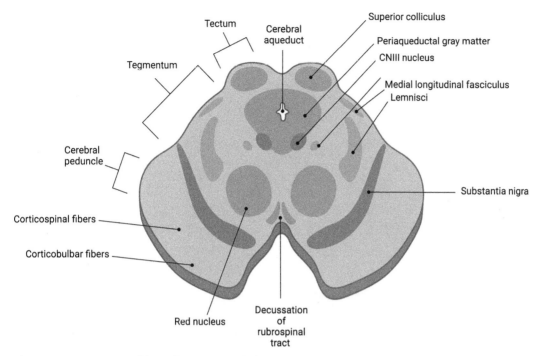

Figure 1.24 Cross-section of the midbrain at the level of the superior colliculus.

artery), which forms a capillary network and a plexus called the hypophyseal portal system. The infundibulum and posterior pituitary gland are supplied by the superior hypophyseal artery, the infundibular artery, and the inferior hypophyseal artery. Both lobes are drained by the anterior and posterior hypophyseal veins.

1.15 Epithalamus

The epithalamus is a dorsal segment of the diencephalon and contains the pineal gland, habenula and stria medullaris. The pineal gland is responsible for secreting melatonin, a hormone involved in the regulation of the circadian rhythm of the body. This gland is supplied by the posterior choroidal arteries (a branch of the posterior cerebral artery) and drains to the internal cerebral veins. The stria medullaris, contains afferent fibers from the septal nuclei and the anterior thalamic nuclei to the habenula, bilateral structures connected by a commissure. The lateral habenula is primarily involved in learning from reward omission and aversive experiences, affect, cognition, and social behavior. The medial habenula may also be involved in fear responses, mood and memory.

1.16 Midbrain

The midbrain (mesencephalon) is part of the brainstem and lies above the pons and below the forebrain (Figure 1.24). It is comprised of two parts: the tectum and the cerebral peduncles (crus cerebra and tegmentum). The tectum houses four colliculi inferior to the pineal gland and superior to the trochlear nerve. The oculomotor nerve exits between the peduncles and the optic tract is found on the superior border.

The cross-section of the midbrain reveals several fiber tracts, and these include the frontopontine fibers, the corticospinal fibers, the corticobulbar tracts, and the temporopontine fibers. The substantia nigra, the tegmentum, and the tectum can be visualized posteriorly. The cerebral aqueduct and the periaqueductal gray matter can be seen in the midline, and the medial longitudinal fasciculus can be seen anteriorly. The red nuclei (which receive input from the cerebral cortex and cerebellum and are involved in coordination of sensorimotor information) and decussation of the rubrospinal tracts (motor control, modulation of flexor muscle tone, reflex activity, and inhibition of antigravity muscles) can be seen at the level of the superior colliculus. The oculomotor nucleus can be seen

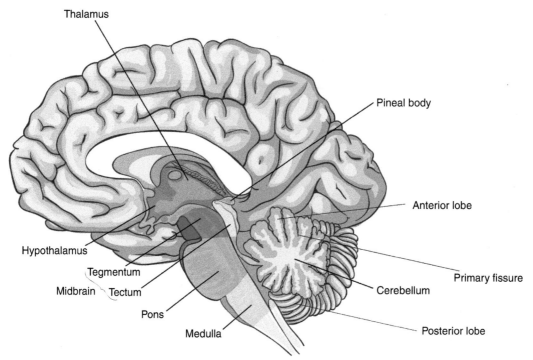

Figure 1.25 Sagittal section of the brain demonstrating the medulla and pons.

with the oculomotor nerve projecting anteriorly (Figure 1.24). The trochlear nerve can be seen at the level of the inferior colliculi.

The blood supply to the midbrain is the basilar artery and its branches (the posterior cerebral artery, the superior cerebellar artery, the posterior choroidal artery, and the interpeduncular branches).

1.17 Hindbrain

1.17.1 Pons

The pons is found below the midbrain and above the medulla (Figure 1.25). It develops from the embryonic metencephalon. The pons is the site of origin for several cranial nerves (Figure 1.26).

The pons is connected to the cerebellum via the middle cerebellar peduncles. Underlying the cerebellum is the fourth ventricle. The angle formed at the junction of the pons, the medulla, and the cerebellum is the cerebellopontine angle. The floor of the fourth ventricle reveals some anatomical landmarks including the medial eminence at the midline, the facial colliculus (containing the abducens nucleus and the facial motor fibers), and the stria medullaris (a part of the epithalamus). The pons is comprised of the ventral pons containing the pontine

nuclei (responsible for coordination of movement), corticospinal and corticobulbar tracts, and the dorsal pons (tegmentum), which forms part of the reticular formation responsible for arousal and attentiveness and which contains cranial nerves and the fourth ventricle.

1.17.2 Vascular Supply

The pons is supplied by the pontine artery (basilar artery branch), the superior cerebellar artery, and the anterior inferior cerebellar artery. The pons drains to the anterior pontomesencephalic vein, and then to the basal and cerebral veins. The inferior aspects drain into the inferior petrosal sinus, which drains into the internal jugular veins.

1.18 Medulla Oblongata

The medulla oblongata contains the ascending and descending tracts and the brainstem nuclei. The inferior margin is marked by the origin of the first pair of cervical spinal nerves as the medulla exits the skull through the foramen magnum.

Several structures can be visualized on the anterior surface. These include the pyramids, the olives, and five cranial nerves (abducens nerve, accessory nerve, hypoglossal nerve,

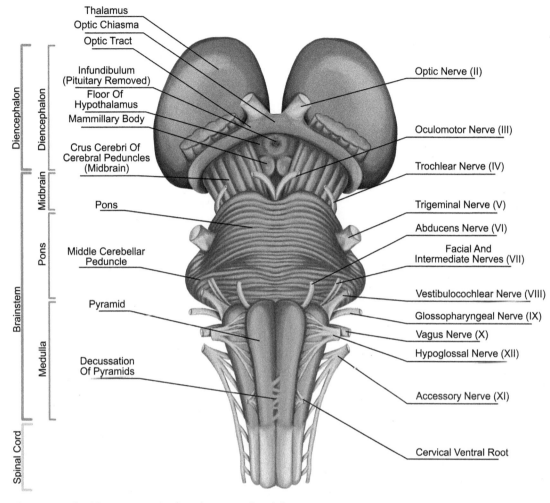

Figure 1.26 Cranial nerves emerging from the pons and medulla.

trochlear nerve, and trigeminal nerve). Posteriorly, the fasciculus gracilis, the fasciculus cuneatus, and the posterior median sulcus can be seen.

The internal structure of the medulla is usually best appreciated in cross-section and is typically discussed at the level of the pyramidal decussation, the medial lemnisci decussation (Figure 1.27), and the level of the olives.

At the level of the pyramidal decussation, we can see the descending motor fibers. The central portion contains the gray matter and the outer portion is made up of white matter, which contains the fasciculus gracilis and the fasciculus cuneatus. Corresponding portions of gray matter extend to these regions and are the nucleus gracilis and nucleus cuneatus, respectively. The spinocerebellar tracts with the lateral spinothalamic tracts in between can

be found laterally, with the trigeminal nucleus found posterior to these tracts.

The decussation of the sensory pathways can be found at the level of the decussation of the medial lemniscus. The medial lemniscus is a bundle of large myelinated axons that function as second-order neurons of the dorsal column–medial lemniscus pathway to transport sensory information. The medial lemniscus is formed by the crossings of the internal arcuate fibers, which are composed of axons of nucleus gracilis and nucleus cuneatus. Centrally the hypoglossal nucleus and laterally the medial longitudinal fasciculus can be seen with the nucleus ambiguus. The medial longitudinal fasciculus controls horizontal eye movements by interconnecting oculomotor and abducens nuclei. The nucleus ambiguus contains

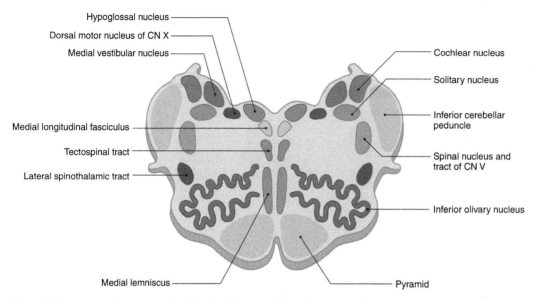

Figure 1.27 Cross-section the medulla at the level of the medial meniscus decussation.

cells bodies of motor nerves involved in swallowing and speaking. The inferior olivary nucleus (ION) is found between the nucleus ambiguus and the pyramids and coordinates signals from the spinal cord to the cerebellum. The climbing fiber axons leave the ION and travel to the cerebellar Purkinje cell.

At the level of the olives, the central canal opens into the fourth ventricle, and at this level the inferior olivary nucleus and inferior cerebellar peduncles can be seen. The vestibular nuclei can be seen in the midline. Laterally, the nucleus of the tractus solitarius (which generates peristaltic activity of the gastrointestinal system during swallowing) can be seen.

1.18.1 Vascular Supply

The vessels that supply the medulla include: the anterior spinal artery, the posterior spinal artery, the posterior inferior cerebellar artery, the anterior inferior cerebellar artery, and the vertebral artery.

1.18.2 Pathways

The ascending tracts refer to the neural pathways by which sensory information from the peripheral nerves is transmitted to the cerebral cortex. In some texts, ascending tracts are also known as somatosensory pathways.

The descending tracts are the pathways by which motor signals are sent from the brain to the lower motor neurons. The lower motor neurons then directly innervate muscles to produce movement, discussed in Chapter 7.

1.19 Cranial Nerves

There are 12 paired cranial nerves that arise from the brain. The first two, the olfactory and optic nerves, originate in the cerebrum and the rest arise in the brainstem.

1.19.1 Olfactory Nerve

This is the first and the shortest nerve. It is derived from the olfactory placode, a thickening of the neural ectoderm, which give rise to the olfactory epithelium of the nose containing the olfactory receptor neurons. These are bipolar cells that gives rise to unmyelinated axons, which are found in bundles and penetrate the cribriform plate of the ethmoid bone. They then enter the cranium and then the olfactory bulb to synapse with neurons called mitral cells, forming the synaptic glomeruli. From here, second-order neurons pass to the olfactory tract, which travels to the optic chiasm and divides into the two stria. The lateral stria carries axons to the primary olfactory cortex in the uncus of the temporal lobe and the medial stria to the anterior commissure, where they meet the olfactory bulb of the opposite side. The primary olfactory cortex sends fibers to the piriform cortex, the amygdala, the olfactory tubercle, and the secondary olfactory cortex.

The olfactory mucosa is found on the roof of the nasal cavity and is made up of pseudostratified columnar epithelium containing basal cells (which form new stem cells), sustentacular cells (for structural support, analogous to glial cells), olfactory receptor cells (bipolar cells consisting of dendrite processes with cilia that react to odors and stimulate olfactory cells), and a central process projecting in the opposite direction through the basement membrane. The mucosa also contains Bowman's glands, which secrete mucus.

1.19.2 Optic Nerve

The optic nerve develops from the optic vesicle. It is a part of the central nervous system (CNS) and is covered by meninges. It is formed by the convergence of axons from the retinal ganglion cells, which in turn receive information from bipolar cells and the photoreceptors of the eye. Each optic nerve leaves its respective orbit via the optic canal, enters the middle cranial fossa, and unite to form the optic chiasm. Here, fibers from the nasal medial half of each retina cross to the contralateral optic tract; however, lateral fibers remain ipsilateral. Therefore, the right optic tract, for example, would contain fibers from the right temporal (lateral) retina but the left nasal retina. The optic tracts then reach the lateral geniculate nucleus (LGN) in the thalamus, which carries visual information in the optic radiation. The upper radiation carries fibers from the superior retinal quadrants (corresponding to the inferior visual field quadrants) through the parietal lobe to reach the visual cortex. The lower radiation carries fibers from the inferior retinal quadrants (corresponding to the superior visual field quadrants), through the temporal lobe, via Meyer's loop, to reach the visual cortex for processing of visual information.

1.19.3 Oculomotor Nerve

The oculomotor nerve originates from the oculomotor nucleus at the level of the superior colliculus in the midbrain of the brainstem. It travels through the dura mater and enters the cavernous sinus. It leaves the cranium via the superior orbital fissure and divides into the superior branch to supply the superior rectus (which elevates the eyeball) and the levator palpabrae superioris (which raises the upper eyelid). It travels with sympathetic fibers that innervate the superior tarsal muscle (which helps to raise the eyelid). The inferior branch supplies the remaining extra ocular muscles (the inferior rectus depressing the eyeball, the medial rectus for adduction, and the inferior oblique for elevation, abduction, and lateral

rotation). The Edinger–Westphal nucleus is dorsal to the oculomotor nuclei and contains preganglionic parasympathetic neurons to the ciliary ganglion. From here, postganglionic parasympathetic fibers supply the ciliary muscles for pupil constriction and the sphincter pupillae for accommodation.

Damage to the oculomotor nerves leads to ptosis, a down-and-out position of the eye and a dilated pupil. This can occur due to raised intracranial pressure, aneurysm of the posterior communicating artery, or damage to the cavernous sinus. It can also be found in other diseases such as multiple sclerosis and myasthenia gravis.

1.19.4 Trochlear Nerve

The trochlear nerve originates from the trochlear nuclei in the midbrain at the level of the inferior colliculus. It has the longest intracranial route because it is the only nerve to emerge from the dorsal brainstem, making it particularly vulnerable to damage. It travels within the cavernous sinus and passes through the superior orbital fissure to innervate the superior oblique muscle, which functions to depress, abduct, and intort the eye. Damage to this nerve leads to double vision and a characteristic head tilt toward the unaffected side.

1.19.5 Trigeminal Nerve

The trigeminal nerve provides sensory and motor innervation to the face. It originates from three sensory nuclei (the mesencephalic, principal sensory, and spinal nuclei) and one motor nucleus extending from the midbrain to the medulla. It has three branches, the ophthalmic, the maxillary, and the mandibular nerves, which arise from the trigeminal ganglion to provide sensory innervation to the face. The mandibular branch also supplies the muscles of mastication. Clinically, the corneal reflex can be performed to test damage to the ophthalmic nerve (which acts as the afferent limb to detect the stimulus) or the facial nerve (which is the efferent limb causing contract of the orbicularis oculi muscle).

1.19.6 Abducens Nerve

The abducens nerve is the sixth paired cranial nerve, with a somatic motor function to the lateral rectus muscle. It arises from the abducens nucleus in the pons, exiting the brainstem at the junction of the pons and the medulla. It then enters the subarachnoid space and pierces the dura mater, and enters the cavernous sinus through the superior orbital fissure. It can be damaged by any space-occupying lesion, which leads to diplopia and unopposed adduction.

1.19.7 The Facial Nerve

The facial nerve is derived from the second branchial arch. The upper motor neuron of the facial nerve is in the primary motor cortex, with its axons descending to the ventral and dorsal facial nucleus in the pons. The dorsal regions supply the muscles of the upper face and receive input from both hemispheres, and the ventral region supplies the muscles of the lower face and receives mainly contralateral inputs. The facial nerve passes through the internal auditory meatus and then on to the facial canal to synapse on the geniculate ganglion. It gives rise to the greater petrosal nerve, supplying the lacrimal gland, and joins the deep petrosal nerve to form the nerve of the pterygoid canal, innervating the pterygopalatine ganglion. It gives rise to the nerve to the stapedius muscle of the ear and the chorda tympani nerve, which supplies the submandibular ganglion and the anterior two thirds of the tongue.

The facial nerve leaves the cranium through the stylomastoid foramen and supplies the external ear, the external auditory meatus, the posterior belly of the digastric, the stylohyoid, the superior and inferior auricular, and the occipitalis muscles. It then travels to the parotid gland, and without supplying it splits into five branches (temporal, zygomatic, buccal, marginal mandibular, and cervical) to supply the muscles of facial expression.

1.19.8 Vestibulocochlear Nerve

The vestibulocochlear nerve has two main sensory divisions: the vestibular and cochlear nerves, which arise from the vestibular nuclei in the pons and medulla, and the cochlear nuclei in the inferior cerebellar peduncle, respectively. They combine at the pons and emerge at the cerebellopontine angle, exiting the cranium via the internal acoustic meatus. The vestibular nerve is responsible for equilibrium and the cochlear nerve is responsible for hearing.

The cochlea contains inner hair cells that respond to vibrations of sound and trigger action potentials from the spiral ganglia. Sound frequency is coded by the position of the activated inner hair cells.

The vestibular hair cells are found in the otoliths (the saccule and the utricle), where they detect linear motion of the head, and the semicircular canals (which detect rotational movement of the head), and coordinate balance. They are also important for the vestibulo-ocular reflex, which allows the stabilization of images on the retina while the head is moving.

Inflammation of the vestibular branch of the nerve can lead to vertigo, nystagmus, loss of equilibrium, and nausea/vomiting. Inflammation of the membranous labyrinth (labyrinthitis) can cause similar symptoms and in addition affect the cochlear nerve, leading to tinnitus.

1.19.9 Glossopharyngeal Nerve

The glossopharyngeal nerve begins in the medulla and leaves the cranium via the jugular foramen. It has mixed sensory and parasympathetic components. The sensory branch innervates the oropharynx via the pharyngeal branch, which merges with the vagus nerve to form the pharyngeal plexus. It forms the afferent limb of the gag reflex (the efferent limb is via the vagus nerve). It supplies the posterior one third of the tongue via the lingual branch and the palatine tonsils via the tonsillar plexus. It also supplies the carotid body and sinus. The tympanic branch of the nerve enters the middle ear and forms the tympanic plexus to supply the middle ear, tympanic membrane, and the eustachian tube. It supplies the stylopharyngeus muscle of the pharynx and provides parasympathetic innervation to the parotid gland.

1.19.10 Vagus Nerve

The vagus nerve extends from the medulla and exits the cranium, where it gives rise to an auricular branch and courses downward into the carotid sheath. At the base of the neck, the right vagus nerve enters the thorax anterior to the subclavian artery and the left vagus nerve passes between the left common carotid and subclavian arteries. In the neck it gives rise to pharyngeal branches (which supply the pharynx and soft palate), the external superior laryngeal nerve (which supplies the cricothyroid muscle), and the internal laryngeal branch (which supplies the laryngopharynx and part of the larynx). The right vagus nerve also gives rise to the recurrent laryngeal nerve (which supplies the intrinsic muscles of the larynx) and then forms the posterior vagal trunk in the thorax. The left vagus nerve forms the anterior vagal trunk. These contribute to the formation of the esophageal plexus innervating the smooth muscle of the esophagus. Cardiac branches to the heart arise in the thorax. The left vagus nerve gives rise to the left recurrent laryngeal nerve under the arch of aorta. The vagal trunks enter the abdomen via the esophageal hiatus in the diaphragm and then terminate into branches to supply the esophagus, the stomach, and the small and large intestines up to the splenic flexure.

1.19.11 Accessory Nerve

The accessory nerve has a somatic motor function and supplies the sternocleidomastoid and trapezius muscles. It contains spinal and cranial components. The spinal components arise from C1 to C6 spinal nerve roots, which merge and enter the cranium via the foramen magnum. After exiting the cranium, it descends to the sternocleidomastoid muscle and then to the posterior neck to supply the trapezius. The cranial component arises in the medulla and exits the cranium via the jugular foramen. It combines with the vagus nerve at the inferior ganglion.

1.19.12 Hypoglossal Nerve

The hypoglossal nerve supplies the extrinsic (genioglossus, hyoglossus, styloglossus) and intrinsic muscles of the tongue. The palatoglossus muscle is innervated by the vagus nerve. The hypoglossal nerve arises from the hypoglossal nucleus in the medulla and exits the cranium via the hypoglossal canal.

1.20 Cerebellum

The cerebellum is derived from the rhombencephalon and is found in the posterior cranial fossa. It is a large structure of the hindbrain with a protruding central vermis, which sits between the cerebellar hemispheres.

On the ventral aspect of the brain, the hemispheres are connected to the pons by the middle cerebellar peduncle. On the ventral aspect of the cerebellum is the flocculus, which is found on the cerebellopontine angle and is important for vestibular function. On each side, close to the medulla, are tonsils, and clinically these are at risk of coning into the foramen magnum when CSF is withdrawn in patients with increased intracranial pressure, resulting in pressure on the vital respiratory and autonomic centers of the medulla.

There are three main lobes of the cerebellum. The anterior lobe extends from the cerebellar peduncle and terminates at the primary fissure and continues as the posterior lobe. The smallest lobe is the flocculonodular lobe and this lies between the posterolateral fissure (inferiorly) and the cerebellar peduncles (superiorly).

1.20.1 Functional Divisions

The cerebellum can be divided into three functional areas: the cerebrocerebellum, the spinocerebellum, and the vestibulocerebellum (Figure 1.28).

The large division is the cerebrocerebellum, which is formed by the lateral hemispheres and is responsible for planning movements and motor learning. It also regulates muscle activation and visually guided movements. It receives inputs from the cerebral cortex and pontine nuclei. The fibers travel through the internal capsule and cerebral peduncles and terminate ipsilaterally in the pons and send their axons to the contralateral middle cerebellar peduncle. The cerebellum also receives information via the ascending spinocerebellar mossy fibers. Fibers from the inferior olive in the medulla form the climbing fibre input via the inferior cerebellar peduncle.

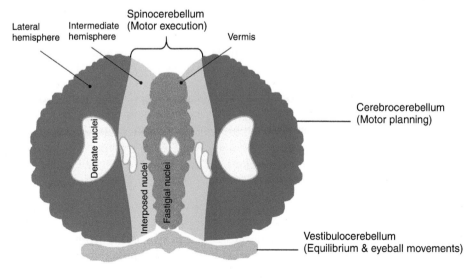

Functional divisions of human cerebellum

Figure 1.28 Functional divisions of the cerebellum.

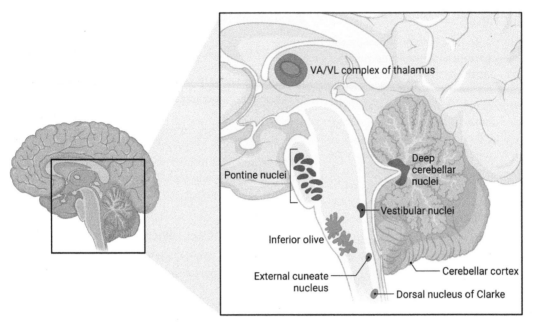

Figure 1.29 Deep cerebellar nuclei.

They are thought to mediate plasticity in the mossy fiber–granule cell–Purkinje cell pathway to coordinate movement. Outputs from the dentate nucleus and the other deep cerebellar nuclei leave the superior cerebellar peduncle and then cross the midline at the lower midbrain, pass through the red nucleus and ascend to terminate in the thalamus. The cerebellum represents ipsilateral movement and sensation.

The spinocerebellum comprises the vermis and intermediate zone of the cerebellar hemispheres. It receives proprioceptive information and regulates body movements by allowing for error correction.

The vestibulocerebellum is the functional equivalent to the flocculonodular lobe. It controls balance and ocular reflexes, and receives inputs from the vestibular system and sends outputs back to the vestibular nuclei.

1.20.2 Deep Cerebellar Nuclei

The cortical output of the cerebellum, which is typically inhibitory, involves the deep cerebellar nuclei (Figures 1.28 and 1.29). There are three nuclei on each side: the dentate nucleus, the nucleus interpositus, and the fastigial nucleus. Some areas, such as the flocculus and the flocculonodular lobe, send outputs to the vestibular nuclei in the medulla. Together, the entire cerebellar output is transmitted to the brainstem descending motor pathways and the motor areas of the cerebral cortex via the thalamus.

1.20.3 The Cerebellar Peduncles

There are three peduncles that connect the cerebellum with the brainstem on each side. The middle peduncle is the largest and the superior peduncle is the major output pathway from the deep nuclei.

1.20.4 Cerebellar Cortex

The cerebellar cortex contains many tightly packed folds (folia). It has three well-defined layers: (i) an outer molecular layer consisting mainly of parallel fibers that run parallel to the folia and dendrites; (ii) the Purkinje cell layer containing large Purkinje cells; and (iii) a granule layer consisting of many small granule cells (Figure 1.30).

The Purkinje cells are the output cells of the cerebellar cortex. They have extensive dendrites and are intersected at right angles by the parallel fibers, allowing each Purkinje cell to receive and make synaptic contact with many parallel fibers along a single folium. The Purkinje cells send axons out of the cortex and inhibit cells in the deep cerebellar nuclei.

1.20.5 Vascular Supply

The cerebellum is supplied by the superior cerebellar, anterior inferior cerebellar, and posterior inferior cerebellar arteries. The venous supply to the cerebellum includes the superior cerebellar veins draining to the

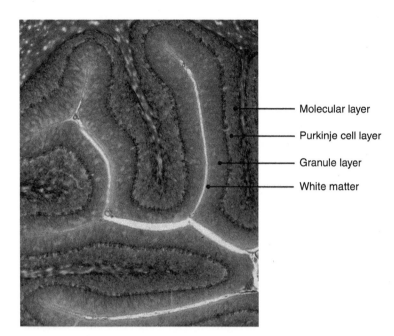

Figure 1.30 Layers of the cerebellum.

Molecular layer

Purkinje cell layer

Granule layer

White matter

straight sinus and internal cerebral veins and inferior cerebellar veins draining to the transverse sinus, superior petrosal sinus, and occipital sinus.

1.21 Spinal Cord

The spinal cord is an organized bundle of nervous tissue extending from the medulla oblongata through the vertebral canal to the L2 vertebral level and terminates as the conus medullaris. Spinal nerves arise from the end of the spinal cord and together are known as the cauda equina. Compression of these leads to the neurosurgical emergency known as cauda equina syndrome and can lead to paralysis. The spinal cord enlarges at the level of C4–T1 (cervical enlargement) and is the site of origin of the brachial plexus. A second enlargement is at the level of T11–L1 (lumbar enlargement), and is where the lumbar and sacral plexi originate.

The spinal cord is surrounded by the spinal meninges (dura, arachnoid, and pia mater) and contains CSF. It is anchored distally to the coccyx by a fibrous band of tissue called the filum terminale. The dura mater extends from the foramen magnum to the filum terminale and is separated from the vertebral canal by the epidural space containing the internal vertebral venous plexus. The dura mater also surrounds the epineurium of spinal nerves that pierce the dura. The arachnoid mater is separated from the pia mater by the subarachnoid space and contains

CSF. The pia mater surrounds the spinal cord, nerve roots, and blood vessels and inferiorly fuses with the filum terminale. The pia mater thickens to form denticulate ligaments which attach to the dura mater, and these help suspend the spinal cord in the vertebral canal.

1.21.1 Neurovascular Supply

The arterial supply to the spinal cord is via the anterior spinal artery (a branch of the vertebral artery) and the two posterior spinal arteries (branches of the vertebral artery or the posteroinferior cerebellar artery), which anastomose in the pia mater. The segmental medullary arteries, of which the largest is the anterior segmental medullary artery (the artery of Adamkiewicz), also supply the spinal cord. Disruption of the blood supply to the spinal cord leads to nerve cell death and signs of weakness, paralysis, and loss of reflexes.

The spinal cord venous drainage includes an extrinsic and an intrinsic network. The extrinsic system includes radicular veins, the pial venous network, dorsal and ventral spinal veins. They are connected to the valveless vertebral venous plexuses, that communicate with the dural venous sinuses and are composed of an external plexus surrounding the vertebral column, internal plexus within the spinal canal (linked together via segmental veins) and basivertebral veins in the vertebral bodies. The intrinsic venous system includes the sulcal (drains to the anterior spinal veins) and radial veins (drains to the posterior spinal veins), linked by the transmedullary anastomotic veins within the parenchyma of the spinal cord.

The spinal nerves originate from the spinal cord and form the peripheral nervous system. They begin as anterior (motor) and posterior (sensory) nerve roots and unite at the intervertebral foramina to form a single spinal nerve, which leaves the vertebral canal via the intervertebral foramina and divides into the posterior and anterior rami (Figure 1.31).

A peripheral nerve has an outer covering called the epineurium. Nerve fibers are organized into bundles called fascicles and each one is covered by the perineurium. Each individual neuron is covered by the endoneurium. Each individual neuron is covered by the endoneurium, a layer of delicate connective tissue around the myelin sheath of each myelinated nerve fiber in the peripheral nervous system (Figure 1.32).

A single spinal nerve innervates a strip of skin known as the dermatome and is used clinically to assess spinal injuries. During embryology the mesoderm adjacent to the neural tube (paraxial mesoderm) differentiates into 31 somites or segments. The ventral part gives rise to the ribs and vertebral column. The dorsal part consists of the dermomyotome. The dermatome forms the dermis, which eventually stretches to create a segmental innervation and the classic dermatome map (Figure 1.33).

1.21.2 Transverse Section of the Spinal Cord

The spinal cord contains inner gray matter surrounded by the white matter. The gray matter is divided into the dorsal horn, the intermediate column, the lateral horn, and the ventral horn. The dorsal horn contains neurons receiving somatosensory information. The ventral horn contains motor neurons that innervate skeletal muscle. The intermediate column and lateral horn contain neurons that innervate visceral and pelvic organs.

1.21.3 Rexed Laminae

The spinal cord can also be visualized in layers or laminae, where cells are grouped according to their structure and function (Figure 1.34). Lamina I contains cells that respond to noxious or thermal stimuli and sends information via the lateral spinothalamic tract. It corresponds to the marginal zone. Lamina II corresponds to the

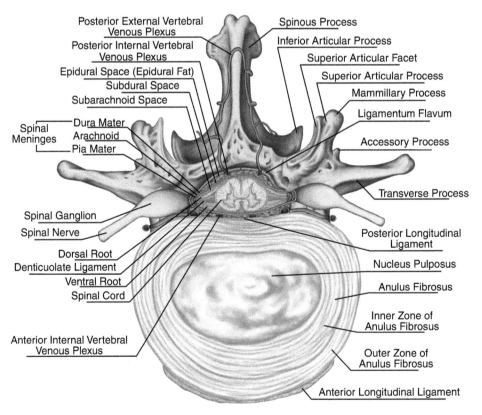

Posterior External Vertebral Venous Plexus
Posterior Internal Vertebral Venous Plexus
Epidural Space (Epidural Fat)
Subdural Space
Subarachnoid Space
Spinal Meninges
Dura Mater
Arachnoid
Pia Mater
Spinal Ganglion
Spinal Nerve
Dorsal Root
Denticuolate Ligament
Ventral Root
Spinal Cord
Anterior Internal Vertebral Venous Plexus

Spinous Process
Inferior Articular Process
Superior Articular Facet
Superior Articular Process
Mammillary Process
Ligamentum Flavum
Accessory Process
Transverse Process
Posterior Longitudinal Ligament
Nucleus Pulposus
Anulus Fibrosus
Inner Zone of Anulus Fibrosus
Outer Zone of Anulus Fibrosus
Anterior Longitudinal Ligament

Figure 1.31 Anatomical relations of a spinal nerve.

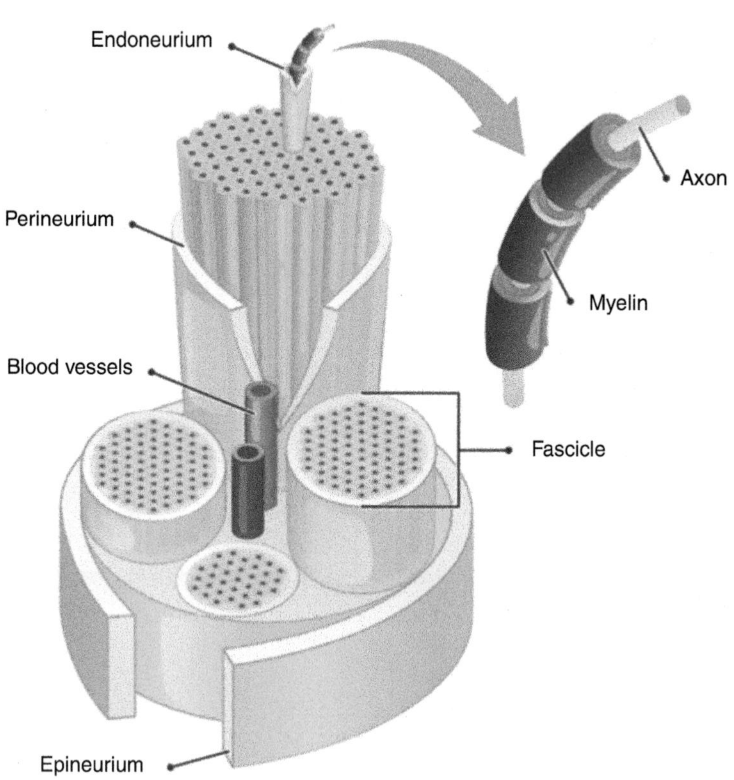

Endoneurium

Axon

Perineurium

Myelin

Blood vessels

Fascicle

Epineurium

Figure 1.32 Layers of a peripheral nerve.

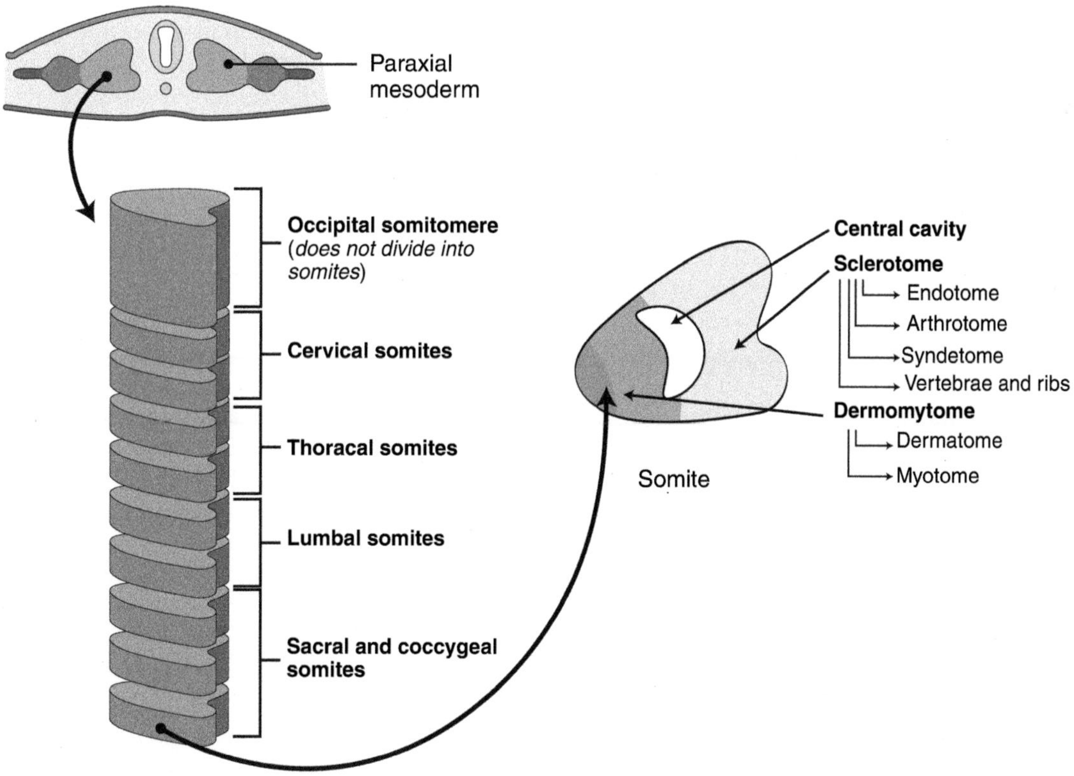

Paraxial mesoderm

Occipital somitomere (*does not divide into somites*)

Cervical somites

Thoracal somites

Lumbal somites

Sacral and coccygeal somites

Somite

Central cavity

Sclerotome
→ Endotome
→ Arthrotome
→ Syndetome
→ Vertebrae and ribs

Dermomytome
→ Dermatome
→ Myotome

Figure 1.33 The development of the dermatome.

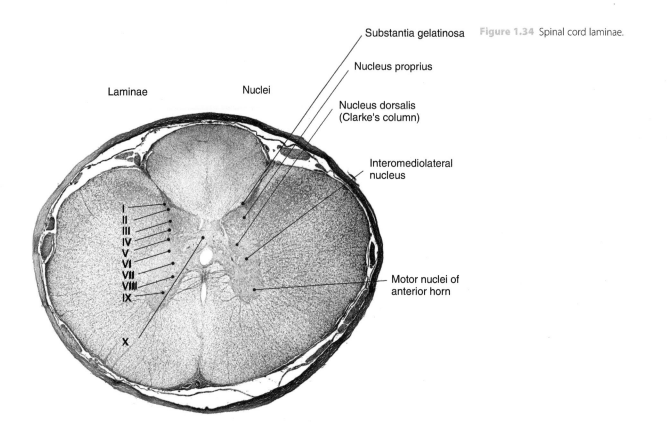

Laminae   Nuclei

Substantia gelatinosa   Figure 1.34 Spinal cord laminae.

Nucleus proprius

Nucleus dorsalis
(Clarke's column)

Interomediolateral
nucleus

Motor nuclei of
anterior horn

I
II
III
IV
V
VI
VII
VIII
IX

X

substance gelatinosa and is involved in sensation of all stimuli and moderates pain sensation. Lamina III is involved in proprioception and light touch sensation. Lamina IV is involved in non-noxious sensory information processing. Lamina V relays sensory information to the brain via the contralateral and spinothalamic tracts, and receives descending information from the brain via the corticospinal and rubrospinal tracts. Lamina VI receives proprioceptive information and sends information to the brain via ipsilateral spinocerebellar pathways and processes spinal reflexes. Lamina VII is a large region and receives information from lamina II to VI and relays motor information to the viscera. Lamina VIII is involved in modulating motor output to skeletal muscle. Lamina IX contains motor neurons innervating striated muscles and muscle spindles. Lamina X, known as the gray commissure, surrounds the central canal of the spinal cord and contains decussating axons.

1.22 Introduction to Neuroembryology

Neuroembryology is the study of the development of the nervous system during embryogenesis. The embryo develops as a zygote following fertilization and subsequently cleaves to become the morula, which reorganizes to form the blastocyst cavity (Figure 1.35). The blastocyst is comprised of two different cell types: the outer cell mass (trophoblast) and the inner cell mass (embryoblast). The trophoblast contacts with the endometrium of the uterus to facilitate implantation and the formation of the placenta. The embryoblast forms the embryo itself and is divided into the hypoblast (which becomes the yolk sac) and the epiblast (which becomes the amniotic cavity). The epiblast contains a groove in its midline called the primitive streak, which helps confer anterior–posterior and dorsal–ventral spatial information to early differentiating cells. The one-dimensional layer of epithelial cells (blastula) reorganizes into a multilayered structure, and this is known as gastrulation. The purpose of gastrulation is to form three germ layers (endoderm, mesoderm, and ectoderm) and this stage is followed by organogenesis. The endoderm develops into the linings of the respiratory and alimentary tracts, the liver, and the pancreas. The mesoderm forms the notochord, somites, and the mesenchyme. The ectoderm develops into skin, the nervous system, and neural crest cells. The neural crest cells give rise to the pharyngeal arches, which

Fertilization and the zygote	Cleavage and the morula	Blastulation

Figure 1.35 The formation of the blastocyst.

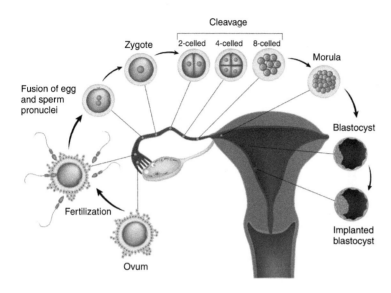

contribute to the development of the facial skeleton. Pharyngeal arches are often used interchangeably with branchial arches (Figure 1.36).

1.22.1 Neurulation (Formation of the Neural Tube)

The embryonic blastocyst develops into a two-layered structure: the epiblast and the hypoblast. In humans, the primitive streak, an opening on the epiblast midline forms ~14 days after fertilization. By the end of the third week, gastrulation occurs and the epiblast and hypoblast develop into the ectoderm and endoderm, respectively. The notochord is a rod of mesodermal cells that extends throughout the entire dorsal plane of the embryo and is responsible for inducing the overlying lateral edges of the ectoderm to form the neural plate (Figure 1.37), which will remodel to form a single closed tube. The notochord arises from a collection of cells called the Spemann–Mangold organizer. The discovery of these cells introduced the concept of induction in embryology where the identity of certain cells influences the development of surrounding cells. Later in development, the cranial and caudal portions of the neural tube form the brain and spinal cord, respectively. Closure of the neural tube is accompanied by accumulation of amniotic fluid in the central canal, which forms the

primitive ventricular system the brain. The ventricular system is lined by the ventricular zone (VZ), which is an embryonic layer containing radial glial cells and is the site of neurogenesis during embryogenesis. The subventricular (SVZ) zone lies adjacent to this area, containing intermediate neuronal progenitor cells that divide into postmitotic neurons.

1.23 Regional Formations in the Brain

Once the formation of the neural tube has been completed, the neural tube continues to differentiate to form different regions of the brain. These regions are the prosencephalon (forebrain), the mesencephalon (midbrain), the rhombencephalon (hindbrain), and the spinal cord (Figure 1.38).

The proper formation of these regions requires the presence of inducing morphogens. The development of the midbrain and hindbrain requires the isthmus organizer, which releases signals that organize the expression of transcription factors.

The forebrain divides into the telencephalon and the diencephalon. The telencephalon includes the olfactory bulbs, hippocampus, and cerebrum. The diencephalon includes the optic nerves, epithalamus, thalamus, and hypothalamus.

The developing hindbrain divides into the metencephalon and the myelencephalon. Coordinating and fine-tuning

39

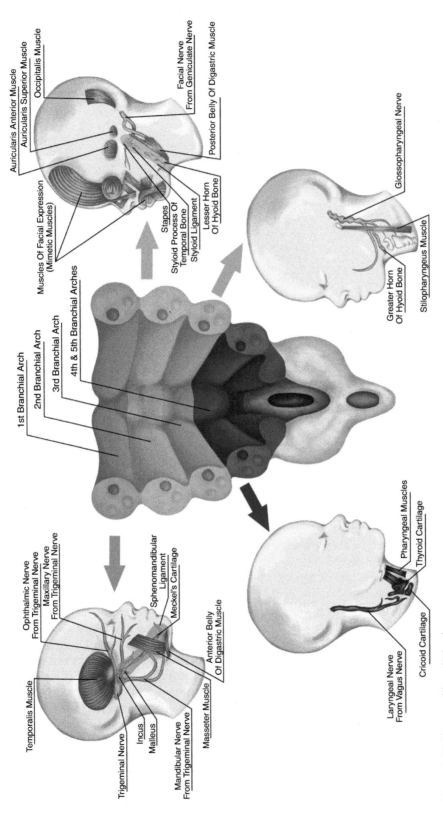

Auricularis Anterior Muscle
Auricularis Superior Muscle
Occipitalis Muscle

Muscles Of Facial Expression
(Mimetic Muscles)

Stapes
Styloid Process Of
Temporal Bone
Styloid Ligament
Lesser Horn
Of Hyoid Bone

Facial Nerve
From Geniculate Nerve

Posterior Belly Of Digastric Muscle

Glossopharyngeal Nerve

Greater Horn
Of Hyoid Bone
Stilopharyngeus Muscle

1st Branchial Arch
2nd Branchial Arch
3rd Branchial Arch
4th & 5th Branchial Arches

Ophthalmic Nerve
From Trigeminal Nerve
Maxillary Nerve
From Trigeminal Nerve

Sphenomandibular
Ligament
Meckel's Cartilage

Anterior Belly
Of Digastric Muscle

Temporalis Muscle

Trigeminal Nerve
Incus
Malleus
Mandibular Nerve
From Trigeminal Nerve
Masseter Muscle

Pharyngeal Muscles
Thyroid Cartilage

Laryngeal Nerve
From Vagus Nerve
Cricoid Cartilage

Figure 1.36 Pharyngeal/branchial arches.

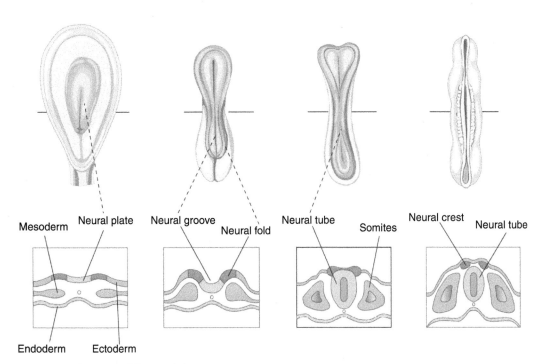

Figure 1.37 Formation of the neural plate.

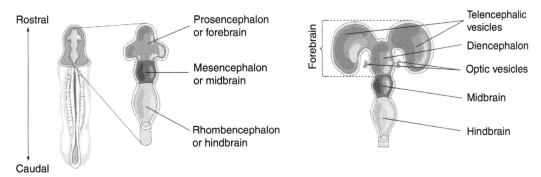

Figure 1.38 Regions of the brain and development of the forebrain.

muscle movements are functions primarily found in the hindbrain, because the cerebellum and pons derive from the metencephalon. The myelencephalon develops the medulla, which relays vital information regarding breathing and heart rate to the brain from the rest of the body and is responsible for involuntary reflex movements, such as sneezing and swallowing.

Three membranous layers cover the CNS: the dura mater (derived from the surrounding mesenchyme), the arachnoid, and the pia mater (both derived from the neural crest cells).

1.24 Neurogenesis

Embryonic neurogenesis refers to the generation of neurons from neural stem cells or neuron progenitor cells. Adult neurogenesis occurs in specialized niches of the brain throughout life, namely in the SVZ of the lateral ventricles and in the subgranular zone (SGZ) of the hippocampal dentate gyrus.

The VZ of the neural tube contains neural precursor cells (NPCs), which become radial glial cells (RGCs). The RGCs oscillate between the basal and apical VZs. They proliferate and symmetrically divide during the cell cycle. This process is known as interkinetic nuclear migration. Progenitor cells also accumulate in the SVZ and continue to expand to give rise to excitatory pyramidal projection neurons and glial cells. They switch to asymmetric cell division and become a postmitotic neuron, which migrates and forms the neocortex or becomes an intermediate progenitor.

RGCs give rise to a six-layered cortex. The earliest neurons become inner layer 6 and the last-born neurons give rise to layer 2. The marginal zone is the external layer (layer 1). RGCs also generate oligodendrocyte and astrocyte progenitors. The oligodendrocytes produce myelin sheath in the CNS. Astrocytes become the most abundant cells in the brain and have several functions including maintenance of the blood–brain barrier (BBB) and metabolism.

There are several transcription factors that play an important role in regulating neurogenesis. The Paired box protein (Pax-6), is involved in neural stem cell proliferation, neuronal specification and migration in the CNS. The Sox family of proteins also have an important role in neuronal fate commitment and differentiation.

Programmed cell death is an evolutionarily conserved trait that is an integral part of the development of the nervous system. It is postulated that up to half of the original neuronal cell population is eliminated as a result of apoptosis. The elimination of superfluous neurons during development is critical for the optimization of synaptic connections, often referred to as the nerve growth factor theory- the idea that targets of innervation supply limiting amounts of neurotrophic factors, which the developing neurons depend on for their survival.

1.25 Neuronal Migration

Neurons can migrate to their target location via radial migration along radial glia fibers in a perpendicular fashion to the ventricular surface. Glutamatergic neurons are made in the VZ and travel to their target zones via radial migration. Radial migration of neurons occurs in several distinct modes, and these include locomotion, somal translocation, and via multipolar migration. Neurons can also migrate to their target location via tangential migration, which involves migration in trajectories parallel to the ventricular surface and orthogonal to the radial glia fibers. Inhibitory GABAergic cortical interneurons travel via tangential migration to the cerebral cortex. Neurons from distinct sites converge and form neural circuits via tangential migration.

1.26 Axon Guidance

The formation of networks following cell division and migration is crucial to normal brain development. The first stage of development of a network is the formation of axonal tracts. Axons project and reach their target through a series of coordinated steps. Axons grow from a region within their terminal called the growth cone.

The growth cone possesses expansions at the tip called lamellipodia and fine processes called filopodia that help move the axon in a certain direction in response to axon cues or guidance molecules such as netrin, semaphorin, Slit–Robo, and Notch. The netrins are large, soluble proteins produced by the VZ and floor plate, which can function as both attractants (via interaction with the Netrin receptor DCC, also known as colorectal cancer suppressor), and repellants via the Slit proteins, which bind to receptors from the round- about (Robo1 - Robo4) family. Midline cells express Slit, thereby controlling axon crossing at the midline and preventing recrossing of axons that have already crossed by interacting with the Robo receptors.

Pioneer axons are the first to grow in a defined region. They are not morphologically different from other axons; however, they facilitate the formation of a navigation path for follower axons. Pioneer axons and follower axons can fasciculate to form a nerve tract. Pioneer axons are aided by guidepost cells, which are specialized populations of neurons or glia that express guidance cues to enable the growth cone to navigate to its destination in a series of short, sequential segments.

1.27 Synapse Formation

The next step in the development process is to form synapses. A growth cone will transform to become a bulbous presynaptic site. This is followed by a rapid increase in intracellular calcium (Ca^{2+}) ion concentration, which causes the shape of the growth cone to change. Various adhesion molecules and factors further contribute to the shape of the cone, and finally the first contact with the postsynaptic membrane is made. Synapse formation is finely regulated and the presynaptic region becomes highly specialized architecturally to allow regulated secretion of neurotransmitters. The postsynaptic region is characterized by clustering of receptors opposite the presynaptic active zone, to allow for efficient transfer of information.. There may also be multiple receptors that bind to the same neurotransmitters, such as GABAA and GABAB receptors, both binding to GABA.

The location of the synapse and its properties will impact the flow of information in the circuit. The synapses formed may be of a specific type – e.g., glutamatergic neurons – and they may also form on specific regions, such as soma or dendritic spines. Those located near the soma or the initial segment of the axons have a greater influence on the firing properties of the action potential. Those in distal dendrites are smaller in nature and must summate to depolarize the membrane.

Synapses also show specificity and can be governed by many factors, such as the Sonic Hedgehog cues expressed by postsynaptic neurons and its receptor Brother of CDO (Boc) in the presynaptic neurons, which aid in the targeted formation of the synapses.

Synaptic maturation is a slower process that continues until the end of adolescence and is designed to refine synaptic connections by elimination and by allowing competition between different inputs. The importance of sensory experience on synapse elimination and stabilization was demonstrated in the classic visual deprivation experiments by Hubel and Wiesel (see section on Ocular Dominance).

1.28 Brain Plasticity

The ability of the nervous system to change structurally and functionally due to various environmental factors is known as plasticity. Structural plasticity includes changes in the cellular architecture and functional plasticity includes changes in function due to changes in the structural components.

Synaptic plasticity includes changes in strength and transmission due to experience or input changes and is particularly pronounced during critical periods of development. Network changes are modifications of neuronal networks composed of linked neuronal populations.

Repetitive firing of adjacent excitatory neurons is known to strengthen synaptic connections or weaken with the firing of inhibitory neurons (Hebb's postulate). This also forms the basis for LTP and LTD models of synaptic plasticity. Spike-timing–dependent plasticity refers to the frequency of presynaptic firing and the order of pre- and postsynaptic firing during a precise time, and this affects the strength of synaptic plasticity. However, some synapses do not follow Hebb's postulate and their strength may be influenced by other factors, such as dendritic depolarization or changes in sensory input. The pruning and formation of synapses leads to various changes, such as spine morphology and neurotransmitter release, with a resultant change in the strength of synaptic connections leading to the modification of neural networks.

Homeostatic plasticity, a major form of non-Hebbian plasticity, refers to cellular and molecular mechanisms that limit the unopposed persistence of activity-dependent synaptic plasticity, which has the inherent risk of inducing extreme neural states and therefore counters the self-reinforcing nature of Hebbian plasticity. It allows neural circuits to achieve functional stability by e.g. equipoise of intrinsic excitability and synaptic strength. Metaplasticity is a higher-order form of synaptic plasticity, and is known as the plasticity of synaptic plasticity. This refers to modulation of synaptic plasticity based on activation history in the same synapse (homo- synaptic metaplasticity) or nearby synapses (heterosy- naptic metaplasticity).

1.29 Critical Period Versus Sensitive Periods

During a critical period, the presence of an experience is needed for the development of a specific circuit. During a sensitive period, sensory experience influences development, but this is not exclusive to a set period. Sensitive periods are important for cognitive abilities, such as learning a language.

1.30 Critical Periods of Brain Development Are Windows of Heightened Plasticity

Critical periods during early brain development are epochs of heightened plasticity, in which sensory experience is required to establish optical cortical representations of the environment. The onset of critical periods is regulated by the balance of excitatory and inhibitory connections. The leading contributor to critical opening in the visual cortex is an increase in GABAergic inhibition, reportedly dependent on brain–derived neurotrophic factor (BDNF) levels. Closure of the critical period is important to ensure that there is sequential consolidation and retention of new and complex perceptual, cognitive, and motor functions. However, if sensory experience is abnormal during this period, there may be permanent detrimental effects. If the abnormal experience occurs after the period has closed, there will be reversible, and less detrimental effects on the brain.

1.31 Critical Periods of Sensory Systems

1.31.1 Ocular Dominance

The neurons in the primary visual cortex of mammals contain monocular neurons in layer 4 and binocular neurons in the remaining layers. Neurons with the same eye preference are grouped together in ocular dominance (OD) columns. In the classic experiments by Hubel and Wiesel (1963), it was demonstrated that monocular deprivation of one eye in kittens during a critical period abolishes the ability of that eye to respond to visual stimulation and shifts the OD columns in favor of the open eye. However, a similar experiment in adult cats had no detrimental effect on vision. In humans, monocular deprivation from conditions such as strabismus can have the same effect, known as amblyopia, and can also lead to problems with depth perception.

1.31.2 Auditory Processing

Neurons in the primary auditory cortex (A1) are topographically arranged by their response to different frequencies. Organization of these tonotopic maps are genetically predetermined but refined in an activity dependent manner, through spontaneous activity and, following hearing onset. During critical periods, heightened plasticity drives maturation of specific features of the auditory system, such as identification of phonemes and language acquisition. However, this period is also exquisitely sensitive to impoverished environmental influences, which may have inadvertent effects on frequency tuning. Similarly, overexposure to pure tones may result in overrepresentation of the tone frequency within the map. Critical periods have also been described for other processes such as binaural hearing, which allows the localization of different sound sources. This can be greatly affected in childhood hearing loss associated with ear infections, with overrepresentation of stimuli to the unaffected ear and weakening of responses to the affected ear, resulting in reduced ability to navigate the auditory scene.

1.32 Plasticity Regulators

As external sensory inputs increase, there is increased cortical activity which guides neural circuit development. This stage is aided by neurotrophic factors that promote plastic changes and simulate neuron growth. However, as inhibitory circuits mature further, these factors decline in number and plasticity regulators prevent further circuit changes to ensure that the cortical representations that have been developed are stable and will not be modified further by passive abnormal sensory inputs. There are several plasticity regulators that are established during the closure of the critical period. These molecular brakes include perineuronal nets (envelops inhibitory neurons) and chemorepulsive cues (restricts axon growth). Axonal growth can be impeded from the binding of axonal growth inhibitors such as Nogo to myelin receptors. There are several plasticity regulators that work in synergy to regulate cortical excitatory/inhibitory (E/I) balance. A high E/I ratio during development is important for remodeling of cortical circuits. However, a high inhibitory tone is important for maintaining stable cortical representations throughout the lifespan. Evidence for this comes from conditions characterized by a downregulation of inhibition, which is associated with impaired sensory processing. During natural aging, there is a reduction in GABA concentration, and this contributes to reduced sensory processing and impaired learning.

Critical period plasticity can be modulated by reopening critical windows in the adult brain or through the premature closure of periods of abnormal plasticity in the developing brain. Approaches that may be used to reset neural networks include for example, the removal of perineuronal nets or manipulation of inhibitory GABAergic circuits.

1.33 Introduction to Comparative Neuroanatomy and Animal Models

Our understanding of the basic function and structure of the nervous system comes largely from studies on a range of species (Figure 1.39). The benefits of comparative neurobiological studies have enabled the discovery of several well-known concepts, such as the squid giant axon and the ionic basis of the action potential by Hodgkin and Huxley, discovery of dendritic spines in the CNS of the chicken by Cajal, and understanding the cellular basic of learning and memory in *Aplysia* by Kandel, to name a few. The examination of the CNS of different species allows us to discern features that are not easily seen in humans. In this section, we discuss the most common species used for neurobiological research.

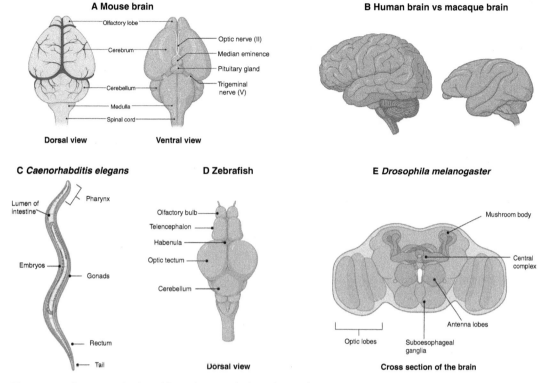

Figure 1.39 Common animal models used in neurobiological research.

1.33.1 Rodents

There are several anatomical differences between human brains and those of rodents. Firstly, it is thought that humans have approximately 86 billion neurons compared to approximately 70 million in mice. The human brain cortex is folded, which increases its surface area, whereas the rodent cortex is smoother. Humans also have highly specialized regions for language and cognition. Rodents, however, have more evolved olfactory bulbs, necessary for their superior sense of smell.

Rats were historically the most popular animals used for neurobiological research due to their genetic and physiological similarities to humans. They are also larger in size than mice and therefore easier to handle and perform procedures on. However, the use of this model has declined largely due to the difficulties in directed manipulation of the rat genome.

Mice are formidable models for research in neuroscience. The ability to manipulate the mouse genome has allowed us to decipher the functions of genes and their role in disease processes. There are several advantages of using mice as models. They are small in size, allowing novel compounds to be delivered in smaller quantities for

testing. They are also relatively cheap to maintain and reproduce quickly. They can also be inbred to yield identical strains, which removes genetic heterogeneity. The gene regulation networks are largely conserved in mice and human, however there are striking differences in gene expression patterns, and equally there are notable differences in immune responses, stress responses and metabolism between mice and humans. This often leads to disappointing results from clinical trials that are spurred on by positive results found in mouse studies. Rodent use in various physiological processes and diseases has been well described in the literature and the reader is directed to these sources for further reading.

1.33.2 Non-Human Primates

The use of non-human primates for basic neuroscience research has provided great insight into brain function and has allowed the testing of several therapeutic strategies used in human disease. Although there are many similarities between the human brain and the primate brain, there are notable anatomical differences. The human brain is 4.8 times bigger in size than it is for a comparable monkey (Figure 1.37). Human neocortex expansion has likely contributed to the higher cognitive abilities of humans. The prefrontal cortex forms a larger part of the human brain with a greater density of neurons compared to macaque brains. Other notable differences include a much smaller or absent fasciculus arcuatus (important for language processing) in non human primates. The consequence of an increase in size means that there is an increase in the number of specialized subregions such as the parietal cortex.

1.33.2.1 Macaque Monkey Model

The most frequently used non-human primates used in brain research are the long-tailed macaque (*Macaca fascicularis*) and the rhesus macaque (*M. mulatta*). Marmosets, squirrel monkeys, and cebus monkeys have also been used, although less frequently.

For ethical reasons, the human brain cannot be easily manipulated. If a particular phenomenon of brain function cannot be studied in other animals, macaques provide a suitable alternative as they are biologically similar to humans. Macaques can be used to systematically investigate the activity of individual neurons and their relation to higher cognition.

The use of deep brain stimulation (DBS) for intractable Parkinson's disease has been mastered in rhesus macaques. It involves the implantation of electrodes in specific regions in the brain, which are then connected to an external neurostimulator. DBS applies intermittent electrical current to the target with higher frequencies than normal firing rates in that region. The most common targets are the STN and the internal globus pallidus and sometimes the ventral intermediate thalamus. The internal globus pallidus is a favored target for gait disturbances, problems with word fluency, and axial symptoms or troublesome dyskinesias. The STN is preferred in patients with higher medication requirements.

Long-tailed macaques have also been used to study Alzheimer's disease as they naturally develop protein deposits in the brain, similar to that in humans. Genetically modified macaques with a mutation of the Huntingtin protein can result in symptoms and signs of Huntington's patients similar to humans.

Brain–machine interfaces (BMIs) are new strategies aimed at restoring mobility in severely paralyzed patients and have been tested in macaques. They involve the insertion of implants into the cortex connected to an electrical stimulator on the spine of a monkey with induced spinal cord injury. The implant records the neuronal activity of regions involved in motor control, interfaced with electrical stimulation in the epidural region of the spinal cord. A computer can recognize the animal's intention to walk and then send signals to the stimulator. This subsequently activates neural circuits in the spinal cord that control the muscle activity involved in walking. The brain–spine interface is therefore able to restore locomotion of the paralyzed leg and has been useful for proof-of-concept studies in humans.

1.33.3 *Drosophila*

The use of *Drosophila* (fruit flies) has been instrumental in furthering advances in neuroscience, with many milestone discoveries made. The advantages and limitations of this model are shown in Table 1.1.

The *Drosophila* brain contains several discrete structures. These include the antennal lobes, important for the olfactory chemosensory pathway, and the mushroom bodies that are involved in olfactory associative learning and memory. A prominent structure in the central brain is the central body complex, which consists of four substructures: the fan-shaped body, the ellipsoid body, the paired nodule, and the protocerebral bridge. The central complex is involved in learning and memory, locomotor control, and courting behavior. The visual neuropils in the *Drosophila* form the optic lobe, which consists of four major substructures: the lamina, medulla, lobula, and the lobula plate. The subesophageal ganglion controls the mouth, salivary glands, and neck muscles (Figure 1.39).

Initial use of *Drosophila* for research was aimed at understanding the principles of heredity. Early studies of this model led to the discovery of balancer chromosomes, allowing the maintenance of mutations in essential genes without the need to genotype the animal for further breeding. Early demonstrations of how x-ray exposure can lead to genetic mutations, with resultant change in the genome, were conducted in *Drosophila*. The discovery of mitotic recombinations, where it was first demonstrated that reciprocal genetic exchange between chromosomes occurred outside the germlines, was first seen in *Drosophila*.

The importance of various genes in nervous system development, segmentation, and pattern formation were discovered using x-ray–induced mutations. The *bithorax* complex of genes and the *polycomb* gene were shown to be important in segmentation in the fruit flies.

Key genes involved in embryonic pattern formation and nervous system development such as *Notch* were first identified in *Drosophila*. The loss of *Notch* leads to the formation of an embryo with hypertrophied regions of the CNS and an underdeveloped ventral hypoderm, leading

Table 1.1 Advantages and limitations of the *Drosophila* model

Advantage	Disadvantage
Limited ethical concerns	Major differences in systems compared to humans limiting translation research e.g. lack of an adaptive immune system.
Ease of genetic manipulation	Difficulty in assessing complex behaviors.
Genetic manipulation is fast and inexpensive (3 months, < $500 per transgene)	Only basic measures of cognitive decline
Plethora of available resources/stocks (e.g., genome-wide RNAi-library)	Need to maintain large breeding stocks due to inability to cryobiologically preserve flies
Short generation time	Less-complex and adaptive immune system than in vertebrates
Fully sequenced and annotated genome	Effects of drugs on the organism might differ (e.g., conversion of pro-toxins to toxins in liver)
Conservation of basic signaling pathways and cellular processes	Fly lines are subject to genetic drift via random mutations complicating genetic research of disease pathways
The availability of balancer chromosomes allowing the maintenance of lethal mutations	

to premature differentiation into neuroblasts. Components of its pathway such as *neuralized* are also important in learning and memory.

Larval *Drosophila* were among the first species to be used as a model for synaptic transmission through the study of their neuromuscular junction (NMJ). Presynaptic and postsynaptic genetic manipulation techniques were used to discover the functions of many proteins, including the roles of synaptotagmin as a calcium sensor.

1.33.4 Zebrafish

The zebrafish has become an instrumental model in answering fundamental questions about the brain and has recently seen many sophisticated applications in investigating clinical diseases. The zebrafish contains many structures that are similar to other vertebrates. Approximately 6 hours post fertilization (hpf), the CNS begins to develop. By 24 hpf, the brain can be distinguished into the forebrain, midbrain, and hindbrain (Figure 1.40). The forebrain further differentiates into the telencephalon, the diencephalon, the hypothalamus, and the retina.

The telencephalon in zebrafish is composed of the subpallium (ventral telencephalon), the pallium (dorsal telencephalon), and the olfactory bulb. The subpallium in the zebrafish serves a similar function as the mammalian basal ganglia. The ventral telencephalon contains the ventral nucleus and a dorsal nucleus. GABAergic and cholinergic neurons are formed in this region. The dorsal telencephalon is composed of a more complex array of regions including the central, lateral, posterior,

and dorsomedial zones. It serves a similar function to that of the hippocampus and amygdala in mammals. The olfactory bulb of the telencephalon receives odor information.

The zebrafish diencephalon is composed of the thalamus, pineal body, and habenula. The habenula connects the forebrain with the midbrain and hindbrain, and is involved in fear modulation, reproductive behavior, and sleep initiation.

The hindbrain is easily visualized in the zebrafish. Numerous motor neurons and those that innervate the branchial arches and the cerebellum originate here. The hindbrain contains reticulospinal neurons including the Mauthner cell, which mediates escape responses.

The zebrafish has several advantages as an animal model, including small size and low maintenance costs. Zebrafish larvae have further advantages in being easily manipulated, permeable to small molecules, rapidly generated, optically translucent, and having non-protected status prior to 5 days post fertilization (dpf). The zebrafish genes are thought to share approximately 70% homology with that of human genes and has high homology to mammalian biology. The zebrafish possesses conserved neural circuits underlying basic behaviors and pathways and is therefore likely to be relevant for translational research. Neurons are accessible during *in vivo* imaging and can therefore be used to investigate how neuronal circuits are involved in complex behavior.

The behavioral repertoire of zebrafish larvae has been exploited to not only understand the functions of distinct regions of the brain but also to test various

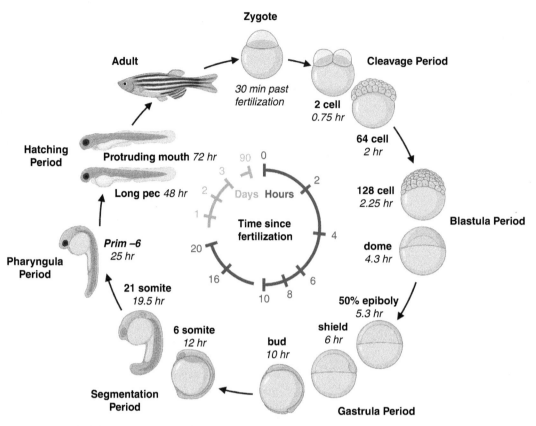

Figure 1.40 Zebrafish developmental timeline.

neuropharmacologic agents. Zebrafish have a developmentally regulated BBB, which is functional at 10 dpf and is therefore ideal for testing drugs. Behavior that is commonly tested in zebrafish includes thigmotaxis (the tendency to move toward the periphery of an environment) for testing anxiety, startle responses to various stimuli, and optomotor responses, an innate visuomotor reflex, initiated by neurons in the pretectum/tectum or through the activation of hindbrain integrator neurons which activate downstream motor commands. Locomotion play an integral role in the feeding, social, and defensive activities of the zebrafish and is produced by reticulospinal neurons of the brainstem along with descending vestibulospinal or neuromodulatory projections. The sleep/wake pattern of the zebrafish is similar to humans and provides great insight into the biology of the circadian rhythms and can be used as a model to study human sleep. Other behavior paradigm tests include habituation (to test non associative learning) and prey capture (decision making and cognition).

The zebrafish has also been used to model various clinical diseases. These include neurodegenerative diseases such as Alzheimer's disease, Parkinson's disease, and Huntington's disease. It has also been used to model brain tumors (Figure 1.41), intracerebral hemorrhage, and arteriovenous malformations.

The use of zebrafish for translational research is still at an infantile stage for many diseases and therefore requires rigorous testing and exploration. For example, although it is exceptional for large scale pharmacologic testing, the route of administration of drugs in zebrafish includes passive exposure in water rather than active administration and therefore may produce differing results in humans.

1.33.5 *Caenorhabditis elegans*

Caenorhabditis elegans is a nematode approximately 1 mm in size. It is a formidable organism for the study of genomes that may otherwise be difficult in mammalian systems. As an animal model it has several advantages, such as a transparent body, a short life cycle, and

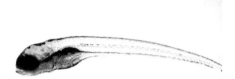

Figure 1.41 Zebrafish larvae at 5dpf showing glioblastoma tumor growth (green)

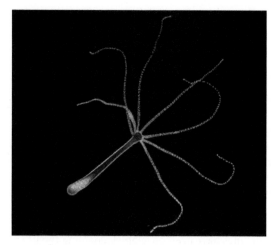

Figure 1.42 Gross structure of the *Hydra*.

fecundity. Furthermore, as they are self-fertilizing hermaphrodites, each progeny represents a genetic clone.

The *C. elegans* lineage is invariant and the complete cell lineage for the 959 cells in the adult has been described. The sequencing of the genome has also demonstrated that approximately 38% of worm genes have a human ortholog and therefore provides opportunity for it to be used as an *in vivo* model for the study of certain human conditions. It also has a compact genome size and therefore genetic screens can be conducted to further elucidate the molecular underpinnings of certain behaviors.

The complete connectome of C. elegans contains 302 neurons for the adult hermaphrodite. It has been used to further our understanding of well-known signaling pathways and study the complexities of the nervous system.

It has been particularly useful for studying memory and learning. These organisms have an ability to quickly make decisions, and this is observed when presented with harmful substances; however, when this is simultaneously presented with attractive odorants, it decides whether to migrate to the attractive odorant or avoid it due to its proximity to the harmful substance. It also possesses long-term memory as evidenced by its enhanced attractive responses to certain odors as adults if it was previously exposed to this at the larval stage.

1.33.6 *Hydra*

Hydra was discovered at the beginning of the eighteenth century. Since then, it has been used as an animal model to improve our understanding of fundamental processes in animal biology (Figure 1.42). In 1744, Trembley published his *Mémoires*, which provided the first description of asexual reproduction by budding, the first controlled experiments in animals on regeneration, the first successful animal grafts, the first study of phototaxis in animals without eyes, and the first vital staining of tissues. Later, Ethel Browne Harvey used *Hydra* in a series of experiments that introduced a new concept in developmental biology, known as the organizer phenomenon. More

specifically, she showed that when grafting the tentacle of one *Hydra* onto the body column of another *Hydra*, one can trigger the growth of a new *Hydra* at the grafting site. This new *Hydra* would develop normally as if it had been the result of budding or asexual reproduction.

Hydra has been studied for more than 300 years, mostly because of how easy it is to culture and manipulate in a laboratory. *Hydra* can grow and shrink by an order of magnitude (from 1 mm to 1 cm) depending on various factors such as food availability and environmental temperature. Consequently, its nervous system is composed of a variable number of neurons from a few hundred to a few thousand depending on the size of the animal. Traditionally, two main types of neurons have been reported: sensory cells, exposed to the external or gastric environment, and ganglion cells, which form a two-dimensional lattice known as a nerve net. Moreover, the nerve net of *Hydra* is made up of two separate components: the endodermal nerve net and the ectodermal nerve net. The morphology of both sensory cells and ganglion cells can vary in terms of the size of their cell body and the ramification of their neurites.

The behavioral repertoire of *Hydra* is quite limited and includes basic behaviors such as periodic contractions of the body column on the longitudinal axis and along its radius, photic response, and feeding.

Establishing links between neuronal activity, anatomy, and behavior in *Hydra* has been challenging because of technical limitations. When it comes to electrophysiology, single-cell recording approaches such as sharp electrode recordings are not possible because *Hydra* neurons are small and spread out. On the other hand, with extracellular recordings (e.g., using suction electrodes) it is difficult to precisely localize their source. For these reasons it has not been possible until recently to measure how many networks exist in the nervous system of *Hydra* and in what behavior each of them participates.

The application of modern methods in molecular biology to *Hydra* has the potential to greatly advance our understanding of its nerve net. The sequencing of the *Hydra* genome makes it possible to study its surprisingly rich repertoire. Indeed, despite its basal metazoan lineage, the *Hydra* genome comprises more than 20,000 genes including a large number of neuronal genes such as sodium, potassium, and calcium channels, and receptors for glutamate, GABA, dopamine, serotonin and a vast array of neuropeptides. Also, methods for creating stable transgenic lines have been developed, enabling the use of a large range of modern molecular tools. Among these tools, genetically encoded calcium indicators are particularly well suited to study the activity of the nervous system of *Hydra* for multiple reasons as they are small, transparent, and contain neurons that are widely scattered.

Figure acknowledgements

The following images were created using a Biorender industrial license: Figure 1.1, 1.4, 1.7, 1.11, 1.15, 1.20, 1.22, 1.24, 1.27, 1.29, 1.39-1.40

The following images were created using a shutterstock license: Figures 1.2–1.3, 1.5–1.6, 1.8, 1.9–1.10, 1.12–1.14, 1.16–1.18, 1.23, 1.25–1.26, 1.28, 1.30–1.38

The following images are credited to the authors of this chapter: Figure 1.19, 1.21, 1.41–1.42

Further Reading

Chapman JA, Kirkness EF, Simakov O, et al. The dynamic genome of *Hydra*. *Nature* 2010;**464**:592–6. https://doi.org/10.1038/nature08830

Cisneros-Franco JM, Voss P, Thomas ME, de Villers-Sidani E. Critical periods of brain development. *Handb Clin Neurol* 2020;**173**:75–88. https://doi.org/10.1016/B978-0-444-64150-2.00009-5. PMID: 32958196.

Darnell D, Gilbert SF. Neuroembryology. *Wiley Interdiscip Rev Dev Biol* 2017;**6**(1):10.1002/wdev.215. https://doi.org/10.1002/wdev.215. Epub 2016 Dec 1. PMID: 27906497; PMCID: PMC5193482.

Ellenbroek B, Youn J. Rodent models in neuroscience research: is it a rat race? *Dis Model Mech* 2016;**9**(10):1079–87. https://doi.org/10.1242/dmm.026120. PMID: 27736744; PMCID: PMC5087838.

Felter D, O'Banion M, Maida M. *Netter's Atlas of Neuroscience (Netter Basic Science)*. Elsevier, 2021.

Ishikawa Y, Yamamoto N, Yoshimoto M, Ito H. The primary brain vesicles revisited: are the three primary vesicles (forebrain/midbrain/hindbrain) universal in vertebrates? *Brain Behav Evol* 2012;**79**(2):75–83. https://doi.org/10.1159/000334842

Kazama H. Systems neuroscience in *Drosophila*: conceptual and technical advantages. *Neuroscience* 2015;**296**:3–14. https://doi.org/10.1016/j.neuroscience.2014.06.035. Epub 2014 Jun 25. PMID: 24973655.

Krebs C, Weinberg J, Akesson E, Dilli E. *Lippincott Illustrated Reviews: Neuroscience*. Wolters Kluwer, 2017.

Passingham R. How good is the macaque monkey model of the human brain? *Curr Opin Neurobiol* 2009;**19**(1):6–11. https://doi.org/10.1016/j.conb.2009.01.002. Epub 2009 Mar 2. PMID: 19261463; PMCID: PMC2706975.

Purves D, Augustine G, Fitzpatrick D, et al. *Neuroscience*. Sinauer Associates, 2017.

Sengupta P, Samuel AD. *Caenorhabditis elegans*: a model system for systems neuroscience. *Curr Opin Neurobiol* 2009;**19**(6):637–43. https://doi.org/10.1016/j.conb.2009.09.009. Epub 2009 Nov 4. PMID: 19896359; PMCID: PMC2904967.

Stewart AM, Braubach O, Spitsbergen J, Gerlai R, Kalueff AV. Zebrafish models for translational neuroscience research: from tank to bedside. *Trends Neurosci* 2014;**37**(5):264–78. https://doi.org/10.1016/j.tins.2014.02.011. Epub 2014 Apr 9. PMID: 24726051; PMCID: PMC4039217.

Trembley, A. *Mémoires pour servir à l'histoire d'un genre de polypes d'eau douce, à bras en forme de cornes*. A Leide, Chez Jean & Herman Verbeek, 1744.

Vieira C, Pombero A, García-Lopez R, Gimeno L, Echevarria D, Martínez S. Molecular mechanisms controlling brain development: an overview of neuroepithelial secondary organizers. *Int J Dev Biol* 2010;**54**(1):7–20. https://doi.org/10.1387/ijdb.092853cv

Wiesel TN, Hubel DH. Single cell responses in striate cortex of kittens deprives of vision in one eye. *J Neurophysiol* 1963;**26**:1003–17. https://doi.org/10.1152/jn.1963.26.6.1003

Chapter 2

Cerebral Autoregulation

Parisa Nikrouz, Xingping Qin, Farhana Akter

2.1 Introduction

The brain and the encased skull constitute an incompressible system that encloses a volume of approximately 1450 mls. Normally, the intracranial volume is made up of 80% brain tissue, 10% cerebrospinal fluid (CSF), and 10% intravascular blood. The basic principle of physics in relation to intracranial content is described by the Monroe–Kellie doctrine. This hypothesis states that the total volume of the brain, CSF, and intracranial blood should be constant. Any increases in the volume of one of the components must be at the expense of the other two to maintain adequate brain function. In the presence of a space-occupying lesion that compromises the compensatory capacity of the brain, dramatic increase of intracranial pressure (ICP) followed by a decrease in cerebral perfusion pressure (CPP) and cerebral blood flow (CBF) will occur, and this may lead to herniation of the brain.

The average brain weight of an adult human is approximately 1400 g or 2% of total body weight. It typically receives 750 mls of blood per minute or 15% of the cardiac output. Cerebral blood flow is the volume of blood that flows per unit mass per unit time in brain tissue and in adults is approximately 50 ml/(100 g/min). It is directly related to CPP and inversely to cerebrovascular resistance (CVR). Cerebral perfusion pressure is the net pressure gradient driving blood into the brain to meet its metabolic demands. It is approximately 80 mm of mercury (mmHg) and is the arithmetic difference between mean arterial pressure (MAP) and ICP. Mean arterial pressure can be estimated as equal to: diastolic blood pressure + 1/3 pulse pressure (the difference between the diastolic and systolic pressure) and is usually around 90 mmHg. When CPP is constant, changes in CBF occur due to changes in CVR. Cerebrovascular resistance is determined by the radius and length of small blood vessels, primarily arterioles, which dilate and constrict in response to

a variety of stimuli. The Hagen–Poiseuille equation can be used to describe CBF and is based on the CPP, the length and caliber of the blood vessels, and the viscosity of blood:

$$CBF = \frac{\Delta P \pi R^4}{8 \eta \mathcal{L}}$$

$\Delta P = CPP$
$R = $ radius of blood vessels
$\eta = $ viscosity of blood
$\mathcal{L} = $ length of blood vessels

Cerebral perfusion pressure must be maintained within the normal autoregulatory range (50–150 mmHg) to prevent cerebral ischemia. Temporary changes in perfusion pressure occur under normal conditions (e.g., during a change in posture). However, more sustained changes due to pathological conditions such as subarachnoid hemorrhage (SAH) can cause dramatic increases in ICP resulting in reduced CPP beyond the limits of autoregulation. The brain possesses a cerebrovascular reserve capacity and can tolerate reductions in flood flow of 30–60% until ischemic symptoms develop. At the upper limits of autoregulation, the brain will no longer be able to maintain vasoconstriction, resulting in disruption of the blood–brain barrier (BBB) and vasogenic edema.

The critical CPP threshold following traumatic brain injury (TBI) has been widely debated. It is generally accepted that following TBI, CPP levels <50 mmHg should be avoided to prevent ischemia; however, dramatic increases in CPP should also be avoided, as they may increase the likelihood of developing acute respiratory distress syndrome (ARDS).

2.2 Optimal Regulation of Cerebral Blood Flow

Cerebral blood flow is regulated by a number of overlapping mechanisms including neuronal regulation, chemoregulation, endothelium-dependent regulation, and autoregulation (Figure 2.1).

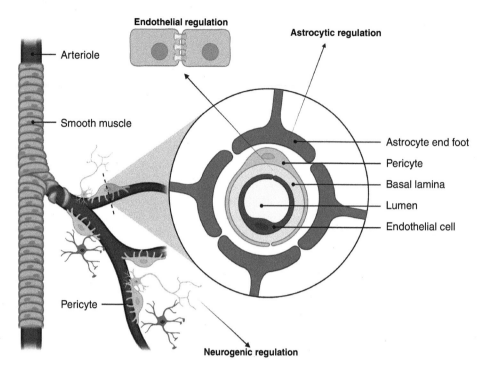

Figure 2.1 Regulation of CBF.

Endothelial regulation

Astrocytic regulation

Arteriole

Smooth muscle

Astrocyte end foot

Pericyte

Basal lamina

Lumen

Endothelial cell

Pericyte

Neurogenic regulation

2.2.1 Chemoregulation and Endothelial Regulation

Cerebral chemoregulation involves vascular changes in response to changes in carbon dioxide (CO_2), partial pressure of oxygen (PaO_2), or oxygen (O_2) content. Reactivity to CO_2 has been the most widely studied and has been shown to elicit dramatic CBF responses due to direct effects on vascular tone. Hypercapnia dilates cerebral arteries and therefore increases blood flow, whereas hypocapnia has the reverse effect.

Endothelium dependent regulation involves changes in vascular tone in response to a plethora of vasoactive factors (e.g. nitric oxide) released from the endothelium as a result of environmental cues such as shear stress, and transmural pressure.

2.2.2 Neuronal Regulation

Neurovascular coupling is a mechanism that affects CBF through transient changes in neural activity. The neuromuscular unit is composed of neurons, astrocytes, and the vascular smooth muscles. Glutamate stimulates neurons and astrocytes, leading to the secretion of vasodilators such as nitric oxide (NO), potassium, adenosine, and prostaglandins. Astrocytes can stimulate vasoconstriction by secreting arachidonic acid or vasodilation by triggering calcium (Ca^{2+}) release, which stimulates pericytes surrounding capillaries, resulting in capillary vasodilation.

Neurometabolic regulation of the brain occurs when glucose enters neurons and is converted to pyruvate during glycolysis, which undergoes oxidative phosphorylation leading to production of adenosine triphosphate (ATP). Astrocytes are also key regulators of neurometabolic coupling. The astrocyte–neuron lactate shuttle (ANLS) pathway is thought to operate under normal physiologic conditions with astrocytes responding to glutamatergic activation by increasing their own rate of glucose utilization, stimulation of glycolysis, and release of lactate, which is subsequently taken up by neurons to be converted to pyruvate (Figure 2.2).

2.2.3 Neurohumoral Factors

The parasympathetic nerves contribute to vasodilation and may play a part in hypotension and reperfusion injury. The stimulation of the sympathetic nervous system causes vasoconstriction and shifts the autoregulation curve (Figure 2.3) to the right in hypertension.

2.2.4 Autoregulation

Cerebral autoregulation (CA) is the inherent ability of blood vessels to keep CBF relatively constant despite changes in CPP. The clinical consequences of failed autoregulation and the mechanisms involved differ

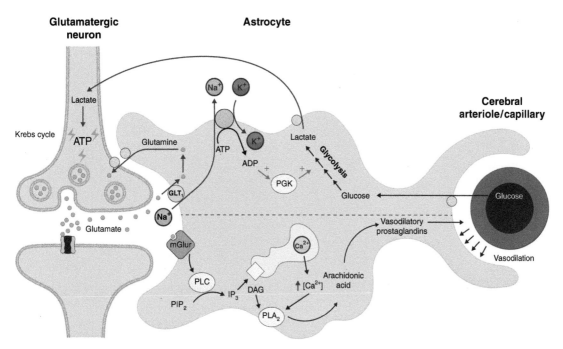

Figure 2.2 The astrocyte–neuron lactate shuttle (ANLS).

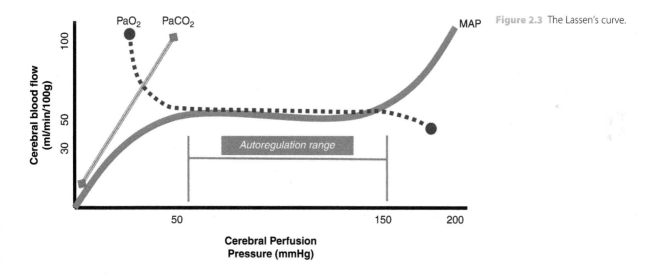

Figure 2.3 The Lassen's curve.

depending on which portion of the autoregulatory curve is affected (Figure 2.3). Failure at the left side of the curve results in hypoperfusion, ischemia, and possibly death. If autoregulatory mechanisms are overwhelmed and fail at the right side of the curve, hyperperfusion, edema due to disruption of the BBB, increased ICP, and death can result. With moderate increases in arterial pressure, elevations in vascular resistance are sufficient to maintain CBF at normotensive levels.

2.2.4.1 Steady-State Cerebral Autoregulation

The steady-state relationship between CBF and blood pressure (BP) under conditions where BP and CBF have independently reached steady state can be thought of as a static state of CA. The classic Lassen's curve

53

demonstrates changes in CBF against a wide range of BP (MAP between ~50 and 150 mmHg), where autoregulation minimizes variations in CBF when there are limited changes in BP (Figure 2.3).

2.2.4.2 Dynamic Cerebral Autoregulation

The ability to respond to rapid changes in BP to minimize large fluctuations of CBF is termed dynamic cerebral autoregulation (dCA). This can be measured using a number of techniques, the most common being the transcranial Doppler ultrasound (TCD), typically of the middle cerebral artery (MCA). Transcranial Doppler ultrasound usually measures blood velocity and not true blood flow. It relies on the assumption that the MCA diameter is constant and, therefore, may not be suitable in older adults who have age-related vascular changes.

In a typical measurement, dCA will be assessed using the thigh-cuff occlusion release technique. Inflation of systolic blood pressures (SBP) for more than 2 minutes before sudden release leads to a dramatic drop in arterial blood pressure (ABP) for approximately 10 seconds before returning to baseline. This is accompanied by a drop in cerebral blood flow velocity (CBFV), which recovers to baseline levels before that of ABP, and this is then measured using TCD. The autoregulatory index (ARI) is used for quantification, with a value of 0 corresponding to an entirely passive autoregulation, and a value of 9 representing the fastest autoregulatory response that can be observed.

2.2.4.3 Transfer Function Analysis

The transfer function analysis (TFA) is a method of evaluating dCA that does not require evoked manipulations of ABP. Transfer function analysis evaluates the relationship between beat-to-beat spontaneous oscillations of MCA velocity and ABP via frequency domain analysis. The spontaneous oscillations of BP that occur at specific frequencies can be quantified. The mathematical concept of coherence allows us to quantify how different BP amplitudes are transferred to CBF. A coherence of 1 indicates that oscillations in CBF occur due to the oscillation of BP, whereas a coherence of 0 suggests no relationship between CBF and BP. Therefore, faster oscillations and higher frequencies are associated with increased coherence. The characteristics between fluctuations in BP and CBF are thought to resemble a high-pass filter, with higher-frequency fluctuations being more linearly transferred to the cerebral circulation (i.e., higher coherence). Transfer function analysis can be used to determine parameters such as gain, i.e., the dampening effect of dCA on the magnitude of BP oscillation and phase difference (the time delay of the CBF response to BP).

2.2.4.4 Cerebral Blood Flow Measurements

The first quantitative method of determining global CBF was described in 1945 by Kety and Schmidt, where the arteriovenous difference of nitrous oxide concentration based on the Fick principle was calculated as an indicator of CBF. However, this technique required repeated blood sampling and overestimated CBF due to recirculation of the gas. Subsequent established methods included the injection of intravenous radioactive agents such as xenon followed by detection of radioactivity decay over time. The hydrogen clearance technique was developed as an invasive technique to measure global and regional blood flow based on the idea that hydrogen ions cause changes in currents and these can be detected by peripheral and brain electrodes as a measure of CBF. Microsphere techniques consist of injection of radioactive dyes into the left atrium followed by calculation of radioactive decay in the brain and the arterial blood. Fluorescent tracers can be used as an alternative to radioactive dyes. Thermal diffusion flowmetry (TDF) is a technique for monitoring CBF that appears to correlate well with regional measurements of brain tissue oxygenation. It was initially developed for the measurement of coronary sinus blood flow and can now also be applied for the measurement of jugular blood flow (JBF) to help estimate CBF at the bedside. It involves the measurement of focal cortical blood flow continuously. In this technique a probe with proximal and distal thermistors is inserted into the region of interest within a catheter. The distal thermistor is heated to generate a constant spherical temperature. The proximal thermistor is outside this heated field and the temperature difference between the thermistors will provide an indication of thermal transfer and a measure of the ability of the tissue to transport heat.

Computed tomography (CT)-based techniques include xenon-enhanced CT, involving the measurement of the clearance rate of xenon, which can diffuse across the BBB. Computed tomography perfusion scans are often used in acute stroke patients. This involves identifying the ischemic penumbra and infarct core by calculating the mean transit time (MTT) or time to peak (TTP) of the tissue, CBF, and cerebral blood volume (CBV), which are related to each other according to the central volume principle (CBF = CBV/MTT). The ischemic penumbra is an area with prolonged MTT, moderately reduced CBF, and normal CBV. However, the infarct core is an area with prolonged MTT, reduced CBF, and CBV.

Positron emission tomography (PET) is the gold standard for the *in vivo* assessment of CBF and brain metabolism. The decay of the radiotracers used with PET scans produces positrons. Single photon emission computed tomography (SPECT) involves the injection of radionuclides, which cross the BBB and emit gamma rays that can be detected to create a 3D representation of CBF. Single photon emission computed tomography scanning is more widely available as it is cheaper than PET. However, PET provides superior image quality and higher diagnostic accuracy.

Magnetic resonance imaging (MRI)-based techniques include phase-contrast MRI, which can be used to derive contrast between flowing blood and stationary tissues by manipulating the phase of magnetization. Spins that are moving toward the magnetic field gradient develop a phase shift that is proportional to the velocity of the spins. A bipolar gradient can be used to encode the velocity of the spins. Stationary spins undergo no net change in phase after the two gradients are applied. However, moving spins experience a different magnitude of the second gradient compared to the first, which results in a net phase shift.

Dynamic susceptibility-weighted imaging involves injection of gadolinium contrast, which can be tracked. This technique is sensitive to compounds that distort the magnetic field, such as deoxyhemoglobin, and therefore can be used to identify hemorrhage or blood products. Arterial spin labeling is a magnetic resonance (MR) perfusion-weighted imaging that does not require an exogenous contrast agent. It allows absolute quantification of CBF by using magnetically labeled arterial blood water as an endogenous tracer.

Other MR-based techniques include magnetic resonance angiography (MRA) and nuclear magnetic resonance spectroscopy (NMRS). Magnetic resonance angiography has been used to provide detailed understanding of cerebral anatomy and determine the total CBF. Nuclear magnetic resonance spectroscopy is a non-invasive method that uses inert radioactive materials to determine CBF. It involves the inhalation of ^{19}F radioactive gas, which diffuses in the brain.

Bedside techniques used to measure CBF include optical modalities such as diffuse correlation spectroscopy (DCS), laser Doppler flowmetry (LDP), optical micro-angiography, and optical imaging of indocyanine green.

Diffuse correlation spectroscopy is an optical modality that enables non-invasive measurements of temporal fluctuations of near-infrared (NIR) light reflected from tissue to understand the motions of tissue constituents such as red blood cells and can therefore be used as a measure of CBF. Laser Doppler flowmetry allows continuous measurements of CBF using Doppler shift principles. It requires the use of a fiberoptic laser probe, which emits photons that will be scattered by the tissue. The signal is processed to give an estimate of the blood flow. However, this technique only measures CBF in a small brain volume and is prone to artifacts due to probe displacement. Optical micro-angiography is an exogenous contrast-free technique that can be used to produce high-resolution maps of dynamic blood perfusion. It can separate intrinsic optical scattering of moving blood cells from scattering of signals by static bulk tissue. Optical imaging of indocyanine green, which emits fluorescent light when stimulated by photodiodes, can be performed to generate CBF maps.

2.2.5 Intracranial Pressure

The maintenance of a normal ICP of 10–20 mmHg is essential in ensuring adequate cerebral perfusion. The Monroe–Kellie doctrine is instrumental to our understanding of the negative impact of raised ICP on the brain. Intracranial pressure values >25 mmHg require treatment and values >40 mmHg indicate life-threatening intracranial hypertension. The resultant decrease in CPP will prevent the brain from compensating adequately, resulting in reduced CBF.

2.2.5.1 Intracranial Pressure Monitoring

Intracranial pressure monitoring is a cornerstone of neuromonitoring as it reflects the consequence of mass effect to cerebral injury. The most common device used for monitoring ICP is the ventriculostomy catheter, which is inserted into the ventricles and connected to an external pressure transducer via fluid-filled tubing. If the ventricles are compressed and cannot be cannulated other devices such as a microsensor transducer or fiberoptic transducer–tipped catheters can be inserted into the subdural space or the brain tissue.

The ICP waveform (Figure 2.4) includes a respiratory component reflecting venous pulsation during respiration and a cardiac component. The cardiac components consist of three peaks: P1 (reflecting arterial pulsations), P2 (reflecting intracranial compliance), and P3 (reflecting aortic valve closure). As the ICP increases the amplitude of P1, P2, and P3 all increase and with severe increase in ICP, P2 is grossly elevated. With significant reduction in intracranial compliance, pathological Lundberg waves can be visualized. Conditions associated with reduced

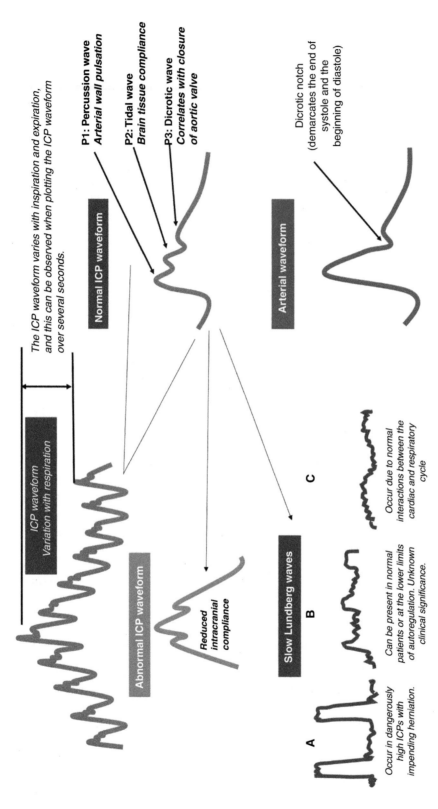

The ICP waveform varies with inspiration and expiration, and this can be observed when plotting the ICP waveform over several seconds.

ICP waveform
Variation with respiration

Normal ICP waveform

P1: Percussion wave
Arterial wall pulsation

P2: Tidal wave
Brain tissue compliance

P3: Dicrotic wave
Correlates with closure of aortic valve

Arterial waveform

Dicrotic notch
(demarcates the end of systole and the beginning of diastole)

Abnormal ICP waveform

Reduced intracranial compliance

Slow Lundberg waves

A

Occur in dangerously high ICP's with impending herniation.

B

Can be present in normal patients or at the lower limits of autoregulation. Unknown clinical significance.

C

Occur due to normal interactions between the cardiac and respiratory cycle

Figure 2.4 ICP waveforms.

CPP and cerebral vasodilation result in A, or plateau, waves, which reflect steep increases in ICP lasting 5–20 minutes and which are associated with poor clinical outcome. B waves are seen with Cheyne–Stokes breathing pattern or during periods of apnea and may appear before A waves. They occur every 30 seconds to 2 minutes. C waves are seen in the normal ICP waveform and are not clinically significant. They have an amplitude of 20 mmHg and a frequency of 4–8 per minute.

Intracranial pressure monitoring provides information about intracranial dynamics and brain compliance using waveform assessment. Intracranial pressure is dynamic and must be considered alongside other factors such as position of the patient and the patient's blood pressure. There are a number of ICP indices that can be used during ICP monitoring. These include pressure–volume compensatory reserve indices such as the cerebrovascular pressure reactivity index (PRx), which reflects the changes in the Pearson correlation coefficient between the ABP and ICP over a short window of time, and is updated frequently to yield continuous monitoring. This allows the estimation of an optimal CPP (CPPopt) by plotting PRx against CPP, producing a U-shaped curve. When PRx is at the lowest value, CA is considered to be at its best and CPP at this PRx value is also considered to be the best. However, this estimation assumes that the calculation period is a stationary process and therefore may not always be reliable. Newer techniques have been developed to reduce these noisy estimates, such as the transform-based wavelet pressure reactivity index (wPRx), which measures the delay between ABP and ICP signals over a range of frequencies followed by characterization of the cross-correlation between the two signals. However, these newer techniques have yet to be widely adopted.

Another parameter for evaluating pressure–volume compensatory reserves involves detecting the amplitude of ICP pulse waves (AMP) generated by heart rate and correlation coefficient between AMP and mean pressure (RAP). Good compensatory reserves are indicated by RAP values of 0 denoting that changes in volume produce very little change in pressure. However, when RAP rises to +1, this indicates that AMP varies directly with ICP and compensatory reserves are low, and any further rises in volume will lead to rapid increases in ICP. Once ICP values have dramatically increased, AMP values will decrease and the RAP index will be closer to –1. This means the autoregulatory capacity of the brain has been exhausted and cerebral arterioles can no longer dilate in response to falling CPPs. This is often associated with irreversible brain damage and potential herniation.

2.2.6 Cerebral Oxygenation

Maintenance of adequate tissue oxygen is a fundamental objective after any form of brain injury. Moderate amounts of hypoxia lead to reduction in CVR, vasodilation, and therefore an increase in CBF. However, the brain lacks fuel stores and requires a continuous supply of glucose and oxygen to maintain brain function and tissue viability.

The human brain consumes 20% of the total O_2 budget and is primarily used by mitochondria to produce ATP. This is often referred to as the cerebral metabolic rate for oxygen, or $CMRO_2$. The amount of O_2 that reaches the brain is the product of local blood flow and the arterial oxygen content (CaO_2). Arterial oxygen content depends on the hemoglobin concentration and how much it is saturated with O_2.

The amount of oxygen that diffuses across the BBB can be calculated using the Fick principle, which states that the uptake of a substance by an organ j (mass/time) is the product of the blood flow to that organ F (volume/time) and the difference between arterial (C_A) and venous (C_V) concentrations of the substance in steady state.

Measures of cerebral oxygenation include jugular venous oxygen saturation ($SjvO_2$), brain tissue oxygen tension ($PbtO_2$), near-infrared spectroscopy (NIRS), and cerebral oximetry.

Jugular venous bulb oximetry measures brain oxygenation by placing a fiberoptic monitor in the jugular bulb and quantifying the percentage saturation of the venous blood returning to the heart ($SjvO_2$), which is a global measure of how much oxygen is being extracted by the entire brain and therefore reflects CBF. $SjvO_2$ desaturation, defined as a value of <50–55% for >10 min, has been associated with poor neurologic outcome. Conversely, $SjvO_2$ >75% is also associated with poor outcome in patients with severe TBI. However, $SjvO_2$ measurements are often subject to artifacts such as the head position and the proximity of the probe to the jugular bulb.

Brain tissue oxygen tension ($PbtO_2$) is the partial pressure of oxygen in the interstitial space of the brain and is a product of CBF and cerebral arteriovenous oxygen tension difference. Normal $PbtO_2$ is in the range of 35–50 mmHg and reflects the local oxygenation of brain tissue, but may not be as useful for determining oxygenation of the whole brain.

Measurement of brain oxygen tension can be performed using an invasive probe with a sensor using polarographic Clarke-type electrode or fiberoptic technology. The Clark electrode consists of two opposing metallic surfaces in an aqueous electrolyte potassium chloride solution. Oxygen then diffuses into the solution, resulting in an electrical potential between the two surfaces. The greater the amount of oxygen that diffuses, the greater the current generated. This process is temperature-dependent, and so a temperature probe is also used alongside the $PbtO_2$ probe. The Licox $PbtO_2$ monitor uses the same principle and is widely used; however, it can take a long time to equilibrate and readings within the first hour of placement may not be accurate. Furthermore, CT scans must typically be performed post insertion to ensure correct placement. Other methods of measuring $PbtO_2$ include the Neurotrend catheter, which uses optical fluorescence technology. However, the readings are not as sensitive and there is a higher rate of catheter malfunction than the Licox system. Newer technologies that have emerged include the Neurovent-PTO, which uses fiberoptic luminescence-quenching properties to measure $PbtO_2$ and simultaneously measures ICP and temperature.

Near-infrared spectroscopy is a cerebral oximetry method based on the optical properties of near-infrared light in tissue, which can be correlated with tissue oxygenation. It can be used to measure the concentration of oxygenated and deoxygenated hemoglobin by detecting the intensity of reflected light emission. An NIRS-based index of cerebrovascular reactivity, called total hemoglobin reactivity (THx), is thought to be comparable to standard measurements of cerebrovascular pressure reactivity (PRx), which requires invasive ICP monitoring. Near-infrared spectroscopy is non-invasive and therefore can be easily used in both operating rooms and ward settings. It also captures high-frequency and continuous data that can be combined with other modalities, such as ABP or end-tidal CO_2.

2.2.7 Microdialysis

Microdialysis is a tool that is used to sample brain extracellular fluid and allows bedside measurement of metabolites such as glucose, lactate, pyruvate, glycerol, glutamate, and pH. Biochemical changes can occur before low CPP is detectable. Microdialysis is therefore a useful tool in guiding management. The measurement of lactate and pyruvate concentrations provides information on the extent of anaerobic glycolysis taking place. The ratio of the two also reflects the intracellular redox state and is a marker of mitochondrial function. Levels of glutamate can be measured to reflect the amount of excitotoxicity following brain injury. However, how much prognostic information this provides is debated, and therefore it is often measured for academic purposes. Levels of glycerol can be used to reflect the amount of tissue hypoxia and cell damage and are usually elevated following abnormal cellular metabolism due to disruption in cell membrane function.

Figure acknowledgements

The following image was created using a Biorender industrial license: Figure 2.1

The following image was created using a Shutterstock license: Figure 2.2

The following images are credited to the authors of this chapter: Figures 2.3–2.4

Further Reading

Akter F, Robba C, Gupta A. Multimodal monitoring in the neurocritical care unit. In Prabhakar H, Ali Z (eds.), *Textbook of Neuroanesthesia and Neurocritical Care.* Springer, 2019.

Cho Won-Sang, Ha Eun, Ko Sang-Bae, Yang Seungman, Kim Hee Chan, Kim Jeong. New Parameters for evaluating cerebral autoregulation and pressure–volume compensatory reserve in neurocritial patients. *J Neurointens Care* 2018;**1**:7–11. https://doi.org/10.32587/jnic.2018.00038.

Czosnyka M, Pickard JD. Monitoring and interpretation of intracranial pressure. *J Neurol Neurosurg Psychiatry* 2004;**75**:813–21. https://doi.org/10.1136/jnnp.2003.033126. PMID: 15145991; PMCID: PMC1739058.

Czosnyka M, Smielewski P, Timofeev I, et al. Intracranial pressure: more than a number. *Neurosurg Focus* 2007;**22**(5):E10. https://doi.org/10.3171/foc.2007.22.5.11. PMID: 17613228.

Ragosta M. *Textbook of Clinical Hemodynamics.* 2nd ed. Elsevier, 2017.

Silverman A, Petersen NH. Physiology, cerebral autoregulation. [Updated 2022 Feb 16]. *StatPearls* [Internet], 2022. www.ncbi.nlm.nih.gov/books/NBK553183/

Steiner LA, Andrews PJ. Monitoring the injured brain: ICP and CBF. *Br J Anaesth* 2006;**97**(1):26–38. https://doi.org/10.1093/bja/ael110. Epub 2006

Wymer DT, Patel KP, Burke WF 3rd, Bhatia VK. Phase-contrast MRI: physics, techniques, and clinical applications. *Radiographics* 2020;**40**(1):122–40. https://doi.org/10.1148/rg.2020190039. PMID: 31917664.

3

Neuroimmune Interactions

Allison Chang

3.1 Basic Immunology

The immune system is a complex network that acts to recognize and eliminate foreign antigens – any protein, carbohydrate, lipid, deoxyribonucleic acid, or small organic molecule that can produce an immune response – from the body, and is divided into two subdivisions: the innate immune system and the adaptive immune system.

3.1.1 Innate Immunity

The innate immune system is often considered to be the first line of defense, and responds quickly and remotely to non-specific, conserved signals characteristic of infection or tissue damage (Medzhitov and Janeway, 2002). Innate immune cells involved in this process include leukocytes – the primary cells of the peripheral innate immune response – as well as tissue macrophages and monocytes, granulocytes (basophils, eosinophils, neutrophils), and natural killer (NK) cells (Figure 3.1). Upon detection of conserved pathogen- or tumor-associated molecules, for example bacterial lipopolysaccharide receptors or tumor-derived heat-shock proteins, the cytotoxic machinery of innate immune cells becomes activated. These mechanisms can then induce the phagocytosis or lysis of virally infected cells, extracellular bacteria, or tumor cells, and are typically accompanied by the release of a range of cytokines – small signaling proteins such as interleukin (IL)-4, IL-6, and tumor necrosis factor (TNF)-α – and inflammatory mediators that include oxygen radicals, nitric oxide, and prostaglandins (Janeway, 1999).

In the central nervous system (CNS), the primary innate immune cells are microglia, tissue-resident macrophages that infiltrate the brain at an early developmental stage and come to comprise around 80% of the immune cell population in the CNS (Korin et al., 2017). Beyond their traditional involvement in the surveillance of tissue homeostasis (Wolf et al., 2017), microglia in their normal state also contribute to numerous developmental processes in the CNS, including synaptic formation, myelination, neuron proliferation, and programmed cell death

(Cunningham et al., 2013; Miyamoto et al., 2016). Ultimately, the combined effects of the innate immune response are essential for the initiation and continuation of the subsequent adaptive immune response as well.

3.1.2 Adaptive Immunity

The adaptive immune response represents the second line of defense against foreign pathogens and tumors, and targets extremely specific antigens based on "memory" of prior incursions. The adaptive immune response requires a longer period of time to produce, and involves four phases to generate effector cells capable of eliminating specific antigens: recognition and activation, proliferation, effector, and memory. Adaptive immune cells are comprised of lymphocytes with B- or T-cell receptors – these are the only cells in the body capable of specific recognition, and can be involved in either humoral or cellular adaptive immune responses depending on the receptor type expressed (Figure 3.1).

3.1.2.1 Humoral Immune Response

The main components of the humoral immune system are B cells, which contain the surface immunoglobulin B-cell receptor, and antibody-secreting plasma cells. When B cells are stimulated by Th2 helper cells, they are able to differentiate into antibody-producing plasma cells; these secreted antibodies are then able to recognize and bind to specific, freely circulating antigens in the body. Antibodies can induce lysis in their targets when: (1) the complement system, a family of serum proteins, binds to antibody-coated targets and causes lysis; (2) antibodies opsonize the particles or cells they coat by attracting phagocytic cells that possess receptors for the Fc portion of the antibody; and (3) leukocytes (monocytes, neutrophils, and NK cells), which also present Fc receptors, are activated and induce lysis upon contact with antibody-coated targets.

As the humoral immune response involves freely circulating antibodies, it is unable to effectively cross the blood–brain barrier (BBB) and is therefore not ideally

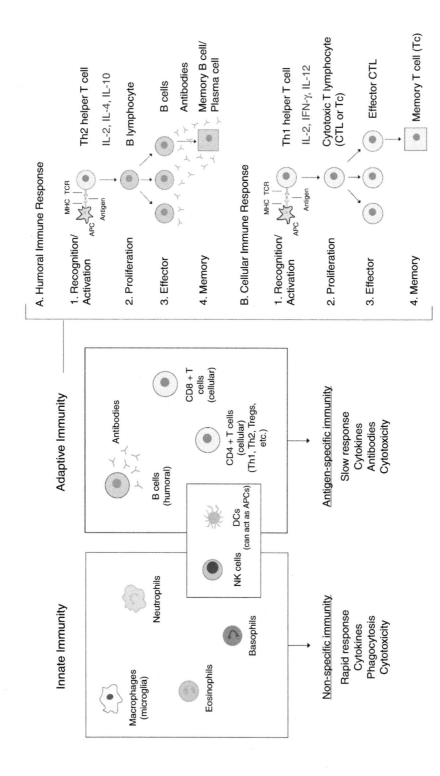

Figure 3.1 The innate and adaptive immune systems. Innate immunity is non-specific and rapid, involving macrophages (microglia in the CNS), neutrophils, eosinophils, and basophils, while adaptive immunity is antigen-specific and slow, involving B cells (humoral) and T cells (cellular). Adaptive immunity is further divided into humoral and cellular immunity; both involve four steps to generate effector cells capable of eliminating specific antigens: recognition and activation, proliferation, effector, and memory.

suited for responding to CNS tumors. However, recent findings indicate that B cells may possess additional antibody-independent methods for T-cell regulation that involve the release of inflammatory cytokines (Bar-Or et al., 2010). These mechanisms are not yet well understood, but may present potential therapeutic targets and help to explain the involvement of B cells in multiple sclerosis–related inflammation (Shen et al., 2014).

3.1.2.2 Cellular Immune Response

There are two major types of T cells involved in the cell-mediated immune response: (1) CD8+ T cells, often called cytotoxic T lymphocytes (CTL), which have the potential to differentiate into effector CTL and lyse infected or tumor cells, and (2) CD4+ T cells, or helper T cells (Th), which secrete a wide array of immune-regulating cytokines and can differentiate into either Th1 or Th2 cells, depending on the stimulus. Th1 cells are involved in cell-mediated immune responses and secrete dendritic cell (DC)-activating cytokines (e.g., IL-2, IL-12, interferon-γ), while Th2 cells are involved with humoral immune responses by secreting B-cell–activating cytokines (e.g., IL-4, IL-10).

Unlike antibodies released by B cells, which are able to detect freely circulating antigens, T cells can only recognize antigens that have been processed and bound to major histocompatibility complex (MHC) proteins on the cell surface. T-cell specificity is further restricted to one of the two MHC types. MHC Class I molecules typically associate with endogenous antigens synthesized by native cells, such as cytoplasmic tumor proteins or viral products, and are recognized by CD8+ T cells (direct pathway). In contrast, MHC Class II molecules usually associate with exogenous antigens, such as tumor surface peptides or bacterial by-products, that have been taken up by macrophages or antigen-presenting cells (APC), which are then recognized by CD4+ T cells (indirect pathway). Naive T cells that have not yet been exposed to antigens circulate throughout the body until they encounter an APC presenting one of their specific target antigens, at which point the T cells differentiate into cytokine-secreting effector T cells and proliferate.

3.2 Central Nervous System–Immune Interactions

3.2.1 Neuroimmune Interactions

While the brain has previously been thought to be an immune-privileged site, recent research – especially the discovery of meningeal lymphatic vessels lining the dural sinuses that contribute to the exchange between cerebrospinal fluid (CSF) and interstitial fluid (ISF in the rest of the body – has continued to reveal its status as a special immune-controlled site. In the adult brain, the BBB, a highly selective border composed of endothelial cell tight junctions at cerebral capillaries, restricts most entry of adaptive immune cells into the CNS (Zhao et al., 2015). However, the CNS remains in constant communication with the immune system through a range of mechanisms, and a number of molecules and cells typically associated with the immune system are also expressed in various CNS regions.

During development, microglia infiltrate the CNS at an early stage and contribute to numerous highly orchestrated developmental processes throughout the brain, including synaptic formation, angiogenesis, proliferation and migration of neurons and glia, programmed cell death, and myelination (Cunningham et al., 2013; Miyamoto et al., 2016; Pang et al., 2013). Although lymphocytes (including T cells, B cells, and NK cells) are scarce in the CNS (Pösel et al., 2016), they also play important roles in development. T cells have been implicated in spatial learning, memory, emotional behavior, stress responsiveness, and other complex brain processes; in particular, CD4+ helper T cells in the brain secrete the anti-inflammatory cytokine IL-4 and induce astrocyte production of brain-derived neurotrophic factor, leading to an improvement in spatial learning and memory (Derecki et al., 2010; Kipnis et al., 2004; Ziv et al., 2006). While the B-cell population declines in number following the neonatal period, it may also indirectly contribute to oligodendrogenesis and myelination by influencing microglia in earlier developmental stages (Tanabe and Yamashita, 2018, 2019).

In the adult brain, immune surveillance involving T cells continues to take place in meningeal compartments at the interface between the brain and the periphery (Korn and Kallies, 2017). Furthermore, neuroimmune reflexes also act as channels for two-way communication between the CNS and the immune system. The main inflammatory reflex involves cooperation in the vagus nerve – the parasympathetic division's main nerve – between the sensory arc responding to cytokines and the motor arc inhibiting cytokines (Tracey, 2002). While afferent sensory neurons modulate and communicate pro-inflammatory signals, including cytokines (IL-1β and TNF; Browning et al., 2017; Ek et al., 1998), from the periphery to the brain through specific vagus nerve activation patterns, efferent vagus nerve cholinergic signaling through autonomic neurons allows the CNS to release catecholamines that inhibit pro-inflammatory cytokine production and contribute to anti-inflammatory functions in a wide range of diseases (Andersson and Tracey, 2012; Levine et al., 2014; Olofsson et al., 2015; Pavlov, 2008). Other neuroinflammatory reflexes have also been identified, with circuits involving dopamine release and associated anti-inflammatory effects (Torres-Rosas et al., 2014), multiple sclerosis (Sabharwal et al., 2014), and post spinal cord injury immunosuppression (Ueno et al., 2016). Spatially, the CNS integrates afferent and efferent vagus nerve activity in two nuclei within the dorsal vagal complex (DVC) of the brainstem (Goehler et al., 2000), and is therefore able to coordinate and provide regulatory control of vagus nerve activity and related neuroimmune activities in response to behavior (Benarroch, 1993; Dampney, 2016).

3.2.2 Neuroinflammatory Mechanisms in Disease

Neuroinflammation, or the response of reactive CNS elements to internally or externally altered homeostasis, is characteristic of all neurological diseases and results in neuroinflammatory responses that may be either helpful or harmful (Figure 3.2). The main reactive CNS elements involved in neuroinflammatory mechanisms include microglia and infiltrating myeloid cells, other neuroglia such as astrocytes and oligodendrocytes, the BBB, and cytokine signaling (Ransohoff et al., 2015).

Although the traditional dichotomies of referring microglia as M1 vs M2 according to their activation states have fallen out of favor, it is worth mentioning due to their predominance in literature. Macrophage and microglial activation have been loosely classified into two opposing states: the pro-inflammatory M1 state, associated with the release of inflammatory cytokines (e.g., IL-6, TNF-α) and reactive oxygen species, and the non-inflammatory M2 state, associated with anabolic factor (e.g., brain-derived neurotrophic factor, or BDNF) release. In the normal CNS, microglia may be more polarized toward the M2 state, but an unbalanced overexpression of M1 markers combined with a decrease in M2 markers during inflammation may initiate destructive events (Tang and Le, 2016). While the transition from a predominantly M2 state to an increased inflammatory M1 form can be observed in the progression of many conditions, including Alzheimer's and postischemic stroke (Shen et al., 2018; Wang et al., 2018), the inappropriate dominance of non-inflammatory M2 markers can also result in the facilitation of glial tumor progression in the brain (Sasaki, 2017). Therapeutic approaches aimed at restoring imbalances of M1 and M2 polarity in the brain have been found promising for diminishing adverse changes associated with Alzheimer's disease–related neuroinflammation, as well as for glioma therapy (Song and Suk, 2017). Astroglia possess the same duality in pro- and anti-inflammatory functions as microglia, although astroglia may be more prone to encouraging neuroinflammation through apparently unprovoked reactive gliosis, and promoting increased pro-inflammatory responses to adverse CNS events and in the aging brain (Norden et al., 2015; Primiani et al., 2014). Astroglial activation has also been implicated in several neurodegenerative diseases including Alzheimer's, Parkinson's, and multiple sclerosis (Sofroniew, 2015; Stephenson et al., 2018), and the suppression of predominantly deleterious reactive astroglia in Alzheimer's disease may offer a promising therapeutic strategy (Ceyzériat et al., 2018).

Moreover, the BBB becomes compromised in neurological disease and allows for the entry of immune cells and pro-inflammatory cytokines and chemokines into the brain from the rest of the periphery (Ransohoff and Engelhardt, 2012). The resulting infiltration of normally peripheral monocytes, cells of the innate immune system that may closely resemble but functionally differ from resident microglia, may result in greater liability for autoimmune attacks on nervous tissues in the CNS (Li and Barres, 2018). Additionally, elements of the adaptive immune system play a role in modulating inflammation in the CNS. Although memory T cells, specifically CD4+ Th cells involved in cell-mediated adaptive immunity, are typically confined to immunosurveillance in the meningeal compartments of the brain (Ransohoff and Engelhardt, 2012), in neuroinflammation they induce the additional release of pro-inflammatory signals, including cytokines, that contribute to chronic neuroinflammation and neuronal death (Ransohoff et al., 2003). In diseases such as multiple sclerosis (MS), B cells involved in humoral adaptive immunity have been shown to express cytokines in abnormal proportions, with an overproduction of pro-inflammatory cytokines (e.g., TNF-α, IL-6) and a deficit in anti-inflammatory cytokines (e.g., IL-10) (Bar-Or et al., 2010). Moreover, B cells may also physically interact with and activate T cells in the context of MS-related neuroinflammation: emerging insight shows that B cells may enter or exit the CNS through the BBB during disease, draining to peripheral lymph nodes where they can be involved with antigen presentation for T-cell differentiation (Stern et al., 2014). Beyond neurological disorders, disease states in non-nervous tissues may also transmit a general inflammatory process from the periphery to the brain through afferent signaling in the vagus nerve via the inflammatory reflex (Tracey, 2009).

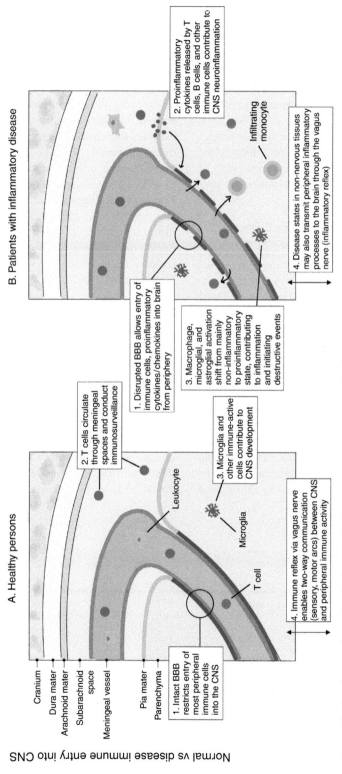

Figure 3.2 Neuroimmune interactions in the CNS in healthy persons versus patients with inflammatory disease.

3.3 The Immune System in Neurosurgical Disease

3.3.1 Brain Tumors

Among primary malignant brain tumors, glioblastoma (GBM) is the most common. In affected individuals, GBM is aggressive and characterized by a fast and infiltrative growth pattern leading to progressive neurologic deterioration and, ultimately, death (Alexander and Cloughesy, 2017). Despite the existence of available therapies, outcomes for patients with GBM remain poor. The need remains for more effective treatment options, and a diverse range of immunotherapies are currently being explored to fight malignant glioma.

3.3.1.1 Interactions Between the Immune System and Gliomas

The main immune mechanism for the precise elimination of tumor cells is cross-presentation, in which APCs process exogenous tumor antigens and display them on MHC Class I (MHC I) molecules in order to induce the lysing of cancerous cells by CD8+ cytotoxic T lymphocytes (Rock, 1996; Figure 3.3). The primary location of glioma antigen cross-presentation is debated, but a number of immune components including microglia, tumor-infiltrating DCs, macrophages, pericytes, and even peripheral pathways may all potentially play roles in antigen presentation (Grauer et al., 2009).

Another observed characteristic of higher-grade gliomas, which are associated with disruption of the BBB and tumor necrosis, is that they tend to have an increased population of tumor-infiltrating leukocytes throughout the tumor bed (Amin et al., 2012). It is important to note, however, that a substantial presence of immune cells infiltrating into the CNS and the glioma does not indicate a more robust immune reaction or a better outcome – instead, tumors may prevent the trafficked immune cells from properly functioning, and/or recruit additional cells with anti-inflammatory capabilities (Safdari et al., 1985).

In order to maintain and promote growth, gliomas possess various immunosuppressive mechanisms that include impairing T-cell proliferation and activity, downregulating MHC I complexes and pro-inflammatory cytokines, and hindering the activation of APCs, NK cells, and CD8+ cells (Grauer et al., 2009; Waziri, 2010; Zagzag et al., 2005). Furthermore, gliomas may recruit anti-inflammatory immune cells such as tumor-associated macrophages (TAMs) through the release of cytokines and growth factors such as vascular endothelial growth factor, or VEGF (Cohen et al., 2009; Johnson et al., 2007).

3.3.1.2 Approaches to Glioma Immunotherapy

The field of cancer immunology has only truly emerged with modern understanding of the innate and adaptive immune systems, and in recent years immunotherapeutic approaches such as checkpoint inhibitors and oncolytic viruses (OVs) have greatly contributed to the care of other cancers in the body (Andtbacka et al., 2015; Garon et al., 2015; Hodi et al., 2010, 2015). Current immunotherapy approaches that have gathered clinical interest include vaccines (peptide, heat-shock protein (HSP), and DC vaccines), OVs, chimeric antigen receptors (CARs), and checkpoint inhibitors.

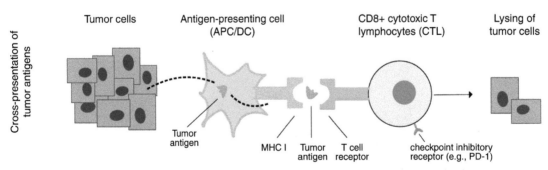

Figure 3.3 Cross-presentation of tumor antigens. Antigen-presenting cells, including dendritic cells (DCs), take in, process, and cross-present tumor antigens (TAs) through the MHC-I presentation pathway in a process known as cross-presentation. CD8+ cytotoxic T lymphocytes are able to recognize cross-presented TAs via their specific T-cell receptors, resulting in the lysis of tumor cells. Checkpoint inhibitors may restrict the lysing ability of CD8+ CTL by binding to checkpoint inhibitory receptors (e.g., PD-1) present on CTLs.

3.3.1.2.1 Vaccines (Peptide, Heat-Shock Protein, Dendritic Cell)

Vaccines, which serve to present antigens expressed by a target particle or organism to the immune system and induce the acquisition of adaptive immunity specific to the target(s), have been explored as potential immunotherapeutic approaches to gliomas.

Peptide vaccines have the benefit of being easy to produce and administer, and several potential tumor-associated peptide targets have been identified (Mitchell and Sampson, 2009). The epidermal growth factor receptor variant III (EGFRvIII) mutation is a tumor-specific antigen expressed in approximately 20–30% of GBMs, and the EGFRvIII-targeting rindopepimut vaccine has progressed through several clinical trials with mixed results, potentially owing to the antigen's heterogeneous expression in tumors (Humphrey et al., 1990; Malkki, 2016). Another promising peptide vaccine targets the IDH1 R132H mutation, which is present in roughly 70% of grade 2 and 3 gliomas and secondary GBMs and, unlike EGFRvIII, is expressed homogeneously throughout the tumor (Hartmann et al., 2009; Schumacher et al., 2014). Several multipeptide vaccine candidates such as the 11-peptide–targeting IMA950 vaccine are also in development, and aim to address the dilemma of immunologic escape by tumors in response to therapy-induced selection pressures (Halford et al., 2014).

Heat-shock proteins are involved in protein regulation and are generated by cells in increased quantity in response to environmental stress; HSP expression has been observed to be upregulated in a myriad of cancers, and several HSP families are associated with tumor growth and apoptosis inhibition in gliomas (Beamann et al., 2014; Ciocca and Calderwood, 2005). HSPs may present a viable vehicle for cancer vaccines due to their ability to bind to soluble proteins taken up by APCs, participate in cross-presentation, and generate cytotoxic T-lymphocyte–driven immune reactions (Zhou et al., 2014). Several HSP vaccines, for example HSPPC-96, are currently in trial – this approach may serve as a pathway to individualized vaccines that include peptides isolated directly from a patient's own brain tumor (Crane et al., 2013).

In contrast to directly administered, general tumor-derived peptide vaccines, DC vaccines involve the extraction of DCs from the individual patient, harvesting and exposure of DCs to tumor lysate or particular tumor antigens, and a return of the processed products to the patient in order to promote a principally T cell–mediated reaction (Dunn-Pirio and Vlahovic, 2017). Since the early 2000s, several DC vaccines have undergone clinical trials to various degrees of success, ultimately catalyzing an ongoing search for methods to produce more significant antitumor effects by enhancing DC migration and lymphocyte activation (Aarntzen et al., 2013; Heimberger et al., 2000). The emergence of recent candidates in Phase 3 trials, including the lysate-pulsed DCVax-L (Polyzoidis and Ashkan, 2014) and the multi-antigen–targeting ICT-107 (Wen et al., 2019), as well as the adoption of supportive measures such as recall antigen administration (Mitchell et al., 2015) and regulatory T cell (Treg) suppression (de la Rosa et al., 2004), promising therapeutic possibilities.

3.3.1.2.2 Oncolytic Viruses

Oncolytic viruses are either inherently or genetically altered to exclusively infect and eliminate cancer cells without harming surrounding tissue – a crucial characteristic for CNS tumor therapies (Dunn-Pirio and Vlahovic, 2017). Beyond these direct oncolytic properties, OVs also induce antiviral and antitumor immune responses through mechanisms that are not yet entirely clear (Kaufman et al., 2015). Several OVs have been tested in clinical trials and these include: (1) adenovirus-based OVs, for example DNX-2401, which were well-tolerated and showed enhanced pro-inflammatory responses in a modest subset of patients (Lang et al., 2014); (2) OVs combining MV, an RNA virus (Allen et al., 2008), with human carcinoembryonic antigen (CEA) that have shown positive tumor responses combined with the absence of viral replication in healthy brain tissue (Galanis et al., 2001; Phuong et al., 2003); (3) poliovirus (PV)-based (Dobrikova et al., 2008; Gromeier et al., 1996, 1999, 2000) OVs that have been rendered incapable of killing neurons while triggering a powerful inflammatory reaction against infected glioma cells (Desjardins et al., 2015, 2016).

3.3.1.2.3 Chimeric Antigen Receptors

A fairly novel category of adoptive T-cell transfer involves extracting T cells from a patient, transducing the cells using a lentiviral vector, and obtaining a hybrid T-cell–expressing CAR that combines both antigen-binding and T-cell–activating functions (Gross et al., 1989). In preclinical experiments, CAR T cells have been able to bypass the BBB and infiltrate the brain tumors, resulting in suppressed tumor growth (Miao et al., 2014). In humans, EGFRvIII-targeted CAR T cells and several other CAR

T-cell candidates are currently being evaluated at various clinical trial stages (Brown et al., 2015; Debinski et al., 1999); however, neuro-oncologists must be aware of and ready to address the cytokine release syndrome (CRS) complication of CAR T-cell therapy, an acute – but reversible – inflammatory reaction driven by excess cytokine release that can lead to multiorgan system failure (Maude et al., 2014).

3.3.1.2.4 Checkpoint Inhibitors

Checkpoint inhibitors allow tumor-suppressed T cells to cause tumor cell death by blocking T-cell–inhibiting checkpoint proteins such as CTLA-4 (Krummel and Allison, 1995) and PD-1. The majority of glioma checkpoint-inhibitor trials are in early phases, but existing checkpoint inhibitors, including nivolumab and ipilimumab, have also been tested in trials, albeit with increased adverse event occurrence seen following combination therapy (Sampson et al., 2015).

3.3.2 Vascular Disorders

Stroke occurs when the blood supply to a particular brain region is compromised, leading to permanent neurological deficits such as weakness, sensory deficits, visual field defects, and aphasia (Musuka et al., 2015). The adaptive and innate immune systems play distinct but synergistic roles in brain injury following ischemia, and the adaptive immune response contributes to poststroke immunodepression while also preventing autoimmunity of the body to CNS antigens that are released into the periphery as a result of stroke-related BBB compromise (Qin et al., 2020). Following an ischemic event, the ischemic cascade is initiated, involving the loss of adenosine triphosphate (ATP) and eventual cell excitotoxicity (Taxin et al., 2014). Dying CNS neurons and other cells then release damage-associated molecular patterns (DAMPs) that activate microglia and other pro-inflammatory mediators contributing to the disruption of the BBB (Gülke et al., 2018); the resulting influx of system inflammatory cells (e.g., monocytes, neutrophils, T and B cells) further exacerbates brain injury.

Cytotoxic CD8+ T cells migrating into the injured region following ischemia may play deleterious roles (Mracsko et al., 2014) and lead to neuronal damage via a number of pathways including the Fas ligand (FasL) pathway (Fan et al., 2020), humoral pathways through the release of inflammatory mediators (e.g., IFN-γ) and pro-inflammatory IL-16 cytokines (Schwab et al., 2001), and direct cytolytic pathways through the release of cytotoxic proteins (e.g., granzymes, perforin; Mracsko et al., 2014). Furthermore, cytotoxic CD8+ T cells may worsen white matter damage and contribute to demyelination in cerebral ischemia (Matute et al., 2013). Considering that IL-2 monoclonal antibody has the ability to affect CD8+ differentiation, it may be a possible therapeutic target for preserving white matter integrity following ischemia (Zhou et al., 2019).

CD4+ T helper cells, further divided into conventional Th cells and Tregs, have also been shown to increase in the infarcted region poststroke, and contribute to the two opposing Th1 and Th2 Th-cell response phenotypes. Whereas Th1 is a cell-mediated pro-inflammatory response characterized by pro-inflammatory IFN-γ cytokine production linked to ischemia-related neurodegeneration (Seifert et al., 2014), Th2 is a humoral-mediated anti-inflammatory response characterized by improved BBB integrity and the release of various ILs such as IL-10 (Grilli et al., 2000). Tregs, which suppress the proliferation of T cells and maintain self-tolerance (Bodhankar et al., 2015), contribute to several neuroprotective mechanisms (Li et al., 2013; Zhang et al., 2014) and the minimization of neurological damage following ischemia (Liesz et al., 2009). Treg expansion thus represents a possible therapeutic approach – the use of IL-2/IL-2 antibody complex (Guo and Luo, 2020), selective serotonin reuptake inhibitors (SSRIs; Ito et al., 2019), and poly ADP-ribose polymerase-1 (PARP-1) inhibitors (Noh et al., 2018) have been shown to potentially improve neurological outcome.

In the hours and days following stroke, the adaptive immune system plays a significant role in poststroke immunodepression and susceptibility to infection. While the shift from a cell-mediated inflammatory Th1-type response to a humoral-mediated anti-inflammatory Th2-type response occurs in order to protect the brain from further damage, this mechanism also suppresses the body's systemic immune system and therefore increases vulnerability to systemic infections (Jin et al., 2018). To compensate for immune-mediated poststroke immunodepression, promising methods to reduce pneumonia, bacterial infections, and other dangerous infections include IFN-γ administration at day 1 after stroke (Dirnagl et al., 2007), inhibition of CD147 (Farris et al., 2019), and targeted inhibition of immunosuppressive sympathetic nervous system and hypothalamic–pituitary–adrenal (HPA) axis signaling (Dirnagl et al., 2007; Walter et al., 2013).

Figure acknowledgements

The following images are credited to the authors of this chapter: Figures 3.1- 3.2.
The following image was adapted from Robert-Tissot and Speiser (2016): Figure 3.3

References

Aarntzen EH, Srinivas M, Schreibelt G, et al. Reducing cell number improves the homing of dendritic cells to lymph nodes upon intradermal vaccination. *OncoImmunology* 2013;**2**(7): e24661. https://doi.org/10.4161/onci.24661.

Alexander BM, Cloughesy TF. Adult glioblastoma. *J Clin Oncol* 2017;**35**(21):2402–09. https://doi.org/10.1200/JCO.2017.73.0119.

Allen C, Paraskevakou G, Liu C, Iankov ID, Zollman P, Galanis E. Oncolytic measles virus strains in the treatment of gliomas. *Expert Opin Biol Ther* 2008;**8**(2):213–20. https://doi.org/10.1517/14712598.8.2.213.

Amin MM, Shawky A, Zaher A, Abdelbary M, Wasel Y, Gomaa M. Immune cell infiltrate in different grades of astrocytomas: possible role in the pathogenesis. *Egypt J Pathol* 2012;**32**(1):175–80. https://doi.org/10.1097/01 .XEJ.0000415777.74514.34.

Andersson U, Tracey KJ. Reflex principles of immunological homeostasis. *Annu Rev Immunol* 2012;**30**(1):313–35. https://doi .org/10.1146/annurev-immunol-020711-075015.

Andtbacka RHI, Kaufman HL, Collichio F, et al. Talimogene laherparepvec improves durable response rate in patients with advanced melanoma. *J Clin Oncol Off J Am Soc Clin Oncol* 2015;**33**(25):2780–8. https://doi.org/10.1200/JCO.2014.58.3377.

Bar-Or A, Fawaz L, Fan B, et al. Abnormal B-cell cytokine responses a trigger of T-cell–mediated disease in MS? *Ann Neurol* 2010;**67**(4):452–61. https://doi.org/10.1002/ana.21939.

Beaman GM, Dennison SR, Chatfield LK, Phoenix DA. Reliability of HSP70 (HSPA) expression as a prognostic marker in glioma. *Mol Cell Biochem* 2014;**393**(1–2):301–07. https://doi .org/10.1007/s11010-014-2074-7.

Benarroch EE. The central autonomic network: functional organization, dysfunction, and perspective. *Mayo Clin Proc* 1993;**68**(10):988–1001. https://doi.org/10.1016/s0025-6196(12) 62272-1.

Bodhankar S, Chen Y, Lapato A, et al. Regulatory CD8+CD122+ T-cells predominate in CNS after treatment of experimental stroke in male mice with IL-10-secreting B-cells. *Metab Brain Dis* 2015;**30**(4):911–24. https://doi.org/10.1007/s11011-014-9639-8.

Brown C, Badie B, Barish M, et al. Bioactivity and safety of IL13Rα2-redirected chimeric antigen receptor CD8+ T cells in patients with recurrent glioblastoma. *Clin Cancer Res* 2015;**21** (18):4062–72. https://doi.org/10.1158/1078-0432.CCR-15- 0428.

Browning KN, Verheijden S, Boeckxstaens GE. The vagus nerve in appetite regulation, mood, and intestinal inflammation. *Gastroenterology* 2017;**152**(4):730–44. https://doi.org/10.1053/j .gastro.2016.10.046.

Ceyzériat K, Ben Haim L, Denizot A, et al. Modulation of astrocyte reactivity improves functional deficits in mouse models of Alzheimer's disease. *Acta Neuropathol Commun* 2018;**6**(1): 104–104. https://doi.org/10.1186/s40478-018-0606-1.

Ciocca DR, Calderwood SK. Heat shock proteins in cancer: diagnostic, prognostic, predictive, and treatment implications. *Cell Stress Chaperones* 2005;**10**(2):86–103. https://doi.org/10 .1379/csc-99r.1.

Cohen MH, Shen YL, Keegan P, Pazdur R. FDA drug approval summary: bevacizumab (Avastin) as treatment of recurrent glioblastoma multiforme. *The Oncologist* 2009;**14**(11):1131–8. https://doi.org/10.1634/theoncologist.2009-0121.

Crane CA, Han SJ, Ahn B, et al. Individual patient-specific immunity against high-grade glioma after vaccination with autologous tumor derived peptides bound to the 96 KD chaperone protein. *Clin Cancer Res Off J Am Assoc Cancer Res* 2013;**19**(1):205–14. https://doi.org/10.1158/1078-0432.CCR-11- 3358.

Cunningham CL, Martínez-Cerdeño V, Noctor SC. Microglia regulate the number of neural precursor cells in the developing cerebral cortex. *J Neurosci* 2013;**33**(10):4216–33. https://doi.org /10.1523/JNEUROSCI.3441-12.2013.

Dampney RAL. Central neural control of the cardiovascular system: current perspectives. *Adv Physiol Educ* 2016;**40**(3): 283–96. https://doi.org/10.1152/advan.00027.2016.

Debinski W, Gibo DM, Hulet SW, Connor JR, Gillespie GY. Receptor for interleukin 13 is a marker and therapeutic target for human high-grade gliomas. *Clin Cancer Res Off J Am Assoc Cancer Res* 1999;**5**(5):985–90.

Derecki NC, Cardani AN, Yang CH, et al. Regulation of learning and memory by meningeal immunity: a key role for IL-4. *J Exp Med* 2010;**207**(5):1067–80. https://doi.org/10.1084/jem .20091419.

Desjardins A, Sampson JH, Peters KB, et al. Oncolytic polio/ rhinovirus recombinant (PVSRIPO) against recurrent glioblastoma (GBM): optimal dose determination. *J Clin Oncol* 2015;**33**(15_suppl):2068–2068. https://doi.org/10.1093/neuonc/ nou209.5.

Desjardins A, Sampson JH, Peters KB, et al. Patient survival on the dose escalation phase of the Oncolytic Polio/Rhinovirus Recombinant (PVSRIPO) against WHO grade IV malignant glioma (MG) clinical trial compared to historical controls. *J Clin Oncol* 2016;**34**(15_suppl):2061–2061. https://doi.org/10.1056 /NEJMoa1716435.

Dirnagl U, Klehmet J, Braun JS, et al. Stroke-induced immunodepression. *Stroke* 2007;**38**(2):770–3. https://doi.org/10 .1161/01.STR.0000251441.89665.bc.

Dobrikova EY, Broadt T, Poiley-Nelson J, et al. Recombinant oncolytic poliovirus eliminates glioma *in vivo* without genetic adaptation to a pathogenic phenotype. *Mol Ther J Am Soc Gene Ther* 2008;**16**(11):1865–72. https://doi.org/10.1038/mt.2008.184.

Dunn-Pirio AM, Vlahovic G. Immunotherapy approaches in the treatment of malignant brain tumors. *Cancer* 2017;**123** (5):734–50. https://doi.org/10.1002/cncr.30371.

Ek M, Kurosawa M, Lundeberg T, Ericsson A. Activation of vagal afferents after intravenous injection of interleukin-1β: role of endogenous prostaglandins. *J Neurosci* 1998;**18**(22):9471–9. https://doi.org/10.1523/JNEUROSCI.18-22-09471.1998.

Fan L, Zhang C-J, Zhu L, et al. FasL–PDPK1 pathway promotes the cytotoxicity of CD8+ T cells during ischemic stroke. *Transl Stroke Res* 2020;**11**(4):747–61. https://doi.org/10.1007/s12975-019-00749-0.

Farris BY, Monaghan KL, Zheng W, et al. Ischemic stroke alters immune cell niche and chemokine profile in mice independent of spontaneous bacterial infection. *Immun Inflamm Dis* 2019;**7** (4):326–41. https://doi.org/10.1002/iid3.277.

Galanis E, Bateman A, Johnson K, et al. Use of viral fusogenic membrane glycoproteins as novel therapeutic transgenes in gliomas. *Hum Gene Ther* 2001;**12**(7):811–21. https://doi.org/10.1089/104303401750148766.

Garon EB, Rizvi NA, Hui R, et al. Pembrolizumab for the treatment of non-small-cell lung cancer. *N Engl J Med* 2015;**372** (21):2018–28. https://doi.org/10.1056/NEJMoa1501824.

Goehler LE, Gaykema RP, Hansen MK, Anderson K, Maier SF, Watkins LR. Vagal immune-to-brain communication: a visceral chemosensory pathway. *Auton Neurosci* 2000;**85**(1–3):49–59. https://doi.org/10.1016/S1566-0702(00)00219-8.

Grauer OM, Wesseling P, Adema GJ. Immunotherapy of diffuse gliomas: biological background, current status and future developments. *Brain Pathol Zurich Switz* 2009;**19**(4):674–93. https://doi.org/10.1111/j.1750-3639.2009.00315.x.

Grilli M, Barbieri I, Basudev H, et al. Interleukin-10 modulates neuronal threshold of vulnerability to ischaemic damage. *Eur J Neurosci* 2000;**12**(7):2265–72. https://doi.org/10.1046/j.1460-9568.2000.00090.x.

Gromeier M, Alexander L, Wimmer E. Internal ribosomal entry site substitution eliminates neurovirulence in intergeneric poliovirus recombinants. *Proc Natl Acad Sci U S A* 1996;**93** (6):2370–5. https://doi.org/10.1073/pnas.93.6.2370.

Gromeier M, Bossert B, Arita M, Nomoto A, Wimmer E. Dual stem loops within the poliovirus internal ribosomal entry site control neurovirulence. *J Virol* 1999;**73**(2):958–64. https://doi.org/10.1128/JVI.73.2.958-964.1999.

Gromeier M, Lachmann S, Rosenfeld MR, Gutin PH, Wimmer E. Intergeneric poliovirus recombinants for the treatment of malignant glioma. *Proc Natl Acad Sci U S A* 2000;**97**(12):6803–8. https://doi.org/10.1073/pnas.97.12.6803.

Gross G, Waks T, Eshhar Z. Expression of immunoglobulin-T-cell receptor chimeric molecules as functional receptors with antibody-type specificity. *Proc Natl Acad Sci U S A* 1989;**86**(24):10024–8. https://doi.org/10.1073/pnas.86.24.10024.

Gülke E, Gelderblom M, Magnus T. Danger signals in stroke and their role on microglia activation after ischemia. *Ther Adv Neurol Disord* 2018;**11**:1756286418774254. https://doi.org/10.1177/1756286418774254.

Guo S, Luo Y. Brain Foxp3+ regulatory T cells can be expanded by interleukin-33 in mouse ischemic stroke. *Int Immunopharmacol* 2020;**81**:106027. https://doi.org/10.1016/j.intimp.2019.106027.

Halford S, Rampling R, James A, et al. Final results from a Cancer Research UK first in man phase I trial of Ima950 (a novel multi peptide vaccine) plus Gm-Csf in patients with newly diagnosed glioblastoma. *Ann Oncol* 2014;**25**:iv364. https://doi.org/10.1093/annonc/mdu342.10.

Hartmann C, Meyer J, Balss J, et al. Type and frequency of *IDH1* and *IDH2* mutations are related to astrocytic and oligodendroglial differentiation and age: a study of 1,010 diffuse gliomas. *Acta Neuropathol (Berl)* 2009;**118**(4):469–74. https://doi.org/10.1007/s00401-009-0561-9.

Heimberger AB, Crotty LE, Archer GE, et al. Bone marrow-derived dendritic cells pulsed with tumor homogenate induce immunity against syngeneic intracerebral glioma. *J Neuroimmunol* 2000;**103**(1):16–25. https://doi.org/10.1016/s0165-5728(99)00172-1.

Hodi FS, O'Day SJ, McDermott DF, et al. Improved survival with ipilimumab in patients with metastatic melanoma. *N Engl J Med* 2010;**363**(8):711–23. https://doi.org/10.1056/NEJMoa1003466.

Hodi FS, Postow MA, Chesney JA, et al. Clinical response, progression-free survival (PFS), and safety in patients (pts) with advanced melanoma (MEL) receiving nivolumab (NIVO) combined with ipilimumab (IPI) vs IPI monotherapy in CheckMate 069 study. *J Clin Oncol* 2015;**33**(15_suppl):9004–9004.

Humphrey PA, Wong AJ, Vogelstein B, et al. Anti-synthetic peptide antibody reacting at the fusion junction of deletion-mutant epidermal growth factor receptors in human glioblastoma. *Proc Natl Acad Sci U S A* 87: 4207–4211. https://doi.org/10.1073/pnas.87.11.4207.

Ito M, Komai K, Nakamura T, Srirat T, Yoshimura A. Tissue regulatory T cells and neural repair. *Int Immunol* 2019;**31** (6):361–9. https://doi.org/10.1093/intimm/dxz031.

Janeway C. *Immunobiology: The Immune System in Health and Disease*. 4th ed. Garland, 1999.

Jin Wei-Na, Gonzales R, Feng Yan, et al. Brain ischemia induces diversified neuroantigen-specific T-cell responses that exacerbate brain injury. *Stroke* 2018;**49**(6):1471–8. https://doi.org/10.1161/STROKEAHA.118.020203.

Johnson BF, Clay TM, Hobeika AC, Lyerly HK, Morse MA. Vascular endothelial growth factor and immunosuppression in cancer: current knowledge and potential for new therapy. *Expert Opin Biol Ther* 2007;7(4):449–60. https://doi.org/10.1517/1471 2598.7.4.449.

Kaufman HL, Kohlhapp FJ, Zloza A. Oncolytic viruses: a new class of immunotherapy drugs. *Nat Rev Drug Discov* 2015;14 (9):642–62. https://doi.org/10.1038/nrd.2016.178.

Kipnis J, Cohen H, Cardon M, Ziv Y, Schwartz M. T cell deficiency leads to cognitive dysfunction: implications for therapeutic vaccination for schizophrenia and other psychiatric conditions. *Proc Natl Acad Sci* 2004;101(21):8180–5. https://doi .org/10.1073/pnas.0402268101.

Korin B, Ben-Shaanan TL, Schiller M, et al. High-dimensional, single-cell characterization of the brain's immune compartment. *Nat Neurosci* 2017;20(9):1300–9. https://doi.org /10.1038/nn.4610.

Korn T, Kallies A. T cell responses in the central nervous system. *Nat Rev Immunol* 2017;17(3):179–94. https://doi.org/10 .1038/nri.2016.144.

Krummel MF, Allison JP. CD28 and CTLA-4 have opposing effects on the response of T cells to stimulation. *J Exp Med* 1995;182(2):459–65. https://doi.org/10.1084/jem.182.2.459.

Lang FF, Conrad C, Gomez-Manzano C, et al. First-in-human phase I clinical trial of oncolytic delta-24-RGD (DNX-2401) with biological endpoints: implications for viro-immunotherapy. *Neuro Oncol* 2014;16(Suppl 3): iii39. https://doi.org/10.1093/neuonc/nou208.61.

Levine YA, Koopman FA, Faltys M, et al. Neurostimulation of the cholinergic anti-inflammatory pathway ameliorates disease in rat collagen-induced arthritis. *PLoS One* 2014;9 (8):e104530–e104530. https://doi.org/10.1371/journal .pone.0104530.

Li P, Gan Y, Sun B-L, et al. Adoptive regulatory T-cell therapy protects against cerebral ischemia. *Ann Neurol* 2013;74(3):458– 71. https://doi.org/10.1002/ana.23815.

Li Q, Barres BA. Microglia and macrophages in brain homeostasis and disease. *Nat Rev Immunol* 2018;18(4):225–42. https://doi.org/10.1038/nri.2017.125.

Liesz A, Suri-Payer E, Veltkamp C, et al. Regulatory T cells are key cerebroprotective immunomodulators in acute experimental stroke. *Nat Med* 2009;15(2):192–9. https://doi.org /10.1038/nm.1927.

Malkki H. Trial watch: Glioblastoma vaccine therapy disappointment in Phase III trial. *Nat Rev Neurol* 2016;12 (4):190. https://doi.org/10.1038/nrneurol.2016.38

Matute C, Domercq M, Pérez-Samartín A, Ransom BR. Protecting white matter from stroke injury. *Stroke* 2013;44 (4):1204–11. https://doi.org/10.1161/STROKEAHA.112.658328.

Maude SL, Barrett D, Teachey DT, Grupp SA. Managing cytokine release syndrome associated with novel T

cell-engaging therapies. *Cancer J* 2014;20(2):119–22. https://doi .org/10.1097/PPO.0000000000000035.

Medzhitov R, Janeway CA. Decoding the patterns of self and nonself by the innate immune system. *Sci Am Assoc Adv Sci* 2002;296(5566):298–300. https://doi.org/10.1126/science .1068883.

Miao H, Choi BD, Suryadevara CM, et al. EGFRvIII-specific chimeric antigen receptor T cells migrate to and kill tumor deposits infiltrating the brain parenchyma in an invasive xenograft model of glioblastoma. *PLoS One* 2014;9(4):e94281. https://doi.org/10.1371/journal.pone.0094281.

Mitchell DA, Batich KA, Gunn MD, et al. Tetanus toxoid and CCL3 improve dendritic cell vaccines in mice and glioblastoma patients. *Nature* 2015;519(7543):366–9. https://doi.org/10.1038 /nature14320.

Mitchell DA, Sampson JH. Toward effective immunotherapy for the treatment of malignant brain tumors. *Neurotherapeutics* 2009;6(3):527–38. https://doi.org/10.1016/j .nurt.2009.04.003.

Miyamoto A, Wake H, Ishikawa AW, et al. Microglia contact induces synapse formation in developing somatosensory cortex. *Nat Commun* 2016;7(1):12540. https://doi.org/10.1038 /ncomms12540.

Mracsko E, Liesz A, Stojanovic A, et al. Antigen dependently activated cluster of differentiation 8-positive T cells cause perforin-mediated neurotoxicity in experimental stroke. *J Neurosci* 2014;34(50):16784–95. https://doi.org/10.1523/ JNEUROSCI.1867-14.2014.

Musuka TD, Wilton SB, Traboulsi M, Hill MD. Diagnosis and management of acute ischemic stroke: speed is critical. *CMAJ* 2015;187(12):887–93. https://doi.org/10.1503/cmaj .140355.

Noh M-Y, Lee WM, Lee S-J, Kim HY, Kim SH, Kim YS. Regulatory T cells increase after treatment with poly (ADP-ribose) polymerase-1 inhibitor in ischemic stroke patients. *Int Immunopharmacol* 2018;60:104–10. https://doi.org /10.1016/j.intimp.2018.04.043.

Norden DM, Muccigrosso MM, Godbout JP. Microglial priming and enhanced reactivity to secondary insult in aging, and traumatic CNS injury, and neurodegenerative disease. *Neuropharmacology* 2015;96:29–41. https://doi.org/10.1016/j .neuropharm.2014.10.028.

Olofsson PS, Levine YA, Caravaca A, et al. Single-pulse and unidirectional electrical activation of the cervical vagus nerve reduces tumor necrosis factor in endotoxemia. *Bioelectron Med* 2015;2(1):37–42.

Pang Y, Fan L-W, Tien L-T, et al. Differential roles of astrocyte and microglia in supporting oligodendrocyte development and myelination *in vitro. Brain Behav* 2013;3(5):503–14. https://doi .org/10.1002/brb3.152.

Pavlov VA. Cholinergic modulation of inflammation. *Int J Clin Exp Med* 2008;1(3):203–12.

Phuong LK, Allen C, Peng K-W, et al. Use of a vaccine strain of measles virus genetically engineered to produce carcinoembryonic antigen as a novel therapeutic agent against glioblastoma multiforme. *Cancer Res* 2003;**63**(10):2462–9.

Polyzoidis S, Ashkan K. DCVax®-L developed by Northwest Biotherapeutics. *Hum Vaccines Immunother* 2014;**10**(11):3139–45. https://doi.org/10.4161/hv.29276.

Pösel C, Möller K, Boltze J, Wagner D-C, Weise G. Isolation and flow cytometric analysis of immune cells from the ischemic mouse brain. *J Vis Exp* 2016;**108**:e53658. https://doi.org/10.3791/53658.

Primiani CT, Ryan VH, Rao JS, et al. Coordinated gene expression of neuroinflammatory and cell signaling markers in dorsolateral prefrontal cortex during human brain development and aging. *PLoS One* 2014;**9**(10):e110972. https://doi.org/10.1371/journal.pone.0110972.

Qin X, Akter F, Qin L, et al. Adaptive immunity regulation and cerebral ischemia. *Front Immunol* 2020;**11**:689. https://doi.org/10.3389/fimmu.2020.00689.

Ransohoff RM, Engelhardt B. The anatomical and cellular basis of immune surveillance in the central nervous system. *Nat Rev Immunol* 2012;**12**(9):623–35. https://doi.org/10.1038/nri3265.

Ransohoff RM, Kivisäkk P, Kidd G. Three or more routes for leukocyte migration into the central nervous system. *Nat Rev Immunol* 2003;**3**(7):569–81. https://doi.org/10.1038/nri1130.

Ransohoff RM, Schafer D, Vincent A, Blachère NE, Bar-Or A. Neuroinflammation: ways in which the immune system affects the brain. *Neurotherapeutics* 2015;**12**(4):896–909. https://doi.org/10.1007/s13311-015-0385-3.

Robert-Tissot C, Speiser DE. Anticancer teamwork: cross-presenting dendritic cells collaborate with therapeutic monoclonal antibodies. *Cancer Discov* 2016;**6**(1):17–9. https://doi.org/10.1158/2159-8290.CD-15-1366.

Rock KL. A new foreign policy: MHC class I molecules monitor the outside world. *Immunol Today* 1996;**17**(3):131–7. https://doi.org/10.1016/0167-5699(96)80605-0.

Rosa M de la, Rutz S, Dorninger H, Scheffold A. Interleukin-2 is essential for CD4+CD25+ regulatory T cell function. *Eur J Immunol* 2004;**34**(9):2480–8. https://doi.org/10.1002/eji.200425274.

Sabharwal L, Kamimura D, Meng J, et al. The Gateway Reflex, which is mediated by the inflammation amplifier, directs pathogenic immune cells into the CNS. *J Biochem Tokyo* 2014;**156**(6):299–304. https://doi.org/10.1093/jb/mvu057.

Safdari H, Hochberg FH, Richardson EP. Prognostic value of round cell (lymphocyte) infiltration in malignant gliomas. *Surg Neurol* 1985;**23**(3):221–6. https://doi.org/10.1016/0090-3019(85)90086-2.

Sampson JH, Vlahovic G, Sahebjam S, et al. Preliminary safety and activity of nivolumab and its combination with ipilimumab in recurrent glioblastoma (GBM): CHECKMATE-143. *J Clin Oncol* 2015;**33**(15_suppl):3010–3010.

Sasaki A. Microglia and brain macrophages: an update. *Neuropathology* 2017;**37**(5):452–64. https://doi.org/10.1111/neup.12354.

Schumacher T, Bunse L, Pusch S, et al. A vaccine targeting mutant IDH1 induces antitumour immunity. *Nature* 2014;**512**(7514):324–7. https://doi.org/10.1038/nature13387.

Schwab JM, Nguyen TD, Meyermann R, Schluesener HJ. Human focal cerebral infarctions induce differential lesional interleukin-16 (IL-16) expression confined to infiltrating granulocytes, CD8+ T-lymphocytes and activated microglia/macrophages. *J Neuroimmunol* 2001;**114**(1):232–41. https://doi.org/10.1016/s0165-5728(00)00433-1.

Seifert HA, Collier LA, Chapman CB, Benkovic SA, Willing AE, Pennypacker KR. Pro-inflammatory interferon gamma signaling is directly associated with stroke induced neurodegeneration. *J Neuroimmune Pharmacol* 2014;**9**(5):679–89. https://doi.org/10.1007/s11481-014-9560-2.

Shen P, Roch T, Lampropoulou V, et al. IL-35-producing B cells are critical regulators of immunity during autoimmune and infectious diseases. *Nat Lond* 2014;**507**(7492):366–70. https://doi.org/10.1038/nature12979.

Shen Z, Bao X, Wang R. Clinical PET imaging of microglial activation: implications for microglial therapeutics in Alzheimer's disease. *Front Aging Neurosci* 2018;**10**:314. https://doi.org/10.3389/fnagi.2018.00314.

Sofroniew MV. Astrocyte barriers to neurotoxic inflammation. *Nat Rev Neurosci* 2015;**16**(5):249–63. https://doi.org/10.1038/nrn3898.

Song GJ, Suk K. Pharmacological modulation of functional phenotypes of microglia in neurodegenerative diseases. *Front Aging Neurosci* 2017;**9**:139–139. https://doi.org/10.3389/fnagi.2017.00139.

Stephenson J, Nutma E, van der Valk P, Amor S. Inflammation in CNS neurodegenerative diseases. *Immunology* 2018;**154**(2):204–19. https://doi.org/10.1111/imm.12922.

Stern JNH, Yaari G, Vander Heiden JA, et al. B cells populating the multiple sclerosis brain mature in the draining cervical lymph nodes. *Sci Transl Med* 2014;**6**(248):248ra107–248ra107. https://doi.org/10.1126/scitranslmed.3008879.

Tanabe S, Yamashita T. B-1a lymphocytes promote oligodendrogenesis during brain development. *Nat Neurosci* 2018;**21**(4):506–16. https://doi.org/10.1038/s41593-018-0106-4.

Tanabe S, Yamashita T. B lymphocytes: crucial contributors to brain development and neurological diseases. *Neurosci Res* 2019;**139**:37–41. https://doi.org/10.1016/j.neures.2018.07.002.

Tang Y, Le W. Differential roles of M1 and M2 microglia in neurodegenerative diseases. *Mol Neurobiol* 2016;**53**(2):1181–94. https://doi.org/10.1007/s12035-014-9070-5.

Taxin ZH, Neymotin SA, Mohan A, Lipton P, Lytton WW. Modeling molecular pathways of neuronal ischemia. In Blackwell KT (ed.), *Progress in Molecular Biology and Translational Science*. Academic Press, 2014: 249–75. www.sciencedirect.com/science/article/pii/B978012397 8974000140

Torres-Rosas R, Yehia G, Peña G, et al. Dopamine mediates vagal modulation of the immune system by electroacupuncture. *Nat Med* 2014;**20**(3):291–5. https://doi.org/10.1038/nm.3479.

Tracey KJ. The inflammatory reflex. *Nat Lond* 2002;**420** (6917):853–9. https://doi.org/10.1038/nature01321

Tracey KJ. Reflex control of immunity. *Nat Rev Immunol* 2009;**9** (6):418–28. https://doi.org/10.1038/nri2566.

Ueno M, Ueno-Nakamura Y, Niehaus J, Popovich PG, Yoshida Y. Silencing spinal interneurons inhibits immune suppressive autonomic reflexes caused by spinal cord injury. *Nat Neurosci* 2016;**19**(6):784–7. https://doi.org/10.1038/nn.4289.

Walter U, Kolbaske S, Patejdl R, et al. Insular stroke is associated with acute sympathetic hyperactivation and immunodepression. *Eur J Neurol* 2013;**20**(1):153–9. https://doi.org/10.1111/j.1468-1331.2012.03818.x.

Wang J, Xing H, Wan L, Jiang X, Wang C, Wu Y. Treatment targets for M2 microglia polarization in ischemic stroke. *Biomed Pharmacother* 2018;**105**:518–25. https://doi.org/10.1016/j.biopha.2018.05.143.

Waziri A. Glioblastoma-derived mechanisms of systemic immunosuppression. *Neurosurg Clin N Am* 2010;**21**(1):31–42. https://doi.org/10.1016/j.nec.2009.08.005.

Wen PY, Reardon DA, Armstrong TS, et al. A randomized double-blind placebo-controlled phase II trial of dendritic cell vaccine ICT-107 in newly diagnosed patients with glioblastoma. *Clin Cancer Res* 2019;**25**(19):5799–807. https://doi.org/10.1158/1078-0432.CCR-19-0261.

Wolf SA, Boddeke HWGM, Kettenmann H. Microglia in physiology and disease. *Annu Rev Physiol* 2017;**79**(1):619–43. https://doi.org/10.1146/annurev-physiol-022516-034406.

Zagzag D, Salnikow K, Chiriboga L, et al. Downregulation of major histocompatibility complex antigens in invading glioma cells: stealth invasion of the brain. *Lab Investig J Tech Methods Pathol* 2005;**85**(3):328–41. https://doi.org/10.1038/labinvest.3700233.

Zhang J, Mao X, Zhou T, Cheng X, Lin Y. IL-17A contributes to brain ischemia reperfusion injury through calpain-TRPC6 pathway in mice. *Neuroscience* 2014;**274**:419–28. https://doi.org/10.1016/j.neuroscience.2014.06.001.

Zhao Z, Nelson AR, Betsholtz C, Zlokovic BV. Establishment and dysfunction of the blood–brain barrier. *Cell* 2015;**163**(5):1064–78. https://doi.org/10.1016/j.cell.2015.10.067.

Zhou YJ, Messmer MN, Binder RJ. Establishment of tumor-associated immunity requires interaction of heat shock proteins with CD91. *Cancer Immunol Res* 2014;**2**(3):217–28. https://doi.org/10.1158/2326-6066.CIR-13-0132.

Zhou Y-X, Wang X, Tang D, et al. IL-2mAb reduces demyelination after focal cerebral ischemia by suppressing CD8+ T cells. *CNS Neurosci Ther* 2019;**25**(4):532–43. https://doi.org/10.1111/cns.13084.

Ziv Y, Ron N, Butovsky O, et al. Immune cells contribute to the maintenance of neurogenesis and spatial learning abilities in adulthood. *Nat Neurosci* 2006;**9**(2):268–75. https://doi.org/10.1038/nn1629.

Anatomy and Physiology of the Neuron

Oluwatobi Ariyo and Farhana Akter

4.1 Introduction

In this chapter we discuss the fundamental units of the nervous system: neurons and supporting cells. All neurons in the cerebral cortex and certain lineages of glia e.g. parenchymal glial cells are produced from radial glial cells, that arise during expansion of the neural tube. These are progenitor cells that extend fibers from the ventricular zone to the pia and act as a scaffold for migrating neurons on route to their final destination in the cortical surface. Neurons are electrically excitable cells and an understanding of basic neurophysiology enables us to decipher how information travels within the nervous system and how neurons communicate with each other through synapses to form networks capable of performing sophisticated and complex tasks.

Our knowledge of the anatomical features of a neuron comes from early methods to distinguish the different types of cells within the nervous system such as the Nissl stain and the Golgi stain (Figure 4.1), which allow us to visualize the cytoarchitecture of the neuron and its components such as the cell body, dendrites, and the axon (Figure 4.2). The use of the electron microscope has allowed us to appreciate that neurons are not continuous structures, contrary to that proposed by Camillo Golgi, but instead are individual units, a theory that was proposed by Raman Cajal.

4.2 Classification of Neurons

Neurons can be classified according to the total number of axons and dendrites (Figure 4.3), the shape of their cell body, according to their function (e.g., sensory, motor), or the type of neurotransmitter that they transport (e.g., glutamate and γ-aminobutyric acid (GABA).

Unipolar neurons are typically sensory and found in the afferent part of the peripheral nervous system (PNS). Bipolar neurons are typically found in the retina and the olfactory system.

Multipolar neurons have multiple (three or more) processes and are the most predominant type of neuron in the central nervous system (CNS). Multipolar neurons include pyramidal neurons and Purkinje neurons. Pyramidal neurons are the most common excitatory neurons and typically send their axons over long distances. They are commonly found in the cerebral cortex, and also in

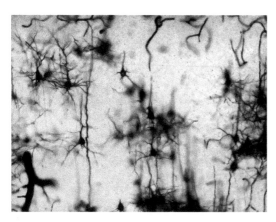

Figure 4.1 Golgi stain.

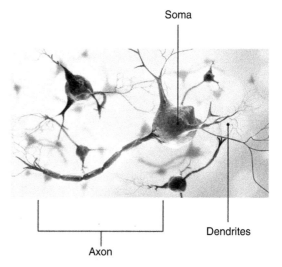

Figure 4.2 A myelinated neuron.

Figure 4.3 Types of neurons.

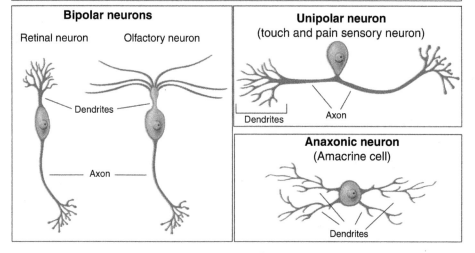

Multipolar neurons

Motor neuron

Pyramidal neuron

Purkinje cell

Dendrites

Dendrites

Dendrites

Axon

Axon

Bipolar neurons

Retinal neuron   Olfactory neuron

Dendrites

Axon

Unipolar neuron
(touch and pain sensory neuron)

Dendrites   Axon

Anaxonic neuron
(Amacrine cell)

Dendrites

subcortical structures such as the hippocampus and the amygdala. They contain triangular somata, from which a single axon, a large apical dendrite and many basal dendrites emanate. The dendrites contain spines that receive excitatory post synaptic potentials. Purkinje neurons are GABAergic inhibitory cells that are responsible for the sole output of the cerebellar cortex. Each Purkinje cell receives direct excitatory input from one climbing fiber (originating in the inferior olivary nucleus of the medulla oblongata) and indirect input via the mossy fibers, which originate from brainstem nuclei and terminate on granule cells in the cerebellar cortex. The granule cell axons bifurcate into parallel fibers that innervate Purkinje cell dendrites. Parallel and climbing fibers also send excitatory synaptic inputs to stellate and basket cells in the molecular layer of the cerebellum. These are GABAergic interneurons and therefore inhibit Purkinje cells. Basket cells, form 'baskets' of axonal arborizations around the Purkinje cells and terminate as pinceaux at the initial segment of axons.

4.3 Soma

The soma (cell body) varies in shape in different regions of the brain. It contains a potassium (K^+)-rich solution that is separated from the outside of the cell by a neuronal membrane. The soma contains numerous organelles that are crucial for the function of the neuron (Figure 4.4). Within the soma can be found the nucleus containing chromosomes and deoxyribonucleic acid (DNA). The presence of ribosomes and rough endoplasmic reticulum (RER) is crucial for protein synthesis, particularly as the

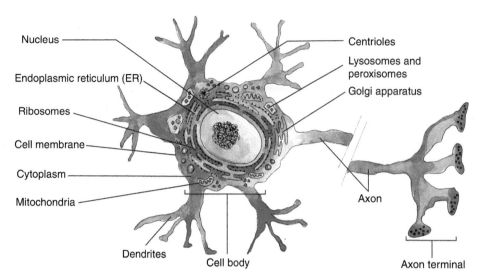

Figure 4.4 The cell body of a neuron.

axons are devoid of ribosomes and rely on the soma for protein synthesis.

4.4 Dendrites

The dendrites of a neuron are outward projections from the soma. Synapses are formed on the dendritic tree of a single neuron and when activated lead to convergence of signal integration in the axon, prior to the generation of an action potential. The integration of inputs in dendrites is essential for understanding neural circuits and behavior and will be discussed in Chapter 8.

Dendrites of many neurons contain protrusions called spines (Figure 4.5). These contain a dense network of cytoskeletal molecules and are the site of most excitatory synaptic signaling in the brain. They typically appear as mushroom-like projections with a head that contains the postsynaptic density (PSD) and a neck that connects the head to the shaft of the dendrite. Postsynaptic densities contain the signaling machinery involved in synaptic transmission. The area of this region is proportional to the size of the spine head, glutamate receptors, and the number of docked vesicles in the presynaptic membrane. Larger spines are therefore indicative of stronger synapses and growth of the spine head is thought to correlate with strengthening of synaptic transmission.

During early development, the majority of the spines are thin filopodia and are gradually replaced by bulbous spines that are more stable and less motile (Figure 4.5). A typical mature spine usually has a single glutamatergic synapse on the head, and therefore measuring the

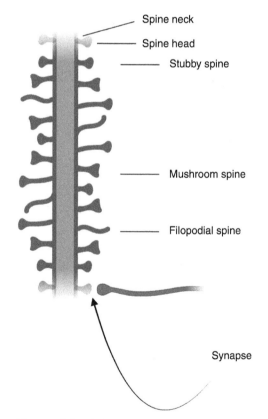

Figure 4.5 Dendritic spine.

number of spines can provide information on the synapse density of a region. Pruning of spines contributes to neural network refinement during development and adulthood and is important for learning.

4.5 Axon

Axons are long, cylindrical protrusions from the soma and are crucial for information transfer from one cell to the next. The initial segment of the axon is the hillock. The internal structure of this segment is characterized by fine granules underneath the plasma membrane, fascicles of microtubules, and a sparse clustering of ribosomes lacking Nissl bodies, which disappear at the end of the initial segment. Functionally, the initial segment is where there is summation of somatic input leading to the initiation of an action potential.

Information is then transferred from the hillock to the main shaft of the axon, where any fluctuations of membrane potential can be integrated. Finally, there is propagation of the action potential to the axon terminal, which forms synapses with other cells and contains several organelles such as the mitochondrion and synaptic vesicles containing neurotransmitters.

In addition to electrical signal transmission, the axon is also responsible for transport of cargo such as mitochondria, lipids, synaptic vesicles along its microtubules, and other organelles along its body to the terminals (anterograde transport), with the aid of the kinesin protein or the motor protein dynein for retrograde transport of cargo such as autophagosomes toward the cell body.

4.6 Supporting Cells

4.6.1 Astrocytes

Astrocytes are glial cells and the major cell types of the brain, outnumbering neurons more than fivefold. Astrocytes play a crucial role in both health and in injury where a process termed "reactive astrogliosis" takes place to limit damage by scar formation or remodeling of cells to modulate regeneration. Astrocytes contain a cytoskeleton made up of intermediate filaments such as glial fibrillary acidic protein (GFAP) and vimentin.

There are two main types of astrocytes: fibrous and protoplasmic astrocytes. Fibrous astrocytes have long processes, contact the nodes of Ranvier, and are found in the white matter. Protoplasmic astrocytes are found in the gray matter, typically enveloping synapses; they possess short processes and allow astrocytes to be exposed to neurotransmitters released from synaptic terminals. The idea of the "tripartite synapse" is that a neurotransmitter is released from the presynaptic terminal and activates the postsynaptic cell and astroglial cell leading to a postsynaptic potential in the neuron and a Ca^{2+} signal in the astrocyte, which in turn signals to the pre- and postsynaptic neuronal cell.

Astrocytes are essential for neuroprotective tasks of the brain including formation and maintenance of the blood-brain barrier (BBB; Figures 4.6 and 4.7). They also play an important role in releasing various transmitters, neurotrophic factors, and molecules such as cholesterol into the extracellular space. In addition, they are responsible for clearing neurotransmitters such as glutamate, which in excess can trigger neuronal cell death, through conversion to glutamine followed by uptake into presynaptic cells.

Astrocytes have a profound impact on synaptic pruning and elimination of exuberant projections and synapses through various secreted and contact-mediated signals. Modulation of homeostatic plasticity in this way is thought to be the cellular basis of learning and memory and therefore astrocytic synaptic regulation may also be important for cognition.

Dynamic astrocytic Ca^{2+} signals propagate within glial cells and through the glial networks, and these are mediated by Ca^{2+} release from intracellular calcium storage organelles.

Although astrocytes themselves do not fire action potentials, they control extracellular potassium ion homeostasis. They increase levels of extracellular K^+ in both physiological and pathological conditions and remove excess K^+ by spatial redistribution or by increasing activity of enzyme pumps.

Another member of the glial cell family is the radial glial cell. These are bipolar cells that possess stem cell–like properties and span the entire developing cerebral wall. They are responsible for the production and final placement of neurons in the developing brain. Neurons that are produced from these cells migrate along the radial glial fibers toward the cortical surface. They persist in the ventricular zone and are used by migrating neurons as a scaffold. They eventually transform into astrocytes and ependymal cells. In the retina, a special type of radial glial cell called Muller glia is found during development and in adults. In the cerebellum, a distinct array of unipolar astrocytes derived from radial glia can be found. These are the Bergmann glia, and they are important during early cerebellum development and for synaptic pruning and gliosis following injury.

4.6.2 Microglia

Microglia, the resident macrophages of the CNS has polarized the scientific community with the use of dichotomies

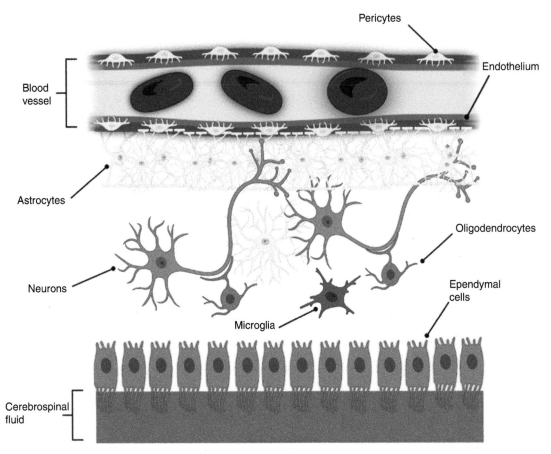

Pericytes

Endothelium

Blood
vessel

Astrocytes

Oligodendrocytes

Neurons

Ependymal
cells

Microglia

Cerebrospinal
fluid

Figure 4.6 Blood–brain barrier.

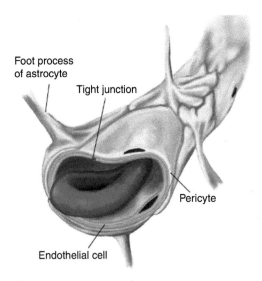

Foot process
of astrocyte

Tight junction

Pericyte

Endothelial cell

Figure 4.7 Foot process of astrocytes.

such as M1/M2 or resting/activated states, however these represent a simplified conceptual framework and research has now entered a fertile era showing that microglial phenotypes are characterized by temporal and spatial evolution. Microglia provide a surveillance and scavenging function, this includes removal of apoptotic cells that release molecules such as Danger- associated molecular patterns (DAMPs) which activate the innate immune system and promote pathological inflammatory responses. Microglia are also crucial for engulfing supernumerary synapses and help refine developing neural circuits.

4.6.3 Ependymal Cells

Ependymal cells are ciliated epithelial glial cells that develop from radial glia along the surface of the ventricles of the brain and the spinal canal. They play a critical role in cerebrospinal fluid (CSF) homeostasis, brain metabolism, and the clearance of waste from the brain.

4.6.4 Pericytes

Pericytes are cells found within the walls of capillaries, near the brain parenchyma. They are a critical component of the neurovascular unit that forms the BBB. Pericytes are important for regional control of cerebral blood flow as they are able to contract or relax in response to changes in the flow. They can modulate the integrity of the BBB and loss of pericytes can affect the tight junctions between endothelial cells, leading to increased permeability. Pericytes also contribute to immune defense mechanisms alongside microglia, astrocytes, and leukocytes.

4.6.5 Oligodendrocytes

Oligodendrocytes (OLGs) are responsible for the myelination of axons in the CNS to ensure efficient signal conduction and axonal transport. Myelin also clusters sodium channels in the node of Ranvier of the axon and is important for saltatory nerve conduction. These cells develop from oligodendrocyte precursor cells (OPCs), a subtype of glial cells that emerge during development initially in the germinal cells and then migrate throughout the CNS. Oligodendrocyte precursor cells divide a limited number of times before terminally differentiating into OLGs. They can also persist as resident, stable cells in the adult brain and are important during a demyelinating insult, when they can differentiate into OLGs to allow remyelination to occur. However, new OLG generation from adult OPCs is limited.

In the PNS, axonal ensheathment by Schwann cells (Figure 4.8) are critical for the integrity and function of nerves. These cells derived from neural crest cells migrate to nerve trunks and populate nascent nerves and this is regulated by various signaling molecules such as the neuronal growth factor Neuregulin (NRG) 1, interacting with ErbB2/ErbB3 tyrosine kinase receptors.

4.7 Electrical Signaling in the Neuron

The nervous system utilizes electrical signals to transmit and store information throughout neurons. Each individual neuron receives, integrates, and propagates signals from the dendrites through the axon to the synapse based on transient changes in the membrane potential. The membrane potential is the electrical potential difference across the neuron cell membrane and is mediated by the flow of ions across the neuron's selectively permeable membrane. The membrane potential of a neuron not actively transmitting information, or the resting membrane potential, is typically negative. When a neuron is excited, an electrical signal known as the action potential transiently changes the negative resting membrane potential to make it positive. Action potentials are propagated along the cell axon to the presynaptic terminals, facilitating the transmission of information between neurons.

4.8 Resting Membrane Potential

4.8.1 Electrochemical Equilibrium

Neurons have a lipid bilayer cell membrane that is impermeable to charged molecules such as ions. Therefore, in

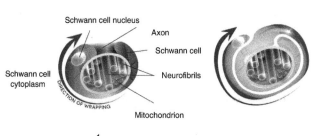

1.
Schwann cell wraps
around the axon in a spiral fashion.

2.
Schwann cell rotates around
the axon forming layers.

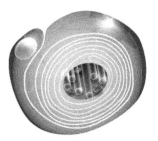

3.
A single myelin sheath is formed by a
Schwann cell (note oligodendrocytes form
multiple myelin sheaths around an axon).

Myelination drives reorganization of axonal
proteins and accumulation of voltage gated
sodium channels at the nodes of Ranvier,
which are separated from potassium
channels by the presence of paranodal
junctions.

Figure 4.8 Myelin sheath formation.

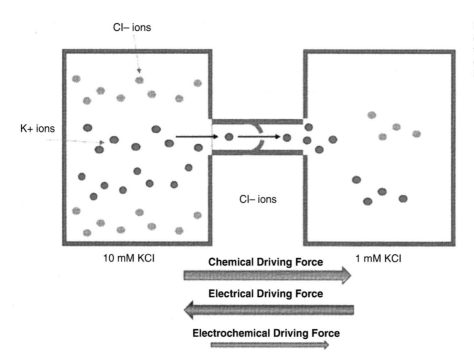

Cl− ions

K+ ions

Cl− ions

10 mM KCl

Chemical Driving Force

1 mM KCl

Electrical Driving Force

Electrochemical Driving Force

Figure 4.9 The balancing of both the chemical and the electrical driving force establishes an electrochemical driving force that directs the flow of ions across the cell membrane.

order to move across the membrane, ions must pass through special transport proteins that span the cell transmembrane. These transport membrane proteins can be divided into two major categories: ion channels and transporters. Ion channels are proteins that have an aqueous pore that allows specific ions to passively flow from areas of higher concentration to lower concentration. Transporters, however, have two separate gates that open and close sequentially in order to move from one side of the membrane to the other.

Active transporters are a type of transporter that uses energy to preferentially move certain ions from a lower to a higher concentrated environment. Therefore, ion channels and active transporters work antagonistically. This antagonistic relationship is what establishes resting potentials and generates action potential.

Molecules separated by a selectively permeable membrane will naturally move through transport proteins from the side with a higher concentration to a lower concentration or down their chemical gradient. Because ions are charged molecules their movement through ion channels and active transporters also creates an electrical gradient – a difference in the electrical potential across the membrane. Therefore, the movement of ions across the cell membrane generates an electrochemical gradient. In the presence of only ion channels, ions will diffuse across the

membrane to balance both the ion concentration (chemical gradient) and ion charge (electrical gradient) (Figure 4.9). At the electrochemical equilibrium both the chemical gradient and electrical gradient are balanced and there is a net ion flow of zero.

For example, imagine two aqueous chambers separated by a lipid bilayer that has only potassium selective ion channels. If one chamber has 10 mM of KCl and the other 1 mM, K^+ ions will diffuse from the higher concentrated chamber to the lower. However, each K^+ ion also carries a positive charge, causing the more concentrated chamber to become more negative. The electrical gradient will work to prevent the difference in charge between the chambers, thus inhibiting the further flow of K^+ down its concentration gradient. These driving forces will work antagonistically until an electrical potential is met where both the chemical gradient and the electrical gradient are balanced and there is no net flow of K^+ ions. This electrical potential at the electrochemical equilibrium is known as the equilibrium potential and can be calculated using the Nernst equation: E_x is the equilibrium potential for X ion, R and F are physical constants, T is the absolute temperature (kelvins), and z is the valence of the ion. The equilibrium for each ion in the neuron is listed in Equation 4.1 and Table 4.1.

Table 4.1 Equilibrium for each ion in a neuron

Extracellular concentration	Intracellular concentration	Ratio (E:I)	Equilibrium potential (37°C)
$[K^+]_o$	$[K^+]_i$	1:20	−80 mV
$[Cl^-]_o$	$[Cl^-]_i$	11.5:1	−65 mV
$[Na^+]_o$	$[Na^+]_i$	10:1	60 mV
$[Ca^{2+}]_o$	$[Ca^{2+}]_i$	10,000:1	120 mV

$$E_{Ion} = -\frac{RT}{zF} \ln \frac{[ion]_o}{[ion]_i} \qquad (4.1)$$

4.8.2 Calculating Resting Membrane Potential

The Nernst equation is useful for calculating the equilibrium potential for one ion. However, in a neuron there exist multiple ions. The resting membrane potential or the electrical potential in a neuron where there is no net flow of ions is determined by the differential membrane permeabilities of each ion. The neuron is most permeable to K^+ ions but is also simultaneously permeable, albeit less so, to Na^+ and Cl^-. The Goldman–Hodgkin–Katz (GHK) equation (4.2) allows us to calculate the resting membrane potential V_m at equilibrium:

$$V_m = \frac{RT}{F} \ln \left(\frac{p_k[K^+]_o + p_{Na}[Na^+]_o + p_{Cl}[Cl^-]_i}{p_k[K^+]_i + p_{Na}[Na^+]_i + p_{Cl}[Cl^+]_o} \right) \qquad (4.2)$$

where p_k, p_{Na}, and p_{Cl} are the permeabilities for K^+, Na^+, and Cl^-, respectively. This equation is similar to the Nernst equation but allows us to account for multiple ions at once. Each ion's independent contribution to the resting potential is weighed by the membrane's permeability to that ion. Because, at rest, the neuron is most permeable to K^+ ions, the resting membrane potential is largely influenced by K^+ equilibrium potential.

4.8.3 Ohm's Law and Voltage-Gated Ion Channels

There is a dynamic relationship between the membrane potential and ion flow. Electrical circuit models can help us to understand this relationship. In an electrical circuit the electric current that passes through can be represented by Ohm's law: I = V/R, where I represents the current, V represents the voltage, and R represents the resistance. The manipulation of this formula can help us to understand

the relationship between potential and ion current: R is equal to the inverse of g, where g represents ion conductance and is similar to permeability in GHK. Therefore, I = gV; V can also represent the electrochemical driving force acting upon an ion, which is the difference between the membrane potential and the ion's equilibrium potential. Thus, the ionic current can now be represented as:

$$I_{ion} = g_{ion}(V_m - E_{ion}).$$

As will be discussed later, it is the rapid change of g_{Na+} and g_{K+} as a function of membrane potential that underlies the generation of action potentials.

In addition to leak channels and ion pumps, the neuron has voltage-gated ion channels. These channels open and close in response to changes in the membrane voltage. It is the sequential opening and closing of voltage-gated Na^+ and K^+ channels that accounts for the changes in Na^+ and K^+ conductance underlying the production of action potentials.

4.8.4 How Resting Membrane Potential Is Established

The resting membrane potential in neurons is established by two main processes: the passive flow of cations through potassium leak channels and the active transport of ions by sodium–potassium pumps (Figure 4.10).

The negative resting membrane potential is due to the increasing concentration of cations in the neuron's extracellular environment compared to its intracellular environment. In neurons, potassium ions are at higher concentrations inside the cell while sodium ions are at higher concentrations outside of the cell. The cell possesses potassium and sodium leakage ion channels that allow the two cations to passively diffuse down their electrochemical gradient. However, neuronal membranes are more permeable to potassium and thus have far more potassium leakage ion channels than sodium leakage ion channels. Therefore, potassium ions leave the cell at a much faster rate than sodium leaks in. This net flow of cations out of

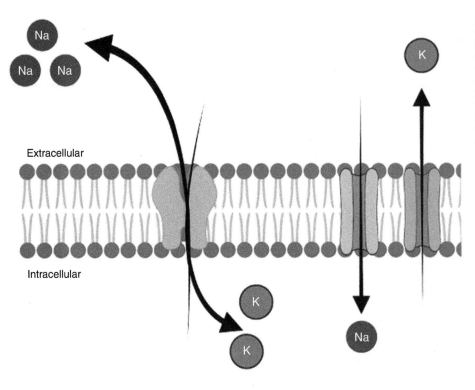

Figure 4.10 Sodium–potassium pump: resting membrane potential is established and maintained by the work of potassium leak channels, which allow the diffusion of K$^+$ ions (positive charge) out of the cell, and Na/K$^+$ pumps, which actively transfer three Na$^+$ ions out and two K$^+$ inside against their concentration gradient for net negative diffusion inside the neuron.

Extracellular

Intracellular

Na$^+$/K$^+$ pump   Na$^+$ channel   K$^+$ channel

the neuron causes the interior of the cell to be negatively charged relative to the outside of the cell, establishing a negative resting membrane potential.

The actions of the sodium–potassium pump are critical in maintaining the resting potential. Sodium–potassium pumps are active transporters that utilize adenosine triphosphate (ATP) to bring two K$^+$ ions into the cell while removing three Na$^+$ ions against their concentration gradient. This is important in maintaining resting potential for two reasons: (1) the movement of two K$^+$ ions into the cell for every three Na$^+$ out creates a net influx of negative charge into the cell, and (2) the movement of Na$^+$ and K$^+$ counteracts the leak of these ions across the membrane and thus maintains their respective intracellular concentrations. Without these pumps a negative resting potential could not be maintained.

4.9 Action Potential

As described earlier, resting membrane potential is the steady state of the neuron, which is regulated by the work of ion leak channels and ion pumps. Without any outside force, the neuron will remain at this negative resting potential. Deviation from this steady state is how the neuron encodes and transmits signals. It is critical for the brain to be able to send signals over long distances extremely quickly in order to react to stimuli promptly.

Action potentials arise from the brief reversal of the resting membrane potential. Action potentials are propagated along the axon and allow for rapid long-range transmission of information. In the action potential there is a cycle of rapid depolarization (Figure 4.11) and rapid hyperpolarization before finally retuning to the resting membrane potential. This cycle is mediated by voltage-gated ion channels and rapid changes in the K$^+$ and Na$^+$ ion current.

4.9.1 Action Potential Steps

The first phase of an action potential is the rising phase, which rapidly depolarizes the neuron (Figure 4.11). Before an action potential occurs, the neuron receives a stimulus that causes local depolarization of the cell. If the stimulus is strong enough and the membrane potential reaches a threshold potential of –55 mV, an action potential will occur. Action potentials are therefore considered "all or nothing" events – an action potential will faithfully occur if the threshold potential is met and will

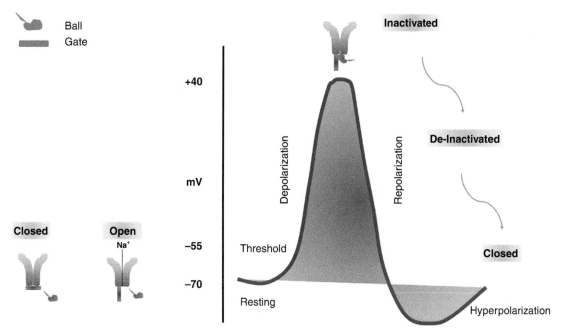

Figure 4.11 A typical action potential.

never occur if it is not. Upon reaching the threshold potential, voltage-gated sodium channels at the axon hillock are opened. Voltage-gated Na^+ channels have two gates: an activation gate and an inactivation gate (ball). Once the voltage-gated Na^+ channel activation gate is open, Na^+ ions rush into the cell and the cell quickly depolarizes as it approaches the equilibrium potential of sodium. This rising phase of action potential is generated by a positive feedback loop. As voltage-gated Na^+ channels open and the neuron is depolarizing, the conductance of Na^+ increases (g_{Na+}), which subsequently leads to the opening up of even more voltage-gated channels and further depolarization. The neuron will continue to depolarize until a membrane potential of approximately +60 mV, at which voltage-gated Na^+ will be inactivated. The inactivation ball will remain closed until the membrane potential returns to the resting potential, allowing depolarization to occur.

As the membrane is depolarizing during the rising phase of action potential, voltage-gated potassium channels also start to open. However, the opening of voltage-gated K^+ channels is delayed. This accounts for the overshoot, or when the neuron is above +0 mV, of the rising phase. Therefore, while g_{Na+} is still increasing, g_{K+} also starts to increase shortly thereafter. The delayed increase of g_{K+} and the subsequent opening of voltage-gated K^+ channels represent a negative feedback loop that works to restore resting potential. At +60 mV when the sodium channels are inactivated g_{Na+} peaks while g_{K+} continues to rise. The voltage-gated K^+ channels finally open, which prompts the repolarization or falling phase of action potential. As K^+ ions quickly flow down their electrochemical gradient out of the cell the membrane potential falls and starts to approach the resting potential. However, the neuron will typically repolarize beyond the resting membrane potential and become even more negative. This is known as hyperpolarization, or the undershoot phase of action potential. This occurs because the voltage-gated K^+ channels are also delayed in closing and cause the g_{K+} to become greater than at rest. The cell will therefore hyperpolarize to approximately –80 mV, approaching E_{K+}. Shortly thereafter, the voltage-gated K^+ channels close and the increased g_{K+} subsides. The resting membrane potential is finally restored, concluding the action potential. All of this takes place within approximately 2 milliseconds.

Action potentials are characterized by refractory periods, or a period of time when it is difficult to generate another action potential. The refractory period is divided into two phases: the absolute refractory period and the relative refractory period. During the absolute refractory period it is impossible to generate another action potential. This is due the inactivation of the voltage-gated Na^+ channels after the rising phase. The inactive conformation of these sodium channels is distinct from its conformation at rest as the channel pore becomes physically obstructed. Without the flow of sodium ions, the cell cannot depolarize and thus cannot generate an action potential. The relative refractory period is when the sodium channels start to leave their inactivated confirmation and revert back to their resting state confirmation. Although the channel's pore is no longer obstructed, the cell is still hyperpolarized during this phase. Therefore, a stronger stimulus than the original one will be needed to initiate action potential. Overall, the refractory period is important because it limits the amount of action potentials a neuron can fire at a given moment while also establishing the unidirectionality of action potentials.

The typical shape of an action potential may vary in different cells. In Purkinje cells, for example, the resulting action potential is composed of complex spikes. These typically have a large-amplitude spike followed by multiple smaller-amplitude spikes, with a total duration longer than a typical action potential, and this is due to the presence of P-type voltage-gated calcium channels, which are much slower to open and close.

4.10 Saltatory Conduction Versus Continuous Conduction

The node of Ranvier contains a high density of sodium channels and is involved in the generation of action potentials at the node, which passes or "jumps" to the next node allowing faster signaling without degradation of the signal. Saltatory conduction is also more energy-efficient as it does not require the Na–ATPase pump to restore normal ion concentrations across the membrane. This is in contrast to continuous conduction in non-myelinated fibers, where an action potential propagates over the surface of the axon. As sodium flows into the cell, nearby regions are depolarized by the opening of sodium channels allowing previously resting areas to reach threshold and depolarize and thereby propagating the action potential along the axon (Figure 4.12).

4.11 Cable Properties

The distance over which local Na$^+$ entry affects the membrane potential and factors that affect attenuation of current can be described by the cable properties of an axon. These

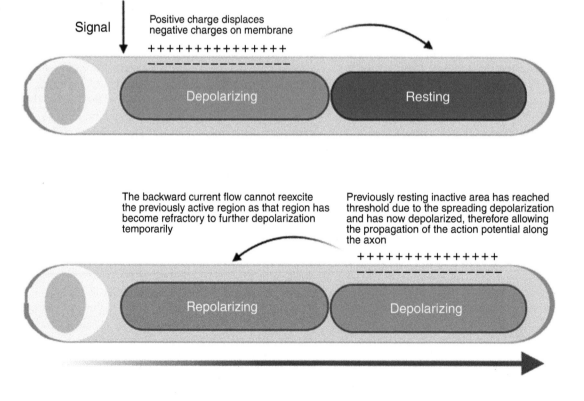

Propagation of action potential

Figure 4.12 Continuous conduction of an action potential in an unmyelinated axon.

factors include axial resistance, membrane resistance, and membrane capacitance. The axial resistance refers to the internal resistance to ionic flow. Axons with greater diameters have lower resistance and therefore a greater opportunity for ions to transmit charge down the axon with less attenuation. Membrane resistance refers to the opposition of ionic flow across the membrane. When more ion channels are open, there is less opposition to ionic flow out of the membrane and therefore greater attenuation of the signal. The membrane capacitance refers to ionic storage capacity. With a larger surface area, there is greater opportunity for the signal to be lost. The lipid membrane increases capacitance and the myelin reduces capacitance.

Figure acknowledgements

The following images were created using a Shutterstock license: Figures 4.1-4.4, 4.7-4.8
The following images were created using a Biorender industrial license: Figures 4.5-4.6
The following images are credited to the authors of this chapter: Figures 4.9-4.12

Further Reading

Daneman R, Prat A. The blood–brain barrier. *Cold Spring Harb Perspect Biol* 2015;7(1):a020412. https://doi.org/10.1101/cshperspect.a020412. PMID: 25561720; PMCID: PMC4292164.

Debanne D, Campanac E, Bialowas A, Carlier E, Alcaraz G. Axon physiology. *Physiol Rev* 2011;**91**(2):555–602. https://doi.org/10.1152/physrev.00048.2009. PMID: 21527732.

Dessalles CA, Babataheri A, Barakat AI. Pericyte mechanics and mechanobiology. *J Cell Sci* 2021;**134**(6):jcs240226. https://doi.org/10.1242/jcs.240226. PMID: 33753399.

Ghosh SK. Camillo Golgi (1843–1926): scientist extraordinaire and pioneer figure of modern neurology. *Anat Cell Biol* 2020;**53**(4):385–92. https://doi.org/10.5115/acb.20.196. PMID: 33012727; PMCID: PMC7769101.

Hartline DK, Colman DR. Rapid conduction and the evolution of giant axons and myelinated fibers. *Curr Biol* 2007;**17**:R29–R35. https://doi.org/10.1016/j.cub.2006.11.042.

Kress GJ, Mennerick S. Action potential initiation and propagation: upstream influences on neurotransmission. *Neuroscience* 2009;**158**(1):211–22. https://doi.org/10.1016/j.neuroscience.2008.03.021.

Major G, Larkman AU, Jonas P, Sakmann B, Jack JJ. Detailed passive cable models of whole-cell recorded CA3 pyramidal neurons in rat hippocampal slices. *J Neurosci* 1994;**14**:4613–38. https://doi.org/10.1523/JNEUROSCI.14-08-04613.1994.

Sofroniew MV, Vinters HV. Astrocytes: biology and pathology. *Acta Neuropathol* 2010;**119**(1):7–35. https://doi.org/10.1007/s00401-009-0619-8.

Wright SH. Generation of resting membrane potential. *Adv Physiol Educ* 2004;**28**(1–4):139–42. https://doi.org/10.1152/advan.00029.2004. PMID: 15545342.

Synaptic Transmission

Katrina Hon, Farhana Akter, and Nigel Emptage

5.1 Introduction

There are in the order of 86 billion neurons within a human brain. Communication between these neurons is achieved at highly specialized junctions called synapses. In this chapter we discuss the basic concepts of synaptic transmission through the two major types of synapses: chemical and electrical synapses.

5.2 Chemical Synapses

A typical chemical synapse is made of two anatomically distinct structures, a presynaptic terminal or bouton and a postsynaptic specialization. The presynaptic terminal is a modified section of axon, held by adhesion molecules in close proximity to the membrane of the postsynaptic target neuron. The two cells do not share cytosolic constituents, but are separated by a physical space, the synaptic cleft (Figure 5.1). The presynaptic terminal contains small, membrane-bound organelles called synaptic vesicles. These contain the *chemical* neurotransmitter. The arrival of an action potential at the presynaptic terminal depolarizes the membrane, which results in the opening of voltage-gated calcium channels (Figure 5.2). Ca^{2+} rapidly diffuses across the membrane into the presynaptic terminal. The rapidity of influx is driven by a steep concentration gradient for Ca^{2+}, where the external Ca^{2+} concentration (approximately 10^{-3} M) is far greater than the internal Ca^{2+} concentration (approximately 10^{-7} M). The influx of Ca^{2+} ions increases the internal Ca^{2+} concentration sufficiently to trigger a Ca^{2+}-dependent fusion process where individual synaptic vesicles become integrated into the presynaptic membrane. This exocytotic process is transient, with the vesicular membrane recovered by a balanced endocytotic process. The significance of vesicular fusion with the plasma membrane is that the vesicle's cargo of neurotransmitter is released into the synaptic cleft. The neurotransmitter is able to diffuse across the synaptic cleft where it binds to protein receptors on the postsynaptic neuron. Activation of these receptors by the neurotransmitter typically results in current flow. The flow of current serves to increase or decrease the probability of an action potential firing in the postsynaptic neuron. Particularly elegant is that different neurotransmitters are able to trigger postsynaptic currents of different type and duration offering considerable opportunity to refine the impact of the neurotransmitter signal on the output of the postsynaptic neuron.

Over 100 types of neurotransmitters have thus far been identified. The first of these was the neurotransmitter *vagusstoff*, or acetylcholine as it is now known. *Vagusstoff* was identified by the German physiologist Otto Loewi (1921), who found that stimulation of the vagus nerve could slow the rate of a frog heart. When the perfusate of a stimulated heart was collected and applied to a second isolated frog heart the beat rate also slowed, leading Loewi to conclude that *vagusstoff* was a chemical agent able to directly act on heart tissue to slow it down. Acetylcholine is now well established as an important neurotransmitter within the autonomic nervous system, as well as the primary neurotransmitter at the neuromuscular junction. Since Loewi's elegant experiment, many different neurotransmitters have been identified and classified. Their variety affords a rich diversity of physiological outcomes. In many instances their complexity of action is enhanced by different neurotransmitters acting together on a single postsynaptic cell.

The precise effect of any neurotransmitter depends upon the type of receptor with which it interacts, and while typically only one neurotransmitter binds to one type of receptor, multiple different classes of receptor can be activated by a single neurotransmitter. Perhaps the best "rule of thumb" remains that provided by Eccles (1976) in his rework of Dale's Principle, where he states that at all of the axonal branches of a neuron there is liberation of the same transmitter substance or substances. This preserves the concept that the identity of the postsynaptic cell is not important in this context while recognizing that on occasion two or more different

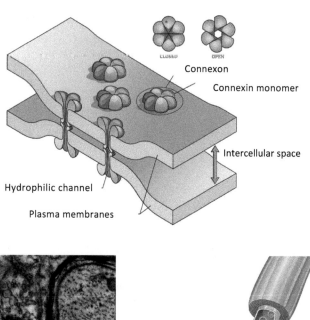

Electrical synapse

Connexon

Connexin monomer

Intercellular space

Hydrophilic channel

Plasma membranes

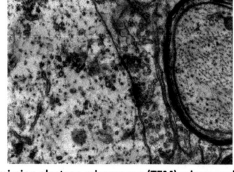

Transmission electron microscope (TEM) micrograph of a chemical synapse

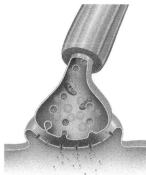

Chemical synapse

Figure 5.1 Transmission electron microscope (TEM) image of a chemical synapse.

neurotransmitters are synthesized and released. This is referred to as co-transmission.

Neurotransmitters can be differentiated into two main types, neuropeptides and small-molecule neurotransmitters. Small-molecule transmitters can be further classified as amino acid transmitters – which are small organic molecules such as glutamate, glycine, and γ-aminobutyric acid (GABA) – and amine transmitters – which include small organic molecules such as acetylcholine, dopamine, and histamine. The neuropeptides are made up of short amino acid chains (3–36 amino acids long), and examples include dynorphin and enkephalin. The vesicular packaging of different transmitters is quite distinct, with small-molecule neurotransmitters packaged into small, clear-core vesicles that are 40–60 nm in diameter located near their site of release, the so-called active zone of the presynaptic terminal. In contrast, neuropeptides are packaged into long, dense-core vesicles that are 90–250 nm in

diameter and are found away from the active zone. In fact, the different storage locations are indicative of the physiological conditions of release of the transmitter, with small-molecule transmitters released with great rapidity and frequency whereas neuropeptide transmitters are released less frequently and typically only after prolonged periods of neural activity.

The location for synthesis of the different transmitters also varies. Small-molecule neurotransmitters are produced within the presynaptic terminal from which they are released, with the enzymes required for their synthesis produced somatically and transported to the terminals where they are localized. Once synthesized, small-molecule neurotransmitters are directly packaged into synaptic vesicles. Packaging the transmitter to a high concentration within a vesicle requires energy. A proton ATPase, located in the membrane of the vesicle, hydrolyzes ATP to generate a proton gradient and in doing so

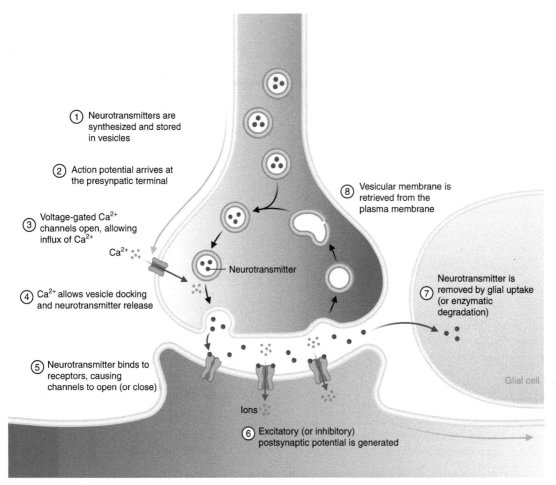

① Neurotransmitters are synthesized and stored in vesicles

② Action potential arrives at the presynpatic terminal

③ Voltage-gated Ca²⁺ channels open, allowing influx of Ca²⁺

Ca²⁺

④ Ca²⁺ allows vesicle docking and neurotransmitter release

Neurotransmitter

⑤ Neurotransmitter binds to receptors, causing channels to open (or close)

Ions

⑥ Excitatory (or inhibitory) postsynaptic potential is generated

⑧ Vesicular membrane is retrieved from the plasma membrane

⑦ Neurotransmitter is removed by glial uptake (or enzymatic degradation)

Glial cell

Figure 5.2 Steps of neurotransmission in a chemical synapse.

reduces the pH of the vesicle lumen to around 5.6. The proton gradient is used to drive transport of the transmitter, with proton–transmitter antiporters mediating the transport of a specific transmitter. Synthesis of neuropeptide transmitters occurs within the cell soma, where they become integrated into the secretory pathways of the neuron. It is here that they are post-translationally modified, often becoming cleaved from a longer precursor protein and then packaged into dense-core vesicles.

Although it is now recognized that the neuromuscular junction (NMJ) is not a "classic" synapse, it has nonetheless proven to be a powerful model system with which to study neurotransmitter release. The NMJ is the site where the lower motor neurons release the neurotransmitter acetylcholine onto skeletal muscle to evoke muscle contraction, what Sherrington called "the final common pathway." The NMJ is large (~30 μm) and achieves extremely reliable transmission, that is, the arrival of an action potential at the axon terminal releases sufficient transmitter to evoke an action potential in the skeletal muscle cell. Bernard Katz, a researcher at University College London, worked with his colleagues throughout the 1950s and 1960s to generate a beautiful set of experiments that transformed our understanding of chemical neurotransmission. The work secured the Nobel Prize in 1970. The approach was to record, with an intracellular microelectrode, the membrane potential of a muscle cell while stimulating the axon innervating the cell. While one component of what they observed was an action potential, the other was a change in membrane potential that preceded the action potential. Careful manipulation of the ionic composition of the extracellular bathing media of the muscle tissue made it possible to have the action potential fail to generate, thereby isolating the potential.

Katz named the potential waveform the end-plate potential (EPP) – after all, it did arise following stimulation of the plate-shaped synaptic terminals upon the muscle cell.

In a subsequent set of experiments Katz and Paul Fatt (1951) found that even in the absence of presynaptic terminal stimulation there were occasionally entirely spontaneous changes in postsynaptic membrane potential. These changes had a waveform similar to the EPPs, except they were much smaller in amplitude (1–2 mV instead of around 50 mV for the EPPs). They were also sensitive to the same pharmacological agents that abolished EPPs, specifically antagonists of acetylcholine receptors. The small, spontaneous events were named miniature end-plate potentials (MEPPs).

Through further analysis, the nature of the relationship between MEPPs and EPPs was clarified. Again, this involved changing the ionic composition of the extracellular bathing medium. By lowering the extracellular Ca^{2+} concentration, muscle contraction can be eliminated and the magnitude of the EPP decreased. In fact, it was observed that as the EPPs became smaller their waveform and size was extremely similar to a single MEPP. Remarkably, the size of EPPs did not change gradually but in a stepwise manner, with the size of each "step" approximately equal to the size of a MEPP. Katz and his colleague Jose del Castillo referred to these steps in potential as *quantal* fluctuations and observed that the amplitude of an EPP could be arithmetically described as the sum of a discrete number of MEPPs. This led to the development of the *quantal* hypothesis, which states that neurotransmitter is released as discrete, quantized packets, the MEPP represents one single packet, and an EPP is the sum of many of these; therefore, the size of an EPP must be an integer of a MEPP. Evidence in support of the hypothesis grew and included the observation that MEPP amplitude declines with distance from the neuromuscular junction, supporting the idea that MEPPs arise at the presynaptic terminal. Miniature end-plate potentials can also be mimicked by puffing acetylcholine at the neuromuscular junction. The quantity required to mimic a MEPP represents about 5,000 molecules of acetylcholine and this is the right order of magnitude to equate with the concentration of acetylcholine found within a single synaptic vesicle.

Following the realization that neurotransmission is quantized, the relationship between vesicles and quanta was explored. Specifically, does the release of the contents of a single vesicle generate the minimal quantal response, i.e., the MEPP? One clue came through the use of electron microscopy, where omega figures, or vesicles in the process of fusing with the plasma membrane, were observed shortly after stimulation of the synapse. The approach was powerfully refined by John Heuser, Tom Reese, and their colleagues during the late 1970s, where they were able to correlate fusion of vesicles with the plasma membrane of the presynaptic cell with quantal responses recorded in the postsynaptic cell. They achieved this by collecting electron micrographic measurements of vesicle fusion alongside electrophysiological measurements of EPPs. By experimentally manipulating the number of quanta released by a single action potential they were able to compare the number of synaptic vesicles fusions with the number of quanta released at the synapse. The correlation was a close one, with single vesicle fusion equating with the generation of a MEPP. These experiments helped support Katz's hypothesis that chemical synaptic transmission was the release of discrete vesicles of transmitter. When vesicles were released concurrently the EPP they produced was sufficient in amplitude to exceed the threshold required for action potential generation.

The importance of Ca^{2+} influx for neurotransmitter release was quickly appreciated by the simple observation that the removal of Ca^{2+} from the extracellular media surrounding the synapse resulted in the abolition of transmitter release. As knowledge of ion channel biology grew, in particular the identification of highly specific channel inhibitors, the presence of voltage-gated Ca^{2+} channels at the presynaptic terminal was robustly confirmed. An analysis of the relationship between vesicular release and Ca^{2+} concentration reveals it not to be linear, with a fourth power relationship reported for the NMJ. Such a relationship helps ensure that even small changes in intracellular Ca^{2+} concentration will lead to vesicle fusion. It is now clear that the role of Ca^{2+} is that of a second messenger, the arrival of an action potential at the terminal depolarizes the membrane and voltage-dependent Ca^{2+} channels open to allow an influx of Ca^{2+}. The influx is rapid, generates a steep rise in the intracellular Ca^{2+} concentration, and triggers extremely rapid vesicular fusion. The rapidity of fusion following Ca^{2+} entry indicates that the Ca^{2+} channels must be located close to synaptic vesicle release sites and that the vesicles must be primed for release at the plasma membrane.

With the concept of vesicle fusion established as the basis of chemical transmission attention turned to understanding the molecular machinery required for the processes to occur. Careful characterization of the proteins decorating synaptic vesicles allowed identification of the proteins with which they were associated in the plasma membrane of the presynaptic terminal. Slowly a picture emerged of proteins with distinct roles including those responsible for corralling vesicles, those responsible for tethering and fusion of vesicles with the plasma membrane, proteins that sensed the Ca^{2+} influx and therefore triggered vesicle fusion, and proteins responsible for the recovery of membrane, the endocytosis step.

While it was clear from electron micrographic data that some vesicles are in close proximity with the plasma membrane, some are not. Ultimately it was established that vesicles are not diffusing at random but were held in distinct regions of the terminal. Some are tethered at the plasma membrane by a SNARE (SNAp REceptors) protein complex and some elsewhere in the terminal within readily releasable and reserve pools. The reserve pool is created by cross-linking vesicles to the cytoskeleton. The linkage is formed by the protein synapsin. Phosphorylation of synapsin by protein kinases, most notably Ca^{2+}/calmodulin-dependent protein kinase type II, allows vesicles to dissociate, permitting movement and ultimately the formation of a SNARE complex. The SNARE complex is a protein bundle comprising synaptobrevin, syntaxin, and SNAP-25. The SNARE proteins syntaxin and SNAP-25 are located within the presynaptic plasma membrane, and synaptobrevin within the synaptic vesicle membrane. The tight association of these proteins secures the vesicle to the plasma membrane. A further vesicle protein, synaptotagmin, is a Ca^{2+} sensor. A rise in cytoplasmic Ca^{2+} concentration produces a conformational change in synaptotagmin that permits it to associate with the SNARE complex. The Ca^{2+}-dependent association is a key step in driving fusion, although the precise way in which fusion occurs is still the subject of some debate (Figure 5.3).

Progress in understanding the role played by the SNARE proteins has been aided by the fact that they are the target of the bacteria *Clostridium botulinum*, the pathogen responsible for botulism. Infection in humans usually occurs as a result of the ingestion of the toxin from eating improperly prepared foods, which results in muscle paralysis and can be fatal. Seven toxin serotypes have been identified, with different serotypes able to selectively cleave synatobrevin, syntaxin, and SNAP-25. Cleavage of any one of these proteins prevents vesicle fusion and thus blocks neurotransmission. Another closely related clostridial toxin, tetanus, also blocks neurotransmission as a result of cleavage of a SNARE protein. While these toxins have proven instructive in the study of neurotransmission, they are also used for a wide variety of medical indications, particularly those associated with muscle disorders, such as post spinal injury spasticity, or muscle clenching conditions. Botulinum toxins are also used for cosmetic purposes (Botox), particularly the reduction of facial wrinkles.

Once vesicle fusion has occurred the vesicular membrane becomes integrated into the plasma membrane of the terminal. One important piece of evidence in support of this comes from the measurement of a change in the capacitance of the plasma membrane of the presynaptic neuron. The change arises as the membrane surface area increases altering the charge storage capacity. The change is all the more interesting as it is extremely transient, suggesting that membrane surface area is reduced almost as soon as it is increased. The process of recovering membrane is known as endocytosis and is mediated by a quite specific set of proteins. Of these, clathrin plays a central role. Adaptor proteins such as AP-2 and AP-180 link clathrin to the plasma membrane. These adaptor proteins, along with amphiphysin, epsin, and Eps-15, help assemble the triskelia that make geodesic domes to form clathrin-coated pits. A GTPase, dynamin, forms a ring-like coil around a lipid stalk that links a coated pit to the plasma membrane, ultimately undergoing a conformational change that pinches off the membrane to separate the coated pit from the plasma membrane. Proteins such as synaptojanin then mediate vesicle uncoating, re-establishing a vesicle for recharging with neurotransmitter and reuse.

Occurring in parallel with the endocytotic process is the recovery of neurotransmitters. The time taken for the transmitter to diffuse across the synaptic cleft is very short, <1 μs, whereas the time taken for the transmitter to diffuse out of the cleft is relatively slow, ~1 ms. Therefore, mechanisms that reduce the duration of neurotransmitter interaction with postsynaptic receptors are in place. When a transmitter is released in large quantities, such as at "fail-safe" synapses like the NMJ, the transmitter action is terminated by enzymatic action. For acetylcholine this is performed by the enzyme acetylcholinesterase, with the breakdown product, choline, recovered back into the presynaptic terminal by a choline transporter. At most synapses transmitters are transported into the presynaptic or postsynaptic cell or into surrounding astrocytes by dedicated membrane transporters. Examples include the excitatory amino acid transporters (EAATs) for glutamate, the serotonin transporters (5HTTs) for serotonin and the dopamine active transporter (DAT) for dopamine.

5.3 Electrical Synapses

Electrical synapses are relatively rare in the mammalian nervous system, at least as compared to their chemical counterparts. Nonetheless, they are widely distributed and

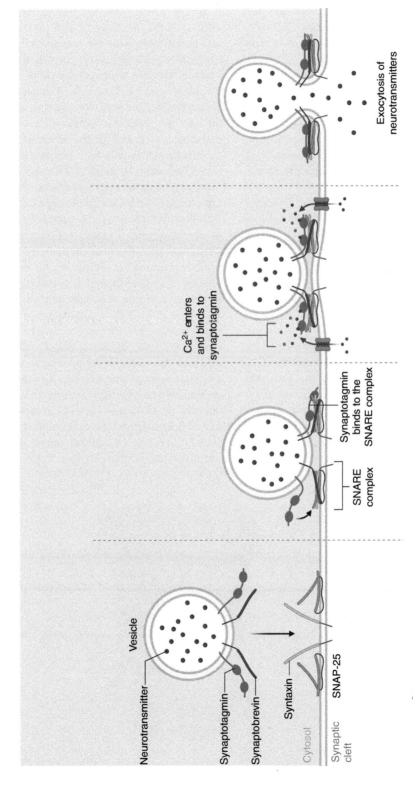

Figure 5.3 Ca²⁺-triggered vesicle fusion and exocytosis of neurotransmitters.

are typically found in circuits where speed, reliability, or synchronization of transmission is of huge importance. Electrical synapses are developmentally regulated and play a role in the early stages of neural development. In adulthood they are found in the brainstem, where they help synchronize breathing; in the thalamus, where they support the genesis of brain waves; and in the medulla oblongata, where they help synchronize action potential discharge during inspiration. They are also found between glial cells.

As their name suggests, electrical synapses function by permitting the direct flow of current from one neuron to another and this facilitates the initiation or inhibition of action potentials. The transmission rate is extremely rapid (<1 ms).

The current is generated by the potential difference that arises due to a presynaptic action potential(s). Current flows from one neuron to another at intercellular specializations called gap junctions. Gap junctions are formed by a group of proteins that align to form a conduit between the two communicating neurons. The pathway is partially selective, the pore diameter determines the limit of flow, which typically means that ions and small molecules may pass. The protein group comprises of connexons (Figure 5.4), specialized membrane channels that connect the two cells at a gap junction.

Connexons are key to understanding the way that electrical synapses work. Connexons are made up of six subunits called connexins, a unique family of ion channel proteins that form connexon channels. Connexins are expressed in many different cell types and their different isoforms have been shown to yield a diverse range of physiological properties. They each have four transmembrane domains, and so far there have been 21 human connexin genes identified (GJA–GJE). The six connexin subunits form the hemi-channel present in both the pre- and postsynaptic neurons, and when aligned form a pore connecting both cells. The pore of the channel exceeds 1 nm in diameter, which is large when compared to a typical voltage-gated ion channel. In consequence, ions, as well as molecules of up to 700 daltons, are able to diffuse through the pore. Such molecules include intracellular metabolites such as ATP as well as second messengers.

Electrical synapses have features that are different to their chemical counterparts. The minimal delay in transmission, due to the absence of vesicle fusion, ensures that information can be passed between cells with great rapidity. Electrical synapses can permit bidirectional current flow, aiding synchronization of electrical activity among a population of neurons, although it is worth noting that some connexons are rectifying and in these cases transmission is unidirectional. This can be important in networks of neurons that generate patterned, oscillatory activity such as central pattern generators. The capacity to permit the passage of second messengers serves in the synchronization of intracellular pathways. Electrical synapses are also able to pass hyperpolarizing current. They are energy efficient, as they do not have ATP-dependent transmission machinery, and are relatively fail-safe. At first sight electrical synapses appear to offer a great deal; however, they are unable to change the "sign" of the current flow from one cell to another and do not support synaptic plasticity (see Section 5.7).

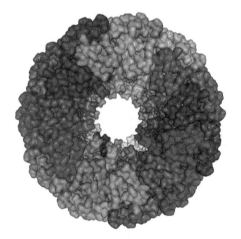
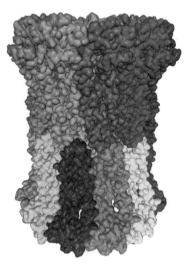

Figure 5.4 Connexon proteins.

5.4 The Postsynaptic Response

As discussed, the neurotransmitter acetylcholine generates an EPP when it is released onto skeletal muscle, but the type of response that a neurotransmitter generates is far more diverse when examined in different cell types. While all neurotransmitters trigger their action by binding to protein receptors, the outcomes vary greatly as the receptors to which they bind can be quite different. Four broad classes of receptor classes have been identified, although it should be noted that each class contains multiple subdivisions. The first are ionotropic receptors (Figure 5.5). These are ligand-gated ion channels that rapidly respond to neurotransmitter binding (<1–5 ms). For this group binding of the ligand induces a conformational change that causes an ion channel, integral to the receptor's structure, to open or close. This changes the permeability of the membrane and most often results in a flow of ions that alters the membrane potential. These receptors are typically formed from two protein domains, an extracellular domain that includes the binding site(s) for the transmitter and a transmembrane domain that forms a channel permissive of ion flux. The second class of receptors are metabotropic receptors, or G-protein-coupled receptors (GPCRs). These receptors have a slower rate of action than ionotropic receptors (many milliseconds to seconds) that involve multiple steps. When a neurotransmitter binds to the GPCR this triggers the dissociation of the G_α subunit from the receptor, which can activate different signaling cascades or second messenger pathways. The ultimate targets of these pathways are diverse and include ion channels, enzymes, and transporter proteins. GPCRs are a large family of integral membrane proteins receptors characterized by a common structure: seven membrane-spanning α-helices that act to regulate intracellular reactions indirectly via the use of second messenger intermediates Their key transducing element is a GTP-binding protein (or G-protein).

The third group of receptors are the enzyme-linked receptors; these too have an extracellular binding site for a chemical ligand, but their intracellular domain is an enzyme that becomes activated when the ligand is bound to the extracellular domain. The intracellular or catalytic domain is activated by a conformational change that arises from ligand binding. These receptors have a membrane-spanning domain that anchors them within the cell membrane. Activity associated with these receptors frequently initiates second messenger cascades. Most common within this group are the protein kinases that phosphorylate intracellular proteins in the target cell. Notable protein kinases include tyrosine kinases, the Trk family of neurotrophin receptors, and growth factors. The fourth group of receptors are the intracellular receptors. These are activated by cell-permeant, lipophilic signaling molecules that pass through the plasma membrane. Signaling molecules frequently bind to a target in or around the cell nucleus where the binding triggers a change in transcription. One common mechanism is where the receptor is linked to an inhibitory protein complex that dissociates when the receptor is bound, which exposes a DNA-binding domain that is able to interact with nuclear DNA, thereby altering cell transcription. Thus, together these four classes of receptor can mediate a vast range of postsynaptic responses that is made even more diverse as a single type of neurotransmitter can activate more than one class of receptor.

Understanding the basis of the electrical events generated in the postsynaptic cell can be achieved in a number of ways. If we again take the NMJ as an example, when the post-junctional membrane potential is hyperpolarized relative to the resting potential the amplitude of the EPP becomes larger, whereas if the membrane potential is depolarized relative to the resting potential, the EPP becomes smaller. Under conditions where voltage-gated Na^+ channels are inactivated or pharmacologically blocked (to prevent action potential generation) it is possible to see that at approximately 0 mV, no EPP is detected, and that further depolarization reverses the potential. The potential where the EPP reverses is known as the reversal potential. At the reversal potential the net flow of ions through the receptor channel is zero. By knowing the value of E_{rev} it is also possible to calculate the ion conductance activated by acetylcholine release at the neuromuscular junction (g_{ACh}). See the following equation, where EPC is the end-plate current:

$$EPC = g_{ACh}(V_m - E_{rev}).$$

What the equation makes very clear is that the polarity and magnitude of the EPC are dependent on the electrochemical driving force acting upon the ions that pass through the receptor channel. Postsynaptic potentials (PSPs) can be either excitatory or inhibitory depending on the direction and charge of ion movement. If the reversal potential of the PSP is more positive than the reversal potential, then the PSP is depolarizing, bringing the membrane potential closer to the threshold for action potential firing. If the reversal potential is more negative than the resting membrane potential, then the PSP is

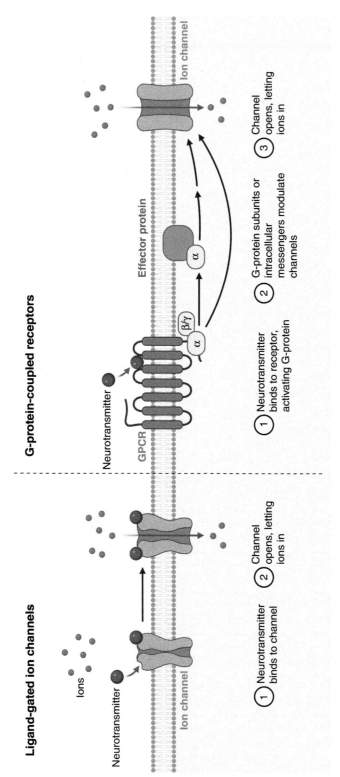

Figure 5.5 Ligand-gated ion channels and G-protein coupled receptors.

hyperpolarizing, bringing the membrane potential away from threshold. Thus, the type of channel coupled to the receptor activated by the neurotransmitter, as well as the concentration of ions inside and outside the cell, determine whether a postsynaptic response is excitatory or inhibitory.

5.4.1 Excitatory Postsynaptic Potentials

Excitatory postsynaptic potentials (EPSPs) increase the likelihood that an action potential will occur; that is, they move the membrane potential closer to threshold. Excitatory ligand-gated ion channels are most commonly found in the NMJ and the central nervous system (CNS). We have seen that acetylcholine is a key excitatory transmitter in the peripheral nervous system; however, within the CNS most excitatory transmission is mediated by the amino acid transmitter glutamate. Fast transmission occurs when glutamate binds to one of three classes of ionotropic receptors, each with unique pharmacology and functional characteristics. The names of these receptors are derived from the specific agonists that activate them: α-amino-3-hydroxy-5-methyl-4-isoxazole propionic acid or AMPA receptors, *N*-methyl-D-aspartate or NMDA receptors and kainate receptors activated by kainic acid. Glutamate also acts upon metabotropic receptors, of which at least eight types have been identified. The functional action of the metabotropic receptors is determined by the second messenger cascade to which they are linked. It is worth noting that rarely, if ever, do all of the different types of glutamate receptor coexist at a single synapse; instead, different combinations are expressed at synapses at different sites within the CNS generating unique properties at these synapses.

5.4.2 Inhibitory Postsynaptic Potentials

Inhibitory postsynaptic potentials (IPSPs) decrease the likelihood that an action potential will occur; that is, they move the membrane potential away from the firing threshold or increase the permeability of the cell membrane such that a larger depolarizing current is required for the neuron to reach threshold. Two neurotransmitters are responsible for the majority of inhibition in the CNS – these are the amino acids γ-aminobutyric acid (GABA) and glycine. GABA is found widely across the CNS including within the cortex, midbrain and cerebellum. GABA binds to three classes of receptor $GABA_A$, $GABA_B$, and $GABA_C$. $GABA_A$ receptors are ligand-gated chloride channels. Activation of $GABA_A$ receptors moves the resting membrane potential toward E_{Cl}. As these channels are permeable almost exclusively to Cl^- ions $E_{rev} = E_{Cl}$. $GABA_B$ receptors are metabotropic; that is, they are G-protein coupled and link to K^+ channels and Ca^{2+} channels. $GABA_C$ receptors are also ligand gated Cl^- channels; they are found primarily in the retina and have pharmacology that is quite distinct from $GABA_A$ receptors. Glycine receptors are also ligand-gated Cl^- channels and are typically found in the spinal cord, brainstem, and retina.

Investigation of the mechanisms that give rise to a postsynaptic response was transformed with the development of the patch-clamp technique. This method has been used to study changes in postsynaptic membrane permeability including those that arise following neurotransmitter release (Figure 5.6). The approach proved so powerful that in 1976 Erwin Neher and Bert Sakmann received the Nobel Prize for their contribution to its development and implementation. Perhaps unsurprisingly, one of first neurotransmitters to be studied was acetylcholine, revealing that it opens ligand-gated ion channels. One of the more remarkable aspects of the work was the discovery that channels are opened or closed, and that when open they have a unitary conductance that is specific to that channel. Channels flicker open and closed in a stochastic manner, even in the absence of neurotransmitter, with binding of neurotransmitter increasing the probability that they open. Although any one ligand-gated ion channel will produce only a small stepwise increase in conductance, the bolus of neurotransmitter released by vesicle fusion will ensure that many channels open in near unison to generate a macroscopic current such as an EPP. It is also relatively straightforward to use the patch-clamp technique to identify which ion species pass through the channel.

5.5 Synaptic Integration

The process of synaptic transmission at single synapses is now well described; however, central neurons receive not one but hundreds and often thousands of individual synaptic inputs. These are most typically a mixture of both excitatory and inhibitory inputs. It is in fact quite rare for one input to exert great influence upon the target neuron's output; instead, the genesis of an action potential usually arises from the combined action of synaptic inputs with a balance being struck between the influence of excitatory and inhibitory inputs. Thus, the role of a neuron goes considerably beyond simply producing an action potential(s) and releasing neurotransmitters, but includes the integration of synaptic input information to produce a response that appropriately reflects the input

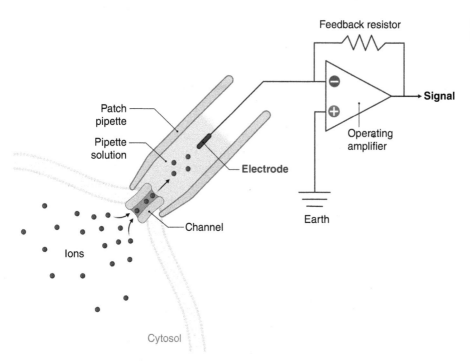

Figure 5.6 Patch-clamp recording principle.

that they receive. In essence, synaptic integration is a complex decision-making process that determines whether a neuron generates no output, a single action potential, or multiple action potentials. In order for an action potential to occur in the target neuron the synaptic inputs must achieve a threshold level of depolarization within the initial segment of the axon, also known as the axon hillock or the trigger zone. As synapses occur at different locations on the neuronal dendritic tree, the electrical events that they generate must propagate through the neuron to the axon hillock, and because of the different synaptic locations this has the predictable impact of creating time delays between inputs and varying levels of signal attenuation. The interplay of how inputs sum together to influence the generation of an action potential lies at the heart of synaptic integration.

As a starting point it is not unreasonable to assume that the larger the excitatory synaptic input, either by virtue of the number of inputs, or the strength of each input, the more likely an output will be generated in the postsynaptic neuron. However, there is a considerable degree of subtlety. As mentioned previously, neurons receive both inhibitory and excitatory synaptic inputs, each showing anatomical specializations that contribute

to their role. While excitatory synapses occur on dendritic shafts and in large numbers on dendritic spines, inhibitory synapses have rich variation, occurring on dendritic shafts, the neuronal soma, the axon initial segment, and upon presynaptic terminals. Dendritic spines appear to be a hallmark of excitatory synapses. Indeed, the functional significance of the structure is a source of much interest, with suggestions that include both electrical and biochemical compartmentalization. The action potential initiation site, the axon initial segment, expresses the highest density of voltage-gated Na^+ channels within the neuron and in consequence has the lowest threshold for action potential generation. Other factors also contribute to a low threshold for action potential initiation that include low membrane capacitance and channel activation characteristics that open the Na^+ channels at potentials more hyperpolarized than those in the soma. While action potentials are most commonly generated at the initial segment of the axon, regenerative events, so-called dendritic spikes, can occur in dendrites under certain conditions. Simultaneous somatic and dendritic patch-pipette recordings have revealed dendritic spikes in the absence of or before "classic" somatic action potentials. Dendritic spikes appear to occur following strong synaptic excitation and are

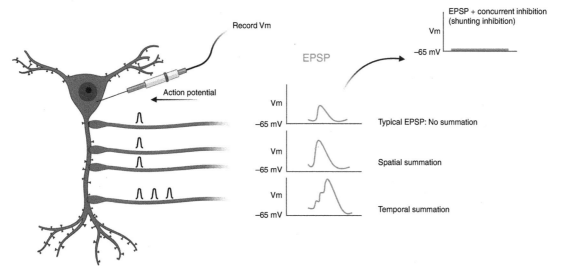

Figure 5.7 EPSP summation.

underpinned by the activation of Na$^+$ channels, Ca^{2+} channels, and NMDA receptors. As there is a large variability in the contribution of each channel class, dendritic spikes vary greatly in shape and duration. However, a dendritic spike is no guarantee that a somatic action potential will be elicited and so once more a complex relationship exists between activity and the final output of neuron – the production of action potential(s).

There are a variety of factors that determine the effectiveness of a synapse in generating an action potential. First, the location of the synaptic input. If we assume that the potential generated by a synapse at any location on the dendritic tree is constant (in reality this is unlikely to be true) the farther the input from the initial segment, or trigger zone, the smaller its impact. This arises due to the "leaky" properties of dendrites, as they have low membrane resistance, high capacitance, and large axial resistance, all of which contribute to the attenuation of signal in amplitude with distance. Signal attenuation is referred to as the length constant (lambda) and is the distance that the signal propagates before it has decreased to approximately 37% of its original amplitude. Membrane resistance reflects the ability of ions to flow across the cell membrane, i.e., the membrane permeability. A reduction in the number of channels in a membrane increases membrane resistance and will reduce signal attenuation – that is, increase the length constant. Membrane capacitance is the ability of a membrane to store electrical charge. The more the membrane stores electrical charge, the more rapidly the signal attenuates. Lastly, axial resistance is the internal

membrane resistance to the flow of charge. The larger the diameter, the lower the axial resistance; therefore, neurons with lower axial resistance will have a longer length constant. The high axial resistance and low membrane resistance of dendrites has a profound impact on the attenuation of synaptic potentials as they pass through them. A second important consideration is that synaptic potentials can sum together (Figure 5.7). Several EPSPs arising at a single synaptic location in response to a burst of presynaptic activity is referred to as temporal summation. During temporal summation the EPSPs do not always add up to the arithmetic sum of the individual potentials, the result is non-linear. Non-linear summation occurs because as the membrane potential becomes more positive, the driving force on the Na$^+$ influx decreases; therefore, each additional input will have a smaller effect on the overall amplitude of the final potential. Synaptic potentials that arise at different locations are also able to sum together, which is referred to as spatial summation. Next we need to consider the contribution of inhibitory inputs. An inhibitory synaptic input arising between an excitatory synaptic input and the axon initial segment can moderate or even completely suppress the level of excitatory depolarization. An inhibitory synapse can shunt the excitatory signal. Finally, inhibitory inputs can change the shape of excitatory signals, changing the degree of temporal summation. Inhibition that is near concurrent with excitation will decrease the membrane resistance, accelerating the repolarization of the EPSP, making it far less likely that summation will occur.

5.6 Synaptic Modulation

A process that modulates the frequency or amplitude of synaptic transmission is referred to as synaptic modulation. Modulatory changes may be transient or longer-lasting and can be produced in ways that are physiological, pharmacological, or pathological. The mechanisms that produce these changes are diverse and range from transient changes in the intracellular ion concentration through to covalent modifications. The distinction between the different forms of presynaptic modulation rests on their time constant of decay, with facilitation and depression decaying rapidly, augmentation over seconds, and short-term potentiation over minutes.

Paired-pulse facilitation of synaptic transmission can be observed when two action potentials arrive at the synaptic bouton in close temporal proximity (within a few tens of milliseconds) The EPSPs generated are not of equal magnitude, but the second of the pair is larger or facilitated. The change in synaptic strength arises due to a change that occurs presynaptically, increasing the number of vesicles released. The increase is thought to occur as a function of "residual calcium," an idea that suggests the concentration of intracellular Ca^{2+} available to trigger vesicle fusion is greater for a second event because the clearance of Ca^{2+} from within the bouton is not fully complete following the influx of Ca^{2+} that occurred during the first action potential. A second short-term form of synaptic modulation is short-term depression. This refers to a decrease in the size of EPSPs following repetitive stimulation. Like paired-pulse facilitation this feature of the synapse also arises presynaptically, in this case a result of a decrease in the availability of readily releasable vesicles at the terminal membrane.

Other forms of presynaptic plasticity include augmentation and short-term potentiation and, these too are linked to the intracellular Ca^{2+} concentration within the bouton impacting upon vesicle fusion. Both forms of modulation are elicited by short bursts of action potentials in the presynaptic neuron. While the exact mechanisms responsible for these types of plasticity are not well understood, it has been proposed that augmentation results from Ca^{2+} enhancing the actions of presynaptic SNARE-regulatory proteins, specifically munc-13, whereas short-term potentiation has been linked to Ca^{2+} activation of presynaptic protein kinases that phosphorylate substrates such as synapsin, and in doing so changing the availability of vesicles for release.

Modulation can also occur at synapses as a result of changes that occur postsynaptically. Two of the most common are receptor saturation and receptor desensitization. Both reduce the size of synaptic events following activity. These changes also have different decay time constants, with saturation impacting transmission during the initial activity and desensitization lasting seconds to near permanence as the transmitter loses functional access to receptors.

5.7 Synaptic Plasticity

Synaptic plasticity is the process by which patterns of neural activity, action potential firing, bring about long-lasting changes in the transmission performance of the synapse. Changes can be days, weeks, and even years, and in consequence are thought likely to be the substrate for the storage of memory. Perhaps unsurprisingly, a change that has the capacity to be of such a long duration is supported by protein synthesis and the upregulation of gene expression. Remarkably, and to the great surprise of many, it appears that there are no unique plasticity proteins or genes; the process instead relies upon using the same synaptic components as in basal transmission but to a greater or lesser degree. From an evolutionary standpoint it is difficult not to be in awe of such an elegant solution.

5.7.1 Habituation and Sensitization

Pioneering experiments performed by Eric Kandel and colleagues in the marine mollusk *Aplysia* paved the way in the study of how synaptic alterations can represent a memory as evidenced by a change in the animal's behavior. Habituation is a form of non-associative conditioning that arises when repeated stimulation manifests as a decrease in the behavioral response to the stimulus. Habituation is seen widely across many animal phyla, and is much in evidence in our everyday lives. One form of habituation in *Aplysia* is seen as a decrease in its gill retraction reflex following a repeated gentle touch to the gill. The withdrawal is a protective response that the animal displays quite naturally. Habituation has been shown to occur as a direct consequence of a decrease in the synaptic response at the glutamatergic synapses between the sensory and motor neurons of the gill. Successive stimuli generate a smaller EPSP between the sensory neuron, which detects the touch, and the gill muscle motor neuron that produces the withdrawal. The magnitude of EPSP reduction directly correlates with the decrease in the extent of gill withdrawal. Quantal analysis at this synapse has revealed that the decrease in EPSP size is a consequence of a change that occurs presynaptically, specifically a decrease in the amount of transmitter released. A second form of non-associative conditioning, sensitization, is also seen for the gill withdrawal reflex of *Aplysia*. Sensitization occurs when the animal encounters a noxious stimulus, this enhances the magnitude of withdrawal. The synaptic mechanism of sensitization is an increase in the size of the EPSP between the sensory and motor neuron, thereby enhancing the magnitude of withdrawal. The mechanism has been shown to be a heterosynaptic one, a process where the sensory neurons detecting the noxious stimulus activate interneurons which release serotonin (5HT) onto the presynaptic terminals of sensory neurons mediating the gill withdrawal. Serotonin enhances transmitter release by activating a GPCR-mediated pathway. GPCR activation of the enzyme protein kinase A (PKA) results in the phosphorylation of a serotonin-sensitive K^+ channel in the gill sensory neuron. Phosphorylation of the channel increases the duration of the presynaptic action potential, allowing a longer period for the opening of more presynaptic Ca^{2+} channels. This enhances the influx of Ca^{2+} and leads to an increase in the amount of transmitter released, hence facilitating the size of the EPSP.

5.7.2 Long-Term Potentiation

The identification of an activity-induced long-lasting change in synaptic transmission within the mammalian CNS came a few years after the initial work in *Aplysia* with the publication of details of long-term potentiation (LTP) by Tim Bliss and Terje Lomo. Long-term potentiation was initially studied in the hippocampus, an area of the brain known to be important in the formation of episodic memories. In subsequent years LTP has been detected at excitatory synapses across many brain areas including different areas of the neocortex, the amygdala, cerebellum, and nucleus accumbens, to name but a few. In part, the ubiquity of LTP across brain areas has helped underscore its prominence as a likely mechanism for the storage of memory in the mammalian brain.

Mechanistic studies of LTP initially focused upon excitatory synaptic connections between the Schaffer collaterals axons of CA3 pyramidal neurons and their monosynaptic target, the CA1 pyramidal neurons of the hippocampus. Here it was shown that brief, high-frequency bursts of activity in the Schaffer collateral axons led to a long-lasting increase in the EPSP amplitude between these cells. The long-lasting nature of the change is not to be understated and can last days, weeks, and even years. Unsurprisingly, the duration of LTP expression

adds further to its suitability as the neural substrate of information storage in the mammalian brain.

As the mechanistic properties of LTP were slowly revealed these too appeared to highlight the suitability of LTP for information storage. One of these is the discovery that LTP requires coincident activity in both presynaptic and postsynaptic neurons. The need for coincident presynaptic and postsynaptic activity was judged particularly significant as Donald Hebb (1949) had reported a theory where he proposed that coordinated activity between a presynaptic and a postsynaptic neuron may be required for strengthening of synaptic connections. There are a number of reasons why this may be desirable in a network of neurons, but one very intuitive one is that such a mechanism affords input specificity. Said another way, the requirement for coincident pre–post activity makes it straightforward to see how it is possible to express LTP at one synapse and yet not be a neighbor on the same dendrite. This important feature of LTP affords neurons the potential of huge information storage capacity as critical data content rests at the synapse, not the cell. Of course, this is not the same as saying that each synapse stores a complete memory, but more akin to the saying that each synapse is like a transistor on a computer chip, with many contributing to form the final output.

Careful investigation of the properties of the principal glutamate receptors at Schaffer collateral-CA1 synapses has revealed a great deal about the underlying mechanisms of LTP. One of the more remarkable observations is the relatively modest extent to which NMDA receptors contribute to basal synaptic transmission. The role of the NMDA receptor is most evident during LTP induction, where it serves as a molecular coincidence detector, requiring both membrane depolarization and glutamate binding in order to activate the receptor. The dependence on these two factors for NMDA receptor activation neatly explains why both presynaptic (glutamate release) and postsynaptic (membrane depolarization) activity are required for LTP induction. The mechanism of NMDA receptor activation on membrane depolarization is elegantly explained by the fact that magnesium (Mg2+) ions restrict the flow of other ions species through the receptor channel at the resting membrane potential. When a neuron is depolarized Mg^{2+} ions become displaced. It is the displacement of Mg^{2+} ions that permits the flow of other ions species through the receptor channel. Of these ions Ca^{2+} is of huge importance, as a second messenger it sets into motion a complex series of events that generate relatively short-term, minutes to hours, covalent modifications, as well as long-term changes that are dependent upon both transcription and translation. The significance of these steps is to generate changes at the synapse that support enhanced synaptic transmission and in consequence a larger EPSP. The ways that this is achieved varies but two common motifs are in evidence; one is a change in AMPA receptor function, the other a change in transmitter release. As AMPA receptors mediate basal transmission any change in their performance will result in a change in transmission performance. Many types of AMPA receptor change have been observed and vary from alterations in the conductance of single receptors through to changing the total number of receptors at the synapse. In some instances AMPA receptors are added to synapses that had previously had only NMDA receptors, this is referred to as the unmasking of "silent synapses." Changes in transmitter release typically take the form of an enhancement in the probability of release. It is not unreasonable to ask why LTP mechanisms have both pre- and postsynaptic variants and why these also take different forms. In truth, the full answer has yet to be revealed, but it is already clear that the patterns of neural activity that induce the different forms of expression are themselves different and so it is reasonable to imagine that ultimately these variations underpin different operational/computational tasks within the network.

5.7.3 Long-Term Depression

Long-term depression (LTD) describes the process through which patterned neural activity, albeit a different pattern to those required to induce LTP, leads to long-lasting decreases in synaptic strength. In many respects the process looks to be the opposite of LTP, weakening synapses, and so it is tempting to imagine that it may equate to memory loss or forgetting. In fact this is unlikely to be the case, not least as experiments where LTD is compromised have been shown to also compromise memory. LTD may represent a different memory mechanism altogether or, as seems perhaps more likely, may work alongside LTP to sculpt the performance of a population of synapses that functional collectively in the formation of the memory.

LTD has also been studied extensively in the hippocampus, and it was found to occur when the Schaffer collaterals are stimulated at a low frequency (1 Hz) for sustained periods of time (10–15 minutes). This leads to a lasting depression of the EPSP, which, like LTP, is input-specific. Just as there are different forms of LTP, there are also different forms of LTD; however, one extensively studied variant is closely related to LTP in that it requires the activation of NMDA receptors and an influx of Ca^{2+} into the postsynaptic cell. The determinant as to whether LTD or LTP is generated is that LTD requires a low concentration of intracellular Ca^{2+} presented over a prolonged period, whereas LTP requires a rise that is large and rapid. The explanation for these differences hinges upon the sensitivity to Ca^{2+} of different enzymatic pathways, the details of which lie beyond the scope of this discussion. Ultimately, at these synapses, the expression of LTD is the converse of LTP, with AMPA receptors either modified or internalized from the postsynaptic membrane or the probability of transmitter release being reduced.

LTD has also been studied in considerable detail in the cerebellum, where a reduction in strength of the excitatory inputs of the parallel fibers onto Purkinje neurons is seen. As in the hippocampus LTD appears to be critical for the formation of memory, in this case the establishment of new motor memories. The mechanism, although not the same as that in hippocampus, does share some similarities. Of these, one is particularly striking: plasticity, as these synapses, although NMDA receptor-independent, do require coincidence detection. Two classes of neuron, climbing fibers and parallel fibers, each fire in close temporal coincidence to trigger the activation of intracellular pathways within the Purkinje neuron. These biochemical pathways ultimately exert their effect by weakening the synapse, LTD, by the internalization of AMPA receptors.

Figure acknowledgements

The following images were created using a Shutterstock license: Figure 5.1, 5.4
The following images were created using a Biorender industrial license: Figures 5.2-5.3, 5.5-5.7

Further Reading

Anderson P, Morris R, Amaral, D, Bliss T, O'Keefe J. *The Hippocampus*. Oxford University Press, 2006.

Cowan M, Cowan WM, Sudhof T. *Synapses*. Johns Hopkins University Press, 2000.

Mtui E, Gruener G, Dockery P. *Fitzgerald's Clinical Neuroanatomy and Neuroscience*. Elsevier, 2015.

Sensory Pathways

Chapter 6

Rachel Chau, Megan Chau, and Farhana Akter

6.1 The Visual System

Our visual system is critical to accessing information and communicating with others. The visual pathway begins with a photon of light traveling through the pupil of the eye to the retinal photoreceptors to induce a signaling cascade responsible for transmitting electrical information to the brain.

Light energy is a form of electromagnetic radiation and exhibits wave-like properties (Figure 6.1). Light waves can be described in terms of their amplitude and this is associated with the intensity of the wave. The distance between two waves is known as the wavelength. The number of wavelengths that pass by a given time point every second is known as the wave frequency (Hertz) One hertz equals 1 wave passing a fixed point in 1 second.

The wave–particle duality theory tells us that a photon of light acts both as an oscillatory wave and a discrete particle. Moreover, the energy in a photon of light varies depending on its frequency, and the higher a photon's frequency, the lower its wavelength, and this can be detected by the retinal cells. When photons between 400 and 780 nm in wavelength enter the eye, they interact with the pigment molecules and induce conformational changes leading to stimulation of intracellular cascades and eventually transmitting electrical signals to the brain. The relationship between energy (E) and wavelength (λ) is best described using Planck's Formula, $E = hc/\lambda$, where energy is transferred in the form of quanta assigned as h, which has a Planck's constant of 6.626×10^{-34} Joule - sec (J/s); c is the velocity of light.

6.2 Anatomy of the Eye

6.2.1 Bony Orbit

The eye sockets are bony orbits that enclose the eyeball. The orbit is formed by seven bones (Chapter 1). Several vessels and nerves enter and leave the orbit through the optic canal (optic nerve, ophthalmic artery), superior orbital fissure (lacrimal, frontal, trochlear, oculomotor, nasociliary and abducens nerves, superior ophthalmic vein), and the

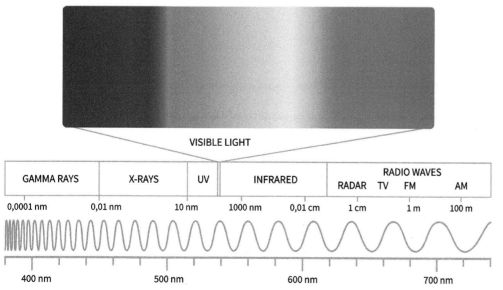

Figure 6.1 The electromagnetic spectrum.

inferior orbital fissure (zygomatic branch of the maxillary nerve, the inferior ophthalmic vein, and sympathetic nerves). Other openings include the nasolacrimal canal (passage for nasolacrimal duct), supraorbital foramen (transmits the supraorbital nerve, artery and vein), and infraorbital canal (transmits the infraorbital nerve and vessels). Orbital fractures usually affect the orbital rim consisting of the maxilla, zygomatic, and frontal bones. Blowout fractures lead to herniation of the orbital contents through one of its walls. The medial and inferior walls are the weakest, with the contents herniating into the ethmoid and maxillary sinuses, respectively. Orbital fractures usually increase intraorbital pressure, causing exophthalmos (protrusion of the eye).

6.2.2 Internal Structure of the Eye

The eyeball is housed in the orbit and is enveloped by a fascial sheath called the Tenon's capsule, which is an attachment site for the extraocular muscles and their tendons. It consists of three layers: the outer fibrous sclera, the vascular choroid and the inner retinal layer, which passes information to the brain via the optic nerve for processing in the cerebral cortex to become visual information (Figure 6.2).

The outer sclera consists of tough white connective tissue and connects external muscles that move the eyeballs within their sockets. The sclera contains three layers: the outer episclera, the middle scleral stroma, and the inner lamina fusca. The episclera is connected to the Tenon's capsule and contains an arterial episcleral plexus formed by the branches of the anterior ciliary arteries.

The scleral stroma is composed of irregular connective tissue and gives the sclera a white color. The lamina fusca contains a large number of melanocytes and overlies the choroid. The sclera is perforated by the optic nerve posteriorly at the posterior scleral foramen. This region is covered by the lamina cribrosa, a mesh-like structure that surrounds the retinal ganglion cells (RGCs) as they form the optic nerve and through which the central retinal artery and central retinal vein pass. The sclera also contains apertures to transmit the anterior ciliary arteries, vortex veins, ciliary vessels, and nerves.

The anterior margin of the sclera is continuous with the transparent avascular cornea, involved in light refraction. It consists of five primary layers: outer stratified corneal epithelium, Bowman's layer consisting of irregular collagen fibers, substantia propria containing parallel collagen fibers, Descemet's basement membrane, and the corneal endothelium.

The other structures involved in refraction of light include the lens, vitreous body, and aqueous humor. The lens is found anterior to the vitreous body and posterior to the iris. It consists of the capsule, epithelium, and lens fibers. The lens is held in place by the zonular ligamentous fibers (suspensory ligament of lens) and helps change the shape of the lens during accommodation. The aqueous humor is a clear fluid located in the anterior chamber produced by ciliary processes in the posterior chamber. This is the space between the lens and the retina and houses vitreous humor, which contains mostly phagocytes that remove unwanted debris. Fluid production and drainage must be constant to ensure adequate blood

Figure 6.2 Anatomy of the eye.

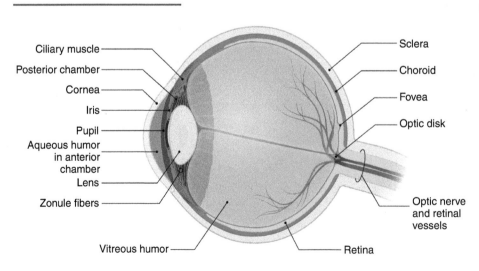

supply to the retinal neurons and maintenance of a constant intraocular pressure.

The middle vascular layer consists of the choroid, the ciliary body, and the iris, collectively known as the uveal tract. The choroid consists of a rich capillary bed that nourishes the eye. Its outer surface is continuous with the inner surface of the sclera and its inner surface is attached to the retina. The choroid is divided into three layers: a vessel layer containing melanocytes and blood vessels, a capillary layer also consisting of melanocytes and some blood vessels, and the Bruch's membrane.

The iris is a structure responsible for contractility of the pupil (an aperture found within its center). The iris consists of melanocytes giving the color of the eyes. It also contains stroma, which is connected to the sphincter and dilator pupillae muscles, allowing constriction and dilation of the pupils, respectively. The outer root of the iris is attached to the sclera and the anterior ciliary body. The root of the iris and the cornea forms an acute iridocorneal angle, which allows the drainage of aqueous humor into the Schlemm's canal (which drains into the episcleral blood vessels) and if obstructed can lead to the development of closed-angle glaucoma.

The inner layer of the eye is known as the retina. Microscopically, the retina consists of the inner neurosensory layer and the outer retinal pigmented epithelium (RPE), which rests on the Bruch's membrane of the choroid. The anatomy and physiology of the inner neurosensory layer is discussed in Section 6.3.

There are two critical landmarks in the retina. One is called the macula lutea, Latin for "yellow spot." This section of the retina contains no blood vessels and houses the fovea centralis, a specialized central shallow pit with a high density of cones that delivers the highest visual acuity. Another region is the optic disc, where the information from the photoreceptors exits the eye through the optic nerve while blood vessels simultaneously enter the eye and branch extensively over the inner surface of the retina. This results in a blind spot. Papilledema refers to swelling of the optic disc that occurs secondary to raised intracranial pressure. The optic disc is the area of the retina where the optic nerve enters and can be visualized using an ophthalmoscope.

6.2.3 Vascular Supply

The ophthalmic artery, a branch of the internal carotid artery, is a major blood supply to the eyes. The central artery of the retina, a branch of the ophthalmic artery supples the internal surface of the retina. Venous drainage of the eyeball is to the superior and inferior ophthalmic veins and these drain into the cavernous sinus.

The major output of the eyeball is the optic nerve (CN II), which develops from the optic vesicle, an outpocketing of the forebrain. It is surrounded by the cranial meninges and not covered by the typical coverings of a nerve.

6.2.4 Eye Movements

The rotation of each eye is controlled by six extraocular muscles: superior rectus, inferior rectus, lateral rectus, medial rectus, superior oblique, and inferior oblique. The medial rectus is responsible for adduction of the eye and the lateral rectus is responsible for abduction. The superior rectus is responsible for intorsion, elevation, and adduction, whereas the inferior rectus depresses, adducts, and extorts the eye. The superior oblique is responsible for intorsion, depression, and abduction. The inferior oblique is responsible for extortion, elevation, and abduction. The abducens nerve supplies the lateral rectus muscle and the trochlear nerve supplies the superior oblique muscle. The remaining muscles are supplied by the oculomotor nerve, which also innervates the levator muscles of the eyelid and carries axons from the Edinger–Westphal nucleus, which provide parasympathetic innervation to the iris sphincter and ciliary muscle, mediating the pupillary light reflex and accommodation, respectively. Damage to the oculomotor nerve therefore leads to impaired eye movements, ptosis, and pupillary dilation.

Motor neurons innervating the eye muscles are found in the oculomotor, trochlear, and abducens nerves, with their nuclei found in the brainstem. The vestibular nuclei and the superior colliculus influence activity of these nuclei. The medial longitudinal fasciculus (MLFs) receive motor commands regarding eye position from the gaze centers in the reticular formation of the pons, which themselves receive information from the superior colliculus and the frontal and parietal eye field of the cortex. The MLFs connect vestibular nuclei to the motor nuclei controlling eye movements and connect the superior colliculus to the cervical motor neurons in the upper spinal cord controlling head movement.

There are a number of eye movements that are clinically relevant. These include saccades, smooth pursuit, the vestibulo-ocular reflex, and the optokinetic reflex.

Saccades are rapid, conjugate eye movements that change the center of gaze from one part of the visual field to another. Saccades may be horizontal, vertical, or oblique, and can range in amplitude. At the onset of a target for a saccade, there is increased firing of excitatory burst neurons in the brainstem, which allows the position of the target with respect to the fovea to be computed. The motor error (the difference between the initial and intended position) is then calculated and converted to a command that activates the extraocular muscles to move appropriately. A new level of tonic innervation is required to keep the eyes in this position. The peak velocity of the saccades is determined by the density of the action potentials. The saccadic movements are predetermined at initiation and cannot respond to changes in target position during an existing movement and are therefore said to be ballistic. Voluntary saccades are largely initiated by the frontal eye fields and involuntary saccades by the superior colliculus of the midbrain. The striatum, part of the basal ganglia, and the cerebellum have also been implicated in saccadic movements. The direction of the saccade is encoded by two gaze centers located in the reticular formation. The horizontal gaze center (including the paramedian pontine reticular formation (PPRF) and the sixth nerve nucleus) is located in the pons, and the vertical gaze center in the midbrain reticular formation. There are a number of disorders that are associated with impaired saccadic eye movements and these include Parkinson's disease, multiple system atrophy, progressive supranuclear palsy, Hungtington's disease, and spinocerebellar ataxia. Saccades is different from nystagmus, a condition that causes the eyes to make repetitive, involuntary, uncontrolled movements leading to reduced vision and depth perception. Smooth pursuits are slower voluntary tracking movements and allow the eyes to keep a moving stimulus on the fovea. Vergence movements align the fovea with targets located at different distances. Vestibulo-ocular movements stabilize the eyes during head movements and help prevent images from slipping on the surface of the retina as the position of the head changes.

6.3 Neural Retina

The neural retina contains six types of cells: photoreceptors, bipolar cells, ganglion cells, horizontal cells, amacrine cells, and supporting cells.

6.3.1 Photoreceptors and Phototransduction

Photoreceptors are specialized neurons found in the retina that convert light into electrical signals. They have a unique morphology consisting of an elongated outer segment with stacked membrane discs designed to contain a high photopigment density allowing a large proportion of light photons to be absorbed. The shape and morphology of the outer segment can be used to distinguish the two most common photoreceptors: the rods and cones (Figure 6.3). The outer segment also contains the proteins necessary for phototransduction. However, protein synthesis occurs in the inner segment and any molecules that need to be

Figure 6.3 Photoreceptors.

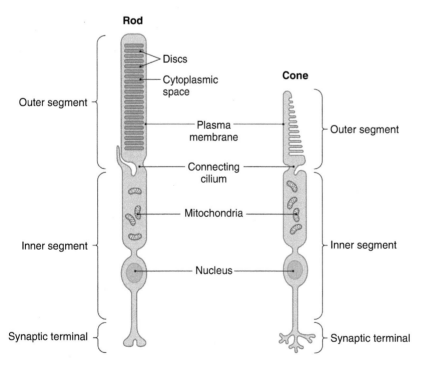

transported to the outer segment travel apically through the connecting cilium. The inner segment has an abundance of mitochondria to provide energy for protein synthesis and phototransduction. The synaptic terminals of photoreceptors are filled with synaptic vesicles and are presynaptic to the bipolar and horizontal cells.

Rods are responsible for vision at low light levels (scotopic vision) and have a LOW spatial acuity. Cones are responsible for color vision and have a higher spatial acuity. There are three types of cones that vary in wavelength.

All photoreceptors possess pigments containing an aldehyde of vitamin A called retinaldehyde (abbreviated to retinal), which forms a covalent bond with an opsin. Rods contain rhodopsin, which absorbs light with a wavelength of 500 nm. However, cone cells contain three different pigments called iodopsins – namely, erythrolabe, chlorolabe, and cyanolabe – which are sensitive to different frequencies of light. Under dark conditions, photoreceptors are in a state of depolarization and continuously release glutamate across the synaptic cleft. When a photon of light hits the retinal molecule, it changes conformation and reverts from its 11-*cis* form to an 11-*trans* state, and dissociates from opsin. The 11-*trans* retinal then binds to guanosine triphosphate (GTP)-binding protein molecules, named transducin, and activates them. Transducin consists of alpha, beta, and gamma subunits. The alpha unit contains guanosine diphosphate (GDP) and becomes dissociated from the rest of the transducin complex by exchanging its GDP for a GTP molecule. The alpha subunit then interacts with the enzyme cyclic guanosine monophosphate (cGMP) phosphodiesterase, which hydrolyzes cGMP to an inactive form, leading to closure of cGMP-gated sodium and calcium channels, resulting in hyperpolarization and less release of neurotransmitter (Figure 6.4).

By default, photoreceptors are depolarized in the dark (Figure 6.5). These dark currents are a result of GTP and cGMP second messenger mechanisms. Guanylyl cyclase converts GTP into cGMP, and cGMP maintains ligand-gated cation channels in an open state. This allows for depolarizing Na^+ and Ca^{2+} influx, resulting in a constant release of glutamate.

6.3.2 Adaptation of Photoreceptors

The phototransduction pathway is reset by deactivating the 11-*trans* retinal back into its *cis*- isomer form via the enzyme rhodopsin kinase, which increases the affinity of arrestin to rhodopsin and therefore inhibits the ability to produce further transducin. High levels of Ca^{2+} ions inhibit guanylate cyclase, reducing the levels of cGMP and therefore providing a negative feedback loop on the transduction cascade. However, Ca^{2+} ions also inhibit phosphorylation of rhodopsin by rhodopsin kinase, and therefore limit recovery and hence also participate in a positive feedback loop.

The sensitivity of the eye can be measured by determining the absolute intensity threshold. This is the minimum luminance of a test spot needed to produce a visual sensation. The Duplicity Theory states that above a certain luminance level (~ 0.03 cd/m^2), cones are primarily involved in mediating photopic (day) vision. Below this level, rods provide scotopic (night) vision. They work together in the mesopic range (twilight vision).

If you see a bright light and then move into a dark room, you may suffer from temporary "blindness." In the dark, vision is primarily mediated by rods, which have greater sensitivity than cones. However, the bright light has already activated rhodopsin in the rods and is now insensitive to further stimulation. As a result, it takes a few minutes to return rhodopsin to its resting state via enzymatic re-association of retinal with opsin. This is known as dark adaptation.

In contrast, light adaptation occurs when moving from a dark room to a bright one. The rods are too sensitive to the light and are overwhelmingly activated. The rhodopsin is "bleached," meaning it will take some time to be inactivated. Thus, a bright light appears to activate less-sensitive cones for a sharper image.

6.3.3 Bipolar Cells and Ganglion Cells

Photoreceptors transmit information to bipolar cells, first-order neurons, which then communicate with ganglion cells. These cells possess an axon on one end and a dendritic tree on the opposite end. Ganglion cells are the second-order neurons in the visual pathway. They synapse with bipolar and amacrine cells containing nonmyelinated axons.

Horizontal cells synapse with rods, cones, and ganglion cells. They function to release the inhibitory neurotransmitter γ-Aminobutyric acid (GABA), which inhibits the ganglion cells. Amacrine cells synapse and stimulate ganglion cells following stimulation by the bipolar cells. Supporting cells include the Müller cells, the most common type of retinal glial cells, retinal astrocytes, perivascular glial cells, and microglial cells (Figure 6.6).

The bipolar cells transmit signals from the photoreceptors to the ganglion cells. Some bipolar cells connect only to cones and others connect only to rods.

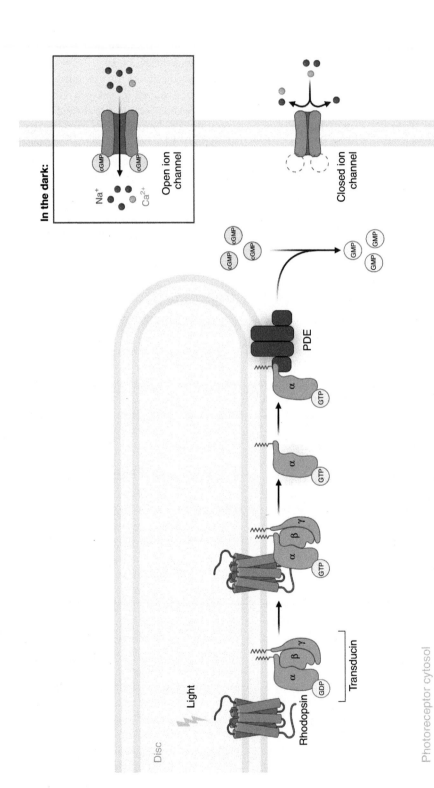

Figure 6.4 The molecular basis of phototransduction within photoreceptors.

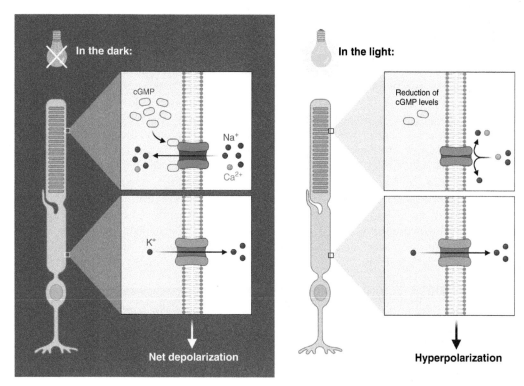

Figure 6.5 The effect of dark and light on membrane potential.

In the dark:

cGMP

Na⁺

Ca²⁺

K⁺

Net depolarization

In the light:

Reduction of
cGMP levels

Hyperpolarization

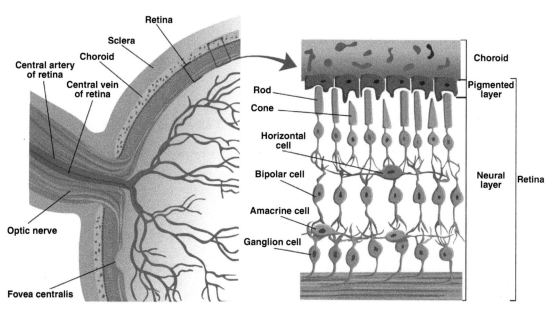

Figure 6.6 Layers and cells of the retina.

Retina

Sclera

Choroid

Central artery
of retina

Central vein
of retina

Optic nerve

Fovea centralis

Rod

Cone

Horizontal
cell

Bipolar cell

Amacrine cell

Ganglion cell

Choroid

Pigmented
layer

Neural
layer

Retina

The chemical mechanisms behind visual processing can be understood in the two retinal pathways: ON and OFF systems. These two pathways respond oppositely in the presence and absence of light, improving image resolution by increasing the brain's ability to perceive contrast at edges or borders.

In the ON pathway, light stimulation hyperpolarizes photoreceptors, resulting in a decrease in glutamate release onto bipolar cells. Because ON bipolar cells have inhibitory glutamate receptors, the light stimulation and consequent decrease in neurotransmitter release results in a depolarized bipolar cell. Specifically, less glutamate binding to metabotropic receptors that cause cGMP breakdown results in less cGMP to be cleaved and more neurotransmitter to be released. The ON bipolar cells thus release more glutamate neurotransmitter that will bind to the ganglion cells, depolarizing them and generating more action potentials.

There is an opposite effect in the OFF pathway. Light stimulation still hyperpolarizes photoreceptors, resulting in a decrease in glutamate release onto bipolar cells. However, because OFF bipolar cells have excitatory glutamate receptors, the light stimulation and consequent decrease in neurotransmitter release results in a hyperpolarized bipolar cell. OFF bipolar cells have ionotropic receptors that serve as non-selective cation channels that depolarize the cell, so less glutamate ligand results in hyperpolarization. As a result, there is less glutamate neurotransmitter released by the hyperpolarized OFF bipolar cells, resulting in hyperpolarized ganglion cells which generate fewer action potentials.

6.4 Visual Pathway From Eye to Brain

With the visual information encoded in neuronal signals, the information can now travel from the retina to the brain. The axons of the ON and OFF ganglion cells will converge and exit the eye through the optic disc, bundling up into the optic nerve. We can describe the side of the retina from which the optic nerve originates. The temporal retina is the half of the retina closest to the temple, while the nasal retina is the half of the retina closest to the nose. Due to its position, the former will always receive visual information from the contralateral visual field. On the other hand, the nasal retina will always receive visual information from the ipsilateral visual field. As a result, the left visual field falls on the left eye's nasal retina and the right eye's temporal retina. The right visual field falls on the right nasal retina and the left temporal retina.

In order to process information from the right and left eyes specifically, the two optic nerves meet at the optic chiasm (Figure 6.7). The bundles of axon after the optic chiasm are now called the optic tract. In humans, approximately 40% of the axons continue along their path, while 60% cross to the opposite side of the brain. Thus, the optic tract contains fibers from both eyes. The decussation or crossing of right and left axons at the optic chiasm allows for similar processing in right and left hemispheres.

As a result, all of the left visual field input will follow the right optic tract to the right lateral geniculate nucleus (LGN) in the thalamus and consequently the right visual cortex. This is able to occur because the left nasal axons continue ipsilaterally, while the right temporal axons will cross over at the optic chiasm. Similarly, all of the right visual field input will follow the left optic tract to the left LGN and left visual cortex.

6.4.1 Lateral Geniculate Nucleus in the Thalamus

The LGN is a region of nuclei in the thalamus that receives visual information from retinal ganglion cells and sends that output to the visual cortex. In humans, the LGN consists of six distinct layers (Figure 6.8).

The layers of the LGN reveal that retinal ganglion cell information is topographically organized and distilled according to the input's cell type and eye of origin. The most ventral layers, layers 1 and 2, are known as magnocellular layers because they contain cells with large somas and receive visual input from large parasol retinal ganglion cells. These cells best respond to objects in motion. However, layer 1 only receives information from contralateral M-type retinal ganglion cells, while layer 2 only receives visual input from ipsilateral M-type retinal ganglion cells.

The dorsal layers, layers 3–6, are known as parvocellular layers because they contain cells with small somas and receive input from small midget retinal ganglion cells. These cells best respond to color, fine details, and still or slow-moving objects. Layers 4 and 6 receive input from contralateral P-type retinal ganglion cells, while layers 3 and 5 receive input from ipsilateral P-type retinal ganglion cells.

Koniocellular cells, critical for processing color, lie between the six prominent layers of the LGN. LGN neurons act similarly to RGCs, but it is unlikely that the LGN serves as a simple relay station between the eye and the visual cortex. Only 10% of neural synapses onto the LGN come from RGCs; 90% of neural synapses to the LGN

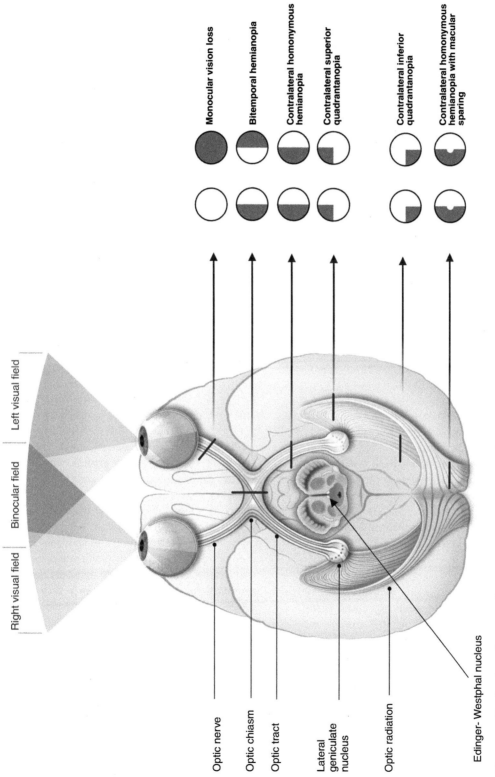

Right visual field | Binocular field | Left visual field

Optic nerve

Optic chiasm

Optic tract

Lateral geniculate nucleus

Optic radiation

Edinger-Westphal nucleus

Monocular vision loss

Bitemporal hemianopia

Contralateral homonymous hemianopia

Contralateral superior quadrantanopia

Contralateral inferior quadrantanopia

Contralateral homonymous hemianopia with macular sparing

Figure 6.7 Visual pathway from eye to brain.

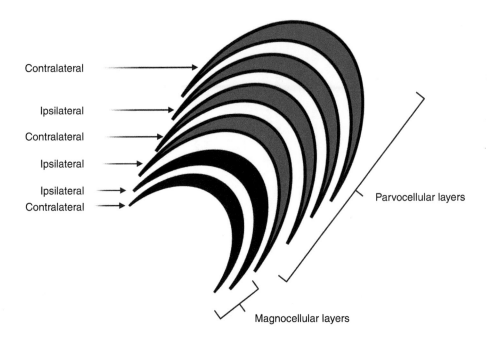

Figure 6.8 Layers of the LGN.

Contralateral

Ipsilateral

Contralateral

Ipsilateral

Ipsilateral

Contralateral

Parvocellular layers

Magnocellular layers

come from cortical, brainstem, or thalamic inhibitory neurons. There is much research being done to understand the complex feedback pathway of the LGN. Nevertheless, it is a critical part of the visual system, as the LGN's optic radiations onto the visual cortex help us process even more information. The upper optic radiation carries fibers from the superior retinal quadrants through the parietal lobe and the lower radiation carries fibers from the inferior retinal quadrants through the temporal lobe via the Meyer's loop to the visual cortex.

The primary visual cortex is also known as V1 and the striate cortex. It receives direct input from the LGN, especially at V1's layer 4. The neurons in layer 4 will synapse onto layers 2 and 3, which will then synapse onto layers 5 and 6 and other areas of the brain.

6.4.2 Receptive Fields

Retinal ganglions cells are the first neurons in the retina that respond with action potentials. Receptive fields are an important characteristic of the visual system (Figure 6.9). They are defined as the region of sensory space that elicits the greatest activity. They always exhibit ON–OFF antagonism. ON cells are stimulated by light at the center region and inhibited by light in the surround. OFF cells are inhibited by light at the center region and stimulated by light in the surround. Receptive fields are useful because they enable cells to detect changes in light in addition to brightness. This allows cells to better detect edges or boundaries between the light and dark.

In the retina, both bipolar cells and RGCs have center/surround receptive fields. This type of receptive field has a straightforward mechanism: the inner circle acts as the center and the outer ring serves as the surround. ON center/surround cells have an ON center that is stimulated by light and an OFF surround that is inhibited by light. On the other hand, OFF center/surround cells have an OFF center that is inhibited by light and an ON surround that is stimulated by light. Neurons in the LGN share a similar center/surround mechanism.

The cells of the visual cortex are unique in that they do not act like RGCs or those in the LGN. The simple cells in the striate cortex have a bar-like, elongated field, allowing these neurons to be tuned to detect lines and edges. Classic experiments on cats performed by Hubel and Wiesel show that V1 neurons are selective for orientation and direction of movement and respond vigorously to bars only near a particular angle on the screen and moving in a particular direction. This demonstrated the importance of visual cortical neurons in encoding features of retinal images (Figure 6.10).

6.4.3 Ocular Dominance Columns

Orientation tuning can result in a simple cell favoring either the right or left eye, and this is known as ocular dominance. This can only occur in binocular neurons, which are responsive to both eyes, unlike monocular neurons. Binocular neurons in the visual cortex exist outside of layer 4 and will order in columns via columnar organization. You can think of these columns as units of neurons

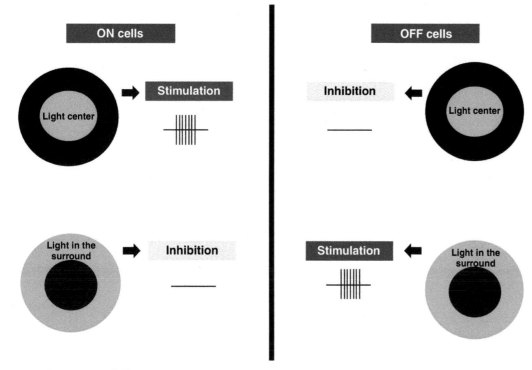

Figure 6.9 Receptive fields.

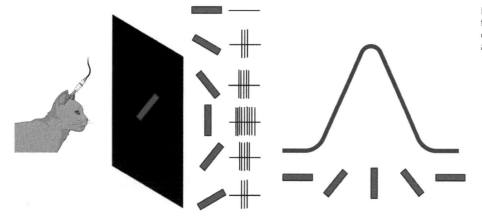

Figure 6.10 Extracellular recording from neurons in the primary visual cortex of a cat to stimuli shown on a screen.

that span multiple layers in the striate cortex. These ocular dominance columns exist all throughout V1 and often alternate in columns of input from the left and right eyes.

In classic experiments performed by Hubel and Wiesel, the concept of ocular dominance was demonstrated in cats. Monocular deprivation in kittens resulted in neurons being responsive to information that came from the non-deprived eye. However, the same manipulation in an adult cat had no effect on the responses of the visual neurons (Figure 6.11).

6.4.4 Dorsal Versus Ventral Processing

Once visual information is processed in the primary visual cortex, it will be sent to one of two destinations. Through a dorsal stream, the information will be sent to the parietal cortex to further analyze where the object is,

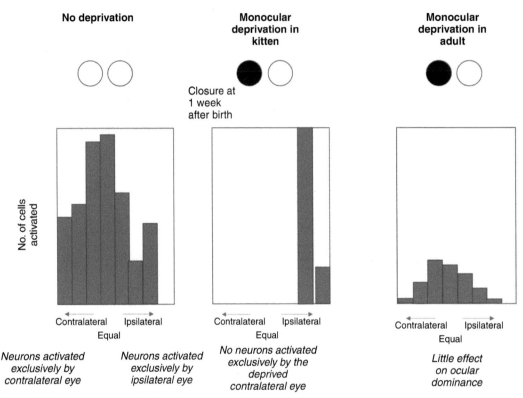

No deprivation

Monocular deprivation in kitten

Closure at 1 week after birth

Monocular deprivation in adult

No. of cells activated

Contralateral — Ipsilateral
Equal

Contralateral — Ipsilateral
Equal

Contralateral — Ipsilateral
Equal

Neurons activated exclusively by contralateral eye

Neurons activated exclusively by ipsilateral eye

No neurons activated exclusively by the deprived contralateral eye

Little effect on ocular dominance

Figure 6.11 Monocular deprivation in early development versus in adults.

focusing on motion and depth. The information may also take a ventral stream to the temporal cortex for analysis of object form and color. These processing pathways are extremely complex and not entirely understood. Increasing evidence has shown that the dorsal and ventral streams are not strictly independent, but do interact with each other.

6.5 Introduction to the Olfactory System

The nose consists of the nasal skeleton and nasal cavity. The cavity functions to humidify inspired air, remove pathogens, allow the sense of smell, drain paranasal sinuses and the lacrimal ducts. The nasal cavity begins with the vestibule of the nose, which surrounds the external opening of the nose. The nasal mucosa contains respiratory epithelium interspersed with mucussecreting goblet cells and the olfactory epithelium.

In the lateral walls of the nasal cavity are found three turbinates (conchae) (Figure 6.12), which increase the surface area of the cavity, disrupting fast laminar airflow to create more time for humidification and create pathways (superior, middle, and inferior meatuses and the spheno-ethmoidal recess) for air to flow.

The nasal cavity is drained by the paranasal sinuses (Figure 6.13). The middle meatus receives the frontal, maxillary, and anterior ethmoidal sinuses. The middle ethmoidal sinuses empty into the ethmoidal bulla and the posterior ethmoidal sinus into the sphenoeth moidalrecess.

6.5.1 Neurovascular Supply

The nose has a rich blood supply from the branches of the external carotid artery (sphenopalatine artery, greater palatine artery, superior labial artery, and the lateral nasal arteries) and the internal carotid artery (anterior and posterior ethmoid arteries). The blood supply to the anterior third of the nose (Kiesselbach area) is particularly rich and the source of most cases of epistaxis.

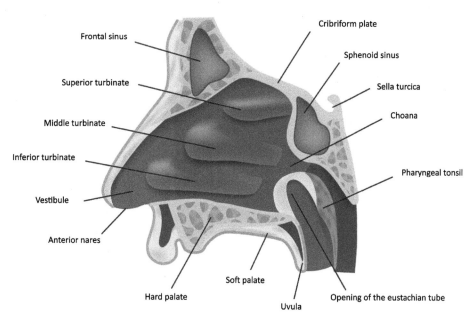

Figure 6.12 Lateral view of the nasal cavity.

Frontal sinus
Superior turbinate
Middle turbinate
Inferior turbinate
Vestibule
Anterior nares
Hard palate
Soft palate
Uvula
Cribriform plate
Sphenoid sinus
Sella turcica
Choana
Pharyngeal tonsil
Opening of the eustachian tube

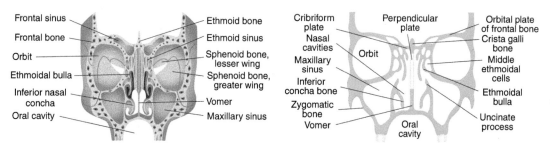

Frontal sinus
Frontal bone
Orbit
Ethmoidal bulla
Inferior nasal concha
Oral cavity
Ethmoid bone
Ethmoid sinus
Sphenoid bone, lesser wing
Sphenoid bone, greater wing
Vomer
Maxillary sinus

Cribriform plate
Nasal cavities
Maxillary sinus
Inferior concha bone
Zygomatic bone
Vomer
Perpendicular plate
Orbit
Oral cavity
Orbital plate of frontal bone
Crista galli bone
Middle ethmoidal cells
Ethmoidal bulla
Uncinate process

Figure 6.13 Paranasal sinuses.

The venous drainage follows the arteries and drains into the pterygoid plexus, facial vein, or cavernous sinus. Nasal veins may also merge with the sagittal sinus and may be a route of infection from the nose to the cranium.

The ability to sense smell is carried out by olfactory nerves, which send branches that travel through the cribriform plate. General sensation to the external nose is through the trigeminal nerve and its branches. Nasal mucosal serous glands are innervated by the parasympathetic fibers of the facial nerve. The sympathetic innervation serves to regulate mucosal blood flow.

6.5.2 Olfaction Transduction

Most odorants stimulate both the olfactory nerve giving the sensation of smell and the trigeminal nerve giving rise to pungent sensations such as tingling. The transduction of olfactory signals occurs in the olfactory cilia. Odorants bind to the specific receptors on the cilia directly or via odorant binding proteins that transport it to the receptor (Figure 6.14). Odorants bind to cilia receptors containing olfactoryspecific guanosine triphosphate (GTP)-binding protein. This leads to increase in cyclic adenosine monophosphate (cAMP), which leads to the opening of Na^+ and Ca^{2+} channels and subsequently depolarization of the olfactory receptor neuron in the olfactory epithelium. There is also amplification of a Ca^{2+}-activated Cl^- current, from the cilia to the olfactory receptor neuron, leading to an action potential transmission to the bulb.

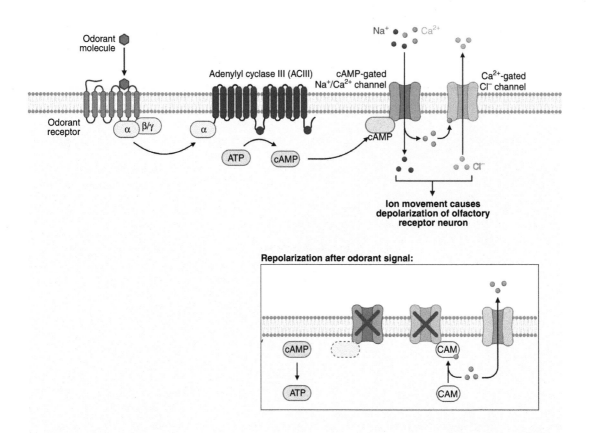

Figure 6.14 Olfactory transduction.

Figure 6.15 Olfactory nerve fibers.

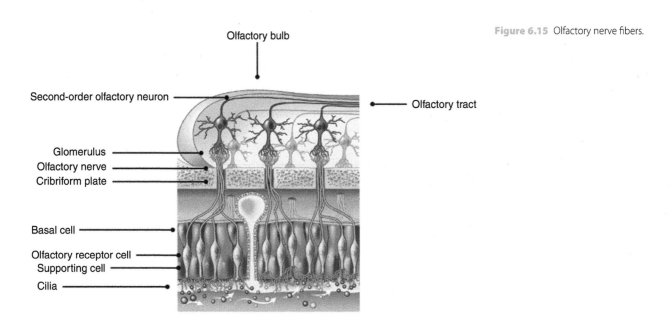

6.5.3 Olfactory Pathway

Olfactory nerve fibers contain bipolar neurons that pass through foramina in the cribriform plate to enter the cranium, where they synapse with the mitral and tufted cells in the glomerulus of the olfactory bulb (Figure 6.15). Axons emerge from here to form the lateral olfactory tract, which then project to the olfactory cortex. This contains several anatomically distinct areas: piriform cortex (largest region), parts of the amygdala (responds to emotionally significant unpleasant odors), anterior olfactory nucleus (important for regulation of flow between regions), olfactory tubercle (forms odor preferences), and the lateral entorhinal cortex (participates in odor discrimination and integration of odor information into associative memories). The piriform cortex, entorhinal cortex and amygdala project to the orbitofrontal cortex, where information about odor identity and the reward value of odors (and other senses) are represented form the lateral olfactory tract, which then project to the olfactory cortex and limbic cortex, including the uncus/pyriform cortex which projects to the amygdala and the entorhinal cortex and the olfactory tubercle which projects to the thalamus, insula, and the orbitofrontal cortex.

6.6 The Auditory System

6.6.1 Anatomy of the Ear

The external ear can be divided into three parts: outer, middle, and inner (Figure 6.16). The outer ear consists of the auricle (pinna) and external acoustic meatus. The auricle contains the cartilaginous helix and is parallel to the antihelix. The external auditory meatus ends at the tympanic membrane, a translucent connective tissue that is susceptible to perforation from trauma or infection.

The external ear is supplied by branches of the external carotid artery and drains to its corresponding veins. The sensory innervation to the skin is from branches of the cervical plexus, mandibular nerve, and facial and vagus nerves. The lymphatic drainage is to the superficial parotid, mastoid, upper deep cervical, and superficial cervical nodes.

The middle ear is divided into the tympanic cavity containing the three ossicle bones (malleus, incus, and stapes) and the epitympanic recess, which is located anterior to the mastoid air cells in the temporal bone. The three ossicles usually respond to sound vibrations in the tympanic membrane allowing passage of sound waves from the external ear to the oval window of the internal ear. The middle ear contains two muscles, the tensor tympani and the stapedius, which contract in response to loud noise by reducing vibrations of the ossicles (the acoustic reflex). The Eustachian tube connects the middle ear to the nasopharynx and equalizes pressure of the middle ear to that of the external auditory meatus. In conditions such as otitis media with effusion (glue ear), the tube cannot equalize pressure, and this creates a negative pressure inside the middle ear, drawing out a transudate from the mucosa of the middle ear.

The Internal ear develops from the otic placode (an ectodermal thickening) at around the fourth week of gestation, which invaginate to form a sphere, the otic vesicle, containing the dorsal and ventral pouch. The

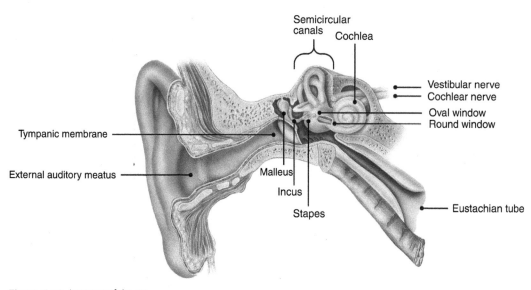

Figure 6.16 Anatomy of the ear.

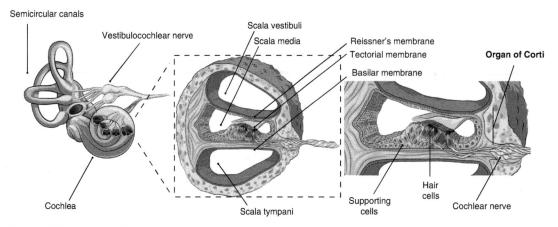

Figure 6.17 Anatomy of the inner ear.

dorsal pouch is responsible for the formation of the vestibular structures and the ventral pouch becomes the cochlea.

The inner ear develops from ectodermal cells by week 4 of gestation. Invagination of the cells forms the otic vesicle containing the dorsal and ventral pouch. The dorsal pouch is responsible for the formation of the vestibular structures and the ventral pouch becomes the cochlea.

The inner ear is composed of the bony labyrinth (cochlea, vestibule, and the semicircular canals) and the membranous labyrinth (cochlear duct, semicircular ducts, utricle, and saccule) filled with endolymph (Figure 6.17). The inner ear is connected to the middle ear by the oval window and the round window.

The cochlea contains the cochlear duct of the membranous labyrinth and separates two chambers filled with perilymph called the scala vestibuli and scala tympani (Figure 6.17). It is separated from the scala vestibuli by the Reissner's membrane and the Scala tympani by the basilar membrane, which contains the epithelial cells of hearing (organ of Corti). The cochlear duct is held in the cochlea by the spiral lamina. The semicircular canals contain the semicircular ducts, which are responsible for balance (along with the utricle and saccule, which also detect motion). The semicircular ducts are located within the semicircular canals. The flow of endolymph in the ducts changes upon head movement and this is detected by sensory receptors in the semicircular canal.

6.6.2 Neurovascular Supply

The bony labyrinth is supplied by branches of the maxillary artery, the middle meningeal artery, and the posterior auricular artery. The membranous labyrinth is supplied by the labyrinthine artery, a branch of either the anterior inferior cerebellar artery or the basilar artery. Venous drainage of the inner ear is through the labyrinthine vein, which empties into the sigmoid sinus or inferior petrosal sinus. The vestibulocochlear nerve supplies the inner ear with the vestibular nerve supplying the utricle, saccular, and the semicircular ducts and the cochlear nerve supplying the organ of Corti.

6.6.3 Cochlea Physiology

Sound waves are transduced into electrical impulses, which can be interpreted as sound frequencies. The spiral shape of the cochlea means that stimulation of specific areas by the vibrations in the endolymph leads to perception of different sound frequencies and therefore creates a tonotopic map.

The sound waves strike the tympanic membrane resulting in vibrations, which are transferred to the middle ear along the ossicle bones. The footplate of the stapes contacts the oval window, which results in transmission of the vibrations to the perilymph. The vibrations then travel to the scala vestibuli and then to the scala tympani, and into the endolymph of the cochlear duct, eventually vibrating inner hair cells in the organ of Corti. These synapse with bipolar spiral ganglion neurons to send afferent nerve impulses back to the brain via the cochlear nerve, to be interpreted as sound frequencies.

The inner hair cells contain stereocilia at the tips, with a tall kinocilium (Figure 6.18). Displacement of the hair cells toward the tallest stereocilia depolarizes the hair cell, while movements parallel to this plane toward the shortest stereocilia cause hyperpolarization. However, displacements perpendicular to the plane do not affect the membrane potential. The resting potential of the hair cell is

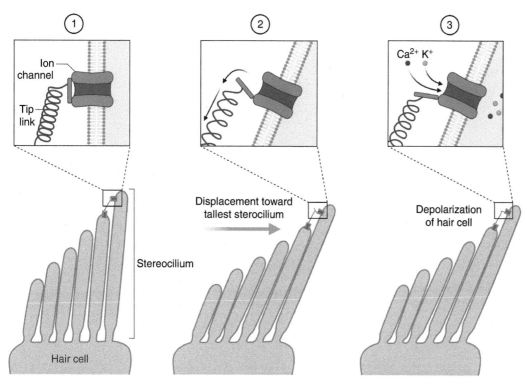

Figure 6.18 Displacement of inner hair cells.

between -45 and -60 mV relative to the surrounding fluid. During depolarization, as more transduction channels open, K^+ enters the cell, followed by opening of the voltage-gated calcium channels leading to calcium (Ca^{2+}) influx, causing transmitter release onto auditory nerve endings.

6.6.4 The Auditory Pathway

The hair cells of the organ of Corti are innervated by the spiral (cochlear) ganglion. Neurons of the spiral ganglion are bipolar and are first in the auditory system to fire action potentials. They make contact with the base of hair cells via their dendrites. There are two types of cells in the spiral ganglion. Type I are bipolar, myelinated neurons, and innervate inner hair cells. Type II are unipolar, unmyelinated cells, and innervate outer hair cells.

They project their axons through the cochlear nerve and then to the dorsal and ventral cochlear nuclei. Most fibers from the dorsal nucleus ascend in the contralateral lateral lemniscus and some fibers ascend in the ipsilateral lateral lemniscus (Figure 6.19). Fibers from the ventral nucleus travel contralaterally to the superior olivary nucleus in the pons. Some fibers ascend in the lateral lemniscus bilaterally. Information then travels to the inferior colliculus, in the tectum of the midbrain, where they converge and project to the medial geniculate body of the thalamus and then to the primary auditory cortex in the superior temporal gyrus.

6.6.5 The Vestibular System

The vestibular system is important for the sense of proprioception. The peripheral vestibular system is comprised of the vestibular labyrinth, vestibular ganglion, and the vestibulocochlear nerve.

6.6.6 Vestibular Labyrinth

This is a bony cavity found in the petrous part of the temporal bone. It is made up of the semicircular canals (which detect angular acceleration of the head) and the utricle and saccule (which detect linear head acceleration and spatial orientation of the head).

6.6.7 Semicircular Canals

These are three membranous channels found in the semicircular ducts of the labyrinth. Each canal dilates to form the ampulla, which contains the cristae ampullaris made

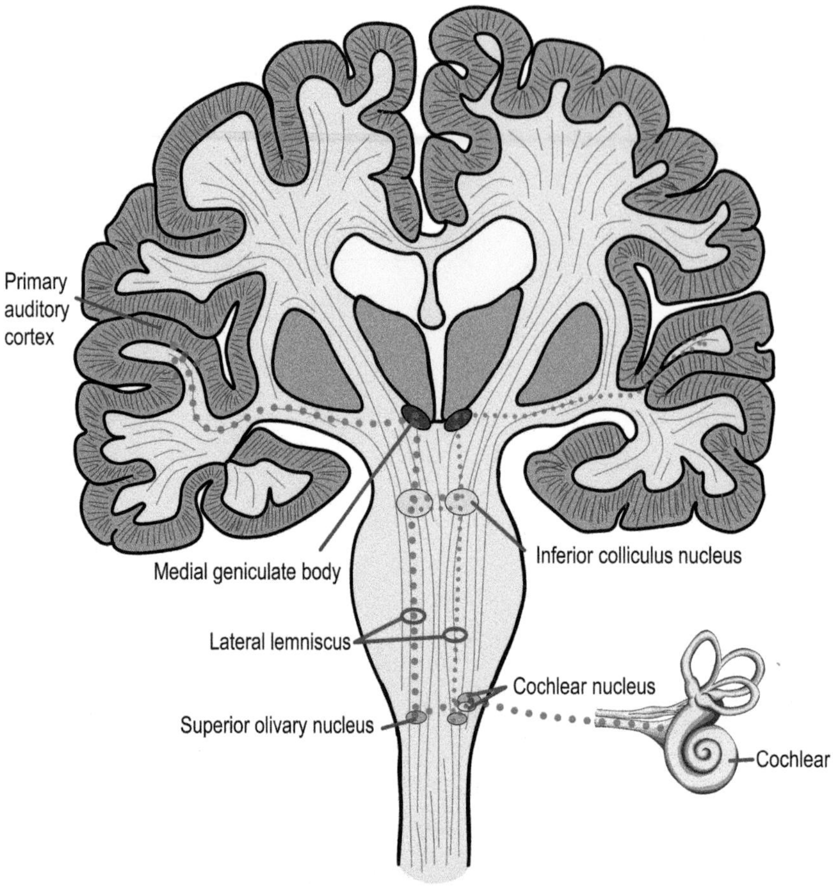

Figure 6.19 The auditory pathway.

Primary auditory cortex

Medial geniculate body

Inferior colliculus nucleus

Lateral lemniscus

Cochlear nucleus

Superior olivary nucleus

Cochlear

up of sensory hair cells. The semicircular canals contain endolymph and any movement of this stimulates the hair cells and in this way the canals can detect head movements. Each hair cell has many stereocilia and one true cilium called a kinocilium. Movement of the head leads to movement of endolymph, which moves the stereocilia toward the kinocilium. These movements lead to transduction followed by cell excitation. The movement of stereocilia in the opposite direction reduces cell activity.

6.6.8 Otolithic Organs (Utricle and Saccule)

These are membranous organs found in the bony vestibule. The utricle lies posteriorly and communicates with the semicircular canals and on the other end forms the utriculosaccular duct with the saccule, which itself communicates with the cochlea.

These organs contain clusters of hair cells called the macula and they are also sensitive to endolymph movement and can detect linear movement of the head in the horizontal plane (utricle), vertical plane (saccular), and its

position in space (Figure 6.20). The cilia in the hair cells of the otoliths require the shearing of the otolithic membrane to be stimulated before firing an action potential.

6.6.9 The Vestibular Pathway

Vestibular information such as body position, gaze stability, linear acceleration (detected by hair cells of otolith organs), and rotational movement (detected by semicircular canals) is transmitted via the bipolar sensory neurons of the vestibular ganglion of Scarpa to the vestibular nerve. Axons of this nerve synapse in the vestibular nuclei on the pontomedullary junction (Figure 6.21). There are four vestibular nuclei (superior, inferior, lateral, and medial). The superior and medial nuclei receive inputs from the cristae ampullaris of the semicircular canals and send axons to the medial longitudinal fasciculus before synapsing with the motor nuclei of the oculomotor, trochlear, and abducens nerves. This is important for controlling reflex activity of the vestibulo-ocular reflex, which is important for adjusting eye movements according to

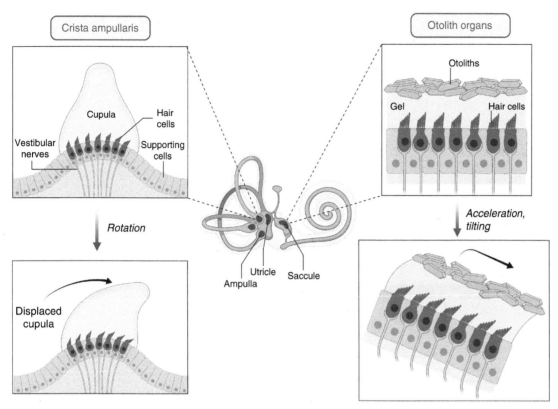

Figure 6.20 Hair cell movement of otolith organs.

head movements and fixing gaze on a static object even while turning the head. The inferior and lateral nuclei receive the remaining fibers from inferior semicircular canals and from the utricle and saccule. Deiters' neurons, located exclusively in the lateral vestibular nucleus sends fibers via the lateral vestibulospinal tract, which synapses with interneurons of the spinal cord and take part in the vestibulospinal reflex, This helps adjust the extensor muscles and body posture according to the vestibular stimulus. The medial and inferior nuclei send their fibers via the medial vestibulospinal tract to the cervical spinal cord and this is important for adjusting the posture of the head and neck (vestibulocervical reflex).

The vestibular nuclei also connect with the cerebellum via the inferior olivary nucleus of the vestibulo-olivary tract and then to the inferior cerebellar peduncle into the ipsilateral cerebellar vermis, flocculus, and nodulus. This is how the cerebellum and vestibular system are both able to modulate balance. Some neurons from the vestibular ganglion also travel via the medial part of the inferior cerebellar peduncle and synapse with the ipsilateral vestibulocerebellum, vermis, and fastigial nucleus. This helps with cerebellar awareness of the vestibular sensation.

The superior and lateral vestibular nuclei send fibers to the ventral posterior nuclei of the thalamus and synapse with the third-order neurons of the vestibular pathway. The thalamus sends information to the primary vestibular cortex of the parietal lobe to integrate vestibular information with other proprioceptive information and then finally sends this information to the primary motor cortex to generate the motor response to the proprioceptive stimulus.

6.6.10 The Gustatory Pathway

Gustation is important for feeding and digestion and involves the activation of various taste pathways. Loss of taste has been reported in many neurological disorders. Sensory taste information is passed from the taste buds to the primary gustatory axons into the brainstem, thalamus, and then to the cerebral cortex. Primary gustatory axons are carried by three cranial nerves (Figure 6.22). The anterior two thirds of the tongue and the palate send axons into the facial nerve, and the posterior third is innervated by the glossopharyngeal nerve. The epiglottis, glottis, and pharynx send axons to the vagus nerve.

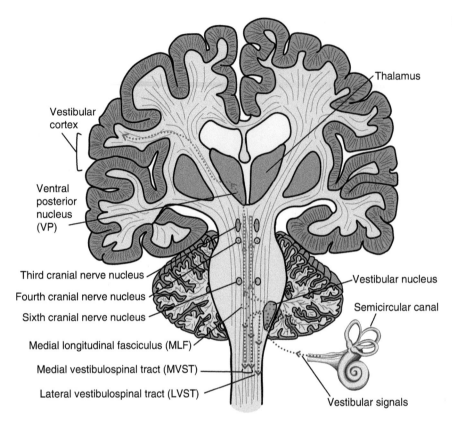

Figure 6.21 The vestibular pathway.

Thalamus

Vestibular cortex

Ventral posterior nucleus (VP)

Third cranial nerve nucleus

Fourth cranial nerve nucleus

Sixth cranial nerve nucleus

Medial longitudinal fasciculus (MLF)

Medial vestibulospinal tract (MVST)

Lateral vestibulospinal tract (LVST)

Vestibular nucleus

Semicircular canal

Vestibular signals

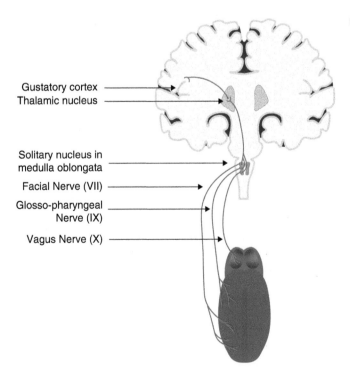

Figure 6.22 The gustatory pathway.

Gustatory cortex
Thalamic nucleus

Solitary nucleus in medulla oblongata

Facial Nerve (VII)

Glosso-pharyngeal Nerve (IX)

Vagus Nerve (X)

Taste Transduction

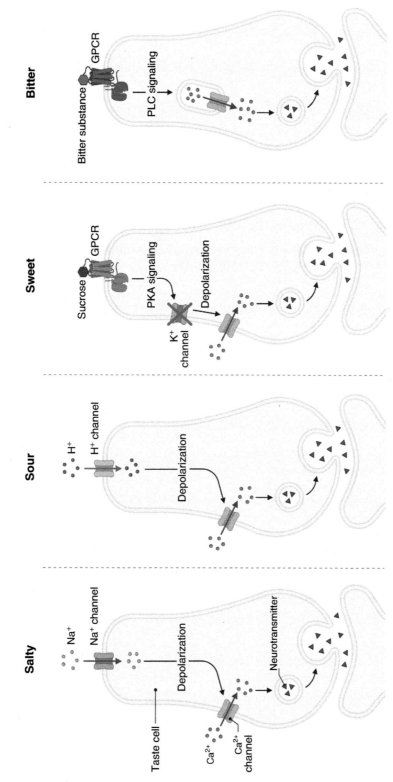

Figure 6.23 Gustatory transduction pathways. GPCR; G-protein-coupled receptor, PKA Protein kinase; PLC; Phospholipase C

These axons enter the brainstem and synapse with the gustatory nucleus, part of the solitary nucleus in the medulla. Gustatory nucleus neurons synapse with neurons in the ventral poster medial nucleus, which then sends axons to the primary gustatory cortex comprised of the anterior insula on the insular lobe and the frontal operculum on the frontal lobe. The taste pathways to the thalamus and cortex are primarily ipsilateral to the cranial nerves that supply them. Some information is also conducted to the hypothalamus, where the lateral and dorsomedial nuclei play an important role in regulating eating behaviors. These nuclei are affected mainly by the hormones leptin and ghrelin, which mediate the balance between satiety and hunger, respectively.

6.6.11 Transduction

The dorsal surface of the mammalian tongue is covered with four kinds of papillae and these are the fungiform, circumvallate, foliate and filiform papillae. Taste buds (gustatory cells) are found on the papillae (except at the filiform papillae). Taste buds consist of columnar cells arranged to form a single taste pore, with surrounding microvilli that contain the taste receptors. These are not neurons; however, they form synapses with endings of the gustatory afferent axons.

Hithero, there are five tastes detected by taste receptor cells (TRCs) - bitter, sweet, umami, sour, and salty. The first three compounds activate TRCs via G-protein coupled receptors (GCPRs), which uses a second messenger system to promote intracellular Ca^{2+} rise followed by ion channel opening and influx of Na+. This leads to depolarization of the cell triggering release of adenosine triphosphate (ATP) activating the purinergic receptors in the taste nerves. An alternative pathway for sweet detection may involve glucose influx via glucose transporters followed by increase of ATP and inhibition of K^+ outflow via the ATPgated potassium (KATP) channels. The kokumi sensation is mediated by the calcium-sensing receptor. Salty and sour compounds both trigger depolarization mediated opening of voltage-gated Na^+ and Ca^{2+} channels, promoting the release of neurotransmitters usually serotonin into the synaptic cleft to bind to afferent taste axons. However salty compounds trigger an initial opening of sodium channels whereas sour tastes involve hydrogenions (proton) entering the cell and triggering the closure of K^+ channels and K^+ efflux.

Figure acknowledgements

The following images were created using a Shutterstock license: Figures 6.1-6.2, 6.6-6.7, 6.12-6.13, 6.15-6.17, 6.19, 6.21, 6.22

The following images were created using a Biorender industrial license: Figures 6.3-6.5, 6.14, 6.18, 6.20, 6.23
The following images are credited to the authors of this chapter: Figures 6.8-6.11

Further Reading

Cheng Z, Gu Y. Vestibular system and self-motion. *Front Cell Neurosci.* 2018;**12**:456. https://doi.org/10.3389/fncel.2018.00456. PMID: 30524247; PMCID: PMC6262063.

Gilbertson TA, Damak S, Margolskee RF. The molecular physiology of taste transduction. *Curr Opin Neurobiol.* 2000;**10**(4):519–27. https://doi.org/10.1016/s0959-4388(00)00118-5. PMID: 10981623.

Howlett M, Smith R, Kamermans M. A novel mechanism of cone photoreceptor adaptation. *PLoS Biology* 2017;**15**(4): e2001210. https://doi.org/10.1371/journal.pbio.2001210.

Iacaruso M, Gasler I, Hofer S. Synaptic organization of visual space in primary visual cortex. *Nature* 2017;**547**(7664):449–52. http://doi.org/10.1038/nature23019.

Khan S, Chang R. Anatomy of the vestibular system: a review. *NeuroRehabilitation* 2013;**32**(3):437–43. https://doi.org/10.3233/NRE-130866. PMID: 23648598.

Kinnamon SC, Finger TE. Recent advances in taste transduction and signaling. *F1000Res* 2019;**8**:F1000 Faculty Rev-2117. https://doi.org/10.12688/f1000research.21099.1. PMID: 32185015; PMCID: PMC7059786.

Lim R, Brichta AM. Anatomical and physiological development of the human inner ear. *Hear Res* 2016;**338**:9–21. https://doi.org/10.1016/j.heares.2016.02.004.

Luo L. *Principles of Neurobiology.* 1st ed. Garland Science, 2015.

Pickles JO. Auditory pathways: anatomy and physiology. *Handb Clin Neurol* 2015;**129**:3–25. https://doi.org/10.1016/B978-0-444-62630-1.00001-9. PMID: 25726260.

Recanzone GH. Perception of auditory signals. *Ann N Y Acad Sci* 2011;**1224**:96–108. https://doi.org/10.1111/j.1749-6632.2010.05920.x.

Simon SA, de Araujo IE, Gutierrez R, Nicolelis MA. The neural mechanisms of gustation: a distributed processing code. *Nat Rev Neurosci* 2006;**7**(11):890–901. https://doi.org/10.1038/nrn2006. PMID: 17053812.

Swienton DJ, Thomas AG. The visual pathway – functional anatomy and pathology. *Semin Ultrasound CT MR* 2014;**35**(5):487–503. https://doi.org/10.1053/j.sult.2014.06.007. Epub 2014 Jun 25. PMID: 25217301.

Usrey W, Alitto H. Visual functions of the thalamus. *Annu Rev Vision Sci* 2015;**1**(1):351–71. https://doi.org/10.1146/annurev-vision-082114-035920.

Widmaier E, Raff H, Strang K. *Vander's Human Physiology.* 13th revised ed. McGraw Hill Higher Education, 2014.

Zhou G, Lane G, Cooper SL, Kahnt T, Zelano C. Characterizing functional pathways of the human olfactory system. *eLife* 2019;**8**:e47177. https://doi.org/10.7554/eLife.47177. PMID: 31339489; PMCID: PMC6656430.

Somatosensory and Somatic Motor Systems

Maria Kaltchenko and Farhana Akter

7.1 The Somatosensory System

The somatosensory system is a network of neurons responsible for conscious perception of touch, pain, pressure, temperature and proprioception. It is a subset of the sensory nervous system that represents the visual, olfactory, auditory, and gustatory pathways discussed in Chapter 6. There are five types of somatosensory receptors: mechanoreceptors, proprioceptors, pain receptors, thermoreceptors, and chemoreceptors.

7.2 Mechanoreceptors

The ability to feel the sensation of touch is due to presence of mechanoreceptors in the skin. There are three classes of mechanoreceptors: tactile, proprioceptors, and baroreceptors. Tactile mechanoreceptors can detect physical deformation and contain mechanically gated ion channels that respond to various stimuli.

There are four types of tactile mechanoreceptors, and these include the Pacinian corpuscle, Meissner corpuscles, Ruffini endings, and Merkel disks (Figure 7.1). Pacinian corpuscles are rapidly adapting and respond to high-frequency vibration. Ruffini endings adapt slowly, respond to stretch and also detect warmth. Meissner corpuscles are sensitive to low frequency vibrations and are involved in fine touch. Merkel disks adapt slowly, sense light touch and contains small receptive fields. The Krause end bulbs were previously thought to be cold receptors, however their full function is unknown. They have been found in the conjunctiva, penile tissue and the clitoris.

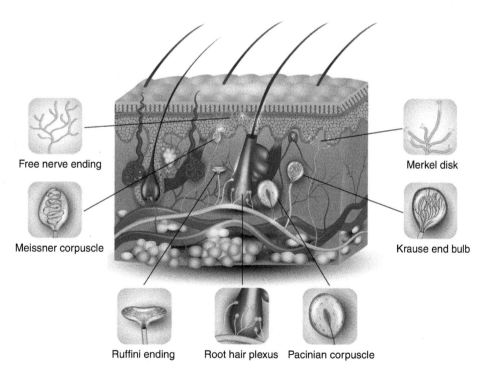

Figure 7.1 Tactile mechanoreceptors of the skin.

Free nerve ending

Merkel disk

Meissner corpuscle

Krause end bulb

Ruffini ending   Root hair plexus   Pacinian corpuscle

7.2.1 Perception of Stimuli

The perception of stimuli is dependent on the distribution of mechanoreceptors and their receptor fields. Nociceptive receptors are typically found near the surface of the skin. The upper layers of the skin also contain the Merkel disks and Meissner corpuscles and are involved in light touch. The deeper layers of skin typically contain the larger Pacinian corpuscles and Ruffini endings and respond to deeper pressure.

A small receptive field allows for precise detection over a smaller region, whereas a larger receptive field allows for detection over a larger area; however, it is less precise. The fingertips typically have densely packed mechanoreceptors with small receptive fields allowing for the detection of fine stimuli. This notable difference is the basis for the two-point discrimination test that can be used to determine the density of receptors and any damage as part of a neurological examination. In this exam, the patient is stimulated with two sharp points and asked to report whether they can feel one or two points. If the patient can detect two separate points, this would suggest that each point is in the receptive field of two separate sensory receptors.

7.3 Nociceptors

Nociceptors, the receptors of pain, are free nerve endings and can be myelinated or unmyelinated. Generally, large-diameter have the greatest conduction velocity followed by Aδ-fibers and finally the C-fibers, which have a small diameter and the slowest conduction velocity (Figure 7.2).

7.4 Thermoreceptors

Thermoreceptors are nerve cells that are sensitive to changes in temperature. These include Ruffini endings,

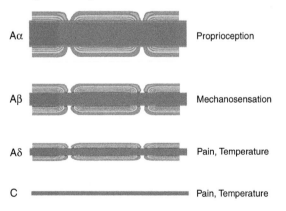

Figure 7.2 Axon fiber types and function.

which detect warmth. There are also warm receptors on free nerve endings that are unmyelinated and cold receptors that are lightly myelinated or unmyelinated.

7.5 Proprioceptors

Proprioceptive stimuli are forces that are generated by the position of a body part. Somatosensory proprioceptive stimuli are combined with vestibular proprioceptive cues and visual cues. There are three types of proprioceptors: muscle spindles in skeletal muscles that signal stretch of muscles; Golgi tendon organs, at the muscles and tendons involved in muscle tension; and joint receptors, in joint capsules.

7.6 Chemoreceptors

Chemoreceptors are specialized sensory receptor cells. They transduce a chemical substance to generate an action potential if the chemoreceptor is a neuron, or activate a nerve fiber if the chemoreceptors are specialized cells such as taste receptors.

7.7 Peripheral Organization of Somatosensory Systems

7.7.1 Primary Afferent Axons

The skin contains axons from the peripheral nervous system (PNS) traveling to the central nervous system (CNS). The morphology of the peripheral somatosensory axon is related to the receptor it innervates and to the sensory information it carries.

Axons bringing information from the somatic sensory receptors to the spinal cord or brain stem are known as the primary afferent axons of the somatic sensory system and enter through the dorsal root ganglion (Figure 7.3). The larger and more heavily myelinated the axon, the greater its conduction velocity. Consequently, the primary afferent axons carrying information required for fine motor control and rapid reflex responses (i.e., those forming body proprioceptors) conduct action potentials rapidly, whereas those carrying information about body and object temperature conduct action potentials at a much slower rate.

7.8 Segmental Organization of the Spinal Cord and Dermatomes

The spinal cord is divided segmentally into cervical, thoracic, lumbar, and sacral divisions. The spinal nerves are named for the level of the spinal cord

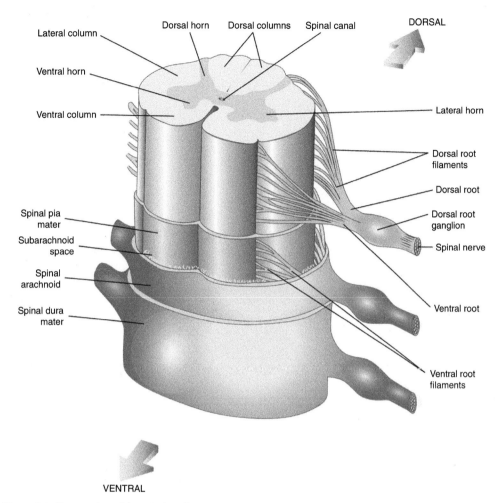

Figure 7.3 Cross-section of the spinal cord.

from which they exit and are numbered from rostral to caudal. The area of the skin that is innervated by the dorsal root of a single spinal segment is called the dermatome (Figure 7.4).

The spinal cord is composed of gray matter surrounded by white matter tracts called columns. The gray matter is separated into horns, with the dorsal horn receiving sensory input from primary afferents (Figure 7.3). Somatosensory neurons are topographically organized so that adjacent neurons represent neighboring regions of the body or face.

7.9 Somatosensory Pathways

The sensory information processed by the somatosensory systems travels along different anatomical pathways depending on the information carried (Figure 7.5).

7.9.1 The Dorsal Column–Medial Lemniscal Pathway

The dorsal column–medial lemniscal (DCML) pathway is important for the passage of information on fine touch, vibration, and proprioception (Figure 7.6). There are three neuronal groups involved in this pathway: first-, second-, and third-order neurons. First-order neurons carry information from the peripheral nerves to the medulla oblongata. Those from lower limb travel in the fasciculus gracilis and then synapse in the nucleus gracilis of the medulla oblongata. Signals from the upper limb travel in the fasciculus cuneatus and synapse in the nucleus cuneatus of the medulla oblongata. The nucleus gracilis and the nucleus cuneatus are the site of origin of second-order neurons, which decussate and travel in the contralateral medial lemniscus before reaching the

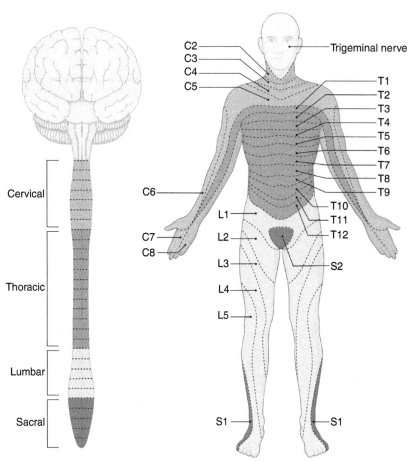

Figure 7.4 Dermatomes.

Sensory Pathways (Ascending)

Figure 7.5 Ascending sensory pathways in cross section.

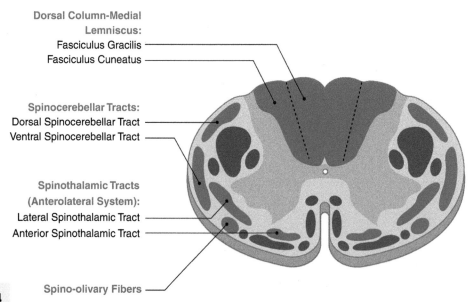

Pathways for the body

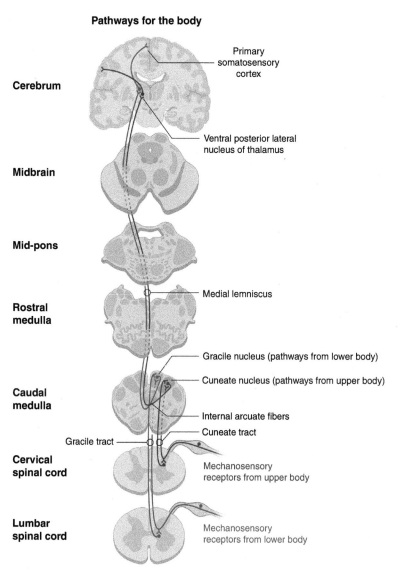

Cerebrum

Midbrain

Mid-pons

Rostral medulla

Caudal medulla

Gracile tract

Cervical spinal cord

Lumbar spinal cord

Primary somatosensory cortex

Ventral posterior lateral nucleus of thalamus

Medial lemniscus

Gracile nucleus (pathways from lower body)

Cuneate nucleus (pathways from upper body)

Internal arcuate fibers

Cuneate tract

Mechanosensory receptors from upper body

Mechanosensory receptors from lower body

Figure 7.6 The dorsal column–medial lemniscal pathway (DCML).

thalamus. The signals from the thalamus travel to the internal capsule and finally to the ipsilateral primary sensory cortex via third-order neurons.

7.9.2 The Trigeminal Touch Pathway

Somatic sensation of the face supplied by the trigeminal nerve enters the brain at the pons. The main sensory trigeminal pathway carries and processes discriminative touch and proprioceptive information from the face. Consequently, it is the cranial homologue of the DCML pathway (Figure 7.7).

7.9.3 The Spinothalamic System

The spinothalamic system is separated into the anterior tract (which transmits the sensation of crude touch and pressure) and the lateral tract (which transmits the sensation of pain and temperature). The first-order neurons travel from the sensory receptors in the periphery to the spinal cord, where they synapse at the substantia gelatinosa of the dorsal horn (Rexed's lamina II) or the marginal zone (lamina I). Information from lamina II is transmitted to second order neurons in laminae IV, V and VI (nucleus proprius); the axons of which cross

Pathway for the face

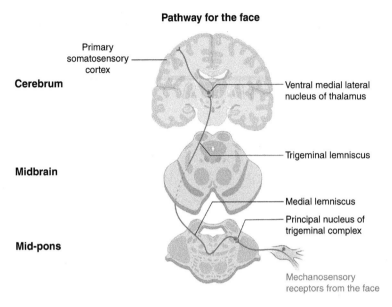

Primary somatosensory cortex

Cerebrum

Ventral medial lateral nucleus of thalamus

Midbrain

Trigeminal lemniscus

Medial lemniscus

Principal nucleus of trigeminal complex

Mid-pons

Mechanosensory receptors from the face

Figure 7.7 The ascending sensory pathway of the face.

midline and ascend to the brainstem and thalamus before decussating into the anterior or lateral tracts. The third-order neurons travel from the thalamus to the ipsilateral primary sensory cortex (Figure 7.8).

7.9.4 The Spinocerebellar Tracts

These tracts carry unconscious information regarding proprioception to the cerebellum. There are four pathways: the posterior spinocerebellar tract (information from the lower limbs to the ipsilateral cerebellum), the cuneocerebellar tract (information from the upper limbs to the ipsilateral cerebellum), the anterior spinocerebellar tract (information from the lower limbs to the ipsilateral cerebellum), and the rostral spinocerebellar tract (information from upper limbs to the ipsilateral cerebellum).

7.10 The Somatic Motor System

The somatic motor system modulates all conscious, volitional movements of the body, in addition to control of involuntary reflex arcs. The somatic motor division of the PNS includes motor axons that connect the CNS to skeletal (striated) effector muscles to initiate voluntary movement, such as lifting a pencil or running, through descending, efferent pathways. Upper motor neurons house their cell bodies in the

cerebral cortex of the brain, including the primary motor cortex, the medial premotor cortex, and the lateral premotor cortex, or in the brainstem, and exert higher-level control of voluntary movement. Axons of the upper motor neurons synapse with local circuit interneurons or directly onto lower motor neurons; upper motor neurons transmit impulses to lower motor neurons through the neurotransmitter glutamate. Lower motor neurons house their cell bodies in the ventral horn of the spinal cord or brainstem motor nuclei and directly innervate skeletal muscles to initiate voluntary movement. Whereas descending pathways from upper motor neurons play a role in the top-down modulation of local circuits in the spinal cord, it is the excitation of lower motor neurons that directly results in the axonal release of acetylcholine at neuromuscular junctions and the initiation of muscular contractions. Local circuits in the spinal cord and brainstem modulate in the activity of lower motor neurons by integrating sensory input and stimulation from upper motor neurons, in the extrapyramidal tracts.

7.11 Descending Motor Pathways

The motor tracts can be divided into the pyramidal tracts, which originate in the cerebral cortex and send fibers to the spinal cord and brainstem, and the extrapyramidal tracts, which originate in the brainstem and carry fibers to the spinal cord (Figure 7.9). Neurons from these tracts

Figure 7.8 Pain pathways to the face and body.

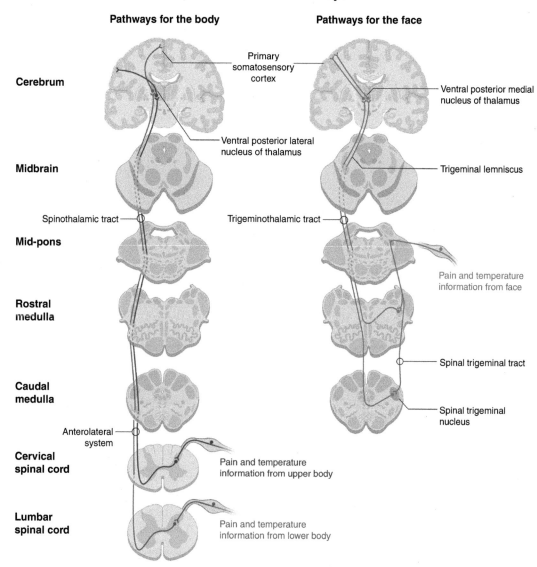

Discriminative Pain Pathways

Pathways for the body

Pathways for the face

Cerebrum

Primary somatosensory cortex

Ventral posterior medial nucleus of thalamus

Ventral posterior lateral nucleus of thalamus

Midbrain

Trigeminal lemniscus

Spinothalamic tract

Trigeminothalamic tract

Mid-pons

Pain and temperature information from face

Rostral medulla

Caudal medulla

Spinal trigeminal tract

Spinal trigeminal nucleus

Anterolateral system

Cervical spinal cord

Pain and temperature information from upper body

Lumbar spinal cord

Pain and temperature information from lower body

(upper motor neurons) synapse with lower motor neurons at their termination.

Two major descending tracts originating from the cerebral cortex include the corticospinal tract, in which upper motor neurons directly synapse with interneurons or lower motor neurons in the spinal cord to control movement of the trunk and limbs, and the corticobulbar tract, in which upper motor neurons synapse with lower motor neurons of the cranial nerves in the brainstem to control the musculature of the head, face, and neck.

Together, the corticospinal tract and the corticobulbar tract comprise the descending pyramidal tracts of the motor system (Figure 7.10).

7.12 Corticospinal Tract

The corticospinal tract is the principal descending pathway in humans and receives inputs from the primary motor cortex, the premotor cortex, and the supplemental motor area. It also receives nerve fibers from the somatosensory area, which regulates activity of the ascending tracts. The

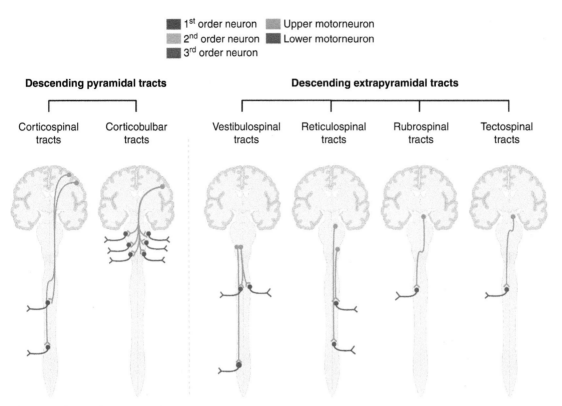

1st order neuron   Upper motorneuron
2nd order neuron   Lower motorneuron
3rd order neuron

Descending pyramidal tracts   **Descending extrapyramidal tracts**

Corticospinal   Corticobulbar   Vestibulospinal   Reticulospinal   Rubrospinal   Tectospinal
tracts   tracts   tracts   tracts   tracts   tracts

Figure 7.9 Descending motor pathways.

fibers descend through the internal capsule to the crus cerebri of the midbrain and the pons, finally emerging as the medullary pyramids in the ventral medulla. They divide into the crossed lateral corticospinal tract and terminate in the ventral horn of all segmental levels of the spinal cord and supply the muscles of the body. The uncrossed ventral corticospinal tract remains ipsilateral, descends in the spinal cord, and terminates in the ventral horn of the cervical and upper thoracic segmental levels.

Damage to the corticospinal tracts commonly at the site of the internal capsule, frequently occurs during a stroke. This leads to contralateral signs including hypertonia, hyperreflexia, muscle weakness, clonus, and the Babinski sign (dorsiflexion of the hallux upon stimulation of the lateral plantar aspect of the foot).

7.13 Corticobulbar Tract

This tract arises from the lateral aspect of the primary motor cortex and receives the same inputs as the corticospinal tract. The output fibers pass through the internal capsule to the brainstem. The neurons terminate on the motor nuclei of the cranial nerves and synapse with lower motor neurons, which carry the motor signals to the muscles of the face and neck. The fibers typically innervate the motor neurons bilaterally and therefore lesions usually lead to mild muscle weakness. However, the facial nerve and the hypoglossal nerve only receive contralateral innervation and, therefore, lesions to the facial nerve lead to spastic paralysis of the muscles in the contralateral lower quadrant of the face. Lesions of the hypoglossal nerve lead to spastic paralysis of the contralateral tongue with deviation to the contralateral side. In a lower motor neuron lesion, the tongue deviates toward the damaged side.

7.14 Extrapyramidal Tracts

The four extrapyramidal tracts begin in the brainstem and carry fibers to the spinal cord, and are responsible for involuntary control of muscle tone, balance, posture, and locomotion. The two ipsilateral tracts, which do not decussate, are the vestibulospinal and reticulospinal tracts, and the rubrospinal and tectospinal tracts provide contralateral innervation.

(a)

Somatic Motor System

**Descending Motor Pathways:
Corticospinal Tract**

Figure 7.10 Pyramidal pathways.

*1. Cell bodies of **upper motor neurons** originate in the cerebral cortex*

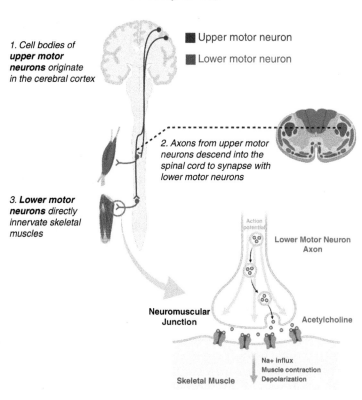

■ Upper motor neuron

■ Lower motor neuron

2. Axons from upper motor neurons descend into the spinal cord to synapse with lower motor neurons

*3. **Lower motor neurons** directly innervate skeletal muscles*

Action potential

Lower Motor Neuron Axon

Neuromuscular Junction

Acetylcholine

Na+ influx
Muscle contraction
Depolarization

Skeletal Muscle

(b)

**Descending Motor Pathways:
Corticobulbar Tract**

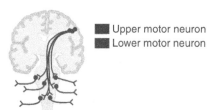

■ Upper motor neuron
■ Lower motor neuron

The corticobulbar tract connects upper motor neurons in the cortex with lower motor neurons in brainstem motor nuclei to control musculature of the face, neck, and head.

7.14.1 Vestibulospinal Tracts

The medial and lateral tracts arise in the vestibular nuclei and convey balance and posture information to the spinal cord. They also control the antigravity muscles (flexors of the arm and extensors of the leg) via lower motor neurons.

7.14.2 Reticulospinal Tracts

The medial reticulospinal tract originates in the pons and controls voluntary movements and increases muscle tone. The lateral reticulospinal tract originates in the medulla and inhibits voluntary movements and reduces muscle tone.

7.14.3 Rubrospinal Tract

The rubrospinal tract originates in the red nucleus, traveling to the spinal cord following decussation. It is thought to play a role in the fine control of hand movements.

7.14.4 Tectospinal Tract

This tract originates in the superior colliculus of the midbrain, which receives input from the optic nerves. The fibers decussate and enter the spinal cord and terminate at the cervical levels to coordinate movements of the head in relation to vision stimuli.

7.15 Lower Motor Neuron

Lower motor neurons house their cell bodies in the brainstem and the ventral horn of the spinal cord, directly projecting their axons to innervate individual extrafusal muscle fibers and initiate muscular contractions. The ventral horn of the spinal cord, which is organized somatotopically, constitutes the gray matter of the spinal cord that holds the lower motor neurons' cell bodies. Lower motor neurons innervating distal muscles are mapped laterally on the ventral horn, while motor neurons associated with axial musculature are mapped medially (Figure 7.11). A single lower motor neuron innervates a set of muscle fibers from a single muscle; together, the lower motor neuron and its associated muscle fibers comprise a motor unit. A motor pool includes all motor units that correspond to a single muscle. Motor neurons with small cell bodies that innervate slow but fatigue-resistant fibers are usually recruited before motor neurons with larger cell bodies which innervate fast, fatigable muscle fibers (known as the Henneman size principle).

Alpha motor neurons are the most numerous of the lower motor neurons and are responsible for the initiation of movements through the excitation of extrafusal muscle fibers. In other words, alpha motor neurons directly mediate force-generating activation of skeletal muscle fibers that results in muscular contractions (thereby altering the length of the muscle and generating force for movement). By contrast, gamma motor neurons innervate intrafusal muscle fibers and are heavily implicated in involuntary motor control related to maintaining muscular tone. Although gamma motor neurons are not directly responsible for the contraction of muscle fibers, they are involved in the maintenance of muscle spindle sensitivity and play a supplementary role in the myotatic stretch reflex by modulating tension in intrafusal muscle fibers within the muscle spindle. Without the supporting role of gamma motor neurons, the activity of the Ia afferent in the myotatic reflex would decrease as the muscle contracts; co-activation of alpha and gamma motor neurons is thus necessary to maintain appropriate levels of excitability of the muscle spindle in the stretch reflex.

7.16 Myotatic Reflex

The myotatic reflex is a monosynaptic reflex arc between Ia afferents and alpha motor neurons that takes place involuntarily at the level of the spinal cord in response to mechanical stretch, without input from the descending pathways of the brain (Figure 7.12). In response to mechanical stretch, proprioceptive receptors of the muscle spindle activate the Ia afferent, which synapses directly with the alpha motor neuron that innervates the homonymous extensor muscle in the spinal cord. The proprioceptive muscle spindle is located in the belly of the muscle and functions to detect changes in muscle length. Composed of intrafusal muscle fibers that are ensheathed by the processes of the Ia axon, the muscle spindle can be thought of as the "transduction apparatus" of the myotatic reflex arc, converting the mechanical stimulus of the tap to an electrical signal via depolarization of the Ia axon. The magnitude of the mechanical stimulus directly correlates with the magnitude of the depolarization of the Ia axon, encoding sensory information (namely stretch intensity) into the amplitude of the corresponding stretch receptor potential.

If the Ia axon is brought to threshold through mechanical stretching of the muscle spindle, the intensity of the mechanical stretch – and by proxy the amplitude of the corresponding receptor potential – is then encoded into the frequency of action potentials that propagate via the Ia axon, through the dorsal root ganglion, into the spinal cord. In the spinal cord, the afferent Ia axon synapses with the alpha motor neuron that innervates the extensor muscle, which in turn releases acetylcholine at the neuromuscular junction. Finally, after a latency of about 20 milliseconds, the extensor muscle extends, completing the myotatic reflex arc and relieving the stretch of the muscle spindle. The comparatively short latency of the myotatic

reflex reflects the local nature of this circuit in the spinal cord, with no input from higher-order neural centers. It is important to note that whereas the monosynaptic reflex arc itself consists of a two-neuron circuit – the Ia afferent and the alpha motor efferent that innervates the extensor muscle – there is simultaneous inhibition of the antagonistic flexor muscle that is mediated by an inhibitory interneuron through a process called reciprocal inhibition. The clinically salient patellar reflex test takes advantage of the monosynaptic reflex arc to assess the proper functioning of the L2, L3, and L4 levels of the spinal cord: a reflex hammer strikes the patellar tendon below the knee, stretching the muscle spindle in the quadriceps. An electric impulse is then propagated via the Ia afferent to the spinal cord, where it synapses with an alpha motor neuron that innervates the quadriceps femoris muscle. Simultaneously, the Ia afferent synapses with an inhibitory interneuron that innervates the antagonistic hamstrings muscle, relaxing it. As a result of this negative feedback loop, the quadriceps muscle contracts and the leg extends, returning the muscle to a physiologically appropriate length.

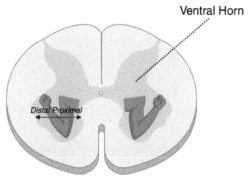

Somatotopic organization of the ventral horn of the spinal cord: lower motor neurons innervating distal muscles are found laterally in the ventral horn, while those innervating proximal muscles are located medially.

Figure 7.11 Somatotopic organization of the ventral horn of the spinal cord.

7.17 Golgi Tendon Organs

Golgi tendon organs are proprioceptive mechanoreceptors found in the collagen fibers of tendons that receive

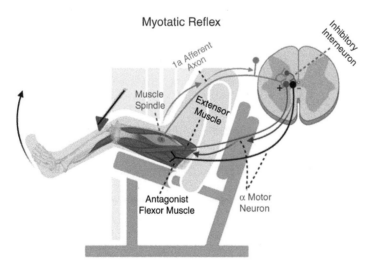

1. Tap of the patellar tendon mechanically stretches the muscle spindle and produces a burst of action potentials in 1a afferent fibers.

2. 1a axons synapse with alpha motor neurons of the same extensor muscle (here, the quadriceps) in the spinal cord, initiating muscular contraction and extension.

3. Simultaneously, 1a axons synapse with inhibitory interneurons that innervate α motor neurons of the antagonist flexor muscle (here, the hamstrings), relaxing it.

Figure 7.12 Myotatic reflex.

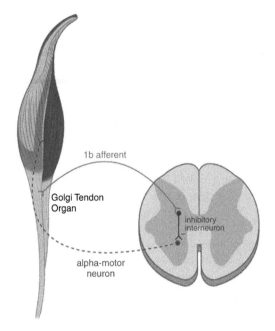

Golgi Tendon Organ: Inverse Myotatic Reflex

1. Sensory information regarding muscular tension is transmitted from Golgi Tendon Organ via 1b afferents.
2. 1b afferents synapse with inhibitory interneurons in the spinal cord.
3. Contraction of the muscle is inhibited through decreased firing of alpha-motor neurons.

Figure 7.13 Golgi tendon organ.

information regarding muscular tension (Figure 7.13). They mediate the Golgi tendon reflex, also known as the inverse myotatic reflex, a negative feedback mechanism that ensures that muscles do not tear from excessive contraction. While the muscle spindle responds to changes in muscular length, the Golgi tendon reflex can be thought of as the force-activated, inhibitory counterpart to the myotatic reflex, inhibiting alpha motor neurons from firing through inhibitory postsynaptic potentials (IPSPs). Sensory information regarding muscular tension is transmitted from Golgi tendon organs via 1b afferents, which synapse with inhibitory local circuit neurons in the spinal cord. Finally, these 1b inhibitory interneurons connect with alpha motor neurons that innervate the homonymous muscle, decreasing its level of activation and thereby preventing it from tearing. While the Golgi tendon organ circuit is localized in the spinal cord, this system can be modulated through descending information from upper neurons, input from muscle spindles, and other sensory receptors.

7.18 Central Pattern Generator

Central pattern generators are neural circuits in the spinal cord and brainstem that produce rhythmic, coordinated contractions of different muscles without input from descending pathways and in the absence of sensory feedback. Highly stereotyped, oscillatory motor behaviors, including respiration and walking, are organized by the local neuronal networks that comprise central pattern generators. These networks include both excitatory and inhibitory neurons that generate patterned motor behaviors.

Figure acknowledgements

The following images were created using a Shutterstock license: Figure 7.1, 7.3
The following image is credited to the authors of this chapter: Figure 7.2
The following images were created using a Biorender industrial license: Figures 7.4-7.13

Further Reading

Bellingham MC. Driving respiration: the respiratory central pattern generator. *Clin Exp Pharmacol Physiol* 1998;**25**(10):847–56.

Binder MD, Kroin JS, Moore GP, Stuart DG. The response of Golgi tendon organs to single motor unit contractions. *J Physiol* 1977;**271**(2):337–49.

Colón A, Guo X, Akanda N, Cai Y, Hickman JJ. Functional analysis of human intrafusal fiber innervation by human γ-motoneurons. *Sci Rep* 2017;**7**(1):17202. https://doi.org/10.1038/s41598-017-17382-2.

Fallon JB, Macefield VG. Vibration sensitivity of human muscle spindles and Golgi tendon organs. *Muscle Nerve* 2007;**36**(1):21–9. https://doi.org/10.1002/mus.20796.

Friese A, Kaltschmidt JA, Ladle DR, Sigrist M, Jessell TM, Arber S. Gamma and alpha motor neurons distinguished by expression of transcription factor Err3. *PNAS* [Internet] 2009 [cited 2021 Feb 8];**106**(32):13588–93. www.pnas.org/content/106/32/13588

Hunt CC, Kuffler SW. Stretch receptor discharges during muscle contraction. *J Physiol* 1951;**113**(2–3):298–315.

Johnson KO. The roles and functions of cutaneous mechanoreceptors. *Curr Opin Neurobiol* 2001;**11**(4):455–61. https://doi.org/10.1016/s0959-4388(00)00234-8. PMID: 11502392.

Lyle MA, Nichols TR. Evaluating intermuscular Golgi tendon organ feedback with twitch contractions. *J Physiol* 2019;**597**(17):4627–42.

Marder E, Calabrese RL. Principles of rhythmic motor pattern generation. *Physiol Rev* 1996;**76**(3):687–717.

Minassian K, Hofstoetter US, Dzeladini F, Guertin PA, Ijspeert A. The human central pattern generator for locomotion: does it exist and contribute to walking? *Neuroscientist* 2017;**23**(6):649–63.

Nielsen JB, Morita H, Wenzelburger R, Deuschl G, Gossard J-P, Hultborn H. Recruitment gain of spinal motor neuron pools in cat and human. *Exp Brain Res* 2019;**237** (11):2897–909.

Pearson K. The control of walking. *Sci Am* 1976;**235**(6):72–4, 79–82, 83–6. https://doi.org/10.1038/scientificamerican1276-72.

Stephens JA, Reinking RM, Stuart DG. Tendon organs of cat medial gastrocnemius: responses to active and passive forces as a function of muscle length. *J Neurophysiol* 1975;**38**(5):1217–31. https://doi.org/10.1152/jn .1975.38.5.1217.

ten Donkelaar HJ, Broman J, van Domburg P. The somatosensory system. In *Clinical Neuroanatomy*. Springer, 2020: 171–255.

Watson C, Kayalionglu G (Eds.). *The Spinal Cord.* Elsevier, 2009.

Windhorst U. Spinal cord and brainstem: motor output, sensors and basic circuits. In Greger R, Windhorst U (Eds.), *Comprehensive Human Physiology: From Cellular Mechanisms to Integration.* Springer, 1996: 987–1006. https://doi.org/10 .1007/978-3-642-60946-6_50.

Chapter 8

Neuron Models

Kumaresh Krishnan

8.1 Spiking Neuron

We are now familiar with the generation of action potentials by neurons. These all-or-nothing events are often referred to as spikes due to their appearance in a sufficiently zoomed-out timescale (Figure 8.1).

However, what information has been transmitted within these spikes and how will this information be further processed? How do neurons represent action potentials at the levels of individual cells or a network of cells? This process is usually termed neural encoding and retrieval of this information from the analysis of an action potential spike train is termed neural decoding.

Reading, interpreting, and writing the neural code is a challenge in neuroscience. This is partly due spiking neuron models only providing information of certain observed phenomena of the brain. Indeed, the information retrieved cannot explain many other unanswered questions about the rest of the brain.

Viewing the neuron as an electrical system gives an easy handle into modeling the generation and transmission of action potentials. In the simplest version of this framework, the entire neuron can be viewed as having a single membrane potential. Models built on this assumption are termed "single-compartment" models. A more detailed assessment of the spatial variation in membrane potential gives rise to "multi-compartment" models. We now look at the basic electrical properties of spiking neurons that are essential to most models.

(i) Membrane potential – The difference in voltage between the outside of the neuronal membrane and the inside. Conventionally, the outside of the neuron is assumed to be at zero volts, so the membrane potential is a measure of how positive or negative the inside of the neuron is with respect to the outside.

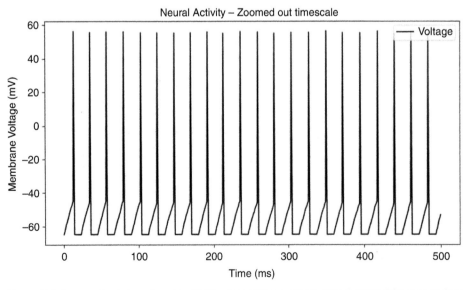

Figure 8.1 A zoomed-out view of a series of action potentials in a neuron. Note the resemblance to "spikes."

(ii) Longitudinal resistance – Axons and dendrites can be thought of as long cables (wires) that allow ions to flow through them. The medium through which these ions move offers a certain resistance to the flow and is termed axial resistance, R_L. This quantity is proportional to the length of the cable and inversely proportional to the cross-sectional area of the cable, πa^2 (Figure 8.2). An intuitive way to understand this is by noting that a greater circumference provides more space for ion flow whereas a thin cable restricts the space available for flow. The constant of proportionality, r_L, is termed "specific resistance," a property of the medium through which the ions travel.

$$R_L = \frac{r_L \cdot x}{\pi a^2}. \tag{Eq. 8.1}$$

(iii) Membrane resistance – When small quantities of current are injected into the membrane of a neuron (e.g., through an electrode), the membrane potential will change by a small amount, ΔV. This difference depends on the resistance of the membrane R_m and follows Ohm's law,

$$\Delta V = R_m \cdot I. \tag{Eq. 8.2}$$

(iv) Membrane capacitance – A capacitor in electrical systems is a device that can accumulate charge. From our knowledge of a neuron's resting potential (around –65 mV), we know that the inside of the neuron has more negative charge compared to the outside. As charges of opposite signs attract, there is a buildup of excess negative charges close to the inner side of the membrane and excess positive charges cluster toward the outer side of the membrane. This setup resembles a capacitor, and the property "capacitance" is a measure of the stored charge in the membrane. The excess charge at the membrane Q is proportional to the membrane potential V. They are related by a quantity C_m, referred to as membrane capacitance.

$$Q = C_m \cdot V. \tag{Eq. 8.3}$$

Electrical current is the flow of charge per unit time and a simple time derivative on both sides of Equation 8.3 yields

$$I \equiv \frac{dQ}{dt} = C_m \frac{dV}{dt}. \tag{Eq. 8.4}$$

Equation 8.4 shows that current of a given magnitude flowing into the cell will change the potential of the membrane at a rate determined by the membrane capacitance C_m. Membrane capacitance is proportional to the surface area A. In this case, the constant of proportionality c_m is termed specific capacitance.

$$C_m = c_m \cdot A. \tag{Eq. 8.5}$$

(v) Membrane time constant – The changes to membrane potential occur on timescales dictated by the membrane capacitance and membrane resistance. The product of the two quantities R_m and C_m has the units of time and is referred to as the membrane time constant (τ_m).

(vi) Conductance – For any quantity indicating resistance, its inverse is termed conductance, g.

(vii) Membrane current – The net current flowing across the membrane is termed membrane current. This includes current through various channels and leakage currents. Conventionally, membrane current is positive when net positive ion flow is out of the cell.

(viii) Equilibrium (reversal) potential – Ions flow through channels in the membrane of a neuron from a region of higher concentration to a region of lower concentration. Excess positive and negative charges line up near the outer and inner sides of the membrane, respectively, which causes an electrical gradient and thereby an electrical potential that opposes the concentration gradient. The value of the electrical potential at which the concentration gradient and electrical gradients are equal and opposite is termed the equilibrium potential, E. This potential depends on the kind of channel, its ion selectivity, etc. The current through any of these channels is proportional to the difference in the membrane potential V and the equilibrium potential for the given channel. The constant of proportionality denoted by g is the conductance of the channel.

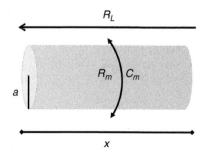

Figure 8.2 A short cable segment of length x with a radius a is shown. The longitudinal resistance R_L is computed along the length of the cable. Membrane resistance R_m and membrane capacitance C_m are computed along the surface area of the cable.

$$I = g(V - E).\qquad\text{(Eq. 8.6)}$$

The difference between membrane potential and equilibrium potential $(V - E)$ is often called *driving force*.

Having defined some basic electrical properties of neurons, we can now formulate a simple single-compartment neuron model.

8.2 Integrate and Fire Neuron

This is one of the earliest proposed models (Lapicque, 1907). The underlying principle is almost self-explanatory – the neuron fires an action potential after reaching a threshold voltage, V_{th}. After firing, the membrane potential returns to a value lower than threshold, V_{reset}. We begin by expressing the total current entering the neuron in terms of the membrane current I_m and injected electrode current I_e. (Remember, membrane current is positive when flowing outward, hence the negative sign for I_m.)

$$I_{net} = -I_m + I_e.\qquad\text{(Eq. 8.7)}$$

Using the expression for I_{net} from Equation 8.4:

$$C_m \frac{dV}{dt} = -I_m + I_e.\qquad\text{(Eq. 8.8)}$$

Making the simplification that all membrane conductances can be bundled as a single "leak" term, we can replace the membrane current by a leak conductance and the corresponding driving force:

$$C_m \frac{dV}{dt} = -g_L(V - E_L) + I_e.\qquad\text{(Eq. 8.9)}$$

This formulation is called the "leaky integrate-and-fire" model. Here, E_L represents a quantity that is similar to the resting potential of the neuron because it houses all the membrane conductances. The equation can be modified by multiplying every term with the membrane resistance T_m, to exploit the fact that the product of R_m and C_m is the membrane time constant τ_m.

$$\tau_m \frac{dV}{dt} = E_L - V + R_m.I_e.\qquad\text{(Eq. 8.10)}$$

We have successfully arrived at the first model of a neuron. The assumptions outlined in the process hold good for some neurons, especially when the conductances are not too sensitive to small fluctuations in the membrane potential. The integrate-and-fire model does not attempt to capture the biophysical mechanisms of action potential generation and treats it as an all-or-nothing event once the threshold voltage is crossed.

Nevertheless, the simplicity of this model allows a quick and cursory analysis of the response of a neuron to injected current. The analytical solution to Equation 8.10 can be used to solve for the membrane potential given an injected current, based on values for other parameters in the equation. For completeness, the analytical solution is given below:

$$V(t) = E_L + R_m.I_e + (V(0) - E_L - R_m.I_e)\exp(-t/\tau_m).\qquad\text{(Eq. 8.11)}$$

Here t denotes time and $V(0)$ is the membrane potential at time $t = 0$.

In the actual biophysics of an action potential, there is a large increase of conductance closer to the spike. This is not accounted for by the passive integrate-and-fire model. The present model is analogous to an electrical circuit with a resistor and capacitor in parallel (Figure 8.3).

We now look at models that attempt to include information about conductance of ion channels that are important for action potentials.

8.3 Hodgkin–Huxley Model

This model was proposed by Alan Hodgkin and Andrew Huxley in 1952. The aim was to include ionic mechanisms behind generation of an action potential. The basis of this formulation differs from the integrate-and-fire (IF) neuron in one key aspect – membrane current. The simple IF neuron bundles the entire membrane current as a single "leak" term. We can break down the current into few key components: (i) sodium current, (ii) potassium current, and (iii) leak current. Two dominant ion channels responsible for the generation of an action potential are the sodium (Na^+) and potassium (K^+) channels. The conductances associated with them see a huge increase closer to the firing of the action potential. Unlike the previous model, the conductance is not constant, but voltage-dependent, which is a crucial aspect for detailed neuron modeling.

The starting point of the model is identical to Equation 8.8:

$$C_m \frac{dV}{dt} = -I_m + I_e.\qquad\text{(Eq. 8.12)}$$

The term denoting membrane current now has three components to be considered – Na^+, K^+, and leak currents. This is incorporated into the equation using the appropriate conductance and driving force.

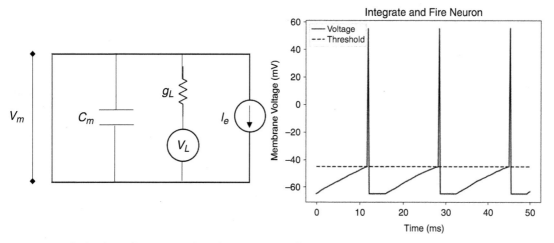

Figure 8.3 Left: The electrical circuit equivalent of an integrate-and-fire neuron including a resistor and current source for leak components, a capacitor for the membrane, and a current source for the injected electrode current. Right: A sample response from a simulation for an integrate-and-fire neuron. The neuron spikes after integrating until a threshold value (–45 mV in this case).

$$C_m \frac{dV}{dt} = -[g_{Na}(V - E_{Na}) + g_K(V - E_K) + g_L(V - E_L)] + I_e.$$

(Eq. 8.13)

A term for leak currents persists, but this now primarily includes the activity of the sodium/potassium pump in neurons and leakage through a small number of ion channels that may be open at rest. While Equation 8.13 provides a reasonably detailed description of the ion channels, it still lacks some essential biophysical details. As the membrane potential nears the threshold voltage, more channels open. At a certain point, the Na$^+$ channels are inactivated, which is a gradual process rather than a switch-like mechanism. Additionally, the K$^+$ channels, which are responsible for bringing the membrane potential back toward rest, take longer to open. Fewer open channels must reflect in the total conductance of the associated ion channel.

To capture these aspects, three quantities called "gating variables" are added to Equation 8.13. They can be interpreted as the extent of opening or inactivation for the specific ion channel. For example, if 50% of the Na$^+$ channels are open, one can naively expect the conductance to also be around 50% of the peak value. Keeping with this idea, the conductance terms in Equation 8.13 represent peak values. The introduction of gating variables m, h, n gives rise to the following equation:

$$C_m \frac{dV}{dt} = -[g_{Na}.m^3 h(V - E_{Na}) + g_K.n^4(V - E_K)$$

$$+ g_L(V - E_L)] + I_e.$$

(Eq. 8.14)

Hodgkin and Huxley used the structure of ion channels to arrive at the appropriate exponent for the gating variables. For example, the K$^+$ channel has four subunits, each of which needs to undergo a specific change in order to facilitate conduction of ions. Hodgkin and Huxley modeled these steps as independent events and noted that the probability of an entire channel to be open can be expressed in terms of the number of subunits and the likelihood of each subunit to be open.

$$P = p^k.$$

(Eq. 8.15)

Here, p refers to the probability of an individual subunit being open, and k is the total number of subunits. In the Hodgkin–Huxley formulation of Equation 8.14, k channels have an associated gating variable n that is raised to the fourth power. The Na$^+$ channels have an inactivation component in addition to opening/closing. In Equation 8.14, the inactivation probability is represented by h and the activation by m. Hodgkin and Huxley found that the structure of Na$^+$ channels and their consequent rates of opening are well captured by Equation 8.15 with $k = 3$.

As a mathematical aside, each of these gating variables is governed by differential equations of a similar form:

$$\frac{dp}{dt} = \alpha_p(V)(1 - p) - \beta_p(V)(p).$$

(Eq. 8.16)

The terms $\alpha_p(V)$ and $\beta_p(V)$ are voltage-dependent terms that describe the rate at which a channel transitions to open and closed, respectively. The probability of opening is denoted by p. The different gating variables m, h, n used by Hodgkin and Huxley differ in the construction of $\alpha_p(V)$ and $\beta_p(V)$. In Equation 8.16, p is a placeholder for m, n, or h. The closed channels at a given instant are the ones that can transition to open and vice versa. This justifies why $\alpha_p(V)$ is multiplied by the probability of closed channels and $\beta_p(V)$ is multiplied by the probability of open channels. The net rate of opening will be a difference between the individual rates of opening and closing.

The evolution of membrane potential in a Hodgkin–Huxley framework along with the changes in gating variables is shown in Figure 8.4. The sudden increase in Na$^+$ conductance near the threshold voltage is mirrored by an increase in m. During this time, the inactivation of Na$^+$ channels decrease, which is reflected in the trace of h. After the peak of the action potential, the inactivation of Na$^+$ channels increases again. The K$^+$ channels, also known as delayed rectifiers, start opening closer to the peak of the action potential and increase as the membrane potential heads toward rest, represented by n. Closer to rest, the K$^+$ channels slowly close, resulting in a lowering of n.

The Hodgkin–Huxley model succeeds in providing a compact description of the non-linear process that is typical of an action potential. It is possible to extend this model to a multi-compartment form as well. At the same time, for cursory analyses, the number of parameters present in the model can be cumbersome. In the simple version outlined in this section, the complicated process of channel dynamics is bundled into just four variables (V, m, n, h). However, the gating variables that treat activation and inactivation of channels as independent events make a simplification that does not necessarily hold true. The Hodgkin–Huxley model matches other formulations (e.g., Markov models that consider the opening of a channel as a transition through different states, each with associated probabilities) when there are many channels. The accuracy dips when considering single-channel dynamics. Nevertheless, the Hodgkin–Huxley formalism provides valuable insight into modeling the biophysical mechanisms of action potential generation.

8.4 Cable Theory

The models addressed up to now have treated the neuron as a single compartment with a uniform membrane potential. In reality, there can be considerable spatial variation in the membrane potential. Voltage gradients allow current to flow in neurons. Typically, voltage decays with distance when traveling along dendritic or axonal cables. Modeling the voltage along these cables now addresses both space and time. For these purposes, the "cables" are assumed to be narrow enough that longitudinal current is a dominant factor and radial current is negligible. The fundamental

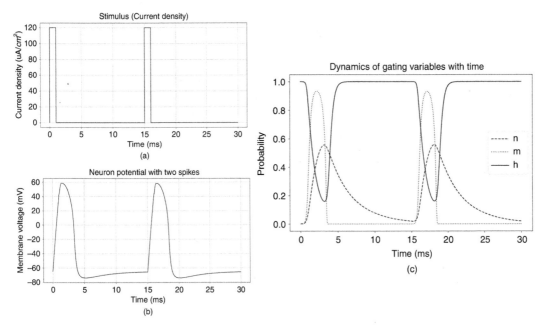

Figure 8.4 (a) Simulation of two action potentials over 30 ms using the Hodgkin–Huxley formulation. (b) The current injection that generates the action potential. (c) The values of gating variables m, n, and h over the 30 ms duration – notice the inversion in h, which represents inactivation of Na channels, whereas m and n are related to activation.

question in cable theory is to determine the voltage $V(x,t)$, where x is the spatial location and t is time.

Treating the cable as a cylinder, the initial step is to compute the resistance of a small segment of the cable (Figure 8.2). Recall from the section on electrical properties of neurons that the longitudinal resistance R_L is

$$R_L = \frac{r_L.x}{\pi a^2}. \tag{Eq. 8.17}$$

In the current framework of a small longitudinal section, we will denote the length of the small cable segment as Δx. The associated voltage drop ΔV across this cable segment can be related to the current I_L using Ohm's law:

$$\Delta V = I_L.\frac{r_L.\Delta x}{\pi a^2}. \tag{Eq. 8.18}$$

Rearranging these terms gives an expression for the longitudinal current through a small cable segment:

$$I_L = -\frac{\pi a^2}{r_L}\frac{\Delta V}{\Delta x}. \tag{Eq. 8.19}$$

The direction of current on a dendrite is toward the soma, whereas the increase in length Δx is away from the soma. Because the convention treats current flowing in the direction of increasing length as positive, a negative sign has been added to the expression in Equation 8.19. By considering an infinitesimally short cable segment ($\Delta x \rightarrow 0$), the expression for current can be turned into a spatial derivative of voltage:

$$I_L = -\frac{\pi a^2}{r_L}\frac{\partial V}{\partial x}. \tag{Eq. 8.20}$$

The cable theory set out to capture $V(x,t)$ and we have currently addressed the spatial variation of voltage. How does time get factored into this analysis? Remember that membrane potential fluctuations due to current flow occur at rates determined by the capacitance of the region. Further, from Equation 8.5, the capacitance of a region can be obtained using the surface area and the specific capacitance c_m. In our consideration of a short cable segment with length Δx, the capacitance of the segment is:

$$C_m = 2\pi a \Delta x c_m. \tag{Eq. 8.21}$$

The current required to change the membrane potential with the above capacitance is obtained with the help of Equation 8.4 (as membrane potential $V(x,t)$ is now varying with space and time, a partial derivative ∂ must be used alongside the temporal component):

$$I = 2\pi a \Delta x c_m \frac{\partial V}{\partial t}. \tag{Eq. 8.22}$$

To formulate the "cable equation," we note that the above current is the net result of all currents entering and leaving the cable segment. These components include (i) current entering from the neighboring segment, (ii) current leaving from the neighboring segment, (iii) membrane current leaving the segment radially outward, and (iv) electrode current injected radially inward. These components are shown in Figure 8.5.

Using the same convention for current – positive in the direction of increasing cable length (away from the soma) – we equate all the current components to the net current changing the membrane potential.

$$2\pi a \Delta x c_m \frac{\partial V}{\partial t} = -\left(\frac{\pi a^2}{r_L}\frac{\partial V}{\partial x}\right)_{left} + \left(\frac{\pi a^2}{r_L}\frac{\partial V}{\partial x}\right)_{right}$$
$$-2\pi a \Delta x (i_m - i_e). \tag{Eq. 8.23}$$

There is a slight deviation from the usual notation for membrane and electrode currents, I_m and I_e, respectively. As this is a short cable segment, the current flowing through it is expressed as "current per unit area" (i_m and i_e) multiplied by the surface area covered by the segment ($2\pi a \Delta x$). Recall that membrane current leaving the neuron and electrode current entering the cell are both positive.

The final form of the generic cable equation is obtained by two modifications on Equation 8.23. First, both sides are divided by $2\pi a \Delta x$. This brings the right side to the following form:

$$\frac{1}{\Delta x}\left[\left(\frac{a}{2r_L}\frac{\partial V}{\partial x}\right)_{left} - \left(\frac{a}{2r_L}\frac{\partial V}{\partial x}\right)_{right}\right]. \tag{Eq. 8.24}$$

Recognize that this term is the difference between the spatial derivative of voltage (V) at two points divided by the space between them – the definition of a derivative if the space between the points is infinitesimally small. Considering infinitesimally short cable segments ($\Delta x \rightarrow 0$), the entire expression can be replaced by a second spatial derivative:

$$\frac{\partial}{\partial x}\left(\frac{a}{2r_L}\frac{\partial V}{\partial x}\right) \equiv \frac{a}{2r_L}\left(\frac{\partial^2 V}{\partial x^2}\right). \tag{Eq. 8.25}$$

The general form of the cable equation can now be expressed as follows:

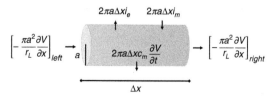

Figure 8.5 A short cable segment with associated labeling for cable theory formulation. The different currents, their direction, and value are indicated on the diagram.

$$c_m \frac{\partial V}{\partial t} = \frac{a}{2r_L}\left(\frac{\partial^2 V}{\partial x^2}\right) - i_m + i_e. \qquad \text{(Eq. 8.26)}$$

This equation allows any model of the membrane current to be substituted as an expression for i_m. The cable equation helps break away from the uniform membrane potential assumption and macroscopic effects to get into the details of individual cables. This is beneficial in understanding the spread of potentials across the dendritic tree and feeds into synaptic integration.

The simplest cable equation solution follows the linear cable theory. This approach approximates the membrane current as $i_m = (V - V_{rest})/r_m$. The resulting equations have standard mathematical procedures to obtain an analytical solution.

Two additional approaches are: (i) constant current injection, which removes the time dependence of the membrane voltage from the cable equation, and (ii) the solution to an instantaneous current pulse that delivers a fixed amount of charge, removing the time dependence of the membrane current. In both of these approaches, the cable is often considered to be infinite in length because current decays with distance in a way that it would be zero at distances far from the site of injection. Qualitatively, the spatial profile of the membrane voltage for the two approaches follows (i) exponential decay on either side of the site of injection for a constant current, and (ii) normal distribution (Gaussian) around the site of injection for a current pulse.

Analytical solutions to the cable equation are dependent on assumptions that simplify the problem. Complexity of the model can be increased by adding complex neuronal structures, detailed descriptions of membrane currents, and most importantly, membrane conductances. In these cases, numerical solutions are the way ahead. These strategies gave rise to multi-compartment neuronal models.

8.5 Multi-Compartment Models

Tractability of the cable equation is often addressed by breaking the analysis into multiple "compartments" (Figure 8.6), each having a specific value of the membrane potential $V(x,t)$ that does not change within the compartment. The number of compartments can be chosen based on the required level of detail. Within each compartment, the starting point is the same as the single-compartment models outlined in this chapter (Equation 8.8). As we are modeling cables, the current flowing through the surface area of the compartment must be factored in. We can replace all the quantities from Equation 8.8 with their "per area" counterparts:

$$c_m \frac{dV}{dt} = -i_m + \frac{I_e}{A}. \qquad \text{(Eq. 8.27)}$$

In a multi-compartment scenario, Equation 8.27 must be augmented with information about current flowing from neighboring compartments. Further, there needs to be a mechanism to identify which of the many compartments is being considered. For this purpose, the subscript μ is used. In the simple case of a cable that has no branches, the following equation holds good:

$$c_m \frac{dV^\mu}{dt} = -i_m^\mu + \frac{I_e^\mu}{A^\mu} + g^{\mu,\mu+1}(V^{\mu+1} - V^\mu)$$
$$+ g^{\mu,\mu-1}(V^{\mu-1} - V^\mu). \qquad \text{(Eq. 8.28)}$$

Note the introduction of a conductance-like term, g. This term is indicative of the transfer of current between compartments due to the resistance between them. For compartments of identical dimensions that have no branches, the value of g is the same between any two compartments. Let us consider any two compartments μ and μ + 1. The current flowing from μ to μ + 1 can be expressed using the

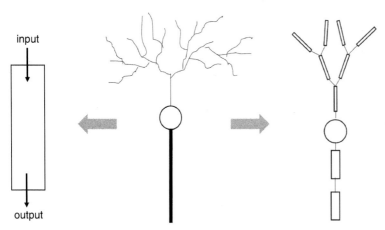

input

output

Figure 8.6 Different levels of abstraction in neuron models. Center: An actual neuron with a long axon and numerous dendrites with a cell body. Left: A single compartment approach where the neuron is treated as a single unit receiving input and sending an output. Right: A multi-compartment approach that breaks the axon and dendrites into a series of linked units which are individually modeled with a cable theory approach.

longitudinal resistance R_L and the difference in voltage between the compartments.

$$I = \frac{(V^{\mu+1} - V^{\mu})}{R_L}. \qquad \text{(Eq. 8.29)}$$

The longitudinal resistance can be expressed in terms of the specific resistance r_L and the cross-sectional area, a substitution that has been repeatedly used in our formulations.

$$I = \frac{\pi a^2}{r_L . L}(V^{\mu+1} - V^{\mu}). \qquad \text{(Eq. 8.30)}$$

Further, the cable modeling strategy expresses currents per unit area. Dividing Equation 8.30 by the surface area $2\pi a L$ yields:

$$i = \frac{a}{2r_L . L^2}(V^{\mu+1} - V^{\mu}). \qquad \text{(Eq. 8.31)}$$

Comparing this expression with the third term of Equation 8.28 immediately translates into an expression for the conductance term $g = a/(2r_L L^2)$. The usefulness of this conductance term is highlighted when compartments have different dimensions. A similar mathematical process can help determine the appropriate value of g between the two compartments.

An important component in neuronal cables is myelination. The effect of myelination can be seen in both the membrane resistance and membrane capacitance. In the current modeling framework, the capacitance term in Equation 8.28 will have to be appropriately modified to incorporate the effect of myelination.

The nature of multi-compartment models allows detailed simulations of individual neurons. This can be especially beneficial in fine study of morphological, pharmacological, and electrical effects. While noting that a macroscopic view may be sufficient in many analyses, the ability to probe the intricate details lends completeness to any study. Neurons receive inputs from numerous others and understanding this interaction requires a model of synaptic conductance and the generation of postsynaptic responses.

8.6 Synaptic Conductances

Earlier sections have provided a handle on understanding the propagation of an electrical signal along a cable. At the synapse, we recognize that postsynaptic channels come into play. The opening and closing of these channels dictated by the binding of neurotransmitters determines the subsequent flow of ions. Recall from the Hodgkin–Huxley model how gating variables were modeled in terms of their probability of opening or closing. A similar formulation can be used for the probability of opening P_S in the case of postsynaptic channels.

$$\frac{dP_s}{dt} = \alpha_s(1 - P_s) - \beta_s P_s. \qquad \text{(Eq. 8.32)}$$

The constant closing rate of the channel is represented by β_S and the neurotransmitter concentration-dependent rate of opening is α_S. Equation 8.32 follows from the logic that closed channels can transition to open and vice versa.

Fast and slow synapses will vary in their values for α_S and β_S. When an action potential arrives at the presynaptic terminal, α_S rises rapidly because the transmitter concentration increases. This rise is significantly larger in magnitude when compared to β_S and it is possible to neglect the contribution of the term $\beta_S P_S$ in Equation 8.32. The mechanisms involving neurotransmitter release and uptake on the presynaptic end cause a rapid decrease in the probability of opening for postsynaptic channels. Now the term $\beta_S P_S$ dominates Equation 8.32 and others can be ignored.

M fast synapses can be approximated as having an instantaneous rise in P_S because the rise in conductance following the arrival of an action potential is rapid. Under this framework, only the decay of P_S needs to be modeled. One way to account for this is:

$$P_s = P_{max} . exp\left(\frac{-t}{\tau_s}\right). \qquad \text{(Eq. 8.33)}$$

From a peak probability of opening P_{max}, there is a decay whose rate is determined by τ_S. A similar strategy can be used to model the postsynaptic channel opening probability for a series of action potentials arriving at the presynaptic side. After every action potential, a new P_S is determined using the equation:

$$P_s \rightarrow P_s + P_{max}(1 - P_s). \qquad \text{(Eq. 8.34)}$$

The motivation for this substitution stems from the observation that an action potential causes a large rise in synaptic conductance and the term $\beta_S P_S$ can be neglected while solving Equation 8.32. The maximum value for P_S in the resulting equation is represented by P_{max}. The starting point of P_S is non-zero after an action potential, which is addressed by the update step in Equation 8.34.

A probabilistic model can also be used to describe neurotransmitter release. This is useful in describing phenomena like short-term plasticity. The framework for modeling release probability P_{rel} follows:

$$\tau_P \frac{dP_{rel}}{dt} = P_0 - P_{rel}. \qquad \text{(Eq. 8.35)}$$

Here, P_{rel} decays at a rate τ_P to a resting value P_0. For plasticity mechanisms like facilitation and depression, P_{rel} must be updated after each action potential at the presynaptic site, much like Equation 8.34.

Synaptic components can be introduced in models like the integrate-and-fire neuron by incorporating terms to describe the current flow due to synaptic inputs. An example (a modification of Equation 8.10) is given in Equation 8.36, where g_S is the maximal synaptic conductance, P_S is the probability of channel opening and E_S is the equilibrium potential associated with the synaptic input

$$\tau_m \frac{dV}{dt} = E_L - V + R_m.I_e - r_m \bar{g}_s P_s (V - E_s). \quad \text{(Eq. 8.36)}$$

Up to this point we have talked about models that treat neurons as a precise entity. In reality, noise and fluctuation frequently accompany activity in the brain. The following section deals with ways to represent information from neuronal activity.

8.7 Coding for Neural Activity

Neurons must create energy- and information-efficient code. In other words, the neural code must combine sparseness and richness. Most neuron models regard neural activity as discrete, independent but identical spike events, and usually a spike train is characterized by a series of all-or-none events in time. The assumptions are that the information is held within the number of spikes within a certain time period (rate code) or the actual timing (temporal code). Characterizing the encoding of known stimuli is one matter; however, decoding information in a spike train to extract information about unknown, varying stimuli is extremely challenging. This process usually requires identifying specific patterns and determining how they correlate with the encoded information. Characterizing the responses of neurons can be performed using various tools such as reverse correlation or spike triggered correlation, which analyses the spikes emitted in response to a stimulus or spike-triggered covariance, using the covariance of a stimulus that elicits spikes from a neuron.

Encountering the same stimulus does not guarantee an exact replication of neuronal responses. This variability can arise due to stochasticity in the firing of neurons. The simplest form of modeling the stochasticity in neural activity is through a Poisson process. This assumes that spike generation is a probabilistic process where the occurrence of any spike is independent from other spikes fired. The distribution uses "average wait time" between events (spikes in this case) as a parameter, which affects the number of spikes generated in any given time interval. From the biological understanding of neuronal activity, we are aware that spikes are not necessarily independent. The refractory period, for example, is a good demonstration of how the timing of two spikes can be related. The Poisson process assumption will fail in situations where this level of detail is required by the modeling.

Nevertheless, our goal is to find ways to capture the salient aspects of neural activity that can best serve the purpose on hand. Extracting this information can come in various flavors. This section broadly outlines a few strategies that have been used to encode neural activity.

8.7.1 Rate Coding

The rate of firing can be an important aspect that can tie neural responses to a stimulus. Counting the number of spikes $c(t)$ in a time interval Δt will yield a firing rate $r(t)$ that is simply:

$$r(t) = \frac{c(t)}{\Delta t}. \quad \text{(Eq. 8.37)}$$

The simplest use of rate coding can be in estimating the changes in firing rate before and after a stimulus of interest is presented. Note that time dependence on the firing rate has been captured as $r(t)$. Typically, rate coding will not have significant fluctuations in a time period of interest. The underlying assumption is that neural activity is a noisy process and a single neuron firing rate may exhibit some fluctuations due to this stochasticity. Generally, firing rates can be averaged across multiple "trials" (repetitions of the same stimulation) to get an average estimate. The rate coding idea was brought to light by Adrian and Zotterman (1926), when they showed that the firing rate recorded from a muscle increased based on the weight hung from it.

However, arguments can be made that this view of neural communication is too simplistic; indeed, the firing rate can increase non-linearly with increasing intensity of the stimulus. Furthermore, averaging across many similar trials can obscure certain temporal features. Trial averaging is also not appropriate when certain physical behavior is not under strict experimental control.

To obtain meaningful data, repeated trials of spike trains are recorded from a single neuron exposed to the same conditions. However, it is common knowledge that even while keeping the same experimental conditions for repeated trials, the measured spike count varies between one trial and the next. This variability of spike trains has generated much thought in the scientific community. At one extreme, the timing of the temporal location of spikes is said to be important. On the other hand, the timing of individual spikes is thought to be due to stochastic forces, occurring due to an underlying continuous driving force, the instantaneous firing rate, with the generation of each spike being independent of other spikes. This led to modeling of spikes as events of an inhomogeneous Poisson process, which are similar to an ordinary Poisson process, except that the average rate of arrivals is allowed to vary with time.

However, there are instances where the independent spike hypothesis is violated, such as during the absolute refractory period when neurons cannot fire another spike or bursting where neurons fire action potentials in clusters.

A common method to study variability given a stationary input is the interspike interval (ISI) distribution. A common assumption under the renewal theory is that the probability of the next event occurring can be predicted by calculating the time that has passed since the last spike, but does not depend on the earlier spikes of the same neuron and the spikes generated in a renewal process occur stochastically. One factor that is intimately related to the renewal process is the signal-to-noise ratio, where a signal transmitted should be stronger than any noise at the same frequency.

The variability of spike trains repressing the length of ISIs can be quantified using the coefficient of variation (CV), which is the ratio of the square root of the variance of the length of the ISIs to their mean.

Modeling spike counts under the Poisson distribution assumes that spike count mean and variance are equal. However, any deviation from this can be characterized by the Fano factor, the ratio of the variance of the number of spikes to the mean. Compared to CV, Fano factor is less dependent on the intervals between spikes but more on the number of spikes in a given time. Therefore, the Fano factor for a Poisson neuron is equal to one. However, neural responses do not always obey a Poisson distribution and the spike count variance changes non-linearly with the mean.

8.7.1.1 Time-Dependent Firing Rate

Here, an experimenter records from a neuron while stimulating with some input sequence. Experimentally, repeated stimulation and the resulting neuronal response can be graphically represented in a Peri-Stimulus-Time Histogram (PSTH) and therefore provides an empirical estimate of the instantaneous firing rate. An inhomogeneous Poisson process can be used to describe the spike density measured in a PSTH. Here, spike events are independent of each other and occur with an instantaneous firing rate.

8.7.2 Temporal Coding

Neural circuits can work with precise timing as well. The onset of a spike and the interval between spikes can play a role in determining the goal achieved by the circuit. Consider a case of 10 spikes arriving in a 1-second interval with uniform spacing. If these 10 spikes were to arrive in pairs, the firing rate will still be the same, but the ISI will be different. If a firing rate were computed in a time window much smaller than 1 second, there would be some significant fluctuations. Temporal coding does not bundle these fluctuations as noise and looks for information contained in these significant rate fluctuations. Localization of sound is an easy situation where timing of neural activity can store critical information.

The temporal coding uses the precise spike timing to convey information in different forms, such as the timing of the first spike (TTFS), which encodes information by the time difference between stimulus onset and the first spike of a neuron (Figure 8.7). Instead of a single reference point, phase coding encodes information in the relative time difference between spikes and a reference oscillation. This is a coding scheme based on the tendency of a neuron to fire action potentials at particular phases of an ongoing local oscillations. Rank-order coding (ROC) is based on the firing order of a population of neurons in relation to a global reference. Temporal code models assume that precise timing of spikes and ISIs carries information. Interspike interval or the time interval between every pair of spikes can be used to distinguish spike trains. True temporal coding takes inspiration from digital computers by encoding information as binary digits, e.g., 1 for a spike and 0 for no spike.

8.7.3 Population Coding

The average activity of a group of neurons within a brain region of interest can often be an informative approach as it reduces variability associated with individual neuron firing rates. Sensory and motor aspects have often been well understood in the population coding regime. This represents how the timing of pairs of neurons in a population encodes information.

In population coding, each neuron has a distribution of responses over some set of inputs, and the responses of many neurons may be combined to determine the value about the inputs. Neurons in a population code display a Gaussian tuning curve with neurons responding strongly to simile near the mean.

For a population with unimodal tuning curves, the precision increases linearly with the number of neurons;

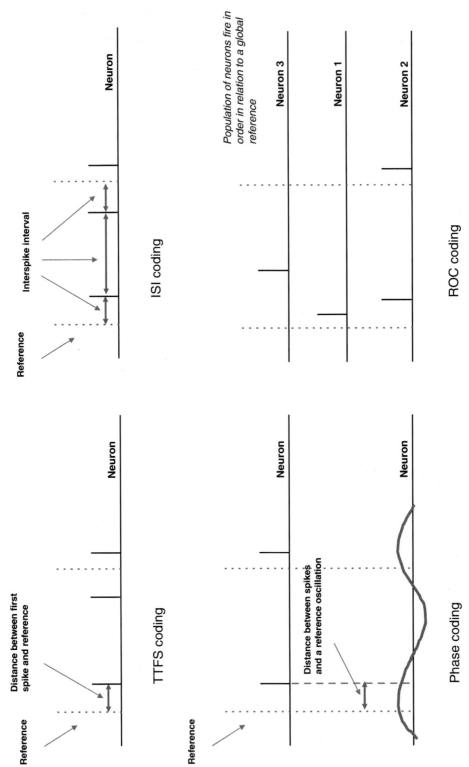

Figure 8.7 Temporal coding models.

however, from multimodal tuning curves with multiple peaks, the precision of the neuronal population increases exponentially with the number of neurons and the number of neurons required for the same amount of precision is less. Therefore, this coding model allows a population of neurons to overcome any limitations of single neuron rate coding.

A well-known population coding brain region is area MT in the visual cortex (Albright, 1984). Here, individual neurons have preferences for a particular direction of motion, but the population activity allows accurate detection of the net direction. For example, diagonal motion to the right would increase the activity of neurons that detect any forward movement as well as neurons that detect any rightward movement. In this way, observing correlations between the population activity of neurons with the stimulus of interest can help tie the two together.

8.7.4   Sparse Coding

Having every neuron be involved in the encoding of every stimulus can be inefficient in many cases. One can think of a subset of neurons that will "encode" a few basic representations (or symbols). Different combinations of these symbols can be used to encode other inputs. The easiest analogy is a language that can be generated from basic phonetics (the alphabet, for example). The sparse coding strategy has biological evidence, for example in the formation of associative memories. Linear generative models are a way of implementing sparse coding. If there are k symbols $b_1 \ldots b_k$, each one has a weight $w_1 \ldots w_k$ associated with it, and they are combined in a linear manner to encode the input.

$$E = \sum_{i=1}^{k} w_i * b_i. \qquad \text{(Eq. 8.38)}$$

8.8   Summary

At this juncture, one can appreciate how the activity of neurons can be described in different levels of detail based on the circumstance. Single- and multi-compartment models along with the cable theory perspective can allow us to either treat the neuron as a processing unit that just integrates inputs or as an aggregation of dendrites and axons that allow electrical impulses to flow through them. Further, we are now equipped with ways to extract information from neural activity through different encoding strategies.

It is important to note that biological processes are inherently variable. A more detailed approach to modeling noise in neuronal activity can be incorporated in the different paradigms considered in this chapter. These styles of modeling noise can be distinguished by isolating whether noise is associated with the input or output of the neuron. Diffusive noise models deal with input noise and escape noise models treat the output of a neuron to be noisy. The details of these models are out of the scope of this chapter and interested readers can find information in Gerstner and Kistler (2002) and Greenwood and Ward (2016).

Figure acknowledgements

The following images are credited to the authors of this chapter: Figures 8.1-8.7

References

Adrian ED, Zotterman Y. The impulses produced by sensory nerve endings: Part 3. Impulses set up by touch and pressure. *J Physiol.* 1926;**61**(4):465–83. https://doi.org/10.1113/jphysiol.1926.sp002308. PMID: 16993807; PMCID: PMC1514868.

Albright TD. Direction and orientation selectivity of neurons in visual area MT of the macaque. *J Neurophysiol.* 1984;**52** (6):1106–30. https://doi.org/10.1152/jn.1984.52.6.1106. PMID: 6520628.

Gerstner W, Kistler WM. *Spiking neuron Models: Single Neurons, Populations, Plasticity.* Cambridge University Press, 2002.

Greenwood PE, Ward LM. Single neuron models. In *Stochastic Neuron Models. Mathematical Biosciences Institute Lecture Series,* vol. 1.5. Springer, 2016. https://doi.org/10.1007/978-3-3 19-26911-5_2

Lapicque L. Recherches quantitatives sur l'excitation e ́lectrique des nerfs traite ́e comme une polarization. *J Physiol Pathol Gen* 1907;9:620–35.

An Introduction to Artificial Intelligence and Machine Learning

Shun Yao, Ye Wu, and Farhana Akter

9.1 Introduction

Artificial intelligence (AI), a term first coined by John McCarthy in the 1950s, is best thought of as the design of intelligent agents that can recognize and process stimuli to make decisions, similar to humans. The use of AI and artificial neural networks (ANNs) in medicine has been widely adopted to improve the efficiency of diagnostic medicine, and these include ANN-based analysis of electrocardiograms, electroencephalograms, radiographs, and automated computerized systems based on ANNs for analysis of cancer data.

In this chapter we will discuss the fundamental concepts of AI, followed by a discussion on machine learning and deep learning using neural networks. The reader is directed to further reading material for in-depth analysis of concepts that are beyond the scope of this chapter.

9.2 Data Science

Data science encompasses a multidisciplinary field that applies machine learning (ML) algorithms and mathematical analysis of large volumes of unstructured data, which is further processed to help with decision making.

9.3 Data Mining

Knowledge discovery in databases (KDD) is the overall process of extracting content implicitly present in data. Data mining, a step in the KDD process, denotes discovery of patterns in datasets, using pre-set rules. This is in contrast to ML whereby computers use algorithms to learn from heterogeneous datasets, without human intervention.

9.4 Machine Learning

Machine learning is a subset of AI that involves the delivery of data to sophisticated machines that have the capacity to analyze data sets and use pattern recognition to make predictions based on certain algorithms. In ML, there are different algorithms (e.g., neural networks) that help to solve problems and these are usually categorized into groups including: supervised learning, semi-supervised learning, unsupervised learning, and reinforcement learning.

9.4.1 Supervised Learning

Supervised learning involves an algorithm that learns from a training data set that has been labeled, i.e., data that have been tagged with the correct answer, to help predict outcomes for unforeseen data. The output from these algorithms is dependent on how good the data labels are.

9.4.1.1 Types of Supervised Learning

Supervised learning can be conducted in the context of two types of problems: classification or regression. Classification involves mapping input to output labels and assigning data into categories, e.g., "disease" versus "no disease." If the algorithm tries to label input into two distinct classes, it is called binary classification. Selecting between more than two classes is referred to as multi-class classification. Outputs always have a probabilistic interpretation, and the algorithm can be regularized to avoid overfitting. Binary classification is commonly performed by algorithms such as logistic regression, decision trees, naive Bayes. Multi-class classification is commonly performed by algorithms such as random forest, k-Nearest neighbors and Naive Bayes.

Regression uses algorithms for mapping input to continuously changing outputs and helps understand the relationship between dependent and independent variables, e.g., "weight." The regression technique predicts a single output value using training data. Examples of regression algorithms include simple linear regression, logistic regression, polynomial regression, and decision tree regression.

9.4.2 Unsupervised Learning

Unsupervised learning models involve validation of output variables without the need for labeled data. Common algorithms are k-means clustering, Principal Component Analysis (PCA), and autoencoders.

9.4.2.1 Types of Unsupervised Learning

Unsupervised learning can be approached through different techniques. These include clustering algorithms, dimensionality reduction (DR) algorithms and association algorithms. Clustering involves grouping together data points into categories depending on their structure/patterns and can therefore be used to understand trends. Hyperparameters can be used to define the overall count of clusters. Methods of clustering include k-means clustering, defined by the distance from the center of each grouping and Gaussian mixture models for probabilistic clustering of data intro groups. DR algorithms can be used reduce noise from data by removing redundant features. Association allows us to understand the relationships between different variables. One method of forming association rules is the Apriori algorithm, which can be used to identify trends based on frequency.

9.4.3 Reinforcement Learning

Reinforcement learning (RL) is the science of decision making and can be positive or negative. Positive reinforcement refers to a stimulus that encourages the desirable behavior, whereas negative reinforcement learning increases the frequency of a specific behavior by avoiding the negative condition. Reinforcement learning can be value- or policy based. Value-based RL is a fundamental concept and estimates how to take the best action in a state to find the optimal value function at any policy. Policy-based RL finds the optimal policy for the maximum future rewards without using the value function. In this approach, the agent tries to apply such a policy that the action performed in each step helps to maximize the future reward.

9.4.3.1 Components of Reinforcement Learning

Reinforcement learning consists of a number of essential components: an agent, policy, rewards, value function, and the environment in which the agent will act.

An agent makes decisions and behaves accordingly in a particular state. State is the information that an agent has about the environment at a given time. The policy, which can be deterministic or stochastic in nature, involves mapping the perceived environmental state to the actions that are taken on these states and therefore defines the behavior of the agent. An optimal policy is one that results in an optimal value function. One policy is better than another

policy if the value function with the policy for all states is greater than the value function with the other policy.

The rewards are the numerical values that the agent receives on performing an action at a state in the environment. The environment will send an immediate signal to the learning agent for each good and bad action. The sum of all rewards that the agent expects to receive is called the returns.

The importance of rewards in the immediate present and the future is known as the discount factor. Here, a value of 0 means the agent is myopic and only learns about actions that will result in an immediate reward. Whereas, a value of 1 indicates that the agent will give more importance to actions that result in future rewards. The agent will attempt to maximize the number of rewards for good actions and therefore may change the policy accordingly to a different action in the future if the reward is low. Therefore, the experience of the agent determines the change in policy.

9.4.3.2 Bellman Equation

The value of a state can be decomposed into an immediate reward combined with the expected future reward and can be calculated using the Bellman equation, which also adds the discount factor to yield the maximum value function (Eq. 9.1). It helps us to determine optimal policies and value functions.

$$V(s) = \max_a (R(s, a) + \gamma V(s')) \qquad \text{(Eq. 9.1)}$$

$V(s)$ is the value for being in a certain state. $V(s')$ is the value for being in the next state that we will end up in after taking action a. $R(s, a)$ is the reward we get after taking action a in state s. γ is the discount factor as discussed earlier.

The value function allows us to estimate how good it is for the agent to be in a particular state and how much reward an agent can expect from an action. The optimal value function is one that gives maximum value compared to all other value functions. The Optimal State- Action Value Function (Q-Function) tells us the maximum reward we will get after committing to a given state- action pair.

The Bellman equation can be solved using a technique called dynamic programming. This is an algorithmic paradigm that involves breaking the problem into simple subproblems followed by computation and storage of each subproblem. A problem can be solved using dynamic programming if it satisfies two properties: optimal substructure that can be divided into subproblems, and overlapping subproblems that can be used to solve other similar subproblems. Finding the value function that will satisfy the Bellman equation allows us to solve a Markov decision process.

9.4.3.3 Markov Decision Process

The mathematical formulation of a RL program is done using a Markov decision process (MDP), which is useful for studying optimization problems solved by dynamic programming. An MDP can be seen as a Markov chain where a network exists with random variables in a sequence with each variable being dependent on its predecessor in a sequence. Therefore, the Markov property states that the future depends only on the present and not on the past.

The MDP can be represented by several elements. Each point in a sequence is called the stage (Figure 9.1). These include the states that the agent will be in, beginning with an initial state s0; actions that the agent can perform by moving states; the probability of moving from one state to another by each state performing an action (transition probability); the probability of a reward acquired by the agent for moving from one state to another state (reward probability); and the discount factor.

9.4.3.4 Model-Free Algorithm

A model-free algorithm in RL is one that does not use the transition probability distribution and the reward function associated with the MDP. This includes the Monte Carlo algorithm, which helps estimate returns by sampling from the environment and policy using a non-bootstrapping method. Another model-free algorithm is Q-learning, which learns the value of an action in a particular state and does not require a model of the environment.

9.5 Reducing Loss of Information

Dimensionality reduction is the process of removing redundant features of data to reduce the complexity of a model and to avoid overfitting. There are two main categories of DR: feature selection, where a subset of original features are selected, and feature extraction, where specific information from a feature is derived to construct a new feature subspace.

9.5.1 Autoencoders

Autoencoders are an unsupervised learning technique that does not need explicit labels to train on. They are composed of the encoder, the code, and the decoder. The encoder and decoder are simple feedforward neural networks, which uses backpropagation algorithms to learn a lower-dimensional representation of higher dimensional data. This method is ultimately lossy in that it is not possible to reconstruct the original data from the compressed version.

The representation of compressed data is also known as latent space representation. This is followed by production of the code, which is a single layer of an ANN. The size of the code, i.e., the number of nodes in the code layer, is a hyperparameter and this must be set before training the autoencoder. Other hyperparameters that need to be set are the layers, and the loss function, for which we can use the mean squared error (MSE) or binary cross-entropy. Keeping the code layer small will result in more compression. Autoencoders can also be modifed by adding random noise to inputs and training the autoencoder to remove the noise. This is known as the denoising autoencoder. Autoencoders can be regularized by using a sparsity constraint to reduce the number of active nodes, allowing the autoencoder to represent each input as a combination of a small number of nodes.

Autoencoders, are limited in that the latent space they convert their inputs to may not be continuous and are non-regularized. The latent spaces of variational autoencoders (VAE) are however continuous and regularized

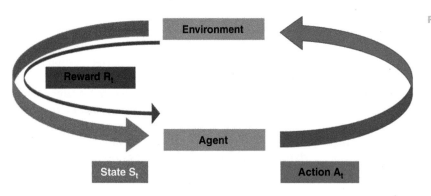

Figure 9.1 Markov decision process.

and has properties enabling a process of generating new content. Here it is trained to minimize the reconstruction error between the encoded -decoded data and the initial data.

The loss function that is minimized when training a VAE and the resultant regularization is expressed as the Kullback–Leibler divergence. Also called relative entropy (see below), it is a measure of how one probability distribution differs from a reference probability distribution.

Other DR Techniques include PCA and Stochastic Neighbor Embedding (t-SNE).

9.6 Information Theory

Information theory is the mathematical study of the quantification and communication of digital information. A key measure in information theory is entropy, a measure of uncertainty, which was introduced as a concept by Claude Shannon in the 1940s. The mathematical definition for information entropy for a single random variable is as follows (Eq. 9.2):

$$H(X) = -\sum_{i=1}^{n} P(x_i)\log_b P(x_i). \qquad \text{(Eq. 9.2)}$$

It measures or quantifies the average uncertainty of X, a random variable and the unit of entropy as the number of bits with x_i possible outcomes. Entropy is dependent on the probability of the random variable and if the value is 0, suggests that no new information will be gained.

Entropy must satisfy a number of criteria. In order to be a good measure of uncertainty, it must achieve its highest values where all the outcomes have the same probability and the uncertainty for one or more events must be the sum of the independent events.

9.6.1 Conditional Entropy

Conditional entropy refers to how much entropy a random variable X has if we have learned the value of a second random variable, Y. It is referred to as the entropy of X conditional on $Y(HY/X)$ (Eq. 9.3).

$$H(Y|X) = \sum_{x \in \chi} p(x)H(Y|X = x). \qquad \text{(Eq. 9.3)}$$

9.6.2 Relative Entropy

Relative entropy, also known as KL-divergence, refers to distributions and not random variables. It is a measure of the distance between two distributions and inefficiency assuming that the distribution is q when the true

distribution is p. It can only have a value of 0 if $p = q$ and is always non-negative (Eq. 9.4).

It can be defined as:

$$D(p\|q) = \sum_{x \in X} p(x)\log\frac{p(x)}{q(x)}. \qquad \text{(Eq. 9.4)}$$

9.6.3 Mutual Information

Mutual information is defined as the reduction in uncertainty of one variable due to the knowledge of the other. It is a measure of the amount of information that one random variable contains about another random variable.

In Equation (9.5), the mutual information $I(X; Y)$ would be the relative entropy between the joint distribution and the product distribution $p(x)p(y)$.

$$\begin{aligned}
I(X; Y) &= \sum_{x \in \chi} \sum_{y \in Y} p(x, y) \log \frac{p(x, y)}{p(x)\, p(y)} \\
&= D(p(x, y)\|p(x)\, p(y)).
\end{aligned} \qquad \text{(Eq. 9.5)}$$

9.6.4 Entropy and Information Gain Using Decision Trees

Decision Trees (DTs) are a non-parametric supervised learning method used for classification and regression. The entropy of the predicted variable is calculated. This is followed by splitting of data into subsets with homogenous values based on entropy. The entropy of the resultant variable is subtracted from the previous entropy value. The core algorithm used is the Iterative Dichotomizer 3 (ID3) algorithm, which uses entropy to calculate homogeneity of a sample. The value is zero if the sample is completely homogeneous and one if it is equally divided. This step is followed by pruning of the data subsets. The process of finding the smallest tree that fits the data with the lowest cross-validated error is called tree selection.

Pruning is the process of removing redundant subtrees. It reduces unnecessary comparisons and results in smaller, less complex pruned trees. There are two approaches to pruning– the pre-pruning approach in which splitting or partition of the tree is halted at a particular node or the post- pruning approach which removes subtrees from the full tree. A subtree pruning involves replacing the branches at a node with a leaf node.

Entropy measures impurity in data and information gain measures reduction in data impurity. The feature that has minimum impurity will be considered the root node. Information gain is used to decide which feature should be used to split a node. The creation of subnodes increases homogeneity, that is, decreases the entropy of these nodes. The more homogenous the child node is, the lower the variance after each split. The information gain of a parent node can be calculated as the entropy of the parent node with the entropy of the weighted average of the child node subtracted.

9.6.5 Cross-Entropy Versus KL-Divergence (Relative Entropy)

Cross-entropy is commonly used in ML as a loss function. It calculates the total entropy between distributions compared to KL-divergence, which calculates the relative entropy between two probability distributions.

9.7 Deep Learning

Deep learning is a subfield of ML, which uses complex multi-layered neural networks where the information is transferred from one layer to another over connecting channels. They are called weighted channels because each has a value attached to it.

All neurons have a unique number called bias. This bias is added to the weighted sum of inputs reaching the neuron, to which an activation function is then applied. The result of the function determines if the neuron becomes activated. Every activated neuron passes on information to the following layers. This continues up to the second last layer. The output layer in an ANN is the last layer that produces outputs for the program.

9.8 Basic Unit of Neural Network

Perceptrons are artificial neurons that retain the biological concept of neurons. A basic unit of a neural network is also known as a single-layer perceptron, which consists of input values integrated with fixed weights to obtain the net weighted sum, bias, and activation function. If the net weighted sum is larger than a given threshold θ, the neuron fires. A neuron that has fired will have an output of one. The initial analogy between biological neurons with binary outputs came from McCulloch and Pitts in 1943, whereas the single-layer perceptron model was first proposed by Rosenblatt in 1957 as an algorithm for supervised learning. Rosenblatt proposed that the patterns used to train the perceptron are drawn from two linearly separable categories that can be converged in an algorithm. An example of a binary output in ML may be the classification of a tumor as malignant or benign.

9.8.1 Components of Perceptrons

A perceptron consists of four parts: input values, weights, bias, and activation function. A perceptron works by combining numerical inputs with weights and a bias. The activation function takes the weighted sum and the bias as inputs and returns a final output node (Figure 9.2).

Let us assume we have a single neuron with three input values [$x1$, $x2$, $x3$] and the output value as Y (0 or 1). Each input value is associated with a corresponding weight [$w1$, $w2$, $w3$]. In order to determine the weight vector for a perceptron we have two approaches: the perceptron training rule and the gradient descent and the delta rule (discussed below). The weight vector and the input vector are taken as input to the target function of a perceptron. Bias is an input to all nodes and always has the value of one. It allows you to shift the result of the activation function to the left or right. It also helps the model to train when all the input features are zero. The target function calculates the linear combination of these vectors and acts accordingly. This is subsequently given to the activation function, which converts the weighted sum to determine the output of the node. The activation functions can be divided into two types: linear activation function and non-linear activation function (Figure 9.3). However, usual data that are fed to the neural networks are not always linear. In that case, you need to use a non-linear activation function. Some of the common non-linear activation functions are shown below.

The equation for a given node (Eq. 9.6) can be expressed as:

$$z = f(b + x \cdot w) = f\left(b + \sum_{i=1}^{n} x_i w_i\right)$$ (Eq. 9.6)

$$x \in d_{1 \times n}, \ w \in d_{n \times 1}, \ b \in d_{1 \times 1}, \ z \in d_{1 \times 1}.$$

This is often simplified as a vector dot product of the weight and input vectors plus the bias.

9.8.1.1 Training Single-Layer Fragments

One method of optimization is to train perceptrons to learn the weights, and this involves iteratively updating the weights to minimize the error function. You begin with randomly initializing the weights for the nodes (step 1) and applying the perceptron to a single data point in a data set (step 2). Finally, you compare the output with the target in the training data and measure the error using a loss function followed by modification of the perceptron weights (step 3). You repeat these steps until the perceptron classifies all training examples

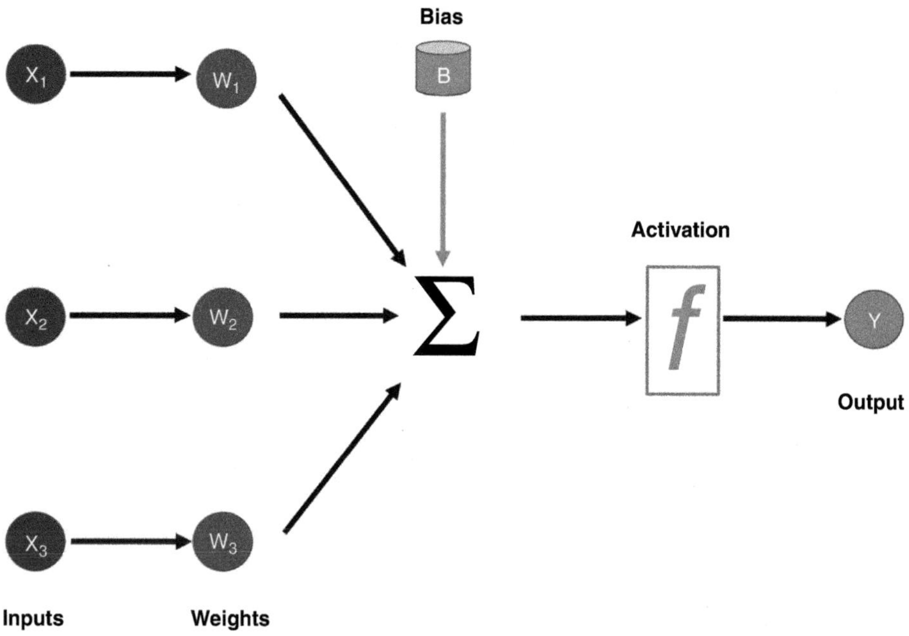

Figure 9.2 Components of perceptrons.

correctly. In order to train our perceptron, we iteratively feed the network with our training data multiple times.

9.8.2 Multi-Layer Perceptrons

The simple single neuron model is limited in not being able to solve nonlinear separable problems. A multi-layer perceptron (MLP), also known as a neural network is therefore used for tasks such as pattern classification, recognition, prediction, and approximation.

Multi-layer perceptrons are supplements of the feed-forward neural networks. With this type of architecture, information flows in only one direction: forward. The input layer receives the input signal to be processed. The required task, such as prediction and classification, is performed by the output layer. The neurons in the MLP are trained with the back-propagation algorithm, which measures how each weight contributes to the overall error (Figure 9.4). However, to optimize the weights to fit the data, an optimization algorithm such as the gradient descent must be used.

9.8.3 Back-Propagation

The end goal of a neural network model is to calculate and minimize the error or loss, i.e., how much the predicted model deviates from the actual values. The process of adjusting the weights in each layer is called back-propagation. To obtain the lowest error values, the weights need to be adjusted to reach the lowest possible error value (Figure 9.5). Each weight's contribution to the error needs to be calculated and the weights are subsequently adjusted. This process is repeated until the desired output is achieved. Once the network has converged to a state where the error is very small, the network is said to have learned the target function.

One algorithm used to minimize this loss, also known as cost function, is called gradient descent (Figure 9.6). It relies on the chain rule of calculus to calculate the gradient backward through the layers of a neural network. Ultimately, the goal is to find the minimum value for the cost function. To do this, we need to know the slope for determining the direction and the magnitude in which to move the coefficient values. We can describe the principle behind gradient descent as "climbing down a hill" until a local or global minimum is reached. At each step, we take a step into the opposite direction of the gradient, and the step size is determined by the value of the learning rate as well as the slope of the gradient.

One common function that is often used to minimize the parameters in the data set is the mean squared error

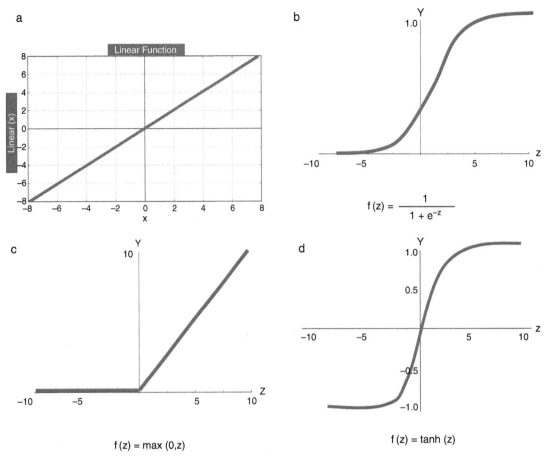

Figure 9.3 Linear versus non-linear activation functions. (a) Linear activation function; (b) sigmoid non-linear activation function; (c) rectified linear unit (ReLU); (d) Tanh.

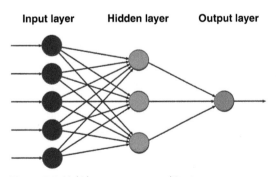

Figure 9.4 Multi-layer perceptron architecture.

(Eq. 9.7), which measures the difference between the predicted and actual values. A limitation of using a standard gradient descent algorithm is that it can be very time-consuming and becomes computationally very expensive to perform. An alternative technique is the stochastic gradient descent, which speeds up the process for large data sets by using select samples at each iteration; however, this does reduce the accuracy of the gradient.

$$J = \frac{1}{n}\sum_{i=0}^{n}\left(y^i - (mx^i + b)\right)^2. \tag{Eq. 9.7}$$

Feed-forward neural networks are useful for data points that are independent of each other. However, when we have data in a sequence that are dependent on each other, the neural network must factor this before the output can be generated. In contrast to feedforward Neural networks, recurrent neural networks (RNNs) can use their internal state (memory) to process sequences of inputs. In RNNs, outputs of neurons from previous time steps are fed as input into a hidden layer in the current time step. This method is therefore useful for short term memory and for sequential data. However, RNNs are subject to a vanishing gradient, whereby previous data from many steps in the past are lost

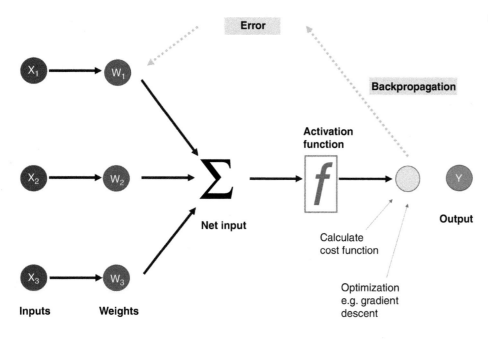

Figure 9.5 Back-propagation.

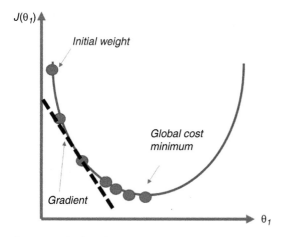

Figure 9.6 Gradient descent.

due to the continuous input of new data and therefore the network becomes more difficult to train.

9.8.4 Recurrent Neural Network

9.8.4.1 Types of Recurrent Neural Networks

A one-to-one RNN has a single input and output and is a traditional neural network. A one-to-many RNN is applied in situations that give multiple outputs for a single input, e.g., generating a musical piece from a single music note. A many-to-one RNN is used when multiple inputs are required to give a single output, such as a movie rating that takes reviews as inputs to subsequently give a rating from one to five. Many-to-many RNNs can refer to input and output layers of the same size or of different sizes. Types of RNNs are shown in Figure 9.7.

9.8.5 Elman and Jordan Networks

Elman and Jordan networks are two of the most popular simple RNNs (Figure 9.8). The Elman network has a hidden layer feeding into a state layer of context nodes that retain memory of past inputs. Jordan networks connect the output layer into the state layer.

9.8.6 The Hopfield Network

Hopfield networks are able to learn (through Hebbian learning) multiple patterns and converge to recall the closest pattern. They are commonly used for optimization tasks, pattern sequence recognition and to model associative memory (Figure 9.9). At initialization, the network is loaded with a partial pattern. Each neuron is then updated until the network converges leading to an output.

Hopfield neurons are binary threshold units but with recurrent instead of feed-forward connections, where each unit is bi-directionally connected to each other. This means that each unit *receives* inputs and

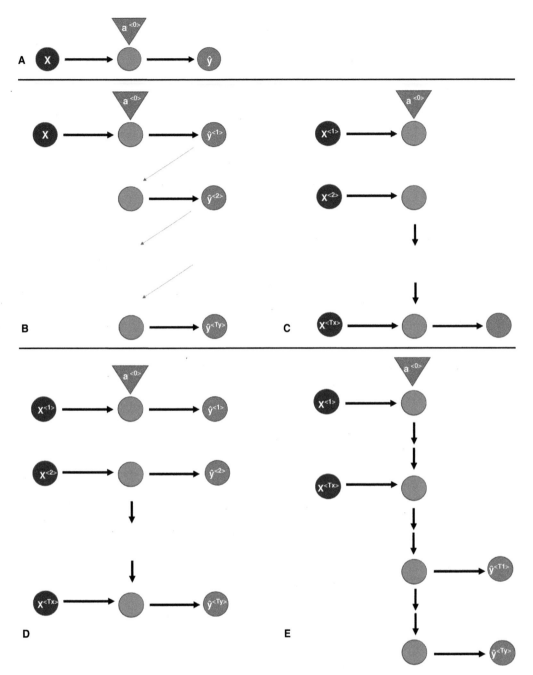

Figure 9.7 Recurrent neural networks. (A) One-to-one network; (B) one-to-many network; (C) many-to-one network; (D, E) many-to-many networks.

sends outputs to every other connected unit. A consequence of this architecture is that weights values are symmetric, such that weights *coming into* a unit are the same as the ones *coming out* of a unit. The value of each unit is determined by a linear function wrapped into a threshold function.

9.8.7 Long Short-Term Memory

Long short-term memory (LSTM) networks (Figure 9.10) are a type of RNN capable of learning order dependence in sequence prediction problems. This is a behavior required in complex problem domains such as speech recognition.

These networks use three gates: input, output, and the forget gate. The latter enables you to "train" individual neurons on what is important and how long it will remain important.

9.8.8 Gated Recurrent Unit

Gated recurrent units (GRUs) are very similar to LSTM. However, they are simpler, faster to train and less prone to overfitting. Just like LSTM, GRU uses gates to control the flow of information (Figure 9.11). GRUs comprise an update gate and a reset gate. The GRU cells takes input from a previous hidden state and an input from the current timestamp. The reset gate determines how much of the previous hidden state to forget to produce a candidate activation vector. How much of this vector will be incorporated into the new hidden state will be determined by the update gate. The final hidden state will be fed into the output layer and this will produce the network's output.

9.8.9 Convolutional Neural Network

A convolutional neural network (CNN) is a feed-forward neural network that is generally used to analyze visual images by processing data with grid-like topology to capture spatial features (Figure 9.12). The building blocks of CNNs are filters, also known as kernels, which can extract relevant features from the input.

Convolutional neural networks are generally composed of the following layers:

1. Convolution layer
2. Rectified linear unit (ReLU) layer
3. Pooling layer
4. Fully connected (dense) layer

The convolution layer is the first step in the process of extracting valuable features from an image. A convolution layer has several filters that perform the convolution operation. Every image is considered as a matrix of pixel values. Once the feature maps are extracted, the next step is to move them to a ReLU layer. The ReLU performs an element-wise operation and sets all the negative pixels to zero. It introduces non-linearity to the network. The generated output is a rectified feature map which goes through a down sampling operation that reduces the dimensionality of the feature map to generate a pooled feature map. The pooling layer uses various filters to identify different parts of the image such as edges, corners, etc.

The next step in the process is called flattening, which is used to convert the two- dimensional arrays from

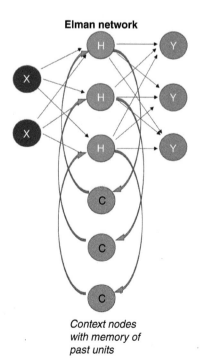

Elman network

Context nodes with memory of past units

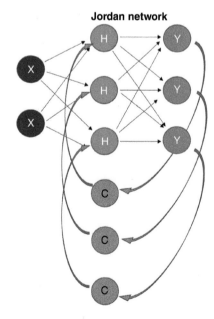

Jordan network

Figure 9.8 Jordan and Elman networks.

155

pooled feature maps into a single long continuous linear vector. The flattened matrix is fed as input to the fully connected (dense) layer to classify the image. These layers are usually found toward the end of CNN architectures and is used for abstract representations of input data.

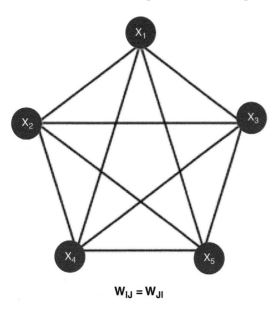

$$W_{IJ} = W_{JI}$$

Figure 9.9 The Hopfield network.

9.8.10 Random Neural Network

The random neural network is a mathematical model, described by analytical equations, for an "integrate and fire" spiking network. Here, neurons interact with each other by probabilistically exchanging excitatory and inhibitory spiking signals, in continuous time. In a steady state, they demonstrate stochastic spiking behaviors and are therefore closer to the biological neuronal network than other neural networks. These networks have been employed for a variety of functions including pattern recognition and image processing.

9.8.11 Modular Neural Network

A modular neural network is one that is composed of more than one ANN connected by an intermediary. Each neural network behaves as a module to independently solve one aspect of a problem. An integrator is then used to combine the responses from each module to generate an overall response. The concepts underpinning modular neural networks were first used to develop a particular type of ML method called ensemble learning, which involves the use of multiple algorithms to obtain better outcomes than what could be achieved by the use of single algorithms.

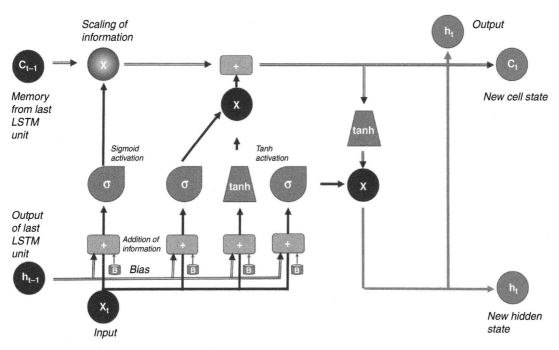

Figure 9.10 Long short-term memory networks.

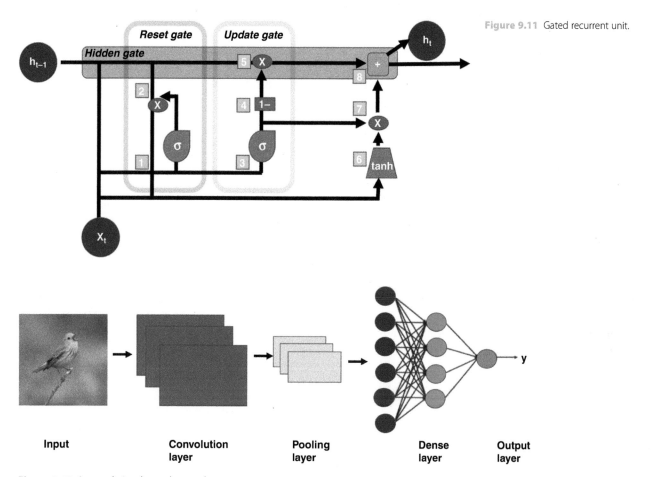

Figure 9.11 Gated recurrent unit.

Figure 9.12 A convolutional neural network.

Figure acknowledgements

The following images are credited to the authors of this chapter: Figures 9.1-9.12

Further Reading

Choi RY, Coyner AS, Kalpathy-Cramer J, Chiang MF, Campbell JP. Introduction to machine learning, neural networks, and deep learning. *Transl Vis Sci Technol* 2020;**9**(2):14. https://doi.org/10.1167/tvst.9.2.14. PMID: 32704420; PMCID: PMC7347027.

McCulloch WS, Pitts W. A logical calculus of the ideas immanent in nervous activity. *Bull Math Biophys* 1943;**5**; 115–33. https://doi.org/10.1007/BF02478259

Rowe M. An introduction to machine learning for clinicians. *Acad Med* 2019;**94**(10):1433–6. https://doi.org/10.1097/ACM .0000000000002792. PMID: 31094727.

Sidey-Gibbons JAM, Sidey-Gibbons CJ. Machine learning in medicine: a practical introduction. *BMC Med Res Methodol* 2019;**19**(1):64. https://doi.org/10.1186/s12874-019-0681-4. PMID: 30890124; PMCID: PMC6425557.

Chapter 10

Artificial Intelligence in Neuroscience

Will Xiao, Mengmi Zhang, and Gabriel Kreiman

Neurosurgeons have the privilege of peeking inside the most precious and the most mysterious device on earth: the human brain (Crick et al., 2004). The human brain is also the most expensive device on earth given that mental health problems constitute the largest health care cost. By deciphering the inner secrets of brain computations, scientists and engineers have taken inspiration to develop smart artificial intelligence (AI) algorithms. These AI algorithms in turn provide much help to understanding brain function and to multiple applications in brain disorders, including neurosurgery.

10.1 From Neural Circuits to Artificial Intelligence

Humanity has long imagined automated machines that can do work for us. The ultimate frontier is to construct machines that can emulate the human brain, or perhaps even surpass human intelligence. The development of AI commenced in the 1950s and has gained momentum in the last decade. Throughout its short history, AI research has been inspired by notions of neuroscience. Visual processing constitutes a paradigmatic example of AI and the links between AI and neuroscience.

Consider a hypothetical algorithm that is capable of taking as input a magnetic resonance image of a subject's brain and detecting the presence of a tumor. At the heart of AI algorithms are neural networks, that is, interconnected neuron-like units that receive inputs and progressively transform those inputs into forms that are more useful to solve the task. The output of the algorithm indicates the probability that the image contains a tumor and its location. A unit in a neural network is a highly simplified model of a neuron: it receives inputs from other units, weighs and sums those inputs, applies a non-linear transformation, and produces a scalar output (McCulloch and Pitts, 1943). Neuronal firing rates are represented by scalar activation values, the strengths of synapses between neurons are replaced by weights, and the biophysics of action

potential generation is captured by a single non-linearity that converts the weighted inputs into an output.

The power of neural networks derives from connecting these simple units into large ensembles that have interesting emergent properties. Here again, AI takes inspiration from the brain. The visual cortex uses a divide-and-conquer strategy by layering neurons in an approximately hierarchical fashion from the retina, to the lateral geniculate nucleus, onto primary visual cortex (V1), onto visual cortical area V2, and so on (Felleman and Van Essen, 1991; Figure 10.1A). A particularly successful computational architecture, known as deep neural networks, follows the same principle by having multiple layers that sequentially transform information (Figure 10.1B).

In the visual cortex, the same image features are extracted at different locations throughout the visual field. For example, each V1 neuron selectively responds to bars of a specific orientation at a specific part of the visual field (Hubel and Wiesel, 1962). The population of V1 neurons tile the entire visual field, with neurons specific to each orientation at, say, the center of gaze and also in the visual periphery. To create an artificial layer with similar properties, computational models recur to a convolution operation, such that units with the same weights are effectively repeated in different locations. Meanwhile, units with different weights account for different orientation tuning. Similarly, features other than orientation are extracted in different units and layers using the convolution operation. The resulting networks are known as deep convolutional neural networks (CNNs). Many other neurobiologically inspired operations are included, such as non-linear pooling of inputs (Riesenhuber and Poggio, 1999) and normalization (Carandini and Heeger, 2011).

Humans learn to recognize cars, chairs, or brain tumors in images. It is generally thought that such learning largely amounts to modifying synaptic strengths in visual cortex. Equivalently, neural networks are trained by modifying the weights between units. Powerful learning algorithms have been developed to modify synaptic weights,

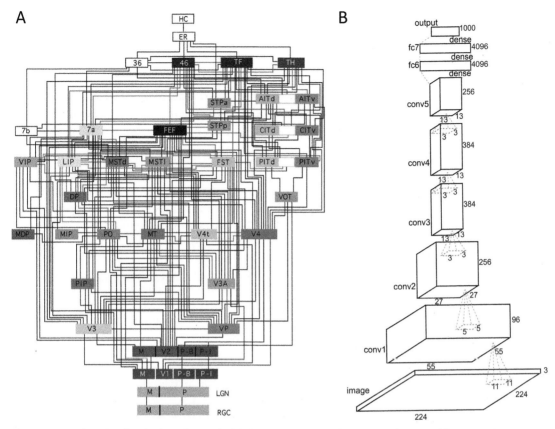

Figure 10.1 Biological and artificial visual networks. (A) Mesoscopic anatomical connections between different visual areas in the macaque cortex (Felleman and Van Essen, 1991). Each colored box shows a brain area and lines represent anatomical connections. The bottom shows the retinal ganglion cells (RGCs). Visual areas are arranged in an approximately hierarchical fashion. This architecture has inspired the idea that information flows in a semi-sequential fashion from the bottom to the top of this diagram. See Felleman and Van Essen (1991) for the definition of each anatomical abbreviation. (B) Example deep convolutional neural network (CNN) architecture known as AlexNet (Krizhevsky et al., 2012). Each solid box represents a layer in a neural network (loosely equivalent to a brain area). The dashed box denotes a unit (neuron) in a layer. The converging dash lines bring information to the next layer (representation of anatomical connections across layers). The input to the model is an image (bottom), the output is a series of numbers, 1000 in this case, which represent the probabilities that the image contains one of 1000 possible object categories. The numbers indicate the dimensions of each layer, "conv" stands for convolutional layer, and "fc" indicates a fully connected layer. See Krizhevsky et al. (2012) for further details.

including back-propagation. Back-propagation is often used in a supervised learning setting: the network produces tentative (initially random) labels for the training examples, and if the output is wrong, the error signal is propagated back throughout the network to modify the weights in the direction that makes the output closer to the correct answer. Trained with many correctly labeled examples, the network can gradually learn to separate, for example, images with or without tumors.

10.2 Artificial Intelligence Contributions to Visual Neuroscience

Just as neuroscientific knowledge inspired advances in AI, so does AI feed back to neuroscience, providing new tools, models, and ways of understanding the brain (see

Hassabis et al., 2017; Richards et al., 2019; Serre, 2019; Zador, 2019 for reviews on the synergisms between neuroscience and AI). We highlight three active research directions in vision that draw on AI as tools and models.

10.2.1 Goal-Driven Convolutional Neural Networks Explain Neuronal Responses Underlying Object Recognition

Object recognition is a well-defined visual process underlying our ability to make sense of the visual world. Clinical case studies exemplify the profound consequences of failures in visual recognition (Sacks, 2002). Neurons along the ventral visual cortex are especially important for visual recognition, as demonstrated by studies in non-human primates (DiCarlo et al., 2012) and using invasive neurophysiological recordings from human neurosurgical patients (Liu et al., 2009). Understanding how these neurons process visual information is of both medical and practical interest. Responses of early visual cortex have been explained by hand-designed models, such as Gabor wavelet filters (Hubel and Wiesel, 1959), or by models based on first-principles such as efficient coding (Olshausen and Field, 1996). However, similar approaches have achieved limited success in describing the responses of neurons in higher-order visual areas, likely because of the complexity of high-level visual features.

In parallel, for a better characterization of visual cortex, CNNs loosely based on neurobiological knowledge were being developed (see previous section). CNNs are image-computable models, meaning that we can show the same images to the models as we show to a monkey or a human. Thus, we can directly compare the responses of artificial units and biological neurons to the same inputs. As described in the previous section, the synaptic weights of the CNNs are adjusted via supervised learning on a computer vision data set created to assess object recognition, notably without using any neural data. One approach to comparing AI units to biological neurons is to use a linear mapping to fit the responses of a biological neuron's response patterns (Yamins et al., 2014). Validation of these models was only possible relatively recently, as AI systems, fueled by several technological advances, became powerful enough to do realistic visual recognition tasks. Remarkably, CNNs as models to quantitatively explain neuronal responses have outperformed all previous models in describing the responses of neurons in the retina, in primary visual cortex, and in other areas along the ventral visual stream, including the top echelons of inferior temporal cortex. For example, the famous AlexNet neural network (Krizhevsky et al., 2012), at its time the best-performing algorithm by far on a challenging image recognition task, has been shown to be a good model of visual neuronal responses, as have later CNNs with increasingly better performance (Schrimpf et al., 2018). Furthermore, CNN models with higher performance on computer vision object categorization tasks tend to better explain neuronal responses in ventral visual cortex. This result suggested that brain-like computations may be specified by brain-related tasks, rather than by neural data directly. Ongoing research highlights the remaining gap in the quantitative description of neuronal responses (Schrimpf et al., 2018), and aims to address deviations of CNNs from biological vision in architecture (Kar et al., 2019; Kubilius et al., 2019; Tang et al., 2018), learning rules (Lillicrap et al., 2020), and behavior (Nguyen et al., 2015; Szegedy et al., 2020).

10.2.2 Convolutional Neural Network-Learned Features Reveal Stimulus Preferences and Organizing Principles in Visual Cortex

As discussed above, visual features learned by neural networks agree well with those used in the brain. In addition, learned features – unlike hand-picked features such as the orientation of a grating, surface texture, shape curvature, or face appearance – apply generally throughout visual areas and types of selectivity. Thus, such visual features can serve as a general framework for defining stimulus preferences and explaining the organizing principles throughout the visual cortex.

A recent study (Ponce et al., 2019) showed that the tuning properties of V1 and inferior temporal (IT) cortex neurons can be discovered using a generative neural network (Goodfellow et al., 2014), without resorting to arbitrary investigator-chosen features like oriented gratings or faces. In a typical CNN, the input is an image and the output is a vector of image features or labels. A generative neural network inverts the process, taking features as inputs and producing images. Combining the generative network with neuronal recordings in a closed loop (Figure 10.2), this method allowed the investigators to discover image features that activated the neurons as well as, and in some cases better than, the best natural images. Notably, although the generative network was trained on natural images, it was not limited to images it has seen. Thus, this approach could discover neuronal tuning in an unbiased fashion, without imposing an investigator's existing notions of what a neuron might be tuned to. Similar approaches have been used to reveal visual neuronal tuning in other areas in monkeys (Abbasi-Asl et al., 2018; Bashivan et al., 2019), mice (Walker et al., 2019), and artificial neural networks (Olah et al., 2017; Zeiler and Fergus, 2014).

An interesting property of the cortex is its topographical organization whereby nearby neurons show similar tuning properties. A recent study (Bao et al., 2020) used CNN-encoded image features to confirm this topographical organization of macaque IT cortex and describe its feature selectivity. The IT cortex contains continuous patches selective for directions of image variation defined by a CNN. Patches selective for different feature directions are arranged in a consistent order, repeated from

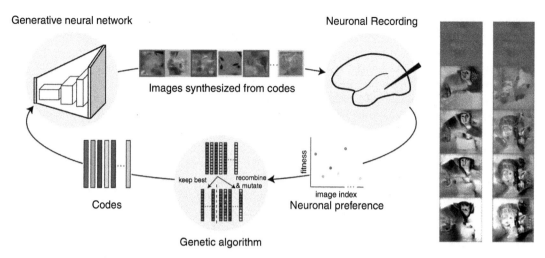

Figure 10.2 Example of how AI has helped advance vision research. A generative neural network coupled to a genetic algorithm can be used in a closed-loop system to uncover neuron selectivity in an automatic and unbiased manner. A generative neural network is an inverted CNN that takes feature codes as inputs and creates images. The synthetic images are presented to a monkey while recording neuronal responses. These neuronal responses are used as a "fitness" function to rank the images from best to worst. Finally, a genetic algorithm mutates and recombines the feature codes to feed back to the image generator. The loop is iterated until the algorithm converges on images that effectively trigger high activation for the neurons (Ponce et al., 2019). The two columns on the right show two example evolutions of preferred images for two face-selective neurons.

posterior to anterior IT cortex. Hearkening to layers in deep neural networks, this organization of the IT cortex is also hierarchical: responses in more anterior patches are more invariant to the same object viewed from different angles. Moreover, previous accounts of IT tuning to faces, size (big–small), and 3D shape can be explained in a common framework based on the CNN-derived features. In fact, although these features partially correlated with semantic categories, CNN-derived features explain neuronal responses better than do semantic categories.

In summary, artificial neural networks can be used to meaningfully interpret the computations along visual cortex and parsimoniously explain neuronal response properties. Such an understanding may one day be used to develop more specific and powerful visual prosthetics (see the last section).

10.2.3 Artificial Intelligence-Based Models Illuminate Complex Visual Behaviors

Artificial intelligence algorithms can now achieve human-level performance on some specialized visual tasks, such as the ImageNet challenge for object recognition (He et al., 2015; Russakovsky et al., 2015) and clinical tasks like detecting whether an image contains a tumor or not (Lotter et al., 2021). Yet, the general visual behaviors of humans are much richer, more complex, and more versatile, and there is still a long way to go for AI systems to

emulate higher-order human vision. Nevertheless, domain-specific AI systems provide useful building blocks for modeling such behaviors. For example, humans can perform efficient visual search. One example is searching for a tumor in a magnetic resonance image. This search is efficient, because humans do not have to exhaustively sample all possible locations; and invariant, because humans can search for objects regardless of their position, scale, illumination, or rotation. In addition, humans can perform a zero-shot search, namely searching for novel objects. In comparison, object detection algorithms in computer vision require extensive training for each object class and extensive sampling of image locations during detection. To start closing the gap, investigators developed a biologically inspired computational model for visual search (Zhang et al., 2018) composed of an object recognition module and an attention module. The model produces a series of eye movements that are specific to the sought target and the search image. Without training on human data, this algorithm approximates human eye movements and search performance. Like humans, this model does not need to be retrained for new search targets or conditions, working out-of-the-box to search for objects in an array on a uniform background, in natural photographs, and in Where's Waldo images. Presumably, this is possible because the underlying object recognition model has learned generally useful visual features and invariances. Similar methods of using simple models as building blocks hold promise for explaining a large range of complex visual behaviors.

The reach of AI algorithms now extends well beyond pure sensory processes. Artificial intelligence-based systems have been used to model a large range of behaviors including reinforcement learning (Dabney et al., 2020), decision making, and game-play. In some cases, AI algorithms have achieved superhuman performance in problems not long ago thought to be still out of reach for machines – including Atari games (Mnih et al., 2015), chess, the ancient Chinese game of Go (Silver et al., 2016, 2017, 2018), video games like StarCraft II (Vinyals et al., 2019), and Texas hold 'em (Brown and Sandholm, 2019).

10.3 Prospects of Artificial Intelligence-Based Tools in Neuroscience and Neurosurgery

The ability of AI systems to perform accurate pattern recognition holds the promise to radically transform many aspects of clinical practice. One of the important domains that has been revolutionized by advances in AI is image-based diagnosis, but AI is also likely to impact many other domains such as the development of better brain–machine interfaces.

10.3.1 Discovering the Unexpected: Disease Diagnosis from Retinal Fundus Photographs With Artificial Intelligence Systems

An example application of CNNs in clinical diagnosis is the analysis of retinal fundus photographs (see also work in cancer detection; Lotter et al., 2021). Such images can be used to diagnose conditions such as diabetic retinopathy (Gulsham et al., 2016; Ting et al., 2017). In the same fashion that a CNN can be trained to discriminate images of chairs versus tables via supervised learning, these neural networks can be fed with multiple examples of fundus photographs with or without diabetic retinopathy. These expert-annotated images are used to train the network (i.e., change the synaptic weights between units). The CNNs excel at this task, and their performance is similar to that of expert ophthalmologists (Poplin et al., 2018). Subsequent work extended CNNs to diagnosing glaucoma and age-related macular degeneration (AMD) using retinal images (Ting et al., 2017).

Surprisingly, CNNs can be trained to accurately predict other information from these images, including a subject's gender or age. Clinicians never knew that there was such information in fundus photographs; after all, gender and age are not particularly interesting variables to decipher from clinical images given that such information is always available to the doctor.

What is even more astounding, CNNs could use fundus photographs to predict smoking status (71% of the time) and systolic blood pressure (11.23 mmHg in mean absolute error). Next, the investigators then asked whether it is possible to predict the risk of cardiovascular disease from the same images. Strikingly, CNNs could estimate the risk of cardiovascular disease as well as the Framingham score, without any information other than the images themselves.

10.3.2 Detecting Spatiotemporal Patterns in Data: Seizure Prediction Using Deep Learning

The success of CNNs in pattern classification from images has encouraged the development of a plethora of other types of deep-learning algorithms that extend beyond image processing, for example, incorporating analysis of temporal information in the classification of video data and other time-varying signals. A noteworthy domain of applications is seizure detection and seizure prediction (Fergus et al., 2016). A recent review paper by Siddiqui et al. (2020) shows that a wide range of machine-learning methods are capable of classifying seizures given a segment of time-series data.

The main challenges in seizure detection and seizure prediction involve the selection of appropriate classifiers and features. The type of CNN architectures discussed in Sections 10.1 and 10.2 do not readily incorporate temporal information. Rather, signals go from one layer to the next in a sequential fashion. In stark contrast, information flow in the brain includes complex dynamics arising from horizontal connections between neurons in a given brain area as well as the interplay of bottom-up and top-down signals (Felleman and Van Essen, 1991). Akin to such biological connectivity, recurrent neural networks (RNNs), which belong to a family of deep-learning models, have shown success in describing dynamic aspects of neural firing in the visual system (Kar et al., 2019; Tang et al., 2018) and in natural-language processing (Vaswani et al., 2017).

Similarly, several studies have started exploring the feasibility and efficiency of applying RNNs in extracting temporal signatures of seizures from time-series data. Cho and Jang (2020) surveyed and compared current deep-learning techniques in seizure classification. These techniques typically take inputs from either of three major classes: 5-s segments of raw time-series data from electroencephalographic (EEG) data, 2D images of raw EEG waveforms, and 2D images in frequency domain using short-term Fourier transform of the waveforms. Seizure classification using AI algorithms achieves high accuracy (99.3% of the time). These results encourage the exploration of the more challenging problem of seizure prediction.

10.3.3 Restoring Vision for the Blind: Artificial Intelligence-Assisted Brain–Machine Interactions

In the famous "frog galvanoscope" experiment of 1781, Luigi Galvani injected electric currents to twitch a frog's legs. Since then, humans have never stopped pursuing the dream of communicating between nervous systems and machines. Until now, courageous and initial efforts have been taken in developing medical implants to treat Parkinson's disease via deep brain stimulation (Cagnan et al., 2019) and neuronal signal decoders to decipher movement intentions in quadriplegic patients (Tam et al., 2019). With the advent of powerful AI tools, major revolutions could come for brain–machine interfaces (BMIs) for a wide variety of clinical applications.

A tantalizing prospect is the development of prosthetics for visual restoration, which could be life-changing for the large number of patients who are blind or have severe visual impairment. Economical yet sophisticated digital cameras that can rapidly capture and transmit visual information are now prevalent in smartphones and wearable devices. Convolutional neural networks can extract meaningful information from such images. The main challenge and missing link is how to transmit this information to a patient's brain. A review paper by Niketeghad and Pouratian (2019) outlines opportunities and challenges of the cortical visual prosthesis under investigation. Two main approaches are taken, based on electrical stimulation of either the retina or V1. Both approaches suffer from the limited number of electrodes and non-uniform arrangement of their ensuing phosphenes in the visual field.

An intriguing alternative would be to use the type of computer vision approaches highlighted in the previous section to preprocess the images and submit to the cortex a digested version of neural codes compatible with brains (Figure 10.3). This highly processed information could then be fed into higher visual centers via electrical stimulation. Instead of eliciting individual phosphenes, this approach may be used to evoke a complete visual precept, by triggering neuronal populations tuned to more complex visual features or even aspects of visual scene understanding. For example, depending on the subject's goals, the AI algorithm could either read text, help avoid obstacles during navigation, identify faces, or even provide a description of the visual scene. A schematic illustration of a hypothetical high-level BMI for the blind is presented in Figure 10.3. One could imagine that AI tools, combined with an understanding of the visual cortex, can enable the "inception" of specific precepts by a neuro-visual prosthesis (Roe et al., 2020).

An even more intriguing alternative is to feed this highly processed information into readily available information channels, such as auditory and somatosensory modalities. For example, the AI algorithms could interpret the scene surrounding a blind subject's environment and then provide explicit directions and instructions via a virtually generated avatar that provides directional verbal commands. Rather than a BMI device, this approach merely requires portable and virtual reality (VR)-compatible headphones that are readily available through the gaming community (Liu et al., 2018).

10.3.4 Artificial Intelligence-Specific Concerns in Neuroscience and Neurosurgery

Artificial intelligence technologies come with risks; they face criticisms including privacy threats, security pitfalls, potential biases, issues of legal liability, as well as other ethical and moral concerns (Grote and Berens, 2020; Rigby, 2019; Vayena et al., 2018). For example, many AI models need access to massive data sets for training. Transferring gigabytes of data across multiple healthcare organizations might lead to data breaches. Moreover, biases intrinsic to the data sets (such as those pertaining to race, gender, or other stereotypes) may become ingrained into the algorithm during training. Even if all privacy and bias concerns were adequately addressed, algorithms can fail to provide the right answer. Of course, clinicians do not always make the correct diagnosis, either. But, if an algorithm fails, who is to blame?

With great power comes great responsibility. As humanity continues to develop and benefit from intelligent machines, researchers and practitioners alike should heed potential ethical concerns, address them proactively, and shape the future of AI.

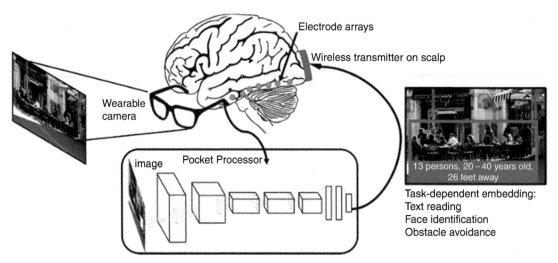

Figure 10.3 Schematic illustration of a hypothetical future high-level brain–machine interface for the blind. A wearable camera sends the visual input to the CNN algorithm for image processing implemented in a pocket processor. The CNN algorithm could extract in real time task-relevant information including reading text, identifying faces, and avoiding obstacles during navigation. The main challenge is how to convey the extracted information to the blind person. This figure illustrates a potential wireless transmitter that communicates with implanted electrodes arrays across multiple levels of ventral visual cortex that would electrically stimulate the brain to pass on the AI-processed information.

Figure acknowledgements

The following images are credited to the authors of this chapter: Figures 10.1-10.3

References

Abbasi-Asl R, Chen Y, Bloniarz A, et al. The DeepTune framework for modeling and characterizing neurons in visual cortex area V4. *bioRxiv* 2018:465534. https://doi.org/10.1101/465534

Bao P, She L, McGill M, and Tsao DY. A map of object space in primate inferotemporal cortex. *Nature* 2020;**583**:103–08.

Bashivan P, Kar K, and DiCarlo JJ. Neural population control via deep image synthesis. *Science* 2019;**364**(6439):eeav9436.

Brown N and Sandholm T. Superhuman AI for multiplayer poker. *Science* 2019;**365**:885–90. https://doi.org/10.1126/science.aay240.

Cagnan H, Denison T, McIntyre C, and Brown P. Emerging technologies for improved deep brain stimulation. *Nat Biotechnol* 2019;**37**:1024–33. https://doi.org/10.1038/s41587-019-0244-6.

Carandini M and Heeger D. Normalization as a canonical neural computation. *Nat Rev Neurosci* 2011;**23**:51–62. https://doi.org/10.1038/nrn3136.

Cho KO and Jang HJ. Comparison of different input modalities and network structures for deep learning-based seizure detection. *Scientific Rep* 2020;**10**:1–11. https://doi.org/10.1038/s41598-019-56958-y.

Crick F, Koch C, Kreiman G, and Fried I. Consciousness and neurosurgery. *Neurosurgery* 2004;**55**:272–82. https://doi.org/10.1227/01.neu.0000129279.26534.76.

Dabney W, Kurth-Nelson Z, Uchida N, et al. A distributional code for value in dopamine-based reinforcement learning. *Nature* 2020;**577**:671–5. https://doi.org/10.1038/s41586-019-1924-6.

DiCarlo JJ, Zoccolan D, and Rust NC. How does the brain solve visual object recognition? *Neuron* 2012;**73**:415–34. https://doi.org/10.1016/j.neuron.2012.01.010.

Felleman D and Van Essen D. Distributed hierarchical processing in the primate cerebral cortex. *Cereb Cortex* 1991;**1**:1–47. https://doi.org/10.1093/cercor/1.1.1-a.

Fergus P, Hussain A, Hignett D, Al-Jumeily D, Abdel-Aziz K, and Hamdan H. A machine learning system for automated whole-brain seizure detection. *Appl Comput Informat* 2016;**12**:70–89. https://doi.org/10.1016/j.aci.2015.01.001.

Goodfellow I, Pouget-Abadie J, Mirza M, et al. Generative adversarial nets. In *Advances in Neural Information Processing Systems*. Curran Associates, Inc., 2014: 2672–80.

Grote T and Berens P. On the ethics of algorithmic decision-making in healthcare. *J Med Ethics* 2020;**46**:205–11. https://doi.org/10.1136/medethics-2019-105586.

Gulshan V, Peng L, Coram M, et al. Development and validation of a deep learning algorithm for detection of diabetic retinopathy in retinal fundus photographs. *JAMA* 2016;**316**:2402–10. https://doi.org/10.1001/jama.2016.17216.

Hassabis D, Kumaran D, Summerfield C, and Botvinick M. Neuroscience-inspired artificial intelligence. *Neuron* 2017;**95**:245–58. https://doi.org/0.1016/j.neuron.2017.06.011.

He K, Zhang X, Ren S, and Sun J. Delving deep into rectifiers: surpassing human-level performance on imagenet classification. In *Proceedings of the IEEE International Conference on Computer Vision*, Santiago, Chile, 2015, pp. 1026–34. https://doi.org/10.1109/ICCV.2015.123.

Hubel DH and Wiesel TN. Receptive fields of single neurones in the cat's striate cortex. *J Physiol* 1959;**148**:574. https://doi.org/10.1113/jphysiol.1959.sp006308.

Hubel DH and Wiesel TN. Receptive fields, binocular interaction and functional architecture in the cat's visual cortex. *J Physiol* 1962;**160**:106. https://doi.org/10.1113/jphysiol.1962.sp006837.

Kar K, Kubilius J, Schmidt K, Issa EB, and DiCarlo JJ. Evidence that recurrent circuits are critical to the ventral stream's execution of core object recognition behavior. *Nature Neuroscience* 2019;**22**:974–83. https://doi.org/10.1038/s41593-019-0392-5.

Krizhevsky A, Sutskever I, and Hinton GE. ImageNet classification with deep convolutional neural networks. In *Advances in Neural Information Processing Systems*. Curran Associates, Inc., 2012:1097–105.

Kubilius J, Schrimpf M, Kar K, et al. Brain-like object recognition with high-performing shallow recurrent ANNs. In *Advances in Neural Information Processing Systems*. Curran Associates, Inc., 2019: 12805–16.

Lillicrap TP, Santoro A, Marris L, Akerman CJ, and Hinton G. Backpropagation and the brain. *Nat Rev Neurosci* 2020;**21**:335–46. https://doi.org/10.1038/s41583-020-0277-3.

Liu H, Agam Y, Madsen J, and Kreiman G. Timing, timing, timing: fast decoding of object information from intracranial field potentials in human visual cortex. *Neuron* 2009;**62**:281–90. https://doi.org/10.1016/j.neuron.2009.02.025.

Liu, Yang, Stiles NRB, Meister M. Augmented reality powers a cognitive assistant for the blind.*eLife* 2018;7:e37841. https://doi.org/10.7554/eLife.37841.

Lotter W, Diab A, Haslam B, et al. Robust breast cancer detection in mammography and digital breast tomosynthesis using annotation-efficient deep learning approach. *Nat Med* 2021;**27**:244–9. https://doi.org/10.1038/s41591-020-01174-9.

McCulloch W and Pitts W. Logical calculus of the ideas immanent in nervous activity. *Bull Math Biophys* 1943;**5**:115–33. https://doi.org/10.1007/BF02478259.

Mnih V, Kavukcuoglu K, Silver D, et al. Human-level control through deep reinforcement learning. *Nature* 2015;**518**:529–33. https://doi.org/10.1038/nature14236.

Nguyen A, Yosinski J, and Clune J. Deep neural networks are easily fooled: high confidence predictions for unrecognizable images. In *Proceedings of the IEEE Conference on Computer Vision and Pattern Recognition*, Santiago, Chile, 2015, pp. 427–36. https://doi.org/10.1109/CVPR.2015.7298640.

Niketeghad S and Pouratian N. Brain machine interfaces for vision restoration: the current state of cortical visual prosthetics. *Neurotherapeutics* 2019;**16**:134–43. https://doi.org/10.1007/s13311-018-0660-1.

Olah C, Mordvintsev A, and Schubert L. Feature visualization. *Distill* 2017;**2**:e7. https://distill.pub/2017/feature-visualization/.

Olshausen BA and Field DJ. Emergence of simple-cell receptive field properties by learning a sparse code for natural images. *Nature* 1996;**381**:607–09. https://doi.org/10.1038/381607a0.

Ponce CR, Xiao W, Schade PF, Hartmann TS, Kreiman G, and Livingstone MS. Evolving images for visual neurons using a deep generative network reveals coding principles and neuronal preferences. *Cell* 2019;**177**:999–1009. https://doi.org/10.1016/j.cell.2019.04.005.

Poplin R, Varadarajan AV, Blumer K, et al. Prediction of cardiovascular risk factors from retinal fundus photographs via deep learning. *Nat Biomed Eng* 2018;**2**:158. https://doi.org/10.1038/s41551-018-0195-0.

Richards BA, Lillicrap TP, Beaudoin P, et al. A deep learning framework for neuroscience. *Nat Neurosci* 2019;**22**:1761–70. https://doi.org/10.1038/s41593-019-0520-2.

Riesenhuber M and Poggio T. Hierarchical models of object recognition in cortex. *Nat Neurosci* 1999;**2**:1019–25. https://doi.org/10.1038/14819.

Rigby MJ. Ethical dimensions of using artificial intelligence in health care. *AMA J Ethics* 2019;**21**:121–4. https://doi.org/10.1001/amajethics.2019.121.

Roe AW, Chen G, Xu AG, and Hu J. A roadmap to a columnar visual cortical prosthetic. *Curr Opin Physiol* 2020;**16**:68–78. https://doi.org/10.1016/j.cophys.2020.06.009.

Russakovsky O, Deng J, Su H, et al. ImageNet large scale visual recognition challenge. *Int J Comput Vis* 2015;**115**:211–52. https://doi.org/10.1007/s11263-015-0816-y.

Sacks O. *The Man who Mistook His Wife for a Hat*. Picador, 2002.

Schrimpf M, Kubilius J, Hong H, et al. Brain-score: which artificial neural network for object recognition is most brain-like? *BioRxiv* 2018:407007. https://doi.org/10.1101/407007.

Serre T. Deep learning: the good, the bad, and the ugly. *Annu Rev Vision Sci* 2019;**5**:399–426. https://doi.org/10.1146/annurev-vision-091718-014951.

Siddiqui MK, Morales-Menendez R, Huang X, and Hussain N. A review of epileptic seizure detection using machine learning classifiers. *Brain Informat* 2020;**7**:1–18. https://doi.org/10.1186/s40708-020-00105-1.

Silver D, Huang A, Maddison CJ, et al. Mastering the game of Go with deep neural networks and tree search. *Nature* 2016;**529**:484–9. https://doi.org/10.1038/nature16961.

Silver D, Hubert T, Schrittwieser J, et al. A general reinforcement learning algorithm that masters chess, shogi, and Go through self-play. *Science* 2018;**362**:1140–4. https://doi.org/10.1126/science.aar6404.

Silver D, Schrittwieser J, Simonyan K, et al. Mastering the game of Go without human knowledge. *Nature* 2017;**550**:354–9. https://doi.org/10.1038/nature24270

Szegedy C, Zaremba W, Sutskever I, et al. Intriguing properties of neural networks. *arXiv* 2013; preprint arXiv:1312.6199. https://doi.org/10.48550/arXiv.1312.6199.

Tam Wk, Wu T, Zhao Q, Keefer E, and Yang Z. Human motor decoding from neural signals: a review. *BMC Biomed Eng* 2019;**1**:22. https://doi.org/10.1186/s42490-019-0022-z.

Tang H, Schrimpf M, Lotter W, et al. Recurrent computations for visual pattern completion. *PNAS* 2018;**28**:8835–40. https://doi.org/10.1073/pnas.1719397115.

Ting DSW, Cheung CYL, Lim G, et al. Development and validation of a deep learning system for diabetic retinopathy and related eye diseases using retinal images from multiethnic populations with diabetes. *JAMA* 2017;**318**:2211–23. https://doi.org/10.1001/jama.2017.18152..

Vaswani A, Shazeer N, Parmar N, et al. Attention is all you need. In *Advances in Neural Information Processing Systems*. Curran Associates, Inc., 2017: 5998–6008. https://doi.org/10.48550/arXiv.1706.03762.

Vayena E, Blasimme A, and Cohen IG. Machine learning in medicine: addressing ethical challenges. *PLoS Med* 2018;**15**:e1002689. https://doi.org/10.1371/journal.pmed.1002689.

Vinyals O, Babuschkin I, Czarnecki WM, et al. Grandmaster level in StarCraft II using multi-agent reinforcement learning. *Nature* 2019;**575**:350–4. https://doi.org/10.1038/s41586-019-1724-z.

Walker EY, Sinz FH, Cobos E, et al. Inception loops discover what excites neurons most using deep predictive models. *Nat Neurosci* 2019;**22**:2060–5. https://doi.org/10.1038/s41593-019-0517-x.

Yamins DL, Hong H, Cadieu CF, Solomon EA, Seibert D, and DiCarlo JJ. Performance-optimized hierarchical models predict neural responses in higher visual cortex. *PNAS* 2014;**111**:8619–24. https://doi.org/10.1073/pnas.1403112111.

Zador AM. A critique of pure learning and what artificial neural networks can learn from animal brains. *Nat Commun* 2019;**10**:1–7. https://doi.org/10.1038/s41467-019-11786-6.

Zeiler MD and Fergus R. Visualizing and understanding convolutional networks. In Fleet D, Pajdla T, Schiele B, Tuytelaars T (Eds.), *Computer Vision – European Conference on Computer Vision 2014*. Lecture Notes in Computer Science, vol. 8689. Springer, 2014: pp. 818–33. https://doi.org/10.1007/978-3-319-10590-1_53.

Zhang M, Feng J, Ma KT, Lim JH, Zhao Q, and Kreiman G. Finding any Waldo with zero-shot invariant and efficient visual search. *Nat Commun* 2018;**9**:1–15. https://doi.org/10.1038/s41467-018-06217-x.

Probability and Statistics

Zachary T. Miller

11.1 Introduction and Motivation

11.1.1 What Is Probability? What Is Statistics?

Probability theory is a mathematical framework that allows us to quantify and study random events and phenomena. By "random," we mean outcomes that could not have been known for certain beforehand. A classic example of a random event is whether a fair coin lands on heads or tails when it is tossed. In fact, many everyday events can be considered random. How long your commute to work takes, whether it will rain today, your chance of winning in a hand of blackjack, these are all examples of random events. Statistics, on the other hand, is the scientific discipline concerned with the study of data. Collecting, analyzing, and presenting data are all different parts of statistics. As we will see throughout this chapter, probability theory and statistics are often used in conjunction with one another.

11.1.2 Why are Probability and Statistics Useful in Neuroscience?

Probability and statistics are useful in any scientific endeavor. Why? Because the scientific method consists of forming a hypothesis and gathering data to either confirm or reject that hypothesis. However, in order to know whether the data that have been gathered support or contradict our hypothesis, we need to use statistics. And to use statistics, we need probability. Returning to the example of tossing a coin, suppose we are studying the properties of a particular coin. Because we know that most coins we have come across are fair (have the same probability of landing on heads or tails when tossed), we may hypothesize that this coin is also fair. To test this hypothesis, we set up an experiment wherein we toss the coin ten times and record our results. But how would we interpret the results of our experiment in the context of

our hypothesis? Does the coin landing on heads exactly five times out of ten confirm our hypothesis? How about six times? Or nine? How much more confident will we be in our conclusion if we toss the coin 100 times instead of ten? The answers to all of these questions can be found using probability and statistics.

In addition to the analysis of scientific data, probability and statistics are commonly used in many models of the nervous system. In fact, probabilistic models are used to describe everything from the firing of individual neurons to neural plasticity to cognitive models of perception. Because the nervous system is so complex, we often use probability and statistics to make simplifying assumptions in a principled way. For example, because it would be infeasible to record the activity of every neuron in the brain, we may instead average over the activity of many neurons in a given region. Probability and statistics can help us understand the merits and limitations of such an approach.

11.2 Random Variables and Probability Distributions

11.2.1 Refresher on What Probabilities Are and Are Not

Probabilities are defined in the language of "experiments," "sample spaces," and "events." Roughly speaking, an *experiment* is some process that maps a set of potential outcomes (the *sample space*) onto some particular outcome or combination of outcomes (the *event*) in a non-deterministic way. That is, if you were to observe the same exact experiment multiple times, you could observe different outcomes. Let's frame this in the context of our coin toss example for concreteness. The sample space of a coin toss is the outcome of heads (H) or tails (T). The experiment is the actual tossing of the coin, which leads to a particular event (the coin landing on H or T). The experiment is non-deterministic because each tossing of the coin can lead to the observation of a different event. Note that if we were to toss the coin twice, we would have four possible outcomes in our sample space (HH, TT, HT, and TH), and an event would be the observation of one of these combinations.

A probability is a number between 0 and 1 (inclusive) that describes how likely a specific event is to occur, with higher values indicating that an event is more likely. Loosely speaking, a probability of 0 means that the given event will definitely not occur. An example of an event with probability 0 could be an event that is not in the sample space, such as a single coin toss resulting in both heads and tails. A probability of 1 means that the given event will definitely occur. For example, if our coin was double-sided heads, then the probability of observing heads would be 1. To describe the probability of some event A, we use the notation $P(A)$. In the case of a fair coin toss, with possible events H or T, we have $P(H) = 0.5$ and $P(T) = 0.5$. We can also describe different combinations of these outcomes as their own events. For example, we can ask the probability of H *or* T, or the probability of H *and* T for a given coin toss. To do this, we use the union ($\cup$) and intersection ($\cap$) symbols, respectively. Thus, we have $P(H \cup T) = 1$ and $P(H \cap T) = 0$ for a single coin toss.

11.2.2 Random Variables

11.2.2.1 What Is a Random Variable?

Random variables are often a source of confusion when learning probability and statistics. However, once it is understood, the random variable is an extremely powerful concept that forms the core of probability and statistics. Simply put, a random variable is a variable that does not have any specific value, but instead has a range of *potential* values that it can take on. We often speak about random variables in the language of events and outcomes, where a random variable represents the range of possible outcomes for a particular event. Returning to our coin-tossing example, the tossing of the coin is the event and the result of the coin toss (heads or tails) is the outcome. If we denote a result of heads with a H, and a result of tails as a T, then we have constructed a random variable, call it X, with potential values H and T. Here, we chose to denote our random variable with a capital letter. This is convention in probability theory and allows us to differentiate random variables from the more familiar algebraic variable, which we denote with a lowercase letter.

Once the event has taken place, the random variable "crystallizes" and takes on an actual value. This value is no longer a random variable, it is a *realization* of a random variable. Returning to our above example, X was the random variable representing the possible outcomes of tossing our coin. However, once the coin has been tossed and we have observed the result, X crystallizes into either a H or a T. We often use the lowercase version of the same letter that denoted a random variable to denote the algebraic variable that represents the realization of that random variable. This way, we can write the equation $P(X = x)$, read as "the probability that the random variable X takes on the value x." In the case of a fair coin toss, we would have $P(X = H) = 0.5$ and $P(X = T) = 0.5$.

11.2.2.2 Probability Distributions

Having added random variables to our probability toolbox, we may want to ask more complicated questions. For example, in the simple case of a random variable representing the outcome of a toss of a fair coin, it is pretty obvious that the outcome of a H and a T are both equally likely, and thus both had a probability of 0.5. However, this becomes more complicated as we move away from our simple example of a fair coin. We could instead consider the probabilities of the potential results of tossing an unfair coin, or of tossing an unfair die, or of recording the number of times a neuron spikes in a specific time interval. In order to account for the probabilities of all these potential outcomes, we could use a function that takes as its input a potential outcome of a random variable, and gives as its output the probability of that outcome. Of course, such a function would have to obey the rules of probability, so the probabilities of all the potential outcomes would all have to be between 0 and 1, and the sum over the probabilities of all the outcomes would have to be 1. Let's denote this function as $p_X(x)$ for some random variable X such that $P(X = x) = p_X(x)$. Here, the subscript of X lets us know that the function $p(x)$ is for the random variable X, which is useful when we are working with problem with more than one random variable. In probability theory, this type of function is called a *probability distribution*. These functions are extremely important because they give us a framework for converting the language of probabilities, events, and outcomes into the language of mathematics. And once in the language of mathematics, we can deal quantitatively with these functions, their properties, and their interactions just as we could with any other mathematical function.

Any function that meets the criteria outlined above can be used as a probability distribution, but there are a few functions that are particularly useful in probability and statistics. In fact, these probability distributions come up so often that they have been given names (some of which you might recognize) like normal (sometimes referred to as Gaussian), binomial, exponential, Poisson, etc. Many of these probability distributions have "scenarios" that they are commonly used to represent, as well as many known mathematical properties that make them nice to work with. Let's take a brief look at the binomial distribution. The binomial distribution is often used when we have some number of independent trials that succeed with probability p and fail with probability $1 - p$, and we want to quantify the probability of having x successes. The number of times a coin lands on heads when the coin is tossed some number of times is a perfect application for the binomial distribution. The equation for the binomial distribution is $P(X = x) = \binom{n}{x} p^x (1 - p)^{n-x}$, where x is the number of successes, n is the total number of trials, p is the probability of success on each trial, and $\binom{n}{x}$ is the binomial coefficient (this is just a more compact notation for $\frac{n!}{x!(n-x)!}$). Don't worry too much if the math looks complicated, just focus on what the terms in the equation mean in the context of our coin-tossing example. x is the

potential outcome we would like to calculate the probability of, and n and p are *parameters* that allow us to alter the form of the function. You can think of n and p as being like little knobs that you can turn to make the above equation fit the specifics of your problem.

As a quick aside on notation, we often write that $X \sim Binom(n,p)$, read as "X is distributed as a binomial, with parameters n and p." This is simply a less tedious way of writing $P(X = x) = \binom{n}{x} p^x (1 - p)^{n-x}$. Most common distributions have a similar shorthand notation. A table of common distributions can be found in Table 11.1.

11.2.2.3 Discrete Versus Continuous Probability Distributions

Thus far, we have only considered a very specific type of random variable that was of a type called *discrete*. Discrete random variables can only take on a specific set of values on some range, and none of the values in between. This is the world of coin tosses, dice rolls, and spiking neurons. For example, our coin toss can result in either a 0 or a 1, but it cannot result in 0.5. However, there is another class of random variables called *continuous* random variables.

Table 11.1 A table of common distributions. The shorthand notation for each distribution is shown under the distribution name.

Distribution Name and Shorthand	Discrete or Continuous	PMF or PDF
Bernoulli $Bern(p)$	Discrete	$P(X = 1) = p$ $P(X = 0) = 1 - p$
Binomial $Bin(n, p)$	Discrete	$P(X = k) = \binom{n}{k} p^k (1 - p)^{n-k}$
Normal or Gaussian $N(\mu, \sigma^2)$	Continuous	$f_X(x) = \frac{1}{\sigma\sqrt{2\pi}} e^{-(x-\mu)^2/(2\sigma^2)}$
Uniform $Unif(a, b)$	Continuous	$f_X(x) = \frac{1}{b-a}$
Poisson $Pois(\lambda)$	Discrete	$P(X = k) = \frac{e^{-\lambda}\lambda^k}{k!}$
Exponential $Expo(\lambda)$	Continuous	$f_X(x) = \lambda e^{-\lambda x}$
Student's t-distribution t_n	Continuous	$f_X(x) = \frac{\Gamma((n+1)/2)}{\sqrt{n\pi}\Gamma(n/2)} (1 + x^2/n)^{-(n+1)/2}$

These are random variables that can take on *any* value within some specified range, not just some subset. Examples of continuous variables include an athlete's time to run 100 meters, the density of a gas, or the time between spikes in a neuron. In all of these examples, there are infinite possible values in any non-zero interval. In the case of the time taken to run 100 meters, it may take an athlete 11 seconds, or 11.1 seconds, or 11.01 seconds, and so on.

Although the difference between discrete and continuous random variables is fairly simple, the differences between their accompanying probability distributions are more complex. To reflect these differences, we break probability distributions into two subtypes. The first is for the probability distributions of a discrete random variable, and is known as a *probability mass function* (PMF). A PMF has all the properties described above: all outputs of the PMF must be between 0 and 1 and all the outputs must all add up to 1 when summed over all possible inputs. Thus, the output value of the PMF for a given input can be directly interpreted as the probability of that value occurring.

The second type is for probability distributions of continuous random variables, and is called a *probability density function* (PDF). Simply put, a PDF is a continuous, positive-valued function that integrates to one, but the value of the PDF at any given point may be greater than one. As such, it has several differences when compared to a PMF. The most important of these differences is the interpretation of the value of the function at any point. Unlike a PMF, where the value for given input is the probability of that input, the value for a given input of a PDF is the *relative likelihood* of that input. Because a continuous random variable can take on an infinite number of possible values, the probability of the random variable taking on any given value is infinitely small. Although this may seem troublesome, in reality we are almost never interested in the probability of a continuous random variable taking on a specific value. Instead, we are usually concerned about the probability of it being within some range of values. Luckily, the probability of a continuous random variable lying within some interval can be easily calculated by taking the integral of the PDF over that interval. Therefore, if we wanted to know the probability of an athlete's 100-meter dash time being between 11.0 and 11.5 seconds, we would simply calculate $\int_{11.0}^{11.5} f_T(t)dt$, where T is the random variable representing the time taken for the athlete to finish the race, and $f_T(t)$ is

the probability density function for T. The same process can be applied in the discrete case using a summation instead of an integral. Notice that, when working with continuous variables, we use the notation f to denote that the function is a PDF rather than a PMF. A visual comparison of discrete versus continuous probability functions can be found in Figures 11.1A and 11.1B.

11.2.3 Properties of Probability

11.2.3.1 Basic Properties

Just as in mathematics, there are some basic axioms upon which the rest of probability theory is built. We will cover these axioms here briefly, and then highlight a couple of important consequences of these axioms. The axioms are as follows:

Axiom 1 *The probability of an event occurring is a real number greater than or equal to 0*

Axiom 2 *The probability of at least one event in the entire sample space occurring is 1*

Axiom 3 *For mutually exclusive events, the probability of at least one of the events occurring is the sum of the probability of each mutually exclusive event occurring*

Although these axioms may seem rather simple, they allow us to derive a few very important rules. Here, we will cover just two of these rules. The first rule we will cover is called the *addition rule of probability*. It states that, for two events A and B, $P(A \cup B) = P(A) + P(B) - P(A \cap B)$. This rule is very useful as it gives us a way for solving any probability question that asks about the probability of one event *or* another occurring. The second rule we will cover here is called the *compliment rule*. Suppose we have a sample space, call it Ω, and an event in that sample space, A. Instead of finding $P(A)$, which is straightforward, we may wish to find $P(A^c)$. A^c is known as the *compliment* of A (usually read as "A compliment"), and it is comprised of all the sample space that does not contain A. For example, if A were the event that the result of rolling a single die once was 1, then A^c would be the event that the result is any of the numbers 2 through 6. The compliment rule states that $P(A^c) = 1 - P(A)$. This result can be extremely useful in cases where it is far easier to find the probability of A than it is to find the probability of all the other possible combinations of events in the sample space.

11.2.3.2 Conditional Probability

When trying to estimate the probability of an event, we may want to incorporate additional information into our

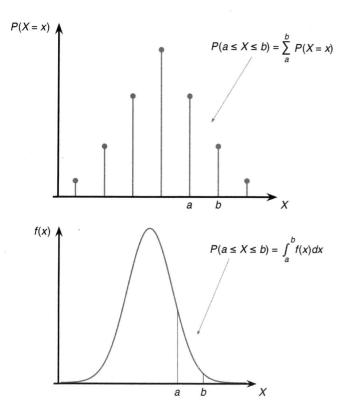

Figure 11.1 Visual depiction of a PMF (A) and a PDF (B).

calculations in order to improve the accuracy of our estimate. For example, suppose we were asked to estimate the probability of a newborn baby growing to be above six feet tall as an adult, denoted by the letter T. Perhaps we create some model and calculate an estimate for $P(T)$ using that model. Now suppose that we are also told that the newborn is female, which we denote with the letter F. Clearly, this new information should change our estimate for $P(T)$, but how can we incorporate it into our calculation? In probability theory, this is a process known as *conditioning*, and yields a *conditional probability*, which we denote as $P(T|F)$ (read as "the probability of the newborn being over six feet tall *given* that the newborn is female"). Conditioning is an extremely important concept in probability and statistics as it gives us a rigorous means for updating our equations based on new information. For two events, A and B, we can calculate the probability of A conditional on B using Equation 11.1:

$$P(A|B) = \frac{P(A \cap B)}{P(B)} \tag{11.1}$$

Equation 11.1 gives us a mathematical way to incorporate new information into probability statements. In our above example of the height of a newborn, we would have $P(T|F) = \frac{P(T \cap F)}{P(F)}$. Equation 11.1 can be manipulated

to obtain a few other important results in conditional probability: Bayes' Theorem and the Law of Total Probability. Bayes' Theorem is given by:

$$P(A|B) = \frac{P(B|A)P(A)}{P(B)} \tag{11.2}$$

Equation 11.2 is useful for solving tough conditional probability problems, as we will see below. Although Bayes' Theorem can be used (and is used often!) to solve any conditional probability problem, it is especially useful when trying to solve conditional probability problems of a particular form in which we have some hypothesis and we are trying to evaluate how probable it is in the face newly collected data. In fact, it is so useful for this kind of problem that the individual terms in Equation 11.2 have their own names in this situation. In this case, we want to know the probability that some hypothesis A is true given some data (sometimes called "evidence") B. The term $P(A|B)$ is called the *posterior*, so-called because it is the probability that our hypothesis is true *after* we have observed the data. The term $P(B|A)$ is often called the *likelihood*, and represents the probability of having observed the data B given that our hypothesis A is true and thus the likelihood of A being true given the observed data. The term $P(A)$ is called the *prior*, it represents the probability that the hypothesis is true *before* we have collected the data B. Finally, the term $P(B)$ is called the *evidence*, and represents the probability of having observed the data B under all possible hypotheses. Example problem 1 should make all of these terms and their relationship to Bayes' Theorem more concrete.

The last equation we will introduce in this section is known as the Law of Total Probability (LOTP). Suppose that we want to calculate the probability of some event B, and we know that one of the events $A_1, \ldots, A_n$ must also occur alongside B. In this situation, the equation for LOTP is given by:

$$P(B) = \sum_{i=1}^{n} P(B|A_i)P(A_i) \qquad (11.3)$$

Note that we can rearrange Equation 11.1 to get the expression $P(A \cap B) = P(A|B)P(B) = P(B|A)P(A)$. We can use this fact to see that the $P(B|A_i)P(A_i)$ terms within the sum of Equation 11.3 are actually just expressing the probability of B and A_i. Now the above equation is actually quite simple, stating that the probability of some event B when one of events $A_1, \ldots, A_n$ must also occur is just the sum of the probabilities of B and each A_i occurring together. This may

---

Example 1: Suppose you are administering a test to see if a given patient has meningitis. The test has a false positive rate of 0.1 and a false negative rate of 0.2. Additionally, you know from previous cases that about 10% of patients with the symptoms presented by this patient actually have meningitis. Let D be the event that the patient has the disease, and let H be the event that the patient does not have the disease. Denote P as the event that the patient tests positive, and N be the event they test negative.

(a) Suppose the test results come back positive, what is the probability that the patient has the disease?

We can express the probability of the patient having the disease given that they tested positive as $P(D|P)$. We could try to use Equation 11.1 to solve this problem, but the resulting equation is very hard to solve. Instead, let's use Bayes' Theorem to express $P(D|P)$ in different terms. Doing this below:

$$P(D|P) = \frac{P(P|D)P(D)}{P(P)}.$$

In the set up above, D is the hypothesis that the patient has the disease, and P is the data (in the form of a positive test result). The likelihood, $P(P|D)$, is just the true positive rate. The true positive rate is given by 1 minus the false negative rate, which is $1 - 0.2 = 0.8$. The prior, $P(D)$, is the probability of the patient having the disease before we knew the test result. As mentioned above, the prior can be tricky and is often subjective. However, in this problem we are told that 10% of patients presenting these symptoms have meningitis, so 0.1 is a good choice. $P(P)$ can be solved for by expanding according to LOTP, which yields $P(P) = P(P|D)P(D) + P(P|H)P(H)$. The first part of this equation, $P(P|D)P(D)$, is the same as the denominator that we already looked at. The second part, $P(P|H)P(H)$, can be solved for again by thinking about what these statements mean. $P(P|H)$ is the false positive rate, 0.1. $P(H)$ is the probability before any test results come back that the patient is healthy, which is $1 - P(D) = 0.9$. Now that we have all the values for the above equation, we simply plug them in and calculate the result:

$$\begin{aligned}
P(D|P) &= \frac{P(P|D)P(D)}{P(P)} \\[2mm]
&= \frac{P(P|D)P(D)}{P(P|D)P(D) + P(P|H)P(H)} \\[2mm]
&= \frac{(0.8)(0.1)}{(0.8)(0.1) + (0.1)(0.9)} \\[2mm]
&= \sim 0.47.
\end{aligned}$$

Now we can see that the probability of the patient having the disease, even if they tested positive, is still less than 50%. Even if it may seem at first glance that this is not such a good test, we note that the physician has more information after the test: the likelihood of the patient having the disease went up from 0.1 to 0.47, which ought to change the way they follow up with respect to further diagnostics and treatment. An interesting example of such a case is a version where the base rate of the disease is very low, say 1 in 100,000, and the false positive rate of the test is also low, say 1 in 1000. In this case the likelihood of having the disease after a positive test is still very low (i.e., 0.01, that is less than 1%), but it nonetheless should change the approach of the physician if the condition is severe.

not seem very useful – why not just calculate the probability of B directly? As we will see in example problem 1, it is often easier to calculate $P(B)$ using the sum on the right-hand side of Equation 11.3. This is especially true when applying Bayes' Theorem, and for this reason LOTP and Bayes' Theorem are often used in conjunction.

11.2.3.3 Independence

Independence is an important idea in probability theory, especially when considering the interactions of two or more random variables. Two random variables are said to be *independent* if the outcome of one of the random variables does *not* affect the outcome of the other. Mathematically, two random variables X and Y are independent if $P(X \cap Y) = P(X)P(Y)$. Alternatively, we can use the language of conditional probability to express independence mathematically as $P(X|Y) = P(X)$, or similarly $P(Y|X) = P(Y)$. As an easy example, if X and Y represent the outcomes of tossing two different coins, then X and Y are independent. However, if X represents the event that the fire alarm is going off, and Y represents the event that the building is currently on fire, then hopefully X and Y are not independent. If they are, we would have to look more carefully into the quality of the fire alarm!

11.2.3.4 Joint Distributions

Thus far, we have only considered the probability distributions of a single random variable. We have also briefly considered the interactions of two or more *independent* random variables. In this section, we will introduce joint distributions. A *joint distribution* (sometimes called a multivariate probability distribution) is any distribution of two or more random variables. These random variables can be independent or dependent (or a mixture), and can be discrete or continuous (or a mixture). In short, a joint distribution gives us a complete framework for working with combinations of random variables and their interactions, just as univariate probability distributions did for single random variables. In this section we will be focusing on joint distributions of two random variables, but the concepts introduced can be applied to joint distributions of higher dimensions as well.

To gain an intuition for what a joint probability distribution is, consider two discrete random variables X and Y. The joint PMF of X and Y, denoted as $p_{X,Y}(x,y)$ (the subscripted variables let us know what variables this PMF is for, which is quite useful when working with PMFs of many variables), is given by $p_{X,Y}(x,y) = P(X = x, Y = y)$. Using this equation, we can find the probability of any particular combination of X and Y using the joint PMF directly, or any range of combinations of X and Y by summing up over all joint PMF values for each combination. In this way, the joint PMF is used in the same way as a regular PMF, just with more dimensions. A visual representation of a discrete joint probability distribution of two random variables is offered by Figure 11.2A.

But what if we wish to recover the probability distribution of just one of the variables in the joint probability distribution, say X for example? All we have to do is sum the joint PMF over all possible values of Y, which gives: $p_X(x) = P(X = x) = \sum_y P(X = x, Y = y)$. Note that this is just the application of LOTP to find the univariate probability distribution of one of our random variables. This process of summing over the variables that you would like to remove from the distribution is known as "marginalizing out" those variables. This term comes from the fact that in the old days when statisticians would work with probability tables, they would literally add up all the values in the row or column of the table and write the results in the margin of the table. A visual intuition for this process is offered by Figure 11.2B.

We may also wish to find the conditional distribution of one of our variables given the value of the other, say the conditional distribution of X given an observed value of Y. To do this, we simply apply Equation 11.1 to the variables in our joint distribution, which yields $p_{Y|X}(y) = P(Y = y|X = x) = \frac{P(X=x,\ Y=y)}{P(X=x)}$, which is a function of y (x is fixed). The visual intuition behind this equation is that you are taking a "slice" of the joint distribution where $X = x$, which is done by the term in the numerator. This "slice" then needs to be re-normalized to sum to one (recall that this is a requirement of a probability distribution), which is accomplished by the term in the denominator. The end result is the probability distribution of Y given that we have observed $X = x$. See Figure 11.2C for an illustration of this process.

You may be wondering why we went through the trouble of introducing a joint probability distribution at all, given that all the operations defined above could just as well have been applied to two random variables considered together without having specifically bundled them into the joint probability distribution. It is true that when the random variables are *independent*, it is easy enough to deal with them as two separate univariate probability distributions. However, when the variables in question are *dependent*, dealing with them separately becomes much more difficult. For example, consider the case where X and Y are independent. In this case,

A

$P(X = x, Y = y)$

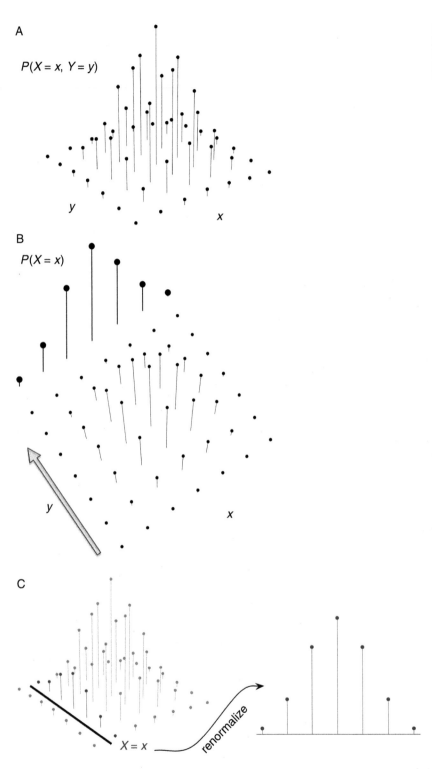

y   x

B

$P(X = x)$

y   x

C

$X = x$ renormalize

Figure 11.2 (A) Visual depiction of a discrete joint probability distribution. Also shown are the processes of obtaining a single variable probability distribution through marginalization (B) and conditioning (C).

$P(X = x, Y = y) = P(X = x)P(Y = y)$, so calculating the probability of X and Y is as simple as multiplying their individual probabilities at the desired values. This is not the case, however, when X and Y are dependent. To see why, think about the definition of dependence: the value of X has a direct effect on the value of Y, and vice versa. Therefore, considering X and Y on their own is not the same as considering them together. For this reason, the joint probability distribution is useful because it gives us a mathematical means of working with X and Y in conjunction while accounting for any dependencies that may exist between them. This is especially useful when considering joint distributions of more than two variables.

In this section, we looked solely at the joint probability distributions between two discrete random variables. However, the principles developed are the same for joint distributions of continuous random variables, although the same differences that existed between continuous and discrete random variables in the univariate case are still present.

11.2.3.5 Expectation and Variance

We often want a more compact and intuitive description of a random variable than the full equation for its distribution. The most common descriptors by far are the expected value and variance of a random variable. The *expected value* of a random variable, sometimes referred to as the "average" or "mean," is a measure of the "middle" of a random variable's probability distribution. In fact, mathematically one can show that the expected value of a random variable is equivalent to the center of mass of its probability distribution. For a random variable X, the expected value is calculated as $E(X) = \sum_x p_X(x)x$ in the discrete case and $E(X) = \int_x f_X(x)x dx$ in the continuous case. Intuitively, this is just taking the sum of each possible outcome times the probability (or relative likelihood, in the case of a continuous random variable) of that outcome.

Another common measure for a distribution is its variance, which measures dispersion of the random variable. One can think of the variance as the square of the expected distance from the mean for all values of a distribution. For random variable X with expected value (mean) μ, the variance is calculated as $Var(X) = \sum_x p_X(x)(x - \mu)^2$ in the discrete case and $Var(X) = \int_x f_X(x)(x - \mu)^2 dx$ in the continuous case. Variance also has a closely related statistic that is often used to measure dispersion called the *standard deviation*. The standard deviation is simply the square root of the variance. The common notation for the expected value, variance, and standard deviation of a random variable are μ, σ^2, and σ, respectively. It is important to note that while the expected value and variance can give some insight into the distribution of a random variable, one must be careful when using these metrics to analyze or present data because they offer an incomplete picture of the distribution. In fact, for a given expected value and variance, one can construct an infinite number of probability distributions that have that expected value and variance.

11.2.3.6 Important Theorems

Probability theory, like any branch of mathematics, has a huge number of important and useful theorems. Here, we will focus on just two of these theorems: the Law of Large Numbers (LLN) and the Central Limit Theorem (CLT). We will not go over the mathematical proofs of these theorems here, but instead discuss their results and consequences.

The LLN is central in the study of probability and statistics. The most basic version of the LLN, sometimes called the "law of averages," states that if a probabilistic process is repeated over many trials, the average over the results of all the trials will tend to get closer to the theoretical average (expected value) as the number of trials increases. This means that, for example, if we repeatedly roll a die and average the results, we should see that the calculated average tends toward the theoretical average (expected value) of 3.5. A more general version of the LLN, known as Borel's Law of Large Numbers, states that if the probabilistic process is repeated many times, then the frequency of the results will tend toward the theoretical probability of obtaining those results on a given trial. Intuitively, this means that we can create an estimate for the probability distribution that we are interested in by repeating the experiment many times. In the die rolling example, we know that each value should have a 1/6 probability of occurring on any given role. And indeed, if we repeatedly roll a die, we will see each number at a frequency that approaches 1/6 as we continue to roll it more and more. Thus, the LLN is significant because it provides a mathematical proof of the relationship between the probability of an event occurring and the frequency at which it occurs, and thus forms the mathematical basis for the frequentist interpretation of probability (discussed more below). One important thing to note is that the LLN says nothing about the rate at which the sample average or frequency converges to the expected value or probability, only that it will converge as more and more trials are repeated. Therefore, it provides no guarantee that the average or frequency will converge to the theoretical value for any finite set of trials, only that it will converge in the limit.

The CLT is another theorem that is used often in probability and statistics when dealing with the sample mean of a large random sample. The CLT tells us that for large sample sizes (usually considered greater than 30 samples), the sample mean will be normally distributed, with sample mean μ^* equal to the population mean μ, and sample variance σ^{2*} equal to $\frac{\sigma^2}{n}$, where σ^2 is the population variance and n is the sample size. This means that if we were to repeatedly draw large random samples from some population and calculate the sample mean, we expect to see that these sample means would be normally distributed with the above parameters. What is amazing about the CLT is that the result holds regardless of the underlying distribution the samples are being drawn from, as long as that distribution has finite variance. As we will see below, the CLT is often used when comparing the sample means of two different distributions to determine how likely they are to be the same or different.

11.2.3.7 Frequentist Versus Bayesian Interpretation of Probability

It may be surprising to learn that there are actually two different interpretations of probability: the *Frequentist* interpretation and the *Bayesian* interpretation. Without going into too much detail, the basic difference between these two interpretations is the following. Frequentists think of probabilities as representing the long-run outcome frequencies of an event if it were to be repeated many times. Under this interpretation, probabilities and parameter values (more on that below) might be unknown, but they are fixed values. Bayesians, on the other hand, take on a much looser interpretation of probability, in which probabilities can be used to represent degrees of belief. In the Bayesian framework, there is nothing wrong with treating probabilities and parameter values as themselves being random variables.

Although the differences mentioned above are largely philosophical, they do have consequences with regard to how the tools of probability and statistics are applied to solve a given problem, and even what kinds of problems these tools can be used to solve. To illustrate these differences, consider the following example. Imagine that you are trying to predict the true probability of a given coin with an unknown bias landing on heads. A frequentist would say that the true probability of the coin landing on heads, although it is unknown to us, is simply a fixed number. It is only the data, the results of a hundred tosses of the coin, that are random. A Bayesian, on the other hand, would treat the unknown probability of the coin landing on heads as a random variable with an accompanying probability distribution. The Frequentist would say nothing about the probability of the true parameter, but would instead talk about the probability of the data given some hypothetical parameter. The frequentist might say "The bias of the coin most likely to have given rise to this data is 0.6," or "The probability of having observed 63 heads given a bias of 0.6 is 85 percent." On the other hand, the Bayesian could make direct claims about the probability of the bias of the coin being a 0.6, because the Bayesian treats the true parameter value itself as a random variable. The Bayesian might say "A bias of 0.6 for heads has the highest probability" or "The probability for the bias being greater than 0.6 is 85 percent."

11.3 Parameter Inference and Hypothesis Testing

In the previous sections, we focused on understanding the basics of probability, random variables, and probability distributions, and even saw how these tools can help us solve real-world problems. However, in these problems we were often given information about the random variables and their distributions and asked to find the probability of observing some outcome. In the following sections we will invert this process: given some outcome (often in the form of data), we want to infer information about the random variables and probability distributions behind those observations.

11.3.1 Data and Sampling

What are data? The term is used so broadly that it is almost impossible to answer that question with a single, coherent answer. However, for the purposes of this chapter we refer to data as characteristics and information collected via observation or experiment for the purpose of answering a question. A patient's test results, recovery time, blood pressure, survey answers, age, race, gender, and diet may all be considered forms of data in the right context. Almost always, we collect data with hopes of answering questions about a population. In statistics, a *population* refers to the group that contains every individual that belongs to that population. This can either be a finite group, such as the population of all the students at a certain medical school in a given year, or it can be a group for which all members cannot be counted, such as the population of all the red blood cells in a patient's body. The latter is sometimes referred to as an *infinite population*. Sometimes a population is small enough that it is feasible to obtain the data of interest on every individual within that population. However, it is more often the case that we can only obtain the desired data on some subset of the population, and then use the data on that subset to try to infer something about the entire population. In statistics, this subset is called a *sample*.

Sampling is an extremely important but often underappreciated part of statistical inference. If you start with a poor sample, your inferences will be incorrect no matter how advanced your analysis methods are and as such cannot be trusted. To illustrate this point, consider the task of trying to estimate the average height of the entire world population. Obviously, it is not feasible to obtain data on the height of every person on earth, so we must use a sample. In our case, it may be tempting to use height data that are already available (this is called *convenience sampling*). For example, there are public height data available on every player in the NBA, but this is clearly not representative of the entire population (the average height of all players in the NBA at the time of this writing is $6'6''$)! Likewise, we might be able to get data from hospitals on patient heights, but these data may be skewed toward overrepresenting infants and the elderly. We have to consider possible height differences that occur as a result of age, gender, race, socioeconomic status, profession, etc. in our sample. To do this, we could employ a number of different sampling strategies including simple random sampling, stratified random sampling, and systemic sampling, to name just a few. The point here is that how you gather your sample is important and must take into account a number of factors.

11.3.2 Inferring Parameters of a Distribution

When dealing with sample data, we often try to use a probabilistic model that explains how those data were generated. That is, we assume the population as existing according to some probabilistic model, and then we try to use our sample data to infer the parameters of that model. Here, we will focus on only one type of probabilistic model: the single variable probability distribution.

The first step in this approach is to pick the probability distribution we think will best be able to fit the distribution of the population we are interested in. This can be done in several different ways. Sometimes, we know that a certain distribution is able to accommodate data that are generated in a certain way, such as data that were generated by taking many independent trials with some probability of success and observing the number of successes, which could be fit by a binomial distribution. In other cases, we know from experience that certain types of data tend to be distributed in certain ways, such as height almost always being normally distributed. We may even look at the shape of our sample data via something like a histogram and try to pick the distribution that seems closest to the shape of our sample data.

Once we have decided on the distribution we will use to model the population, we treat our sample data as being made up of independent draws from that distribution. This is, of course, a strong assumption, but if sampling has been done well then it is usually justifiable. Now that we have a probability distribution in one hand, and a data set that we assume to have been generated by that model in the other, we ask the core question of statistical inference: how can I use these data to learn more about the probabilistic model that generated them? Below, we will focus on how we can create estimates for key parameters of the distribution in question.

11.3.2.1 Point Estimates

Often, we wish to find the best estimate of a parameter of interest for our distribution model. Knowing the parameters of our distribution model can help us gain insight into some of the characteristics of the population, such as its mean and standard deviation. The easiest way to estimate the parameter value is known as a *point estimate*, which is simply a number that represents our best estimate of the true parameter value (known as the *estimand* – what we are trying to estimate). Here, we will introduce two popular methods for obtaining point estimates, the maximum likelihood estimate (MLE) and the maximum a posteriori estimate (MAP).

The MLE is perhaps the most commonly used estimator because it is (usually) simple to calculate and has many desirable theoretical properties. The maximum likelihood estimate does exactly what its name suggests – it picks the most likely parameter value by maximizing the likelihood function, which is the same idea of "likelihood" that we introduced in the section on Bayes' Theorem. The MLE is calculated as follows. Given our data, $\vec{x}$ (which is a vector because it contains many data points), a parameter of interest, θ, and a probability distribution model with unspecified θ, $f_X(x)$, we seek to find the parameter value for our distribution model that maximizes the probability of the observed data having occurred under that model. That is, we wish to maximize the function $f_X(\vec{x}|\theta)$, which is often called the *likelihood function*. To gain some intuition for what this means, think about what we were doing in the probability section of this chapter. There, we learned how to calculate $f_X(\vec{x}|\theta)$ for some known θ. In that section, we were used to treating θ as fixed and $\vec{x}$ as variable. Now, $\vec{x}$ is fixed and θ is variable, and we want to find the value of θ at which $f_X(\vec{x}|\theta)$ is largest. In effect, we want to calculate $f_X(\vec{x}|\theta)$ for every possible value of θ and pick the value that leads to the largest, and thus most likely, result. Luckily, we can use calculus to do precisely that, which is called finding the *argmax* of the function for θ (denoted as argmax$_\theta$). Recall that the minimum or maximum of a function has a derivative of 0. Therefore, if we find where the derivative of the function $f_X(\vec{x}|\theta)$ is zero, then we know that point is either a maximum or a minimum. Then, we can check whether the second derivative of the function is positive or negative, which tells us whether the point is a minimum or maximum, respectively. Putting this all together, we want to find the value of θ for which $\frac{d}{d\theta}f_X(\vec{x}|\theta) = 0$ and $\frac{d^2}{d\theta^2}f_X(\vec{x}|\theta) < 0$, which can be more compactly written as argmax$_\theta f_X(\vec{x}|\theta)$. This is just calculus work, and there are a few assumptions behind this approach that we have not explicitly mentioned (such as the function being convex), but the important part is to understand the intuition behind what the MLE is calculating. It is finding the value of θ that is *most likely* to have generated the observed data.

Another common method for finding a point estimate for a parameter is MAP. As we will see shortly, MAP shares many connections with the MLE method. In fact, one can think of MAP as the Bayesian version of the frequentist-based MLE, and we can even show that the MLE is just a special case of MAP. As with any good Bayesian method, we start with Bayes' Theorem. Our goal is still to find the value of θ that maximizes the probability of having observed the data we did, except now we do so under the Bayesian framework, so we get argmax$_\theta \frac{f_X(\vec{x}|\theta)g_\theta(\theta)}{f_X(\vec{x})}$, where $g_\theta(\theta)$ is the probability distribution that we choose to be the prior for θ. Notice that $f_X(\vec{x})$ is just a number and does not depend on θ, so when we are trying to maximize with respect to θ we can ignore this term. Thus, we get argmax$_\theta f_X(\vec{x}|\theta)g_\theta(\theta)$ Now we can see that the MAP approach ends up being the same as the MLE, except that we have the option to have a prior for θ. Just as we saw on the section on Bayes' Theorem, we can use this prior to represent our prior beliefs as to what θ might be. If we have no strong beliefs about θ, we can choose a uniform prior. A uniform prior considers all values of θ equally likely, and thus $g_\theta(\theta)$ becomes a constant and can be dropped from the optimization just like $f_X(\vec{x})$ was. Thus, in the case of a uniform prior we end up with argmax$_\theta f_X(\vec{x}|\theta)$, which yields the exact same answer as the MLE.

11.3.2.2 Confidence Intervals

Point estimates can be very useful, but sometimes we would rather find a plausible range of values that θ could be rather than an estimate of the most plausible value. In these situations, we can turn to something known as a *confidence interval*. However, before jumping into how to construct a confidence interval, we need to understand exactly what a confidence interval is and how it is interpreted. Recall that under the frequentist interpretation of probability, the true value of θ is fixed, not random. The only randomness in our problem comes from the process of sampling from the population: if we were to repeat this process many times, we could obtain different sample results each time. When we construct a confidence interval, we are trying to construct it in such a way that if we were to repeatedly obtain a sample from population and calculate the interval based on that sample data, the interval would contain the true parameter value some percentage of the time. That percentage is known as our *confidence level*. For example, if we picked out confidence level to be 95%, then we would expect about 95% of our confidence intervals to contain the true parameter value if we repeated the process of sampling from the population and constructing the interval many times. Notice that this is distinctly different from saying that the confidence interval "has a 95% chance of containing the true parameter value," which would be incorrect.

To better illustrate how a confidence interval is calculated, let's look at a specific example. Suppose we want to calculate a confidence interval for the mean θ of the time it takes to perform a certain type of surgery. For simplicity's sake, assume that we know the standard deviation of the time it takes to perform the surgery is σ. The first step in constructing a confidence interval for θ is to choose our confidence level. In this example, let's say we want our confidence level to be 95%. Next, we collect our sample data, $\vec{x}$. Recall that, according to the CLT, when the sample size n is large enough, the sample mean $\bar{x}$ will be approximately normally distributed with mean θ and with standard deviation $\sigma/\sqrt{n}$ Therefore, we can treat our sample mean $\bar{x}$ as having been drawn from a normal distribution with those parameters. To construct our 95% confidence interval, all we have to do is find the interval around the center of that normal distribution that contains 95% of its probability. The boundaries of that interval then become the boundaries of our confidence interval. In practice, there are look up tables or computers for calculating this value.

11.3.2.3 Full Bayes for Parameter Distribution Estimates

If we are approaching the problem from a Bayesian perspective, we may wish to find the posterior probability distribution for $f_X(\theta|\vec{x})$. To do so, the approach is very similar to the approach taken when finding the MAP. We start with Bayes' Theorem, which gives $\frac{f_X(\vec{x}|\theta)g_\theta(\theta)}{f_X(\vec{x})}$. Unlike in the case of MAP, we cannot simply drop $f_X(\vec{x})$ from our equation because we are trying to get an equation for $f_X(\theta|\vec{x})$, not just its maximum. However, $f_X(\vec{x})$ is hard to calculate as is because the calculation relies on the value of the very parameter we are trying to estimate! Luckily, we can use the continuous form of the LOTP to rewrite $f_X(\vec{x})$ as $\int_\theta f_X(\vec{x}|\theta)g_\theta(\theta)d\theta$. Regardless of what form it is in, the denominator of the equation is just a normalizing constant, and we can rewrite the whole equation as $f(\theta|\vec{x}) = c \times f(\vec{x}|\theta)g(\theta)$, where c is the aforementioned normalizing constant. Solving this equation can be a bit tricky, and sometimes requires the use of numerical approximation techniques. For this reason, we will not cover the different methods used to solve such an equation here. However, the key takeaway is that this fully Bayesian method gives you much more than just a single value or interval of values for your estimate. Instead, you get the entire probability distribution function, which may reveal important information about the probability of different parameter values. For example, you might find the probability distribution you calculate is bimodal (meaning it contains two peaks) with peaks of a similar height. In such a case, a confidence interval or point estimate would have left out important information about the parameter.

11.3.3 Hypothesis Testing

Often, we are interested in estimating a parameter not for its own sake, but rather to test some hypothesis about the value of the parameter. As an example, let's return to the example of determining whether a given coin is fair ($P(H) = 0.5$) or not ($P(H) \neq 0.5$). In this example, say that we are going to toss the coin some number of times and record the results, and that we hope to show that the coin is not fair. Below, we will discuss the basics of statistical hypothesis testing in the context of this example. Note that here we will be focusing on only one type of hypothesis test, although the principle behind what the test is doing is the same as most other types of hypothesis tests.

11.3.3.1 Hypothesis and Error Types

When performing a hypothesis test, the first step is to frame the test in terms of a null hypothesis and an alternative hypothesis. The *null hypothesis* can be thought of as the hypothesis that we are trying to "disprove" with our experiment. This hypothesis, often denoted H_0, is most often the currently accepted hypothesis or the one that is assumed *a priori*. Conversely, the *alternative hypothesis* can be thought of as the hypothesis we are trying to "prove" with our experiment. The alternative hypothesis is often denoted H_1, and usually represents the hypothesis of the researchers performing the experiment. The nature of our null and alternative hypothesis will determine whether we perform a one- or two-sided hypothesis test. If our alternative hypothesis is that some parameter of interest, call it θ, is either higher or lower than some value proposed under the null hypothesis, then we will have a two-sided hypothesis test. However, if our alternative hypothesis is only that θ is higher than some range of values proposed under the null hypothesis, then we perform a one-sided test. The same is true if we only cared about θ being smaller than the range of values held under the null hypothesis.

Connecting this back to the case of our coin-tossing example, let's assume a binomial model of the coin tosses where tosses resulting in heads are valued with a 1 and tosses resulting in tails are valued with a 0. Thus, if X is a random variable that represents the sum of the results when the coin is tossed n times, we have $X \sim Binom(n,\theta)$. Here, θ is the probability of a coin toss landing on heads. In our case, the null hypothesis is that the coin is fair, stated as H_0: $\theta = 0.5$. Our alternative hypothesis is that the coin is unfair, without regard to whether heads or tails is more likely. Therefore, our alternative hypothesis is stated as H_1: $\neq 0.5$. Because this means that the null hypothesis is wrong in the case that either $\theta > 0.5$ or $\theta < 0.5$, we have a two-sided hypothesis test. If instead we had had the hypothesis H_0: $\theta \leq 0.5$ and H_1: $\theta > 0.5$, we would have had a one-sided hypothesis test.

When we perform our hypothesis test, we will either find that the data are strongly in favor of the alternative hypothesis and thus *reject the null hypothesis*, or we will not find strong enough evidence to reject the null hypothesis and thus *fail to reject the null hypothesis*. Notice that we never make a claim that we "accept the alternative hypothesis" or "accept the null hypothesis" because we are not trying to *prove* that one hypothesis or the other is correct, but rather to show that the data either do or do not challenge the null hypothesis.

Fundamentally, there are two kinds of mistakes that we could make in this kind of analysis. We could reject the null hypothesis when that hypothesis is in fact true, or we could fail to reject the null hypothesis when that hypothesis is in fact false. These are referred to as *type one* and *type two* errors, respectively. In our coin-tossing example, rejecting the null hypothesis that the coin is fair when the coin really is fair is a type one error. On the other hand, failing to reject the null hypothesis that the coin is fair when the coin is actually biased in some way is a type two error. In any analysis, there is some probability of committing a type one error and a type two error. The probability of committing a type one error is denoted by the symbol α, and the probability of committing a type two error is denoted by the symbol β. α is often called the significance level, and it controls the probability that you will commit a type one error. Statistical power, calculated as $1 - \beta$, controls the probability of correctly rejecting the null hypothesis when it is false. Ideally, we would like to have the lowest significance level and the highest statistical power level as possible. Both the significance level and the statistical power of an analysis will depend on the size of the sample and the effect size. The effect size can be thought of as "how wrong" the null hypothesis is, if it is indeed wrong. Obviously, a smaller effect size is much more difficult to detect than a large effect size. In our coin example, it would be much easier to detect that the coin actually lands on heads 70% of the time than 51% of the time. For a smaller effect size, we will need more samples to detect that effect size at a given level of significance and statistical power. The process of calculating the relationship between the significance level, the statistical power, the sample size, and the effect size is called *power analysis*. Although we will not cover this process here, it is important to understand that these factors all affect each other. To ensure that an analysis has the desired properties and can support the conclusions the researcher wants to be able to make, should the data allow, one must perform power analysis *before* running an experiment. As the great statistician Ronald Fisher once said, "To consult the statistician after an experiment is finished is often merely to ask him to conduct a post mortem examination. He can perhaps say what the experiment died of."

11.3.3.2 The *t*-Test

Perhaps the most widely known method used for hypothesis tests is Student's *t*-test, often just called the *t*-test. It is usually either to test whether a population has a mean specified by a null hypothesis (called a one-sample *t*-test), or to compare two different population means under the null hypothesis that their means are equal (called a two-sample *t*-test). Here, we will focus on the case of a single-sample *t*-test, although the principle behind evaluating a test statistic's value using its known distribution under the null hypothesis is the same in the two-sample case.

At the heart of the *t*-test, and most other statistical hypothesis tests for that matter, is something called a *test statistic*. A test statistic is a function of the data that we construct such that we know the distribution of its output under the null hypothesis. For a single-sample *t*-test, we use the test statistic $t = \frac{\bar{x} - \mu_0}{\hat{\sigma}/\sqrt{n}}$, where $\bar{x}$ is the sample mean, μ_0 is the mean under the null hypothesis, $\hat{\sigma}$ is the sample standard deviation, and n is the number of data points in our sample. When a few basic assumptions are met, it can be proved (although we will not do it here) that our test statistic t follows a t-distribution (hence the name) with $n - 1$ degrees of freedom, which is similar to a normal distribution but with longer tails. Note that, if we knew the true value of σ (and thus did not have to estimate it), t would instead be normally distributed, and we would be performing what is called a Z-test. The difference between the two is only in the distribution of the test statistic, the rest of the procedure is the same. The fact that using an estimate of the standard deviation leads to a distribution with heavier tails reflects the extra uncertainty when using an estimate instead of the true value. The *t*-test relies on a few assumptions in order to work, the most important of which is that the sample mean of the data is normally distributed. This assumption is met when the data are normally distributed, or when the sample size is large enough that the sample mean is approximately normally distributed by the CLT.

Once we have calculated our test statistic, we can use the fact that we know the distribution of that statistic under the null hypothesis to ask the question "What is the probability of obtaining a value for t that is at least this extreme, given that the null hypothesis is true?" To do this, we simply calculate the area under our t-distribution for all values more extreme than our calculated value of t. If we are performing a two-sided hypothesis test, then we do this calculation for both "tails" of the distribution. If we are instead doing only a one-sided hypothesis test, then we only do this calculation for the tail on the side of interest. The resulting value will be a number between zero and one, called a *p*-value. By construction, the *p*-value represents the probability that we would have observed a test statistic at least as extreme as the one we observed under the assumption that the null hypothesis is true. Now that we have our *p*-value, we can draw our conclusion about whether or not to reject the null hypothesis. To do this, we compare the p-value to our significance level α. If our p-value is less than α, then we reject the null hypothesis in favor of the alternative hypothesis. If our p-value is greater than α, then we fail to reject the null hypothesis. Check that, in the context of what the p-value and α mean, you understand why this procedure makes intuitive sense.

As a final note on statistical hypothesis tests, one should be aware that there are many different tests available. These tests differ in both the assumptions they rely on to work and the purpose of the test. In general, one should always try to pick the test for which the assumptions are most reasonable in the context of the problem at hand.

11.3.3.3 A Word on *p*-Values

p-values are one of the most misunderstood concepts within science and statistics, so in this section we will discuss briefly what p-values are and are not. The correct interpretation of a p-value can be read aloud as follows: "The p-value is the probability that we would have observed a test statistic *at least* as extreme as the one we have observed, given that the null hypothesis is true." Notice that this is not making a statement about the probability of either of our hypotheses being correct. Nor does it tell us anything about the effect size of our finding. It is simply a measure of the likelihood of having observed a test statistic at least as extreme as the one we did if the null hypothesis is true. When the p-value is lower than our desired level of significance, we reject it only because we are saying that it is unlikely (but not impossible!) that the model assumed under the null hypothesis would have produced the data it did. Additionally, we must keep in mind that the p-value is only as good as the data, models, and assumptions that have gone into calculating it. Sloppy data collection, poorly chosen tests, and unmet assumptions can lead to p-values that give a misleading reflection of the suitability of different hypothesis.

11.3.3.4 Bayesian Hypothesis Testing

The t-test and other related statistical hypothesis tests are built upon a frequentist framework. As usual, however, one can also approach the problem from a Bayesian perspective. As with the set of frequentist hypothesis tests, there are many different methods available. Here, we will briefly cover just one of these methods that uses something called *Bayes' Factor*. Say we are trying to choose between two different hypotheses, H_1 and H_2, to explain a data set D. As with the t-test, these hypotheses might represent two different

parameter values for the same model, or notably could even represent entirely different models that we want to compare. Here, instead of trying to calculate the probability of the data under just one of these hypothesis as we did with the t-test, we will calculate the probability of the data under both models and look at the ratio of those probabilities (which is our Bayes' Factor, K), as is shown below:

$$
\begin{aligned}
K &= \frac{P(H_1|D)}{P(H_2|D)} \\[2mm]
&= \frac{\dfrac{P(D|H_1)P(H_1)}{P(D)}}{\dfrac{P(D|H_2)P(H_2)}{P(D)}} \\[2mm]
&= \frac{P(D|H_1)P(H_1)}{P(D|H_2)P(H_2)}
\end{aligned}
$$

Above, we started by asking what the probability of each hypothesis was given the data. This is what we want to know, but we do not know how to calculate it, so we used Bayes' Theorem to rewrite both the numerator and denominator of our starting fraction. Finally, we cancelled out $P(D)$ because it was present in both the numerator and denominator, and ended up with the final equation. Note that the terms $P(H_1)$ and $P(H_2)$ allow us to put assign a prior probability to each model. We may choose to favor one over the other. The final equation is something we can easily calculate, because all we have to do is find the probability of the data we have under each model, which we have been doing throughout this chapter. The value of K gives us insight into how strongly we favor the model in the numerator over the model in the denominator. Although different tables for how K should be interpreted have been put forth, it is generally accepted that $K < 1$ is evidence for the model in the denominator, $1 < K < 3.2$ is weak evidence for the model in the numerator, $3.2 < K < 10$ is substantial evidence, $10 < K < 100$ is strong evidence, and $100 < K$ is decisive evidence. As one would do with α in a t-test, one should choose the level of K that will be considered significant before running an analysis. Finally, one should calculate the ratio for the reciprocal as well in order to evaluate evidence for both H_1 over H_2 and H_2 over H_1. This was only a brief overview of how Bayes' Factor can be used to perform hypothesis testing, and the interested reader should see the further reading suggestions at the end of this chapter.

Example 2: Suppose that you are asked to evaluate whether a new surgical technique cuts down on the time taken to perform a particular surgical procedure. The old procedure is known to take an average of 4.2 hours. To see if the average time taken to perform the surgery using the new technique is less than the standard technique, you are given a data set containing the times taken to perform the new technique in 20 different operations. In your data set, the sample mean is 3.8 hours and the sample standard deviation is 1.2 hours. Assume that the time taken to perform the surgery using either technique is normally distributed.

(a) Calculate a 95% confidence interval for the average time taken to perform the surgery using the new technique.

Answer: Because we are told that the data are normally distributed, but we are using sample estimates for the mean and standard deviation, we should use a t-distribution to calculate our confidence interval. Our confidence interval will be of the form $\bar{x} \pm t\frac{\hat{\sigma}}{\sqrt{n}}$. We already know $\bar{x} = 3.8$, $\hat{\sigma} = 1.2$, and $n = 20$ from the data set, so all we have to do is calculate the value of our t-statistic. For a t-distribution with $n - 1 = 19$ degrees of freedom, the interval around the center of the distribution that contains 95% of the probability is 0 ± 2.09, so our critical value is $t = 2.09$. Therefore, we can plug all our values back in find that the 95% confidence interval is 3.8 ± 0.562, or [3.238,4.362].

(b) Set up the null and alternative hypotheses of a statistical hypothesis test to determine whether the new technique has a lower mean time than the previous technique with a significance level of 95%. Additionally, provide the α value for a test at this significance level.

Answer: Because we only care if the new technique takes *less* time than the old one, we have a single-sided hypothesis test. Our null hypothesis should be that the new technique takes the same time or longer than the old technique, expressed as $H_0 : \mu \geq 4.2$, and our alternative hypothesis should be that the new technique takes less time than the old one, expressed as $H_1 : \mu < 4.2$. Because we want our test to have a significance level of 95%, we want to ensure that our type one error rate is at most 5%, so we set $\alpha = 0.05$.

(c) Given the confidence interval you calculated in part (a), do you have enough information to say whether you will reject the null hypothesis if you run your hypothesis test? Why or why not?

Answer: No, the confidence interval was calculated using both tails of the t-distribution, but our hypothesis test is a one-sided test and thus only looks at one tail. However, if we were running a two-sided hypothesis test with $H_0: \mu = 4.2$ and $H_1: \mu \neq 4.2$, then we would be able to see that we would fail to reject the null hypothesis because the 95% confidence interval contains the value proposed by the null hypothesis.

(d) Perform the statistical hypothesis test you set up in part (b) and interpret the results.

Answer: The first step in performing our statistical hypothesis test is to calculate our test statistic, $t = \frac{\bar{x} - \mu_0}{\hat{\sigma}/\sqrt{n}}$. We are given $\bar{x}$, $\hat{\sigma}$, and n in the problem description. We also know μ_0 from our null hypothesis $H_0 : \mu \geq 4.2$, which suggests that we should set $\mu_0 = 4.2$ because that is the value that lies on the boundary between our null and alternative hypotheses. Plugging in, we calculate our test statistic to be $t = -1.49$. For a t-distribution with $n - 1 = 19$ degrees of freedom, the probability contained only to the left side of that value is 0.076, and therefore our p-value is 0.076. As our p-value is greater than our $\alpha = 0.05$, we fail to reject the null hypothesis. As a result, we find that there is insufficient evidence to support the claim that the decrease in time taken to perform the new surgical technique versus the old one is statistically significant with an α of 0.05. However, note that $\alpha = 0.05$ is an arbitrary choice, and we should keep in mind that if we had chosen a significance level of 90% then a p-value of 0.076 would allow us to reject the null hypothesis.

(e) What piece of information would you have needed to perform a Z-test instead of a t-test?

Answer: If we had known the true value of σ rather than having relied on its estimate $\hat{\sigma}$, then our test statistic would have been normally distributed and thus allowed us to use a Z-test.

(f) Can you think of any problems with data collection that may have impacted your analysis?

Answer: Yes. Not having been involved with the data collection and design of the experiment from the beginning makes it much harder to be certain of our results. For example, if all of these surgeries were done by the same surgeon, then that individual surgeon's mean time to perform the surgery may have affected our results. If that surgeon was significantly slower than average, for example, then our failure to reject the null hypothesis may have had more to do with that individual surgeon's ability than the surgical technique itself. In general, the person who will be doing the analysis of the data set should be present in the experiment design and data collection process whenever possible.

11.4 Selected Topics in Modern Statistics

Many of the statistical techniques used today were developed in the early 1900s, long before computers were commonplace. Therefore, all the calculations being performed as part of the techniques had to be completed by hand, which in turn required the math involved in these statistical techniques to be easily solved or approximated by hand. As a result, many of these techniques rely disproportionately on well-known distributions and equations with nice mathematical properties. However, real-world data often fail to take the form of these nice distributions and can be far messier. In the early 1900s, you did your best to make your techniques robust to deviations from their underlying assumptions and made the most of what you had. However, the advent of computers has given us the ability tackle real-world deviations from these assumptions using their ability to do thousands of calculations per second. For example, in Bayesian statistics we often use something called a conjugate-prior to avoid nasty integrals when calculating the distribution of the posterior. However, modern methods like Markov Chain Monte Carlo (often abbreviated as MCMC) utilize the calculation speed of computers to create extremely accurate approximations to these integrals, and thus the posterior distribution. This means that we need not limit ourselves to the set of distributions available as conjugate-priors in a particular problem if we don't think the conjugate-prior is a good choice for the situation at hand. As another example, a main assumption of the t-test is that the data are normally distributed, as was the case in the hypothesis-testing example problem in this chapter. When this assumption is violated in a major way on a small data set, the theoretical guarantees of the t-test can begin to break down. If we have a data set that does not seem to meet this assumption, we may choose to do something called bootstrapping. Bootstrapping involves repeatedly sampling with replacement from the data set and calculating the statistic of interest from that sample (in the case of the t-test example, the sample mean). Doing this thousands of times gives one an idea of the distribution of the statistic of interest, which can then be used to make inferences about that statistic. Of course, these computational methods have drawbacks of their own, namely the requirement of more time and computing power. However, like any tool in our statistical toolbox, it is not the tool but how you use it. When applied properly, these tools can be very useful in solving a set of problems that would otherwise be intractable or require bad assumptions. Although we will not cover these methods in detail here, it is important to be aware of their existence.

Figure acknowledgments

The following images have been adapted from Blitzstein and Hwang (2019), with permission: Figures 11.1-11.2

Further Reading

Blitsztein JK, Hwang J. *Introduction to Probability*. CRC Press, 2019.

MacKay DJC. *Information Theory, Inference and Learning Algorithms*. Cambridge University Press, 2003.

Wasserman L. *All of Statistics*. Springer, 2004.

12

Glioma

David M. Ashley and Justin T. Low

12.1 Introduction

Gliomas are primary tumors of the central nervous system (CNS). They are so named due to their morphological resemblance to glial cells from which they are thought to arise and are divided into astrocytic, oligodendroglial, and ependymal tumors based historically on histologic resemblance to these respective glial subtypes. In recent years, much has been learned regarding the molecular underpinnings of each of these subtypes. In 2021, the World Health Organization (WHO) published an updated classification of CNS tumors that combined genetic markers with histology to create an integrated diagnosis (Louis et al., 2021). Each subtype is assigned a WHO grade, ranging from 1 to 4, that approximates clinical behavior, with grade 1 representing the least aggressive and 4 the most aggressive tumor. Grades 3 and 4 are classified as high-grade gliomas, while grades 1 and 2 are low-grade gliomas. Low-grade gliomas are usually treated initially with surgery; additional systemic chemotherapy or radiation therapy may be employed after careful consideration of patient-specific clinical, histopathologic, and molecular data. In contrast, high-grade gliomas are usually treated, with postoperative radiation therapy and systemic chemotherapy, most commonly with the alkylating agent temozolomide.

In addition to their WHO grade, gliomas are divided into two broad categories: circumscribed gliomas that have well-demarcated borders and can be completely resected surgically; and diffusely infiltrating gliomas whose borders are poorly delineated and cannot be completely removed surgically. Circumscribed gliomas are mostly low-grade tumors that are clinically indolent. On the other hand, diffusely infiltrating gliomas, which include astrocytic tumors and oligodendroglial tumors, may be low or high grade and are generally more clinically aggressive. Despite optimal treatment, tumor progression is inevitable and durable long-term survival of diffusely infiltrating high-grade gliomas is rare.

Although glioma cells can be detected in the systemic circulation (Sullivan et al., 2014), gliomas uncommonly metastasize outside the CNS and consequently are not assigned a stage. A description of gliomas as benign or malignant is commonly made as synonymous with low and high grade, respectively, although this distinction is poorly defined and can be somewhat of a misnomer. "Benign" low-grade gliomas may result in significant morbidity and death due to factors unrelated to histologic grade, such as a critically located surgically inaccessible pilocytic astrocytoma, while certain high-grade "malignant" tumors, such as grade 3 oligodendrogliomas, may exhibit a relatively more indolent clinical course. Therefore, we will avoid the benign/malignant descriptors in favor of the more precise WHO grade and circumscribed/diffuse distinction.

In this chapter we begin with an introduction to each of the major categories of gliomas. Next we describe the key molecular pathways that are disrupted in gliomas. Finally, we review the physiologic principles of gliomas that underlie their unique clinical manifestations.

12.1.1 Diffusely Infiltrating Gliomas

Diffusely infiltrating gliomas are divided into adult-type and pediatric-type diffuse gliomas. Here we will focus on the adult-type diffuse glilomas. These tumors are traditionally graded based on histology and included astrocytic and oligodendroglial tumors. Recent advances in our understanding of the molecular underpinnings of these glioma subgroups have led to increased reliance on molecular information, particularly the status of the IDH mutation and the presence of 1p/19q codeletion, that has resulted in the re-classification and simplification into three groups: astrocytoma, glioblastoma, and oligodendroglioma (Figure 12.1).

12.1.2 Astrocytoma

Diffuse astrocytomas are graded from 2 to 4 reflecting a spectrum of increasingly aggressive clinical behavior.

(Figure 12.1). Astrocytomas were historically further characterized based on the mutational status of the IDH enzyme.

Independently of tumor grade, IDH mutations confer a more favorable clinical prognosis (Gorovets et al., 2012; Sanson et al., 2009). The IDH enzyme catalyzes the reversible conversion of isocitrate to α-ketoglutarate in the citric acid cycle. IDH mutations in gliomas are heterozygous and likely drive tumorigenesis via aberrant production of 2-hydroxyglutarate, which acts as a competitive inhibitor of α-ketoglutarate at multiple enzymes, including histone and DNA demethylases (Dang et al., 2009). This induces the glioma CpG island methylator phenotype (G-CIMP) whereby widespread hypermethylation of gene promoters results in silencing of important cell differentiation signals (Turcan et al., 2012). This may maintain glioma cells in a less-differentiated stem cell–like state conducive to tumorigenesis.

As of the 2021 classification, the presence of an IDH mutation now defines astrocytomas, with IDH wildtype astrocytic tumors now reclassified as a separate category of glioblastoma. The descriptors "diffuse", and "anaplastic" are no longer used, having been replaced by grades 2 and 3, respectively. Glioblastoma was previously considered a grade 4 astrocytoma, and was divided into primary glioblastoma (IDH wildtype) presenting de novo, and secondary glioblastoma (IDH mutant) that arises from lower grade astrocytoma. While histologically indistinguishable, these secondary glioblastomas were noted to be clinically less aggressive than primary glioblastomas and are now classified as grade 4 astrocytomas. Primary glioblastomas are now simply termed glioblastomas, which are defined by the absence of an IDH mutation.

Lower-grade tumors harbor an inevitable tendency for progressive transformation to their higher-grade counterparts. Histologically they are characterized, in order of increasing aggressiveness, by cellular atypia, mitotic activity, endovascular proliferation, and necrosis. Grade 2 astrocytomas diffuse display cellular atypia; grade 3 astrocytomas anaplastic display both atypia and marked mitotic activity; and grade 4 (glioblastoma) additionally demonstrate endovascular proliferation and/or necrosis. Epidemiologically, lower-grade tumors tend to be diagnosed at younger ages, with grade 2 astrocytomas most commonly diagnosed in the mid-30s (Reuss et al., 2015) and glioblastoma showing a peak incidence in ages 55–85 (Ostrom et al., 2014). Overall median survival at diagnosis decreases with increasing grade, being approximately 5–10 years for grade 2 astrocytomas, 3–5 years for grade 3 astrocytomas, and about 1–2 years for glioblastoma (Dong et al., 2016; Reuss et al., 2015).

12.1.3 Glioblastoma

Glioblastomas were first identified and named over a century ago. The suffix -blastoma in its original name glioblastoma multiforme reflects the presumption that these tumors arise from embryologically primitive glial precursor cells, while multiforme alludes to their marked histological heterogeneity. Despite these early observations, our understanding of gliomagenesis and the glioma cell of origin remains incomplete. Recent work has found that only a subset of glioma cells possess the capacity for regenerating complete tumors upon transplantation (Galli et al., 2004; Kroonen et al., 2011; Singh et al., 2004). In analogy to the pluripotency of stem cells, these have been called glioma stem cells (recently reviewed by Ma tarred on a and Pastor, 2019). As the phylogenetic origin of these cells remains controversial, an alternative term is tumor-initiating cells. These cells are resistant to current therapies, and their ability to regenerate likely underlies the treatment resistance that inevitably develops in glioblastomas (Bao et al., 2006; Liu et al., 2006). Glioma stem cells may arise from neural stem cells in the subventricular zone (SVZ) of the lateral ventricles (Alcantara Llaguno et al., 2009; Sanai et al., 2004). Interestingly, approximately half of primary glioblastoma patients harbored mutations in known cancer driver genes in the tumorfree SVZ, suggesting that these cells may be the glioblastoma cell of origin (Lee et al., 2018).

12.1.4 Oligodendroglioma

The histologic hallmarks of oligodendroglial tumors are clear perinuclear halos surrounding round uniform nuclei that are said to resemble fried eggs; and a "chicken-wire"–appearing dense capillary network. Oligodendroglioma exhibit a much more indolent clinical course than their astrocytic counterparts, and are consequently assigned a grade of 2 or 3, with no grade 4 designation. Like lower grade astrocytomas, oligodendrogliomas have a tendency to ultimately transform to higher grade tumors. Median survival estimates vary widely, likely due in part to recent changes in diagnostic criteria, but generally are about 10–15 years for grade 2 oligodendroglioma and about 5–10 years for grade 3 (anaplastic) oligodendroglioma (Cairncross et al., 2013; Ohgaki and Kleihues, 2005; Olson et al., 2000). The molecular hallmarks are concurrent IDH mutations and codeletion of chromosomes 1p and 19q. Indeed, since the 2016 WHO classification, these molecular features are required for the diagnosis of oligodendroglioma (Reifenberger and Louis, 2003).

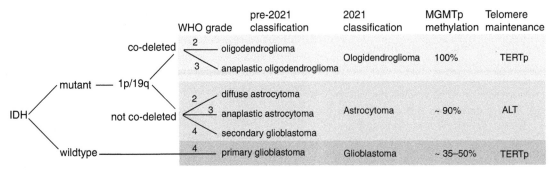

Figure 12.1 Simplified classification of adult-type diffuse gliomas, including both pre-2021 and post-2021 nomenclature. The approximate percentages of MGMT promoter methylation and predominant mechanism of telomere maintenance are also shown.

12.1.5 Diffuse Midline Glioma

Diffuse midline glioma (DMG) is a particularly aggressive diffuse glioma that primarily affects children and young adults. Previously termed diffuse intrinsic pontine glioma (DIPG), DMG is most commonly found in the brainstem but may also arise in other midline structures including the thalamus, cerebellum, and spinal cord. The diagnosis is defined by the presence of the key histone H3 K27M mutation (Schwartzenruber et al., 2012; Wu et al., 2012). This mutation results in loss of K27 trimethylation, a key epigenetic transcriptional regulation signal (Fontebasso et al., 2013). Diffuse midline gliomas carry a very poor prognosis and are consequently designated as grade 4 tumors based on the presence of the H3 K27M mutation, regardless of histopathologic features.

12.1.6 Circumscribed Gliomas

12.1.6.1 Pilocytic Astrocytoma

Pilocytic astrocytomas are grade 1 tumors that occur predominantly in children and young adults. They may arise throughout the neuraxis, but are most common in the cerebellum, brainstem, hypothalamic region, and optic pathway (optic nerves and chiasm). Histologically they are characterized by long, eosinophilic, intracytoplasmic inclusions known as Rosenthal fibers, eosinophilic granular bodies, and microcysts. Long-term survival is usually very good, and unlike diffuse astrocytomas they rarely transform into higher-grade tumors. In fact, regressive changes whereby neoplastic features are lost over time are common. Alterations that activate the mitogen-activated protein kinase (MAPK) pathway are the genetic hallmark of this disease, most commonly large-scale duplications that result in KIAA 1549–BRAF fusion proteins (Jones et al., 2008,

2013). Mutations in neurofibromin (NF-1), which inhibits the MAPK pathway, are commonly encountered in pilocytic astrocytomas (Zhang et al., 2013). Patients with neurofibromatosis type 1 account for the majority of pilocytic astrocytomas involving the optic pathway and hypothalamus.

12.1.6.2 Ependymomas

Ependymal tumors are classified by histology, molecular characteristics, and anatomic location. They include supratentorial ependymomas, posterior fossa ependymomas, spinal ependymomas, and subependymomas. Subependymomas are grade 1 tumors that occur most commonly in middle-aged adults. They have a very favorable prognosis with surgery alone. Supratentorial ependymomas are classified by the presense of either ZFTA (C11orf95) or YAP1 fusions. ZFTA fusion positive supratentoral ependyomas have poorer prognosis and most commonly involving a fusion between ZFTA and RELA. (Parker et al., 2014). *RELA* is a member of the NF-κB transcription factor family and this fusion disrupts NF-κB signaling. The *RELA* fusion forms as a result of *chemothripsis*, which is a shattering and then aberrant reassembly of the chromosome, typically induced by a catastrophic cellular event (Stephens et al., 2011). Posterior fossa ependymomas are divided into groups A and B by methylation profiling. Posterior fossa group A ependymomas occur predominantly in infants and children, with a median age of 3; posterior fossa group B ependymomas occur in young adults, with a median age of 30. Spinal ependymomas occur most commonly in adults and have a favorable prognosis, with progression-free survival of 70-90% in the first 5-10 years, although late relapses are common (Benesch M et al., Childs Nerv Syst 2012; 28: 2017-28; Gomez DR et al., Neuro Oncol. 2005; 7: 254-9). A minority of spinal ependymomas harbor amplifications of the proto-oncogene MYCN and are much more clinically aggressive. Myxopapillary ependymoma is a grade 2 disease that affects young adults and occurs in the conus medularis, cauda equina, and filum terminale.

12.2 Molecular Pathogenesis

Diffuse gliomas generally contain several concurrent classes of mutations: (1) activation of growth factor pathways that promote cell division; (2) disruption of the cell cycle checkpoints that control cell division; and (3) inappropriate maintenance of telomeres (Cancer Genome Atlas Research Network, 2008). Activation of oncogenes, which promote growth and progression through the cell cycle, and inactivation of tumor suppressor genes, which regulate these processes, are involved in all these processes (Nadi and Rutka, 2015). Additionally, epigenetic processes that modulate gene expression without changing the DNA sequence play important roles in glioma biology.

12.2.1 Growth Factor Pathway Activation

Growth factors and their corresponding receptors commonly upregulated in gliomas include epidermal growth factor (EGF), platelet-derived growth factor (PDGF), transforming growth factor-α (TGF-α), and insulin-like growth factor (IGF). Binding of an extracellular growth factor to its cell surface receptor typically activates intracellular signaling such as the Ras–Raf–MAPK, PI3K/Akt–PKB, or PLC-γ/PKC pathway (Figure 12.2). These pathways activate transcription factors such as NF-κB and modulate translation, with the end result being the promotion of growth, proliferation, and differentiation. Phosphatase and tensin homolog (PTEN) acts as a tumor suppressor by inhibiting the PI3K/Akt–PKB pathway and is frequently lost or mutated in glioblastoma (Verhaak et al., 2010). NF-1 acts as a tumor suppressor by inhibiting the Ras–Raf–MAPK pathway and is commonly mutated in pilocytic astrocytoma. Glioblastomas frequently contain amplifications of EGFR, often associated with the EGFRvIII gene rearrangement that results in constitutive activation of EGF signaling (Wikstrand et al., 1998).

12.2.2 Cell-Cycle Checkpoint Dysregulation

The eukaryotic cell cycle is composed of four distinct phases: G1 (gap 1), during which the cell grows; S (synthesis) when DNA is replicated; G2 (gap 2), another growth phase; and M (mitosis) when duplicated chromosomes are separated via mitosis and cellular components divided into two daughter cells through cytokinesis. Cell-cycle checkpoints ensure

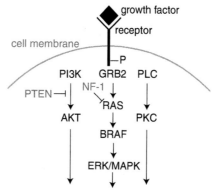

Figure 12.2 Growth factor pathways activated in gliomas. Binding of an extracellular growth factor to receptor tyrosine kinases results in phosphorylation of the receptor and activation of PI3K/Akt, Ras/MAPK, or PLC/PKC signaling cascades. Tumor suppressors PTEN and NF-1 are colored gray. The end result of such activation is the activation of transcription factors that promote cell growth, proliferation, and differentiation.

that progression between phases occurs only if the prior phase was completed appropriately. This ensures that incorrectly replicated cells that could contain cancer-causing mutations are not allowed to proceed through the cell cycle. Tumor suppressors retinoblastoma (Rb) and p53 help to maintain the G1-S and G2-M checkpoints. These tumor suppressors and their related regulators are commonly mutated in gliomas (Figure 12.3). The E2F transcription factor is necessary for progression from G1 to S. Retinoblastoma inhibits this progression by sequestering E2F. The cyclin D1–CDK4/6 complex promotes Rb phosphorylation and release of E2F. The tumor suppressor CDKN2A (p16INK4a) inhibits the cyclin D1–CDK4/6 complex and thus permits Rb-dependent sequestration of E2F. p53 is known as the "guardian of the genome" for its crucial role in regulating the G1-S and G2-M checkpoints and promoting DNA repair or programmed cell death (apoptosis). p53 is inhibited by MDM2, which is in turn inhibited by the tumor suppressor p14ARF. Most IDH-mutant astrocytomas contain loss-of-function mutations in p53 (Reifenberger et al., 1996; Watanabe et al., 1997).

12.2.3 Telomere Maintenance

Chromosomes are protected at either end by a repetitive DNA sequence known as the telomere. Each cell division results in progressive shortening of the telomere due to the

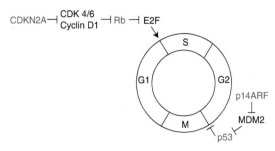

Figure 12.3 Cell cycle with key components of the G1–S and G2–M checkpoints highlighted. Tumor suppressors are colored gray.

lack of an available primer at the end of lagging strand synthesis. This problem can be overcome by the ribonucleoprotein telomerase, which lengthens the 3′ end of telomeres. However, normal somatic cells generally do not express telomerase (Shay and Bacchetti, 1997). This imposes a limit, termed the Hayflick limit, on the number of replications a somatic cell may undergo before entering a senescent phase. Cancer cells attain immortality by mechanisms that maintain telomere length with each replication and thus evade the Hayflick limit. In gliomas, two common mechanisms have been described (Figure 12.1). In IDH-wildtype glioblastoma and oligodendroglioma, activating promoter mutations of the telomerase reverse transcriptase (TERT), a catalytic subunit of telomerase, result in aberrant TERT expression and telomerase activity (Arita et al., 2013). TERT promoter mutations are not found in IDH-mutant astrocytoma. Instead, these tumors contain mutations in *ATRX* that result in aberrant telomere maintenance through a process termed alternative lengthening of telomeres (ALT; Heaphy et al., 2011).

12.2.4 Epigenetic Alterations

Glioma biology is influenced by alterations that do not involve mutations of the DNA sequence itself, but rather of the regulatory mechanisms that control gene expression. Collectively these are termed epigenetic alterations (Gusyatiner and Hegi, 2018; Kreth et al., 2014). Here we will discuss DNA methylation, which is the most well-studied of these modifications. Other epigenetic alterations important for glioma biology include post-translational histone modifications, such as in the case of H3 K27M mutations described above in diffuse midline glioma; and regulation of RNA transcripts (recently reviewed in Peng et al., 2018 and Shi et al., 2017).

DNA methylation typically involves methylation of cytosine residues at CG-rich regions known as CpG islands to form 5-methylcytosine. 5-Methylcytosine does not affect nucleic acid base-pairing and thus genetic integrity is maintained. Methylation patterns are preserved through cell division by specific DNA methyltransferases. Methylation patterns are modulated in gliomas by both increased and decreased methylation, and these patterns may be useful in the classification of glioma subtypes (Capper et al., 2018; Ceccarelli et al., 2016). Aberrant methylation of CpG sites in regulatory regions such as gene promoters alters gene expression, typically through protein binding interactions such as methyl-CpG-binding domain (MBD) proteins. Hypermethylation of gene promoters most commonly results in downregulation of gene expression and is a common mechanism of tumor suppressor silencing in cancer (Portela and Esteller, 2010).

In gliomas with IDH mutations, the oncometabolite 2-hydroxyglutarate is produced at high concentrations and competes with α-ketoglutarate at multiple enzymes, including those involved in DNA and histone methylation. Inhibition of TET family demethylases results in the G-CIMP, which causes widespread hypermethylation of CpG islands across the glioma genome (Figueroa et al., 2010; Turcan et al., 2012; Figure 12.4A). The consequences of such global methylation changes are manifold and remain incompletely understood. The G-CIMP is very common in IDH-mutant low-grade gliomas and likely drives carcinogenesis through disruption of cell-cycle regulation and antitumor innate immunity. Recently, hypermethylation has also been found to drive oncogenesis by directly disrupting DNA topology. Specific DNA sequences containing the CCCTC motif are recognized by CCCTC-binding factors (CTCF) that serve to organize the tertiary structure of DNA and insulate gene regulatory elements such as enhancers and potential oncogenes from each other. Methylation of these motifs abrogates CTCF binding and can allow for the juxtaposition of gene enhancers and oncogenes in three-dimensional space that would normally be far apart in the primary linear sequence (Flavahan et al., 2016; Figure 12.4A).

Hypermethylation of the *O*-6-methylguanine-DNA methyltransferase (MGMT) promoter, a DNA repair enzyme, is a specific epigenetic modification with significant clinical implications in gliomas. *O*-6-methylguanine-DNA methyltransferase promoter methylation silences MGMT expression and renders the cancer cell less able to repair chemotherapy-induced damage, thus improving response to treatment with alkylating agents (Hegi et al., 2005; Figure 12.4B). MGMT promoter methylation is extremely common in IDH-mutant glioma (>90%), and is also found in a significant minority of IDH-wildtype glioblastomas (Gusyatiner and Hegi, 2018; ~35–50%).

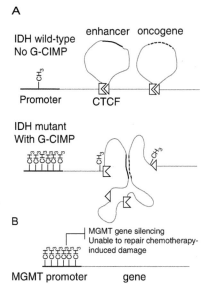

A

IDH wild-type
No G-CIMP

enhancer   oncogene

Promoter   CTCF

IDH mutant
With G-CIMP

B

MGMT gene silencing
Unable to repair chemotherapy-
induced damage

MGMT promoter   gene

Figure 12.4 Epigenetic alterations in diffuse gliomas. Isocitrate dehydrogenase mutations may induce the glioma CpG island methylator phenotype that results in methylation of gene promoters and CTCF binding sites (A). This can silence tumor suppressor gene expression and modulate DNA structure, allowing enhancers (solid black line) to come into close proximity to and activate potential oncogenes (dashed line). MGMT promoter methylation silences expression the MGMT DNA repair enzyme, rendering the tumor more sensitive to alkylating chemotherapy (B).

12.3 Clinical Manifestations and Principles

The clinical manifestations of gliomas depend both on their anatomic location as well as physiologic principles unique to gliomas and their interaction with the CNS environment. In this section we discuss key concepts of glioma physiology that contribute to their clinical presentations, focusing on those aspects that distinguish gliomas from other intracranial pathologies.

12.3.1 Mass Effect and Edema

Space-occupying lesions in the brain generally result in focal neurologic signs. The Monro–Kellie doctrine posits that the total volume of the brain parenchyma, cerebrospinal fluid (CSF), and blood compartments is fixed on account of the fixed volume of the cranial cavity. Given the relatively incompressible nature of CSF and blood, a mass lesion would therefore be expected to compress surrounding parenchyma and cause an increase in intracranial pressure (ICP). However, because gliomas are more gradual in onset as compared to an acute neurologic

event such as a stroke, compensatory mechanisms permit compression of the brain parenchyma while maintaining cerebral function, thus attenuating neurologic deficits and an increase in ICP until the mass is large enough to overcome these mechanisms (Ropper et al., 2019).

The growing tumor mass results in surrounding cerebral edema, which may be both directly symptomatic and compress surrounding normal parenchyma. Cerebral edema is generally described as either vasogenic or cytotoxic. In vasogenic edema, intravascular fluid moves into the extracellular space via defective tight junctions in the endothelium. In cytotoxic edema, acute cellular toxicity results in failure of ATP-dependent ion pumps and an increase in intracellular osmolarity, resulting in movement of fluid from the extracellular into the intracellular space. The cerebral edema associated with brain tumors is primarily vasogenic. Higher-grade gliomas are associated with increased levels of vascular endothelial growth factor (VEGF), which promotes the formation of "leaky" fenestrated neovasculature and enhances endothelial permeability. Vasogenic edema is further exacerbated by increased capillary pressure resulting from local venule compression by the tumor mass (Papadopoulos et al., 2004; Stummer, 2007).

12.3.2 Seizures

Focal-onset seizures are very common in patients with supratentorial gliomas, particularly those in epileptogenic regions such as the frontal and temporal lobes. Many factors contribute to intrinsic epileptogenesis in gliomas, including mechanical disruption of surrounding cortical structure and its inherent electrical networks due to mass effect and edema, and the accumulation of excitatory neurotransmitters and epileptogenic compounds (Samudra et al., 2019). In particular, multiple mechanisms conspire to increase the extracellular glutamate concentration (Pallud et al., 2013). Glutamate both contributes to tumor growth and is the primary excitatory neurotransmitter in the brain (Takano et al., 2001). Seizures are more common in lower-grade as opposed to higher-grade gliomas. Interestingly, the oncometabolite generated by mutant IDH, 2-hydroxybutyrate, is structurally similar to glutamate and may also be directly epileptogenic (Chen et al., 2017; Liubinas et al., 2014).

12.3.3 Systemic Complications

Although gliomas rarely metastasize outside the CNS, they can have significant systemic complications. Clinically important complications include immune suppression and hypercoagulability. Immunosuppression in the glioma microenvironment likely contributes to its poor responses to immunotherapy (Fecci and Sampson, 2019). Additionally, gliomas are associated with systemic immune dysregulation, including peripheral lymphopenia, and dysfunction of T-cells, natural killer (NK) cells, and myeloid cells (Grabowski et al., 2021).

The risks of pulmonary embolism and deep venous thrombosis (DVT) are increased in cancer in general and are especially high in brain cancers (Baron et al., 1998; Walker et al., 2012). Approximately 20% of brain cancer patients develop DVTs or PEs per year (Horsted et al., 2012). Venous thromboembolic risk is likely mediated through the production of tissue factor (TF), which activates thrombin and the coagulation cascade (Mandoj et al., 2019). Tissue factor production is elevated in glioblastoma, particularly those with EGFR amplifications; TF production is relatively lower in IDH-mutant and low-grade gliomas.

12.4 Concluding Remarks

The 2021 WHO classification marked a significant milestone in integration of recent molecular discoveries with long-recognized histologic and clinical observations. Our understanding of gliomagenesis, mechanisms of resistance, epigenetic modulation, and interactions with the immune microenvironment continue to evolve rapidly. Further reliance on molecular categorization is likely in future editions of the WHO diagnostic criteria as we incorporate these advances. Hopefully, such knowledge will ultimately enable us to exploit treatment vulnerabilities in this particularly challenging class of neurologic disease.

Figure acknowledgments

The following images are credited to the authors of this chapter: Figures 12.1-12.2, 12.4
The following image has been adapted from Nadi and Rutka (2014): Figure 12.3

References

Alcantara Llaguno S, Chen J, Kwon C-H, et al. Malignant astrocytomas originate from neural stem/progenitor cells in a somatic tumor suppressor mouse model. *Cancer Cell* 2009;**15**(1):45–56. https://doi.org/10.1016/j.ccr.2008.12.006.

Arita H, Narita Y, Fukushima S, et al. Upregulating mutations in the TERT promoter commonly occur in adult malignant gliomas and are strongly associated with total 1p19q loss. *Acta Neuropathol* 2013;**126**(2):267–76. https://doi.org/10.1007/s00401-013-1141-6.

Bao S, Wu Q, McLendon RE, et al. Glioma stem cells promote radioresistance by preferential activation of the DNA damage response. *Nature* 2006;**444**(7120):756–60. https://doi.org/10.1038/nature05236.

Baron JA, Gridley G, Weiderpass E, Nyrén O, Linet M. Venous thromboembolism and cancer. *Lancet* 1998;**351**(9109):1077–80. https://doi.org/10.1016/S0140-6736(97)10018-6.

Cairncross G, Wang M, Shaw E, et al. Phase III trial of chemoradiotherapy for anaplastic oligodendroglioma: long-term results of RTOG 9402. *J Clin Oncol* 2013;**31**(3):337–43. https://doi.org/10.1200/JCO.2012.43.2674.

Cancer Genome Atlas Research Network. Comprehensive genomic characterization defines human glioblastoma genes and core pathways. *Nature* 2008;**455**(7216):1061–8. https://doi.org/10.1038/nature07385.

Capper D, Jones DTW, Sill M, et al. DNA methylation-based classification of central nervous system tumors. *Nature* 2018;**555**(7697):469–74. https://doi.org/10.1038/nature26000.

Ceccarelli M, Barthel FP, Malta TM, et al. Molecular profiling reveals biologically discrete subsets and pathways of progression in diffuse glioma. *Cell* 2016;**164**(3):550–63. https://doi.org/10.1016/j.cell.2015.12.028.

Chen H, Judkins J, Thomas C, et al. Mutant *IDH1* and seizures in patients with glioma. *Neurology* 2017;**88**(19):1805–13. https://doi.org/10.1212/WNL.0000000000003911.

Dang L, White DW, Gross S, et al. Cancer-associated *IDH1* mutations produce 2-hydroxyglutarate. *Nature* 2009;**462**(7274):739–44. https://doi.org/10.1038/nature08617.

Dong X, Noorbakhsh A, Hirshman BR, et al. Survival trends of grade I, II, and III astrocytoma patients and associated clinical practice patterns between 1999 and 2010: a SEER-based analysis. *Neurooncol Pract* 2016;**3**(1):29–38. https://doi.org/10.1093/nop/npv016.

Fecci PE, Sampson JH. The current state of immunotherapy for gliomas: an eye toward the future. *J Neurosurg* 2019;**131**(3):657–66. https://doi.org/10.3171/2019.5.JNS181762.

Figueroa ME, Abdel-Wahab O, Lu C, et al. Leukemic *IDH1* and *IDH2* mutations result in a hypermethylation phenotype, disrupt TET2 function, and impair hematopoietic differentiation. *Cancer Cell* 2010;**18**(6):553–67. https://doi.org/10.1016/j.ccr.2010.11.015.

Flavahan WA, Drier Y, Liau BB, et al. Insulator dysfunction and oncogene activation in *IDH* mutant gliomas. *Nature* 2016;**529**(7584):110–4. https://doi.org/10.1038/nature16490.

Fontebasso AM, Liu X-Y, Sturm D, Jabado N. Chromatin remodeling defects in pediatric and young adult glioblastoma:

a tale of a variant histone 3 tail. *Brain Pathol* 2013;**23**(2):210–6. https://doi.org/10.1111/bpa.12023.

Galli R, Binda E, Orfanelli U, et al. Isolation and characterization of tumorigenic, stem-like neural precursors from human glioblastoma. *Cancer Res* 2004;**64** (19):7011–21. https://doi.org/10.1158/0008-5472.CAN-04-1364.

Gatta G, Botta L, Rossi S, et al. Childhood cancer survival in Europe 1999–2007: results of EUROCARE-5 – a population-based study. *Lancet Oncol* 2014;**15**(1):35–47. https://doi.org/10.1016/S1470-2045(13)70548-5.

Gorovets D, Kannan K, Shen R, et al. *IDH* mutation and neuroglial developmental features define clinically distinct subclasses of lower grade diffuse astrocytic glioma. *Clin Cancer Res* 2012;**18**(9):2490–501. https://doi.org/10.1158/1078-0432.CCR-11-2977.

Grabowski MM, Sankey EW, Ryan KJ, et al. Immune suppression in gliomas. *J Neurooncol* 2021;**151**(1):3–12. https://doi.org/10.1007/s11060-020-03483-y.

Gusyatiner O, Hegi ME. Glioma epigenetics: from subclassification to novel treatment options. *Semin Cancer Biol* 2018;**51**:50–8. https://doi.org/10.1016/j.semcancer.2017.11.010.

Heaphy CM, de Wilde RF, Jiao Y, et al. Altered telomeres in tumors with *ATRX* and *DAXX* mutations. *Science* 2011;**333** (6041):425. https://doi.org/10.1126/science.1207313.

Hegi ME, Diserens A-C, Gorlia T, et al. *MGMT* gene silencing and benefit from temozolomide in glioblastoma. *N Engl J Med* 2005;**352**(10):997–1003. https://doi.org/10.1056/NEJMoa043331.

Horsted F, West J, Grainge MJ. Risk of venous thromboembolism in patients with cancer: a systematic review and meta-analysis. *PLoS Med* 2012;**9**(7):e1001275. https://doi.org/10.1371/journal.pmed.1001275.

Jones DTW, Hutter B, Jäger N, et al. Recurrent somatic alterations of *FGFR1* and *NTRK2* in pilocytic astrocytoma. *Nat Genet* 2013;**45**(8):927–32. https://doi.org/10.1038/ng.2682.

Jones DTW, Kocialkowski S, Liu L, et al. Tandem duplication producing a novel oncogenic *BRAF* fusion gene defines the majority of pilocytic astrocytomas. *Cancer Res* 2008;**68** (21):8673–7. https://doi.org/10.1158/0008-5472.CAN-08-2097.

Kreth S, Thon N, Kreth FW. Epigenetics in human gliomas. *Cancer Lett* 2014;**342**(2):185–92. https://doi.org/10.1016/j.canlet.2012.04.008.

Kroonen J, Nassen J, Boulanger Y-G, et al. Human glioblastoma-initiating cells invade specifically the subventricular zones and olfactory bulbs of mice after striatal injection. *Int J Cancer* 2011;**129**(3):574–85. https://doi.org/10.1002/ijc.25709.

Lee JH, Lee JE, Kahng JY, et al. Human glioblastoma arises from subventricular zone cells with low-level driver mutations.

Nature 2018;**560**(7717):243–7. https://doi.org/10.1038/s41586-018-0389-3.

Liu G, Yuan X, Zeng Z, et al. Analysis of gene expression and chemoresistance of CD133+ cancer stem cells in glioblastoma. *Mol Cancer* 2006;**5**:67. https://doi.org/10.1186/1476-4598-5-67.

Liubinas SV, D'Abaco GM, Moffat BM, et al. *IDH1* mutation is associated with seizures and protoplasmic subtype in patients with low-grade gliomas. *Epilepsia* 2014;**55**(9):1438–43. https://doi.org/10.1111/epi.12662.

Louis DN, Perry A, Reifenberger G, et al. The 2016 World Health Organization Classification of Tumors of the Central Nervous System: a summary. *Acta Neuropathol* 2016;**131** (6):803–20. https://doi.org/10.1007/s00401-016-1545-1.

Mandoj C, Tomao L, Conti L. Coagulation in brain tumors: biological basis and clinical implications. *Front Neurol* 2019;**10**:181. https://doi.org/10.3389/fneur.2019.00181.

Matarredona ER, Pastor AM. Neural stem cells of the subventricular zone as the origin of human glioblastoma stem cells. Therapeutic implications. *Front Oncol* 2019;**9**:779. https://doi.org/10.3389/fonc.2019.00779.

Nadi M, Rutka J. Molecular markers and pathways in brain tumorigenesis. In Bernstein M, Berger MS (Eds.), *Neuro-Oncology: The Essentials*, 3rd ed. Thieme Verlag, 2015, pp. 35–46.

Ohgaki H, Kleihues P. Population-based studies on incidence, survival rates, and genetic alterations in astrocytic and oligodendroglial gliomas. *J Neuropathol Exp Neurol* 2005;**64** (6):479–89. https://doi.org/10.1093/jnen/64.6.479.

Olson JD, Riedel E, DeAngelis LM. Long-term outcome of low-grade oligodendroglioma and mixed glioma. *Neurology* 2000;**54**(7):1442–8. https://doi.org/10.1212/wnl.54.7.1442.

Ostrom QT, Gittleman H, Liao P, et al. CBTRUS statistical report: primary brain and central nervous system tumors diagnosed in the United States in 2007–2011. *Neuro Oncol* 2014;**16**(Suppl 4):iv1–63. https://doi.org/10.1093/neuonc/nou223.

Pallud J, Capelle L, Huberfeld G. Tumoral epileptogenicity: how does it happen? *Epilepsia* 2013;**54**(Suppl 9):30–4. https://doi.org/10.1111/epi.12440.

Papadopoulos MC, Saadoun S, Binder DK, Manley GT, Krishna S, Verkman AS. Molecular mechanisms of brain tumor edema. *Neuroscience* 2004;**129**(4):1011–20. https://doi.org/10.1016/j.neuroscience.2004.05.044.

Parker M, Mohankumar KM, Punchihewa C, et al. C11orf95–RELA fusions drive oncogenic NF-κB signalling in ependymoma. *Nature* 2014;**506**(7489):451–5. https://doi.org/10.1038/nature13109.

Peng Z, Liu C, Wu M. New insights into long noncoding RNAs and their roles in glioma. *Mol Cancer* 2018;**17**(1):61. https://doi.org/10.1186/s12943-018-0812-2.

Portela A, Esteller M. Epigenetic modifications and human disease. *Nat Biotechnol* 2010;**28**(10):1057–68. https://doi.org/10.1038/nbt.1685.

Reifenberger G, Louis DN. Oligodendroglioma: toward molecular definitions in diagnostic neuro-oncology. *J Neuropathol Exp Neurol* 2003;**62**(2):111–26. https://doi.org/10.1093/jnen/62.2.111.

Reifenberger J, Ring GU, Gies U, et al. Analysis of *p53* mutation and epidermal growth factor receptor amplification in recurrent gliomas with malignant progression. *J Neuropathol Exp Neurol* 1996;**55**(7):822–31. https://doi.org/10.1097/00005072-199607000-00007.

Reuss DE, Mamatjan Y, Schrimpf D, et al. IDH mutant diffuse and anaplastic astrocytomas have similar age at presentation and little difference in survival: a grading problem for WHO. *Acta Neuropathol* 2015;**129**(6):867–73. https://doi.org/10.1007/s00401-015-1438-8.

Ropper AH, Samuels MA, Klein JP, Prasad S. Intracranial neoplasms and paraneoplastic disorders. In: *Adams and Victor's Principles of Neurology*, 11th ed. McGraw-Hill Education, 2019.

Samudra N, Zacharias T, Plitt A, Lega B, Pan E. Seizures in glioma patients: an overview of incidence, etiology, and therapies. *J Neurol Sci* 2019;**404**:80–5. https://doi.org/10.1016/j.jns.2019.07.026.

Sanai N, Tramontin AD, Quiñones-Hinojosa A, et al. Unique astrocyte ribbon in adult human brain contains neural stem cells but lacks chain migration. *Nature* 2004;**427**(6976):740–4. https://doi.org/10.1038/nature02301.

Sanson M, Marie Y, Paris S, et al. Isocitrate dehydrogenase 1 codon 132 mutation is an important prognostic biomarker in gliomas. *J Clin Oncol* 2009;**27**(25):4150–4. https://doi.org/10.1200/JCO.2009.21.9832.

Schwartzentruber J, Korshunov A, Liu X-Y, et al. Driver mutations in histone H3.3 and chromatin remodelling genes in paediatric glioblastoma. *Nature* 2012;**482**(7384):226–31. https://doi.org/10.1038/nature10833.

Shay JW, Bacchetti S. A survey of telomerase activity in human cancer. *Eur J Cancer* 1997;**33**(5):787–91. https://doi.org/10.1016/S0959-8049(97)00062-2.

Shi J, Dong B, Cao J, et al. Long non-coding RNA in glioma: signaling pathways. *Oncotarget* 2017;**8**(16):27582–92. https://doi.org/10.18632/oncotarget.15175.

Singh SK, Hawkins C, Clarke ID, et al. Identification of human brain tumor initiating cells. *Nature* 2004;**432**(7015):396–401. https://doi.org/10.1038/nature03128.

Stephens PJ, Greenman CD, Fu B, et al. Massive genomic rearrangement acquired in a single catastrophic event during cancer development. *Cell* 2011;**144**(1):27–40. https://doi.org/10.1016/j.cell.2010.11.055.

Stummer W. Mechanisms of tumor-related brain edema. *Neurosurg Focus* 2007;**22**(5):E8. https://doi.org/10.3171/foc.2007.22.5.9.

Sullivan JP, Nahed BV, Madden MW, et al. Brain tumor cells in circulation are enriched for mesenchymal gene expression. *Cancer Discov* 2014;**4**(11):1299–309. https://doi.org/10.1158/2159-8290.CD-14-0471.

Takano T, Lin JH, Arcuino G, Gao Q, Yang J, Nedergaard M. Glutamate release promotes growth of malignant gliomas. *Nat Med* 2001;**7**(9):1010–5. https://doi.org/10.1038/nm0901-1010.

Turcan S, Rohle D, Goenka A, et al. *IDH1* mutation is sufficient to establish the glioma hypermethylator phenotype. *Nature* 2012;**483**(7390):479–83. https://doi.org/10.1038/nature10866.

Verhaak RGW, Hoadley KA, Purdom E, et al. Integrated genomic analysis identifies clinically relevant subtypes of glioblastoma characterized by abnormalities in *PDGFRA, IDH1, EGFR,* and *NF1*. *Cancer Cell* 2010;**17**(1):98–110. https://doi.org/10.1016/j.ccr.2009.12.020.

Walker A, West J, Card T, Crooks C, Grainge M. Rate of venous thromboembolism by cancer type compared to the general population using multiple linked databases. *Thrombosis Res* 2012;**129**:S155–6.

Watanabe K, Sato K, Biernat W, et al. Incidence and timing of *p53* mutations during astrocytoma progression in patients with multiple biopsies. *Clin Cancer Res* 1997;**3**(4):523–30.

Wikstrand CJ, Reist CJ, Archer GE, Zalutsky MR, Bigner DD. The class III variant of the epidermal growth factor receptor (EGFRvIII): characterization and utilization as an immunotherapeutic target. *J Neurovirol* 1998;**4**(2):148–58. https://doi.org/10.3109/13550289809114515.

Wu G, Broniscer A, McEachron TA, et al. Somatic histone H3 alterations in pediatric diffuse intrinsic pontine gliomas and non-brainstem glioblastomas. *Nat Genet* 2012;**44**(3):251–3. https://doi.org/10.1038/ng.1102.

Yan H, Parsons DW, Jin G, et al. *IDH1* and *IDH2* mutations in gliomas. *N Engl J Med* 2009;**360**(8):765–73. https://doi.org/10.1056/NEJMoa0808710.

Zhang J, Wu G, Miller CP, et al. Whole-genome sequencing identifies genetic alterations in pediatric low-grade gliomas. *Nat Genet* 2013;**45**(6):602–12. https://doi.org/10.1038/ng.2611.

Chapter 13

Brain Metastases: Molecules to Medicine

Ethan S. Srinivasan, Vadim Tsvankin, Eric W. Sankey, Matthew M. Grabowski,
Pakawat Chongsathidkiet, and Peter E. Fecci

13.1 Introduction

Brain metastases are the most common intracranial tumors in adults, affecting up to 20% of all cancer patients (Ostrom et al., 2018). Due to improvements in population health, systemic cancer therapies, and screening tools, the incidence of brain metastases is expected to increase; as such, examining the process of metastasis is valuable for the practicing neurosurgeon to project future directions in research and management within this growing field.

The most common primary tumor sites to develop brain metastases are lung, breast, and melanoma skin cancer, with additional significant contributions from renal cell carcinoma and colorectal cancers (Berghoff et al., 2016). The progression of these lesions follows a pattern similar to the traditional metastatic cascade, with essential differences specific to the unique structural, cellular, and immunologic parameters of the central nervous system (CNS). This chapter will discuss the process of metastasis to the brain and the development of mature, clinically relevant tumors. The temptation to discuss brain metastases as a monolith is an apparent hazard that overlooks the substantial heterogeneity within the tumor subtypes; thus, our particular aim will be to highlight key shared pathways, mechanisms, and molecular actors. Much of the available research has been completed in breast and lung models, and so integrated codification of these results across a broader range of primary tumor sites remains a notable limitation. In several domains, particularly regarding the tumor microenvironment (TME) and immune consequences, brain metastases remain relatively underinvestigated compared to primary brain tumors. Therefore, some discussion of the results in primary tumors with supporting evidence for analogous findings in metastases will be presented as appropriate; these areas in particular suggest opportunities for further investigation. Several excellent reviews that covers aspects of this chapter can be found in the references section (Achrol et al., 2019; Ciminera et al., 2017; Farber et al., 2016; Fecci et al., 2019; Lambert et al., 2017).

13.2 Metastatic Cascade

Broadly, the process of metastasis begins with the establishment of a premetastatic niche by secreted factors, local invasion at the primary tumor site, intravasation of tumor cells into blood vessels with survival in the circulatory system, extravasation at the CNS, proliferation of micrometastases in a perivascular niche, and progression to clinically relevant macrometastases with co-option of the surrounding CNS architecture and cellular components. The full biomolecular mechanics of each step are beyond the scope of this chapter and remain active areas of investigation. Study of these processes in the context of brain metastasis is unique due to the boundary of the blood–brain barrier (BBB) and the complex bidirectional interplay between invading tumor cells and the resident CNS components, as well as subsequent infiltrating immune effectors. Anatomic components that under physiologic circumstances sequester the brain from potential hazards in systemic circulation are hijacked in the setting of brain metastasis to facilitate the colonization and reorganization of the CNS into a pro-tumorigenic environment; indeed, it selects for development of progressive metastatic cell phenotypes derivative of but distinct from the primary tumor.

13.2.1 Premetastatic Niche

The premetastatic niche describes changes in the CNS vasculature and parenchyma induced by a fleet of cytokines, chemokines, angiogenic factors, and exosomes secreted from the primary tumor and circulating tumor cells (CTCs; Liu and Cao, 2016). These changes precede metastasis, and indeed serve to prime possible metastatic sites. CNS colonization is promoted through the upregulation of cell adhesion mediators on endothelial cells, loosening of tight junctions within the BBB, accumulation of pro-inflammatory myeloid cells, and local cultivation of a pro-inflammatory microenvironment (Bohn et al., 2017; Li et al., 2013; Liu et al., 2013; Soto et al., 2014).

Although investigation of the premetastatic niche within the brain remains limited relative to other sites, several recent studies merit discussion. Secreted factors identified to increase the permeability of the BBB include vascular endothelial growth factor receptor (VEGFR) and angiopoietin-2 in breast cancer, and placental growth factor (PLGF) in small cell lung cancer (Bohn et al., 2017; Li et al., 2013). Tumor exosomes, which are secreted extracellular vesicles containing lipids, proteins, and nucleic acids, have also been implicated in establishing the premetastatic niche (Théry et al., 2002). A subset of these vesicles has been shown to specifically localize to the brain and its vasculature based on their integrin profiles, with $ITG\beta_3$ and $ITG\alpha_v$ identified as key mediators in models of metastatic breast cancer (Hoshino et al., 2015; Wu et al., 2012). Once targeted to the brain, the exosomes are capable of influencing the immediately accessible endothelial cells as well as migrating through the BBB by transcytosis to reprogram the underlying CNS components (Morad et al., 2019). For example, exosomal miRNAs miR-181c and miR-122 have been demonstrated to facilitate BBB disruption and astrocyte metabolic reprogramming in breast cancer models, along with upregulated production of inflammatory mediators caused by exosomal cell migration-inducing and hyaluronan-binding protein (CEMIP) in both breast and lung metastatic models (Fong et al., 2015; Rodrigues et al., 2019; Tominaga et al., 2015). The role of CTCs has also been supported with the induction of increased cellular adhesion molecules (CAMs), selectins, and integrins on brain endothelial cells soon after the administration of brain-seeking metastatic breast cancer cells into the circulatory system (Soto et al., 2014). Although only a small percentage of the full suite of involved factors has so far been described, evidence from clinical samples with confirmatory data in preclinical knock-out and knock-down studies, in addition to potential pharmacologic agents, highlights the potential for pre-emptive targeting of these metastatic pathways.

13.2.2 Local Invasion, Intravasation Into Blood Vessels, and Survival

Selective pressures at each stage of the metastatic cascade induce tumor cell adaptation, resulting in a series of phenotypically distinct intermediates spanning the primary tumor site and eventual metastasis. Invasive growth and subsequent intravasation into the circulatory system at the primary location are driven largely by a suite of reversible reprogramming pathways collectively referred to as the epithelial to mesenchymal transition (EMT; Kalluri and Weinberg, 2009). Physiologically, this phenotype is typically observed during embryogenesis; in the context of malignancy, it permits degradation of the surrounding extracellular matrix, potentiating cell mobility and promoting tumor-initiating abilities similar to cancer stem cells (CSCs; importantly, both EMT-related and CSC-like features have been observed to increase resistance to cytotoxic therapies; Eckert et al., 2011; Jolly et al., 2019; Leong et al., 2014; Mani et al., 2008; Qin et al., 2005).

The EMT is a heterogeneous process that encompasses a range of adaptations present along a spectrum within individual tumor cells, significantly coordinated by transcription factors including the SNAIL, ZEB, and TWIST families (Cano et al., 2000; Gregory et al., 2011; Pastushenko et al., 2018; Yang et al., 2004). Both single-cell and cell-cluster models of migration integrate an element of the EMT and lead to eventual intravasation to the circulatory system, either directly or through lymphatics (Yu et al., 2013). Upon egress from the primary tumor environment, the vast majority of CTCs rapidly succumb to stressors including mechanical shear, improper adaptation to the loss of attachments, and an active immune response frequently mediated by natural killer (NK) cells (Hanna and Fidler, 1980; Regmi et al., 2017). To cope, CTCs have been observed to parasitize other circulating cellular components, notably platelets, which can support CTCs through essential signaling pathways, mediation of adherence to vascular endothelial cells, mechanical protection from fluid forces, and camouflage against immune attack (Labelle et al., 2011; Menter et al., 1987; Palumbo et al., 2005). Eventually these cells are arrested in the dense microvasculature of the CNS and the next stage of the metastatic cascade commences (Kienast et al., 2010).

13.2.3 Extravasation in the Central Nervous System

At this point, the predominant obstacle to entering the CNS is the BBB. Composed of tight junctions between endothelial cells with support from underlying astrocytes and pericytes, the BBB barricades the CNS against the peripheral circulation. The primary mechanism for CNS seeding is thought to be direct traversal of the BBB, either by paracellular or transcellular routes, although

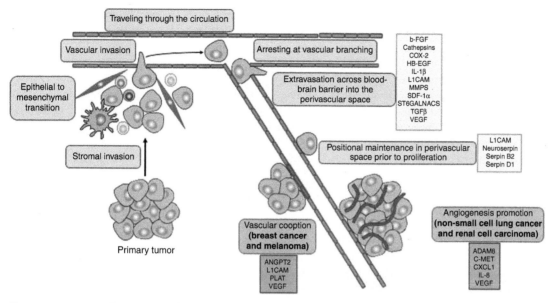

Figure 13.1 Cancer cell dissemination from primary tumor to brain metastasis.

additional mechanisms have been suggested including travel along bridging vessels or through the recently described glymphatic circulation (Louveau et al., 2017; Yao et al., 2018).

While the complete pathway remains to be elucidated, key steps and a number of important factors have been identified. Single-cell studies of CTCs in preclinical models have demonstrated that the larger, relatively rigid shape of tumor cells leads to slowed progress and arrest within the microcapillary network of the brain, where degradation of the BBB ensues (Kienast et al., 2010). This process is summarized in Figure 13.1. A number of gene expression changes, surface molecules, and soluble factors have been implicated in increasing the adhesion to and permeability of the BBB, many within the general categories of selectins, integrins, CAMs, cadherins, proteases, and various chemokines and cytokines, along with associated ligands and substrates. Of note, despite substantial overlap, the significant heterogeneity of these findings across primary tumor types suggests a multiplicity of mechanisms likely defined by predilections of the primary tumor tissues. Specifically identified mediators of this step include the upregulation of adhesive membrane proteins ST6GALNAC5 and CD44, upregulation of COX2, CXCR4, HBEGF, EREG expression, increased secretion of VEGF, angiopoetin-2, PLGF, and S100A4, increased secretion of proteases including cathepsin S and multiple matrix metalloproteinases, various upregulated CAMs, increased melanotransferrin expression

in melanoma, and increased rho kinase signaling in small cell lung cancer (Bohn et al., 2017; Bos et al., 2009; Herwig et al., 2016; Lee et al., 2003; Lee et al., 2004; Li et al., 2006, 2013; Liu et al., 2012; Rolland et al., 2009; Sevenich et al., 2014; Yang et al., 2012). Preclinical models inhibiting many of these mediators have shown success in reducing the incidence of brain metastases, supporting potential treatment strategies that target essential actors in the extravasation pathway.

In addition to its role in the process of metastatic spread, the BBB and subsequent blood–tumor barrier (BTB) are also key actors in limiting treatment efficacy within the CNS. While strict filtering is beneficial in the nonpathologic state, the BBB/BTB presents a hurdle to the CNS access of systemic therapies. Thus far, several strategies have been investigated to increase the permeability of this boundary for delivery of immune- and chemotherapeutic agents, including focused ultrasound, radiation, magnetic nanoparticles, convection-enhanced delivery, and laser interstitial thermal therapy (LITT) (Curley et al., 2017; Liu et al., 2010; Nakamura et al., 2011; Salehi et al., 2002; Tabatabaei et al., 2015; Yuan et al., 2006).

13.2.4 Proliferation of Micrometastases

Once past the BBB, the vast majority of metastatic cells still fail to establish a foothold within the CNS, and fewer still progress from the micrometastatic phase to clinically relevant macrometastases – they enter an inhospitable environment distinct from the primary site, and in which the accumulated adaptations promoting CTC survival are of dubious benefit (Kienast et al., 2010). Moreover, despite the canonical "immune privilege" of the CNS, circumvention of local antitumor immunity is a necessary and critical step to metastatic progression (see Farber et al., 2016, for a detailed review of the BBB and its role in mediating antitumor immunity).

The development of a complex and evolving microenvironment begins as the tumor cell both modifies and is modified by the cellular and non-cellular components of its surroundings. Studies in murine models suggest that these initial metastatic seeds remain in a perivascular location at the abluminal surface of the blood vessel where the developing tumor can meet its immediate and growing need for oxygen and nutrients (Kienast et al., 2010). The initial tumor seed is quickly encircled by reactive astrocytes likely activated through the damage-associated molecular patterns (DAMPs) pathway. These astrocytes first produce tissue plasminogen activators (TPAs), generating resultant plasmin that eliminates most neoplastic cells through subsequent FasL-mediated activation of apoptotic signalling (Lorger et al., 2010; McFarland and Benveniste, 2019). The gene *SERPINI1*, responsible for the plasminogen activator (PA) inhibitor neuroserpin, along with others in the class, has been identified as a tumor cell defense mechanism in both lung and breast metastatic models that enables resistance to this initial antitumor response of astrocytes (Valiente et al., 2014).

For the metastatic cells that survive, this perivascular niche remains an important location within the TME, similar to that of primary brain tumors. As the tumor needs expand beyond the supply of nutrients available from the native vascular architecture, the metastatic cells manipulate their surroundings through either co-option of existing vessels (common in breast and melanoma metastases) or directed angiogenesis (typical in non-small cell lung carcinoma [NSCLS] and renal cell carcinoma); these processes are mediated through VEGF, integrins, and CAMs (in particular ITG$\alpha_v\beta_3$, ITGβ_1, and L1CAM) (Berghoff et al., 2013; Lorger et al., 2009; Yano et al., 2000). Further colonization of the adjacent brain parenchyma occurs as the tumor evolves via complex cross-talk between the metastatic cells and native cellular components, in part also mediated by L1CAM and a set of metabolic reprogramming patterns discussed below (Er et al., 2018; Hoj et al., 2019).

Promising preclinical data support targeting a number of these mechanisms through small molecule inhibitors and monoclonal antibodies. The VEGF inhibitor bevacizumab, in particular, acts at multiple stages of the metastatic cascade and has demonstrated success in murine models of brain metastases (Bohn et al., 2017; Ilhan-Mutlu et al., 2016). Notably, studies with the monoclonal antibody have also shown clinical efficacy when paired with standard-of-care chemotherapy for extending survival in brain metastases from non-small cell lung cancer (Besse et al., 2015; Bohn et al., 2017).

13.3 Establishment of the Tumor Microenvironment

Establishment of co-dependency between tumor cells and local CNS componentry is integral to our understanding of brain metastases, and results in a pro-tumorigenic, treatment-resistant TME. Current understandings point to both shared characteristics and a range of diversity within the metastatic niche across primary tumor sources, with additional work needed to fully elucidate these similarities and differences.

The cellular components of the TME consist primarily of the metastatic cells, reactive astrocytes, endothelium, pericytes, neurons, microglia and bone-marrow-derived macrophages (collectively called tumor-associated macrophages [TAMs]), and tumor-infiltrating lymphocytes [TILs]). Although significant work has been invested in describing the evolution of TME in primary CNS malignancies, less is currently understood about the interactions within metastatic lesions. Thus far, studies have primarily focused on the relationship between metastatic cells, reactive astrocytes, and TAMs, with significant evidence to suggest the development of a cooperative and intimate relationship between the local glial and metastatic tumor cells after the initial anti-tumor response (see Figure 13.2; Achrol et al., 2019). This dynamic TME presents multiple potential therapeutic targets, either through inhibition of CNS metastasis-specific biologic processes or reversal of the immunosuppressive and pro-tumorigenic effects on TAMs, TILs, and astrocytes. Further investigation and extension of the work in primary CNS tumors is a promising basis of research to both build our understanding of these important relationships and to generate translational results for clinical implementation.

13.3.1 Astrocytes

The association between metastatic cells and reactive astrocytes is likely the most intimate of the TME, with evidence in breast cancer metastasis of gap junctions forming between the two (Chen et al., 2016). Signaling

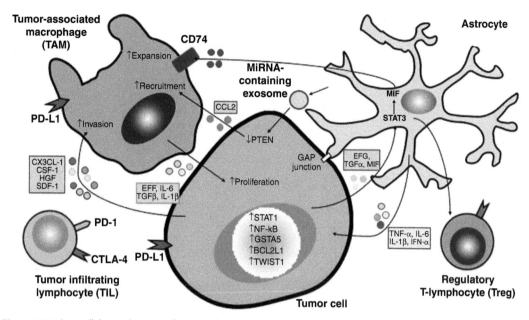

Figure 13.2 Intercellular mechanisms of communication within the metastatic tumor microenvironment.

through this avenue, along with additional paracrine loops including signaling molecules and miRNA-containing tumor-derived exosomes, induces the reactive astrocytes to secrete inflammatory mediators such as tumor necrosis factor-α (TNF-α), interleukin-6 (IL-6), IL-1β, and interferon-α (IFN-α) (Seike et al., 2011). These inflammatory mediators subsequently stimulate tumor cell proliferation and chemoresistance through the upregulation of genes including *STAT1*, NF-κB, *GSTA5*, *BCL2L1*, *TWIST1*, and loss of phosphatase and tensin homolog (*PTEN*), accelerating a flywheel of pro-tumorigenic positive feedback loops (Kim et al., 2011; Zhang et al., 2015). The full spectrum of interactions between metastatic cells and reactive astrocytes across the range of primary tumor sources is an area with substantial opportunity for further investigation. A few of the findings thus far described have identified numerous genetic and secreted mediators involved in these loops, including estrogen, HGF, BDNF, TGF-β2, and endothelin secretion, as well as c-Met, Notch, ANGPTL4, and Reelin expression changes in breast cancer models (Choy et al., 2017; Gong et al., 2019; Jandial et al., 2017; Kim et al., 2014; Sartorius et al., 2016; Xing et al., 2013, 2016; Zhang et al., 2015). Similar interactions have been identified in melanoma and lung cancer, as well as evidence of an induced STAT3-dependent expression profile in reactive astrocytes that contributes to local

immunosuppression via inhibition of CD8+ T cell and TAM antitumor activity (Klein et al., 2015; McFarland and Benveniste, 2019). Notably, interruption of this signaling cascade with the drug silibinin inhibited metastatic brain tumor growth in both mouse and human subjects, in a manner specific to its effect on the TME. This encouraging result provides proof of concept for such strategies aimed at disrupting the pro-tumorigenic interactions within the CNS (Priego et al., 2018).

13.3.2 Tumor-Associated Macrophages and Tumor-Infiltrating Lymphocytes

The interactions between metastatic tumor cells and TAMs (microglia and infiltrating bone marrow-derived macrophages) have been less thoroughly investigated. These two macrophage populations are arguably indistinguishable experimentally and comprise up to 30% of the total tumor mass (Sevenich et al., 2014). In primary brain tumors, TAMs have been identified as key players in the pro-tumorigenic TME, with roles in angiogenesis, immunosuppression, and tumor promotion mediated through TGF-β, MMPs, and cathepsins (Wagner et al., 1999). In metastatic models, the classical anti-inflammatory M2 profile TAM has also been show to exhibit decreased cytotoxicity while promoting local immunosuppression, tumor proliferation and parenchymal invasion, and extracellular matrix remodeling. These effects have been found to be regulated by WNT, CXCR4, and PI3K pathway signaling, with tumor-secreted neurotrophin-3 and miR-503 implicated in breast cancer models (Andreou et al., 2017; Blazquez et al., 2018; Choy et al., 2017; Chuang et al., 2013; Pukrop et al., 2010; Xing et al., 2018). Work remains to be done to further map the key pathways in metastatic lesions, and the reversal of pro-tumorigenic TAM polarization offers another potential therapeutic target for investigation.

A later arrival to the TME, CD4$^+$ T cells, CD8$^+$ T cells, and regulatory T cells (Treg) have been shown to extensively infiltrate brain metastases, particularly in strongly immunogenic tumors such as melanoma (Berghoff et al., 2015). Interestingly, a significant range of heterogeneity in both density and profile of TILs has been shown across primary tumor sources, as well as within brain metastases compared to their paired primary tumor (Berghoff et al., 2015; Kudo et al., 2019). In particular, characterization of immune-checkpoint expression (PD-L1, PD-L2, and IOD1) found significantly higher levels in lung cancer samples compared to breast and colorectal cancers (Harter et al., 2015). Paired samples of non-small cell lung cancer and their primary tumor sources demonstrated lower concentrations of infiltrating immune cells with the ratio skewed significantly toward M2-polarized TAMs, suggesting an immunosuppressed TME that is both permissive to and accelerative of metastatic tumor growth (Kudo et al., 2019). A number of processes appear to parallel findings in primary brain tumors: chemokine production and local induction of Tregs, systemic immune suppression, and sequestration of functional T cells in patient bone marrow (Chongsathidkiet et al., 2018; Lowery and Yu, 2017; Sampson et al., 2020). Preclinical data suggest common pathways and targets for treatment approaches, and consideration of these factors along with immune-licensing therapies presents an avenue forward in treatment approaches for a variety of pathologies concomitantly as discussed further below.

13.4 Metabolomics

Similar to adaptations in response to the structural and cellular elements, brain metastases show heterogeneous metabolic adaptations, matching their needs to substrate availability within the CNS – specifically, the interstitial fluid of the CNS has relatively low concentrations of glucose, and is relatively enriched in glutamine and branched chain amino acids (BCAAs) (Ciminera et al.,

2017; Dolgodilina et al., 2016; Silver and Erecińska, 1994; Sperringer et al., 2017).

The metabolic profile of metastases is typically interrogated using spectroscopy to analyze metabolite substrates and intermediates, with time-course experiments using stable isotope tracers permitting analysis of flux through various metabolic pathways. Broadly, metabolic reprogramming is a hallmark of cancer evolution, traditionally discussed as the "Warburg effect" (Liberti and Locasale, 2016; Warburg, 1925): a transition from oxidative phosphorylation to aerobic glycolysis (reviewed in detail in Lambert et al., 2017). This shift is driven by mutations in metabolic enzymes and tumor suppressor genes, and includes upregulation of traditional oxidative phosphorylation enzymes as well as increased utilization of non-glucose alternative substrates, aerobic glycolysis, and lipid metabolism (Jung et al., 2015; Sjøbakk et al., 2007, 2013; Tiwary et al., 2018). The alternative substrates include acetate, glutamine, and BCAAs; the neurotransmitter gamma aminobutyric acid (GABA) has been co-opted as a metabolic substrate by metastatic breast cancer cells (Chen et al., 2015; Mashimo et al., 2014; Neman et al., 2014).

In addition to internal metabolic reprogramming, brain metastases may reorganize the metabolic landscape of the TME – metastatic breast cancer cells have been shown to inhibit glucose utilization of surrounding astrocytes (Fong et al., 2015). Similarly, the Notch signaling pathway has been identified as an important mediator of metabolic shifts in melanoma and breast cancer cells, and is heavily influenced by local astrocyte secretions (Bi and Kuang, 2015; Nam et al., 2008; Xing et al., 2013).

13.5 Genomics

The genetic and molecular features responsible remain incompletely understood and are an active area of investigation. Human epidermal growth factor receptor (HER) 2-positive and triple-negative (estrogen-receptor, progesterone-receptor, and HER2 negative) subtypes of breast cancer, ALK-rearranged and EGFR-mutant non-small cell lung cancer, and PTEN-depleted melanoma have particular predilections for the brain (Bucheit et al., 2014; Eichler et al., 2010; Kim et al., 2011; Pestalozzi et al., 2006). Meanwhile, bidirectional TME interactions result in distinct genetic and epigenetic changes within the metastatic tumor cells themselves, distinguishing it from its progenitor primary tumor (see Table 13.1; Brastianos et al., 2015; Hohensee et al., 2013). A recent study of matched brain metastases and primary tumors found clinically

Table 13.1 Molecular alterations in brain metastases and primary tumors

Histology type	Shared between primary tumors and brain metastases	Unique to brain metastases
Non-small cell lung cancer	↑**EGFR**, **ALK**, KRAS	↓LKB1
Breast carcinoma	↑ERBB2, AKT1	↑ATAD2, BRAF, DERL1, DNMT3B, EGFR, KRT5, MYC, PROM1, NEK2A, NES
	↓CDKN2A, CDKN2B, PTEN	↓ATM, CRYAB, HSPB2
Melanoma	↑**AKT1**	↑TBX2
	↓CDKN2A, PTEN	↓CDH13, PLEKHA5
Renal cell carcinoma		↑PIK3CA
	↓CDKN2A	↓PTEN
Colorectal carcinoma	↑**KRAS**, **PIK3CA**	↑**NRAS**

*__Bold__ = have been associated with increased brain metastases.

meaningful genetic alterations not found in the primary tumors in 53% of the metastatic samples, with common differences in the PI3K/AKT/mTOR, CDK, and HER2/EGFR pathways (Brastianos et al., 2015). These mutations conferred increased sensitivity to appropriated targeted inhibitors, highlighting a potential mechanism for lesion-specific responses to systemic therapies and targets for brain metastasis–specific treatment plans (Brastianos et al., 2015). Separate matched sample studies demonstrated changes in the pathways of cell proliferation, growth, and survival, specifically with mutations in *CDKN2A*, *PIK3CA*, *TP53*, *DSC2*, loss of *PTEN*, and amplification of *ERBB2* and *KRAS*, as well as alterations in pathways for axonal guidance and angiogenesis signaling (Lee et al., 2015, 2016; Tyran et al., 2019; Wang et al., 2019). It is unknown whether these mutations develop within the primary tumor or at the metastatic site.

13.6 Treatment Implications and Strategies

A diagnosis of cancer metastatic to the brain, previously considered an imminent death sentence, now invites the possibility of ever-advancing treatment strategies aimed at extending life and improving quality of life. The typical mainstays of surgical resection, radiation, and chemotherapy are complemented by advances in systemic treatments, targeted therapies, and immunotherapies – and insights into the mechanisms and ontogeny of brain metastases suggest rational combinations that optimize the efficacy of any given component (Fecci et al.,2019; Moravan et al., 2020). Beyond therapeutics, innovation in surgical treatment, including the use of LITT for recurrent metastases, presents another future direction with promising results in survival and quality of life metrics (Kim et al., 2020; Sharma et al., 2016).

The preceding sections have mentioned a host of appealing targets for investigators, and several targeted therapies including small molecule inhibitors and monoclonal antibodies have gained attention in brain metastases with driver mutations – particularly those directed at well-characterized mutations such as HER-2, ALK, EGFR, MAPK, AXL, ABL, and BRAF (Achrol et al., 2019). Various traditional chemotherapeutics have also been explored and are in use, including platinum-based agents, taxanes, alkylating agents, folate antimetabolites, and topoisomerase inhibitors, with limited and heterogeneous success across primary tumor sources. The challenge of administering effective systemic therapies across the BBB has been met not only with bypassing it through direct, local administration of agents (such as convection-enhanced delivery), but by harnessing windows in which the BBB is temporarily "opened" by local treatments – surgery, radiosurgery, or LITT (Leuthardt et al., 2016; Nakamura et al., 2011; Qin et al., 2001; van Vulpen et al., 2002). Similarly, evidence suggests the BBB may sustain targeted disruptions by focused ultrasound and drugs including regadenoson (Jackson et al., 2016; Liu et al., 2010). Well-coordinated, multidisciplinary clinical trials are critical in establishing and optimizing the interplay between multiple modalities of treatment.

No discussion of systemic therapy is complete without mention of immunotherapy; although clinical success in brain metastases has yet been limited to robustly immunogenic subtypes such as melanoma and lung cancer, the marked successes in these diseases have buoyed investigational interest across multiple subtypes (Chen et al., 2018; Gaudy-Marqueste et al., 2017; Rizvi et al., 2015). Thorough discussion of immunotherapeutic mechanisms is beyond the scope of this chapter, but in general the current generation includes a number of agents aimed at disrupting tumor-induced inactivation of effector immune cells. These agents are termed "checkpoint inhibitors" and include anti-CTLA-4, anti-PD-1, and PD-L1 monoclonal antibodies (Di Giacomo et al., 2019). While the potently immunosuppressive environment of brain metastases presents a key challenge to broad implementation of immunotherapies, the rapidly progressing development of novel strategies is cause for optimism.

The clinical trials of such checkpoint inhibitors in melanoma and non-small cell lung cancer brain metastases have yielded striking results. While previous median overall survival in patients with melanoma brain metastases was just 4.7 months, clinical trials of immunotherapies have radically shifted that prognosis (Davies et al., 2011). One study of patients with melanoma brain metastases treated with ipilimumab (targeting CTLA-4) showed 24% disease control in asymptomatic patients and 10% in symptomatic at 3 months, while long-term follow-up of ipilimumab plus fotemustine showed a 3-year survival rate of 27.8% and a median overall survival of 12.7 months (Di Giacomo et al., 2015; Margolin et al., 2012). The combination of ipilimumab and nivolumab (targeting PD-1) demonstrated an even greater benefit, with intracranial response in 46% of patients with melanoma brain metastases, compared to 20% in the nivolumab alone cohort, and complete intracranial responses in 17% and 12%, respectively (Long et al., 2018). A similar study that continued combination therapy until progression or intolerable toxicity demonstrated an intracranial benefit in 57% of patients, 26% complete, with an overall survival of 92.3% at 6 months and 82.8% at 9 months (Tawbi et al., 2018). While exploration in other primary tumor sources is ongoing, another trial tested pembrolizumab (targeting PD-1) in patients with melanoma or PD-L1 positive NSCLC brain metastases and showed intracranial response in 22% and 33%, respectively, with durable responses lasting up to the date of analysis in 27% of the NSCLC patients (Goldberg et al., 2016). Notably, investigators have also identified an abscopal effect induced by radiotherapy of brain metastasis, and small studies have shown this to be further potentiated by immunotherapies (Grimaldi et al., 2014; Lin et al., 2019; Pfannenstiel et al., 2019). These encouraging results are currently being pursued through a number of ongoing and upcoming clinical trials to expand the use of immunotherapeutic strategies and identify their optimal integration with surgery and radiotherapy (see Table 13.2).

More recent developments in the realm of immunotherapy present other early but promising avenues forward. While adoptive cell therapies, such as chimeric antigen receptor T cells (CAR T cells), have shown the most success in hematologic malignancies, their application in brain metastases is an interesting area of investigation. In one study of metastatic melanoma, patients receiving melanoma antigen-targeting CAR T cells who were retrospectively found to have brain metastases showed radiographic responses in 64% of cases, 35% of which were complete by the Response Evaluation Criteria in Solid Tumors (RECIST) criteria (Hong et al., 2010). Ongoing trials targeting brain metastases of HER2+ breast cancer (NCT03696030) and CD19+ B cell malignancies (NCT04287309) with CAR T cells will be interesting proofs of concept for this strategy, and as the technology continues to evolve there are sure to be further opportunities for implementation.

13.7 Conclusion

Brain metastases represent a clinically challenging and growing segment of neurosurgical practice. While the process of brain metastasis shares many characteristics with systemic spread elsewhere, the unique structural and cellular elements of the CNS create unique barriers to investigation and treatment. Once within the CNS, the metastatic cells adapt, reorganize, and reprogram the native architecture and cellular components to generate a microenvironment that supports and accelerates tumor proliferation and resists treatment. Continued research into the mechanisms of CNS penetration and exploitation of the native cellular components will identify novel strategies to target this pernicious disease process.

Table 13.2 Key clinical trials evaluating targeted therapy and immunotherapy in brain metastases

Primary disease	Trial number	Name	Phase	Interventions	Status	Locations	Available key findings	Reference
Melanoma	NCT02039947	COMBI-MB	II	Dabrafenib, Trametinib	Completed – has results	Multicenter (Australia, Canada, France, Germany, Italy, Spain, USA)	This study demonstrates 40–60% intracranial response rates in patients with BRAF V600-mutant melanoma brain metastases using targeted molecular therapies on the BRAF (Dabrafenib) and MAPK/ERK (Trametinib) pathways combined	PMID: 28592387
	NCT01266967	Break MB	II	Dabrafenib	Completed – has results	Multicenter (Australia, Canada, France, Germany, Italy, USA)	Dabrafenib shows 30–40% intracranial response rates and an acceptable safety profile in patients with V600E BRAF-mutant melanoma and brain metastases including those who were treated for brain metastases and had disease progression and those who are untreated	PMID: 23051966
	NCT01253564		II	Vemurafenib	Completed – has results	Lausanne and Zurich, Switzerland	Vemurafenib (BRAF kinase inhibitor) shows significant tumor regression in patients with advanced symptomatic melanoma and brain metastases. An overall partial response (PR) at both intracranial and extracranial lesions was achieved in 42% of recruited patients. Of patients with measurable intracranial disease, 37% achieved >30% intracranial tumor regression. Other signs of improvement included reduced need for corticosteroids and enhanced performance status	PMID: 24295639
	NCT01378975		II	Vemurafenib	Completed – has results	Multicenter (Australia, Canada, France, Germany, Israel, Italy, Netherlands, Spain, UK, USA)	This study demonstrates clinically meaningful response rates of melanoma brain metastases to vemurafenib. The intracranial best overall response rate (BORR) was 18% in patients who had not received any treatments for brain metastases. Extracranial BORR was 33% in untreated for brain metastases cohort and 23% in previously treated cohort. Drug safety profile was acceptable and without significant CNS toxicity	PMID: 27993793

Table 13.2 (cont.)

Primary disease	Trial number	Name	Phase	Interventions	Status	Locations	Available key findings	Reference
	NCT00623766		II	Ipilimumab, corticosteroids	Completed – has results	Multicenter (USA)	Ipilimumab (anti-CTLA-4) shows disease control in some patients with advanced melanoma and brain metastases, particularly when metastases are small and asymptomatic. In this study, patients were enrolled in either cohort A (neurologically asymptomatic and were not receiving corticosteroid treatment at study entry) or cohort B (symptomatic and on a stable dose of corticosteroids); 18% in cohort A exhibited disease control, as did 5% in cohort B. When the brain was assessed alone, 24% in cohort A and 10% in cohort B achieved disease control. No unexpected toxic effects were reported	PMID: 22456429
	NCT01654692	NIBIT-M1	II	Ipilimumab, Fotemustine	Completed	Multicenter (Italy)	Long-term analysis of this trial shows the efficacy of ipilimumab combined with fotemustine in patients with metastatic melanoma. With a median follow-up of 39.9 months, median overall survival and 3-year survival rates were 12.9 months and 28.5% for the whole study population, and 12.7 months and 27.8% for patients with brain metastases, respectively. The absolute increase from baseline to week 12 in "memory" but not in "naïve" T cells matched patients with a better survival. The neutrophil/lymphocyte ratio correlated with a significantly better survival at early time points. BRAF status did not correlate with clinical outcome. Fotemustine does not impair the immunologic effect of ipilimumab	PMID: 25538176
	NCT02097732		II	Ipilimumab induction in patients receiving SRS	Active, not recruiting	University of Michigan Rogel Cancer Center, Ann Arbor, MI, USA		DOI: 10.1200/j co.2015.33.15 _suppl .tps9079 *Journal of*

NCT number	Acronym	Phase	Intervention	Status	Location	Description	Citation
NCT02374242	ABC	II	Nivolumab, Ipilimumab	Active, not recruiting	Multicenter (Australia)	Nivolumab (anti-PD-1) combined with ipilimumab and nivolumab monotherapy shows some efficacies in melanoma patients with brain metastases. Patients with asymptomatic brain metastases with no previous local brain therapy were randomized to cohort A (nivolumab plus ipilimumab) or cohort B (nivolumab). Patients with brain metastases in whom local therapy had failed, or who had neurological symptoms, or leptomeningeal disease were enrolled in non-randomized cohort C (nivolumab). At the data cutoff (Aug 28, 2017), with a median follow up of 17 months, intracranial responses were achieved by 46% of patients in cohort A, 20% in cohort B, and 6% in cohort C. Intracranial complete responses occurred in 17% of patients in cohort A, 12% in cohort B, and none in cohort C. No treatment-related deaths occurred	*Clinical Oncology* 33, no. 15_suppl PMID: 29602646
NCT02320058	CheckMate204	II	Ipilimumab, Nivolumab	Active, not recruiting	Multicenter (USA)	Nivolumab combined with ipilimumab shows clinically meaningful intracranial efficacy, concordant with extracranial activity, in melanoma patients who had untreated brain metastases. With a median follow-up of 14.0 months, the rate of intracranial response was 57% (the rate of complete response was 26%, the rate of partial response was 30%), and the rate of stable disease for at least 6 months was 2%. The rate of extracranial clinical response was 56%. Treatment-related grade 3 or 4 adverse events were reported in 55% of patients, including events involving the CNS in 7%. One patient died from immune-related myocarditis. The safety profile of the regimen was similar to that reported in patients with	PMID: 30134131

Table 13.2 (cont.)

Primary disease	Trial number	Name	Phase	Interventions	Status	Locations	Available key findings	Reference
							melanoma who do not have brain metastases	
	NCT02716948		I	Nivolumab, SRS	Recruiting	Johns Hopkins University/ Sidney Kimmel Cancer Center, Baltimore, MD, USA		
	NCT03728465		II	Nivolumab, Ipilimumab	Recruiting	Multicenter (Germany)		
	NCT03175432		II	Atezolizumab, Bevacizumab, Cobimetinib	Recruiting	MD Anderson Cancer Center Houston, TX, USA		DOI: 10.1200/J CO.2018.36.15 _suppl .TPS9598 *Journal of Clinical Oncology* 36, no. 15_suppl
	NCT03563729	MEMBRAINS	II	Pembrolizumab, Ipilimumab, Nivolumab, Encorafenib, Binimetinib, Dabrafenib, Trametinib	Recruiting	Multicenter (Denmark)		
	NCT03340129	ABC-X	II	Ipilimumab, Nivolumab, SRS, Salvage therapy	Recruiting	Multicenter (Australia)		DOI: 10.1200/J CO.2019.37.15 _suppl .TPS9600 *Journal of Clinical Oncology* 37, no. 15_suppl
NSCLC	NCT00871923		II	Erlotinib, WBRT	Completed	MD Anderson Cancer Center Houston, TX, USA	Erlotinib (EGFR inhibitor) in combination with WBRT shows a favorable response rate in NSCLC patients with brain metastases. The overall response rate was 86%. No increase in neurotoxicity was reported. At a median follow-up of 28.5 months, median survival time was 11.8 months.	PMID: 23341526

NCT ID	Trial name	Phase	Status	Intervention	Location	Results	PMID
NCT01801111		I, II	Completed – has results	Alectinib	Multicenter (16 countries)	This pooled analysis (together with NCT01871805) demonstrates that alectinib (ALK inhibitor) has a meaningful efficacy in patients with advanced, ALK+ NSCLC who previously failed treatment with crizotinib (ALK and ROS1 inhibitor). Patients who received alectinib had a median overall survival (OS) of 29.1 months. Median OS for patients with CNS metastases at baseline was 28.5 months compared with 29.9 months in patients without baseline CNS metastases. No new or unexpected safety findings were observed. Of those patients with known EGFR status, median survival time was 9.3 months for those with wild-type EGFR and 19.1 months for those with EGFR mutations	PMID: 31706099
NCT00096265		III	Terminated – has results	Erlotinib, 3D conformal radiation therapy, SRS, Temozolomide	Multicenter (Canada, USA)	The addition of temozolomide or erlotinib to WBRT and SRS in NSCLC patients with 1–3 brain metastases did not improve survival and possibly had a deleterious effect. Of note, this study was terminated early due to accrual limitations	PMID: 23591814
NCT02296125	FLAURA	III	Active, not recruiting – has results	Osimertinib, Erlotinib, Gefitinib	Multicenter (30 countries)	Untreated patients with advanced NSCLC with an EGFR mutation who received Osimertinib (EGFR inhibitor) had longer overall survival (38.6 months) than those who received a comparator EGFR-TKI (erlotinib or gefitinib) (31.8 months). The safety profile for osimertinib was similar to that of the comparator EGFR-TKIs (erlotinib or gefitinib), despite a longer duration of exposure in the osimertinib group	PMID: 31751012
NCT02075840	ALEX	III	Active, not recruiting – has results	Alectinib, Crizotinib	Multicenter (30 countries)	Alectinib shows superior efficacy and lower toxicity in primary treatment of ALK-positive NSCLC when compared with crizotinib. During a median follow-up of 17.6 months (crizotinib) and 18.6 months (alectinib), an event of disease progression or death occurred in 41% in the alectinib group and 68% in the crizotinib group. The rate of 12-	PMID: 28586279

Table 13.2 (cont.)

Primary disease	Trial number	Name	Phase	Interventions	Status	Locations	Available key findings	Reference
							month progression-free survival was significantly higher with alectinib (68.4%) than with crizotinib (48.7%); hazard ratio for disease progression or death, 0.47 ($P < 0.001$). 12% in the alectinib group had an event of CNS progression, as compared with 45% in the crizotinib group. Grade 3 to 5 adverse events were less frequent with alectinib (41%) vs. crizotinib (50%)	
	NCT02737501	ALTA−1 L	III	Brigatinib, Crizotinib	Active, not recruiting	Multicenter (19 countries)	Brigatinib (ALK inhibitor) shows superior efficacy than crizotinib in NSCLC patients with ALK-positive who had not previously received an ALK inhibitor. At the first interim analysis, the median follow-up was 11.0 months in the brigatinib cohort and 9.3 months in the crizotinib cohort. Estimated 12-month progression-free survival, 67% (brigatinib) vs. 43% (crizotinib); hazard ratio for disease progression or death, 0.49 ($P < 0.001$). The confirmed objective response rate and intracranial response rate was 71% and 78% (brigatinib) vs. 60% and 29% (crizotinib), respectively. No new safety concerns were reported	PMID: 30280657
	NCT02978404		II	Nivolumab, SRS	Active, not recruiting	Quebec, Canada		
	NCT02696993		I, II	Ipilimumab, Nivolumab, SRS, WBRT	Recruiting	MD Anderson Cancer Center Houston, TX, USA		
	NCT03325166		II	Pembrolizumab	Recruiting	OHSU Knight Cancer Institute Portland, OR, USA		
Melanoma and NSCLC	NCT02085070		II	Pembrolizumab	Completed	Smilow Cancer Center at Yale New Haven Hospital, CT, USA	Pembrolizumab (anti-PD-1) demonstrates some efficacies in melanoma and NSCLC with brain metastases with an acceptable safety profile. An intracranial response was achieved in 22% of melanoma patients and 33% of NSCLC patients with NSCLC	PMID: 27267608

Cancer type	NCT number	Trial name	Phase	Treatment	Status	Location	Description	PMID
	NCT02858869		I	Pembrolizumab, SRS	Recruiting	Emory University/Winship Cancer Institute, Atlanta, GA, USA		
	NCT02681549		II	Pembrolizumab, Bevacizumab	Recruiting	Smilow Cancer Hospital at Yale New Haven, CT, USA and Moffitt Cancer Center, Tampa, FL, USA		
Breast cancer	NCT00967031	LANDSCAPE	II	Lapatinib, Capecitabine	Completed	Centre Leon Berard, Lyon, France	The combination of lapatinib (dual tyrosine kinase inhibitor which inhibits both the HER2/neu and EGFR pathways) and capecitabine is an option as first-line treatment of brain metastases from HER2-positive breast cancer. With a median follow-up of 21.2 months 65.9% of patients whom are assessable for efficacy in this study had an objective CNS response. 31% patients had at least one severe adverse event; treatment was discontinued due to toxicity in 10%. No deaths were reported as adverse events	PMID: 23122784
	NCT01494662		II	Neratinib, Ado-Trastuzumab Emtansine, Capecitabine	Recruiting	Multicenter (USA)		PMID: 31558424

Abbreviations: ALK, anaplastic lymphoma kinase; CNS, central nervous system; EGFR, epidermal growth factor receptor; ERK, extracellular signal-regulated kinase; MAPK, mitogen-activated protein kinase; NSCLC, non-small cell lung cancer; SRS, stereotactic radiosurgery; WBRT, whole brain radiotherapy.

Figure acknowledgements

The following images are credited to the authors of this chapter: Figures 13.1-13.2

References

Achrol AS, Rennert RC, Anders C, et al. Brain metastases. *Nat Rev Dis Primer* 2019;5:1–26. https://doi.org/10.1038/s41572-018-0055-y.

Andreou KE, Soto MS, Allen D, et al. Anti-inflammatory microglia/macrophages as a potential therapeutic target in brain metastasis. *Front Oncol* 2017;7:251. https://doi.org/10.3389/fonc.2017.00251.

Berghoff AS, Fuchs E, Ricken G, et al. Density of tumor-infiltrating lymphocytes correlates with extent of brain edema and overall survival time in patients with brain metastases. *Oncoimmunology* 2015;5(1):e1057388. https://doi.org/10.1080/2162402X.2015.1057388.

Berghoff AS, Rajky O, Winkler F, et al. Invasion patterns in brain metastases of solid cancers. *Neuro Oncol* 2013;15:1664–72. https://doi.org/10.1093/neuonc/not112.

Berghoff AS, Schur S, Füreder LM, et al. Descriptive statistical analysis of a real life cohort of 2419 patients with brain metastases of solid cancers. *ESMO Open* 2016;1:e000024. https://doi.org/10.1136/esmoopen-2015-000024.

Besse B, Moulec SL, Mazières J, et al. Bevacizumab in patients with nonsquamous non–small cell lung cancer and asymptomatic, untreated brain metastases (BRAIN): a nonrandomized, phase II study. *Clin Cancer Res* 2015;21:1896–903. https://doi.org/10.1158/1078-0432.CCR-14-2082.

Bi P, Kuang S. Notch signaling as a novel regulator of metabolism. *Trends Endocrinol Metab* 2015;26:248–55. https://doi.org/10.1016/j.tem.2015.02.006.

Blazquez R, Wlochowitz D, Wolff A, et al. PI3 K: a master regulator of brain metastasis-promoting macrophages/microglia. *Glia* 2018;66;2438–55. https://doi.org/10.1002/glia.23485.

Bohn KA, Adkins CE, Nounou MI, Lockman PR Inhibition of VEGF and angiopoietin-2 to reduce brain metastases of breast cancer burden. *Front Pharmacol* 2017;8:193. https://doi.org/10.3389/fphar.2017.00193.

Bos PD, Zhang XH-F, Nadal C, et al. Genes that mediate breast cancer metastasis to the brain. *Nature* 2009;459:1005–09. https://doi.org/10.1038/nature08021.

Brastianos PK, Carter SL, Santagata S, et al. Genomic characterization of brain metastases reveals branched evolution and potential therapeutic targets. *Cancer Discov* 2015;5:1164–77. https://doi.org/10.1158/2159-8290.CD-15-0369.

Bucheit AD, Chen G, Siroy A, et al. Complete loss of PTEN protein expression correlates with shorter time to brain metastasis and survival in stage IIIB/C melanoma patients with BRAFV600 mutations. *Clin Cancer Res* 2014;20:5527–36. https://doi.org/10.1158/1078-0432.CCR-14-1027.

Cano A, Pérez-Moreno MA, Rodrigo I, et al. The transcription factor Snail controls epithelial–mesenchymal transitions by repressing E-cadherin expression. *Nat Cell Biol* 2000;2:76–83. https://doi.org/10.1038/35000025.

Chen J, Lee H-J, Wu X, et al. Gain of glucose-independent growth upon metastasis of breast cancer cells to the brain. *Cancer Res* 2015;75:554–65. https://doi.org/10.1158/0008-5472.CAN-14-2268.

Chen L, Douglass J, Kleinberg L, et al. Concurrent immune checkpoint inhibitors and stereotactic radiosurgery for brain metastases in non-small cell lung cancer, melanoma, and renal cell carcinoma. *Int J Radiat Oncol* 2018;100:916–25. https://doi.org/10.1016/j.ijrobp.2017.11.041.

Chen Q, Boire A, Jin X, et al. Carcinoma–astrocyte gap junctions promote brain metastasis by cGAMP transfer. *Nature* 2016;533:493–8. https://doi.org/10.1038/nature18268.

Chongsathidkiet P, Jackson C, Koyama S, et al. Sequestration of T cells in bone marrow in the setting of glioblastoma and other intracranial tumors. *Nat Med* 2018;24:1459–68. https://doi.org/10.1038/s41591-018-0135-2.

Choy C, Ansari KI, Neman J, et al. Cooperation of neurotrophin receptor TrkB and Her2 in breast cancer cells facilitates brain metastases. *Breast Cancer Res* 2017;19:51. https://doi.org/10.1186/s13058-017-0844-3.

Chuang H-N, van Rossum D, Sieger D, et al. Carcinoma cells misuse the host tissue damage response to invade the brain. *Glia* 2013;61:1331–46. https://doi.org/10.1002/glia.22518.

Ciminera AK, Jandial R, Termini J. Metabolic advantages and vulnerabilities in brain metastases. *Clin Exp Metastasis* 2017;34:401–10. https://doi.org/10.1007/s10585-017-9864-8.

Curley CT, Sheybani ND, Bullock TN, Price RJ. Focused ultrasound immunotherapy for central nervous system pathologies: challenges and opportunities. *Theranostics* 2017;7:3608–23. https://doi.org/10.7150/thno.21225.

Davies MA, Liu P, McIntyre S, et al. Prognostic factors for survival in melanoma patients with brain metastases. *Cancer* 2011;117:1687–96. https://doi.org/10.1002/cncr.25634.

Di Giacomo AM, Ascierto PA, Queirolo P, et al. Three-year follow-up of advanced melanoma patients who received ipilimumab plus fotemustine in the Italian Network for Tumor Biotherapy (NIBIT)-M1 phase II study. *Ann Oncol* 2015;26:798–803. https://doi.org/10.1093/annonc/mdu577.

Di Giacomo AM, Valente M, Cerase A, et al. Immunotherapy of brain metastases: breaking a "dogma". *J Exp Clin Cancer Res* 2019;38:419. https://doi.org/10.1186/s13046-019-1426-2.

Dolgodilina E, Imobersteg S, Laczko E, Welt T, Verrey F, Makrides V. Brain interstitial fluid glutamine homeostasis is controlled by blood–brain barrier SLC7A5/LAT1 amino acid transporter. *J Cereb Blood Flow Metab* 2016;36:1929–41. https://doi.org/10.1177/0271678X15609331.

Eckert MA, Lwin TM, Chang AT, et al. Twist1-induced invadopodia formation promotes tumor metastasis. *Cancer Cell* 2011;**19**:372–86. https://doi.org/10.1016/j.ccr.2011.01.036.

Eichler AF, Kahle KT, Wang DL, et al. EGFR mutation status and survival after diagnosis of brain metastasis in nonsmall cell lung cancer. *Neuro Oncol* 2010;**12**:1193–9. https://doi.org/10.1093/neuonc/noq076.

Er EE, Valiente M, Ganesh K, et al. Pericyte-like spreading by disseminated cancer cells activates YAP and MRTF for metastatic colonization. *Nat. Cell Biol* 2018;**20**:966–78. https://doi.org/10.1038/s41556-018-0138-8.

Farber SH, Tsvankin V, Narloch JL, et al. Embracing rejection: immunologic trends in brain metastasis. *Oncoimmunology* 2016;**5**:e1172153. https://doi.org/10.1080/2162402X.2016.1172153.

Fecci PE, Champion CD, Hoj J, et al. The evolving modern management of brain metastasis. *Clin Cancer Res* 2019;**25**:6570–80. https://doi.org/10.1158/1078-0432.CCR-18-1624.

Fong MY, Zhou W, Liu L, et al. Breast-cancer-secreted miR-122 reprograms glucose metabolism in premetastatic niche to promote metastasis. *Nat Cell Biol* 2015;**17**:183–94. https://doi.org/10.1038/ncb3094.

Gaudy-Marqueste C, Dussouil AS, Carron R, et al. Survival of melanoma patients treated with targeted therapy and immunotherapy after systematic upfront control of brain metastases by radiosurgery. *Eur J Cancer* 2017;**84**:44–54. https://doi.org/10.1016/j.ejca.2017.07.017.

Goldberg SB, Gettinger SN, Mahajan A, et al. Pembrolizumab for patients with melanoma or non-small-cell lung cancer and untreated brain metastases: early analysis of a non-randomised, open-label, phase 2 trial. *Lancet Oncol* 2016;**17**:976–83. https://doi.org/10.1016/S1470-2045(16)30053-5.

Gong X, Hou Z, Endsley MP, et al. Interaction of tumor cells and astrocytes promotes breast cancer brain metastases through TGF-β2/ANGPTL4 axes. *npj Precis Oncol* 2019;**3**:1–9. https://doi.org/10.1038/s41698-019-0094-1.

Gregory PA, Bracken CP, Smith E, et al. An autocrine TGF-β/ZEB/miR-200 signaling network regulates establishment and maintenance of epithelial–mesenchymal transition. *Mol Biol Cell* 2011;**22**:1686–98. https://doi.org/10.1091/mbc.e11-02-0103.

Grimaldi AM, Simeone E, Giannarelli D, et al. Abscopal effects of radiotherapy on advanced melanoma patients who progressed after ipilimumab immunotherapy. *OncoImmunology* 2014;**3**:e28780. https://doi.org/10.4161/onci.28780.

Hanna N, Fidler IJ. Role of natural killer cells in the destruction of circulating tumor emboli. *J Natl Cancer Inst* 1980;**65**:801–09. https://doi.org/10.1093/jnci/65.4.801.

Harter PN, Bernatz S, Scholz A, et al. Distribution and prognostic relevance of tumor-infiltrating lymphocytes (TILs) and PD-1/PD-L1 immune checkpoints in human brain metastases. *Oncotarget* 2015;**6**:40836–49.

Herwig N, Belter B, Pietzsch J. Extracellular S100A4 affects endothelial cell integrity and stimulates transmigration of A375 melanoma cells. *Biochem Biophys Res Commun* 2016;**477**:963–9. https://doi.org/10.1016/j.bbrc.2016.07.009.

Hohensee I, Lamszus K, Riethdorf S, et al. Frequent genetic alterations in EGFR- and HER2-driven pathways in breast cancer brain metastases. *Am J Pathol* 2013;**183**:83–95. https://doi.org/10.1016/j.ajpath.2013.03.023.

Hoj JP, Mayro B, Pendergast AM. A TAZ-AXL-ABL2 feed-forward signaling axis promotes lung adenocarcinoma brain metastasis. *Cell Rep* 2019;**29**:3421–34. https://doi.org/10.1016/j.celrep.2019.11.018.

Hong JJ, Rosenberg SA, Dudley ME, et al. Successful treatment of melanoma brain metastases with adoptive cell therapy. *Clin Cancer Res* 2010;**16**:4892–8. https://doi.org/10.1158/1078-0432.CCR-10-1507.

Hoshino A, Costa-Silva B, Shen T-L, et al. Tumour exosome integrins determine organotropic metastasis. *Nature* 2015;**527**:329–35. https://doi.org/10.1038/nature15756.

Ilhan-Mutlu A, Osswald M, Liao Y, et al. Bevacizumab prevents brain metastases formation in lung adenocarcinoma. *Mol Cancer Ther* 2016;**15**:702–10. https://doi.org/10.1158/1535-7163.MCT-15-0582.

Jackson S, Anders NM, Mangraviti A, et al. The effect of regadenoson-induced transient disruption of the blood–brain barrier on temozolomide delivery to normal rat brain. *J Neurooncol* 2016;**126**:433–9. https://doi.org/10.1007/s11060-015-1998-4.

Jandial R, Choy C, Levy DM, Chen MY, Ansari KI. Astrocyte-induced Reelin expression drives proliferation of Her2+ breast cancer metastases. *Clin Exp Metastasis* 2017;**34**:185–96. https://doi.org/10.1007/s10585-017-9839-9.

Jolly MK, Somarelli JA, Sheth M, et al. Hybrid epithelial/mesenchymal phenotypes promote metastasis and therapy resistance across carcinomas. *Pharmacol Ther* 2019;**194**:161–84. https://doi.org/10.1016/j.pharmthera.2018.09.007.

Jung YY, Kim HM, Koo JS. Expression of lipid metabolism-related proteins in metastatic breast cancer. *PLoS One* 2015;**10**:e0137204. https://doi.org/10.1371/journal.pone.0137204.

Kalluri R, Weinberg RA. The basics of epithelial–mesenchymal transition. *J Clin Invest* 2009;**119**:1420–8. https://doi.org/10.1172/JCI39104.

Kienast Y, von Baumgarten L, Fuhrmann M, et al. Real-time imaging reveals the single steps of brain metastasis formation. *Nat Med* 2010;**16**:116–22. https://doi.org/10.1038/nm.2072.

Kim AH, Tatter S, Rao G, et al. Laser ablation of abnormal neurological tissue using robotic neuroblate system (LAANTERN): 12-month outcomes and quality of life after brain tumor ablation. *Neurosurgery* 2020;**87**:E338–46. https://doi.org/10.1093/neuros/nyaa071.

Kim S-J, Kim J-S, Park ES, et al. Astrocytes upregulate survival genes in tumor cells and induce protection from chemotherapy. *Neoplasia* 2011;**13**:286–98. https://doi.org/10.1593/neo.11112.

Kim SW, Choi HJ, Lee H-J, et al. Role of the endothelin axis in astrocyte- and endothelial cell-mediated chemoprotection of cancer cells. *Neuro Oncol* 2014;**16**:1585–98. https://doi.org/10.1093/neuonc/nou128.

Klein A, Schwartz H, Sagi-Assif O, et al. Astrocytes facilitate melanoma brain metastasis via secretion of IL-23. *J Pathol* 2015;**236**:116–27. https://doi.org/10.1002/path.4509.

Kudo Y, Haymaker C, Zhang J, et al. Suppressed immune microenvironment and repertoire in brain metastases from patients with resected non-small-cell lung cancer. *Ann Oncol* 2019;**30**:1521–30. https://doi.org/10.1093/annonc/mdz207.

Labelle M, Begum S, Hynes RO. Direct signaling between platelets and cancer cells induces an epithelial-mesenchymal-like transition and promotes metastasis. *Cancer Cell* 2011;**20**:576–90. https://doi.org/10.1016/j.ccr.2011.09.009.

Lambert AW, Pattabiraman DR, Weinberg RA. Emerging biological principles of metastasis. *Cell* 2017;**168**:670–91. https://doi.org/10.1016/j.cell.2016.11.037.

Lee B-C, Lee T-H, Avraham S, Avraham HK. Involvement of the chemokine receptor CXCR4 and its ligand stromal cell-derived factor 1alpha in breast cancer cell migration through human brain microvascular endothelial cells. *Mol Cancer Res* 2004;**2**:327–38.

Lee JY, Park K, Lee E, et al. Gene expression profiling of breast cancer brain metastasis. *Sci Rep* 2016;**6**:28623. https://doi.org/10.1038/srep28623.

Lee JY, Park K, Lim SH, et al. Mutational profiling of brain metastasis from breast cancer: matched pair analysis of targeted sequencing between brain metastasis and primary breast cancer. *Oncotarget* 2015;**6**:43731–42. https://doi.org/10.18632/oncotarget.6192

Lee T-H, Avraham HK, Jiang S, Avraham S. Vascular endothelial growth factor modulates the transendothelial migration of MDA-MB-231 breast cancer cells through regulation of brain microvascular endothelial cell permeability. *J Biol Chem* 2003;**278**:5277–84. https://doi.org/10.1074/jbc.M210063200.

Leong HS, Robertson AE, Stoletov K, et al. Invadopodia are required for cancer cell extravasation and are a therapeutic target for metastasis. *Cell Rep* 2014;**8**:1558–70. https://doi.org/10.1016/j.celrep.2014.07.050.

Leuthardt EC, Duan C, Kim MJ, et al. Hyperthermic laser ablation of recurrent glioblastoma leads to temporary disruption of the peritumoral blood brain barrier. *PLoS One* 2016;**11**:e0148613. https://doi.org/10.1371/journal.pone.0148613.

Li B, Wang C, Zhang Y, et al. Elevated PLGF contributes to small-cell lung cancer brain metastasis. *Oncogene* 2013;**32**:2952–62. https://doi.org/10.1038/onc.2012.313.

Li B, Zhao W-D, Tan Z-M, Fang W-G, Zhu L, Chen Y-H. Involvement of Rho/ROCK signalling in small cell lung cancer migration through human brain microvascular endothelial cells. *FEBS Lett* 2006;**580**:4252–60. https://doi.org/10.1016/j.febslet.2006.06.056.

Liberti MV, Locasale JW. The Warburg effect: how does it benefit cancer cells? *Trends Biochem Sci* 2016;**41**:211–8. https://doi.org/10.1016/j.tibs.2015.12.001.

Lin X, Lu T, Xie Z, et al. Extracranial abscopal effect induced by combining immunotherapy with brain radiotherapy in a patient with lung adenocarcinoma: a case report and literature review. *Thorac Cancer* 2019;**10**:1272–5. https://doi.org/10.1111/1759-7714.13048.

Liu H, Kato Y, Erzinger SA, et al. The role of MMP-1 in breast cancer growth and metastasis to the brain in a xenograft model. *BMC Cancer* 2012;**12**:583. https://doi.org/10.1186/1471-2407-12-583.

Liu H-L, Hua M-Y, Chen P-Y, et al. Blood–brain barrier disruption with focused ultrasound enhances delivery of chemotherapeutic drugs for glioblastoma treatment. *Radiology* 2010;**255**:415–25. https://doi.org/10.1148/radiol.10090699.

Liu Y, Cao X. Characteristics and significance of the pre-metastatic niche. *Cancer Cell* 2016;**30**:668–81. https://doi.org/10.1016/j.ccell.2016.09.011.

Liu Y, Kosaka A, Ikeura M, et al. Premetastatic soil and prevention of breast cancer brain metastasis. *Neuro Oncol* 2013;**15**:891–903. https://doi.org/10.1093/neuonc/not031.

Long GV, Atkinson V, Lo S, et al. Combination nivolumab and ipilimumab or nivolumab alone in melanoma brain metastases: a multicentre randomised phase 2 study. *Lancet Oncol* 2018;**19**:672–81. https://doi.org/10.1016/S1470-2045(18)30139-6.

Lorger M, Felding-Habermann B. Capturing changes in the brain microenvironment during initial steps of breast cancer brain metastasis. *Am J Pathol* 2010;**176**:2958–71. https://doi.org/10.2353/ajpath.2010.090838.

Lorger M, Krueger JS, O'Neal M, Staflin K, Felding-Habermann B. Activation of tumor cell integrin alphavbeta3 controls angiogenesis and metastatic growth in the brain,. *PNAS* 2009;**106**:10666–71. https://doi.org/10.1073/pnas.0903035106.

Louveau A, Plog BA, Antila S, Alitalo K, Nedergaard M, Kipnis J. Understanding the functions and relationships of the glymphatic system and meningeal lymphatics. *J Clin Invest* 2017;**127**:3210–9. https://doi.org/10.1172/JCI90603.

Lowery FJ, Yu D. Brain metastasis: unique challenges and open opportunities. *Biochim Biophys Acta* 2017;**1867**:49–57. https://doi.org/10.1016/j.bbcan.2016.12.001.

Mani SA, Guo W, Liao M-J, et al. The epithelial–mesenchymal transition generates cells with properties of stem cells. *Cell* 2008;**133**:704–15. https://doi.org/10.1016/j.cell.2008.03.027.

Margolin K, Ernstoff MS, Hamid O, et al. Ipilimumab in patients with melanoma and brain metastases: an open-label, phase 2 trial. *Lancet Oncol* 2012;**13**:459–65. https://doi.org/10.1016/S1470-2045(12)70090-6.

Mashimo T, Pichumani K, Vemireddy V, et al. Acetate is a bioenergetic substrate for human glioblastoma and brain metastases. *Cell* 2014;**159**:1603–14. https://doi.org/10.1016/j.cell.2014.11.025.

McFarland BC, Benveniste EN. Reactive astrocytes foster brain metastases via STAT3 signaling. *Ann Transl Med* 2019;**7**. https://doi.org/10.21037/atm.2019.04.17.

Menter DG, Hatfield JS, Harkins C, et al. Tumor cell-platelet interactions in vitro and their relationship to in vivo arrest of hematogenously circulating tumor cells. *Clin Exp Metastasis* 1987;**5**:65–78. https://doi.org/10.1007/BF00116627.

Morad G, Carman CV, Hagedorn EJ, et al. Tumor-derived extracellular vesicles breach the intact blood–brain barrier via transcytosis. *ACS Nano* 2019;**13**:13853–65. https://doi.org/10.1021/acsnano.9b04397.

Moravan MJ, Fecci PE, Anders CK, et al. Current multidisciplinary management of brain metastases. *Cancer* 2020;**126**:1390–406. https://doi.org/10.1002/cncr.32714.

Nakamura T, Saito R, Sugiyama S, Sonoda Y, Kumabe T, Tominaga T. Local convection-enhanced delivery of chemotherapeutic agent transiently opens blood–brain barrier and improves efficacy of systemic chemotherapy in intracranial xenograft tumor model. *Cancer Lett* 2011;**310**:77–83. https://doi.org/10.1016/j.canlet.2011.06.018.

Nam D-H, Jeon H-M, Kim S, et al. Activation of notch signaling in a xenograft model of brain metastasis. *Clin Cancer Res* 2008;**14**:4059–66. https://doi.org/10.1158/1078-0432.CCR-07-4039.

Neman J, Termini J, Wilczynski S, et al. Human breast cancer metastases to the brain display GABAergic properties in the neural niche. *PNAS* 2014;**111**:984–9. https://doi.org/10.1073/pnas.1322098111.

Ostrom QT, Gittleman H, Truitt G, Boscia A, Kruchko C, Barnholtz-Sloan JS. CBTRUS statistical report: primary brain and other central nervous system tumors diagnosed in the United States in 2011–2015. *Neuro-Oncol* 2018;**20**:iv1–iv86. https://doi.org/10.1093/neuonc/noy131.

Palumbo JS, Talmage KE, Massari JV, et al. Platelets and fibrin(ogen) increase metastatic potential by impeding natural killer cell–mediated elimination of tumor cells. *Blood* 2005;**105**:178–85. https://doi.org/10.1182/blood-2004-06-2272.

Pastushenko I, Brisebarre A, Sifrim A, et al. Identification of the tumour transition states occurring during EMT. *Nature* 2018;**556**:463–8. https://doi.org/10.1038/s41586-018-0040-3.

Pestalozzi BC, Zahrieh D, Price KN, et al. Identifying breast cancer patients at risk for central nervous system (CNS) metastases in trials of the International Breast Cancer Study Group (IBCSG). *Ann Oncol* 2006;**17**:935–44. https://doi.org/10.1093/annonc/mdl064.

Pfannenstiel LW, McNeilly C, Xiang C, et al. Combination PD-1 blockade and irradiation of brain metastasis induces an effective abscopal effect in melanoma. *OncoImmunology* 2019;**8**: e1507669. https://doi.org/10.1080/2162402X.2018.1507669.

Priego N, Zhu L, Monteiro C, et al. STAT3 labels a subpopulation of reactive astrocytes required for brain metastasis. *Nat Med* 2018;**24**:1024–35. https://doi.org/10.1038/s41591-018-0044-4.

Pukrop T, Dehghani F, Chuang H-N, et al. Microglia promote colonization of brain tissue by breast cancer cells in a Wnt-dependent way. *Glia* 2010;**58**:1477–89. https://doi.org/10.1002/glia.21022.

Qin D, Ou G, Mo H, et al. Improved efficacy of chemotherapy for glioblastoma by radiation-induced opening of blood–brain barrier: clinical results. *Int J Radiat Oncol* 2001;**51**:959–62. https://doi.org/10.1016/S0360-3016(01)01735-7.

Qin Y, Capaldo C, Gumbiner BM, Macara IG. The mammalian Scribble polarity protein regulates epithelial cell adhesion and migration through E-cadherin. *J Cell Biol* 2005;**171**:1061–71. https://doi.org/10.1083/jcb.200506094.

Regmi S, Fu A, Luo KQ. High shear stresses under exercise condition destroy circulating tumor cells in a microfluidic system. *Sci Rep* 2017;**7**:39975. https://doi.org/10.1038/srep39975.

Rizvi NA, Mazières J, Planchard D, et al. Activity and safety of nivolumab, an anti-PD-1 immune checkpoint inhibitor, for patients with advanced, refractory squamous non-small-cell lung cancer (CheckMate 063): a phase 2, single-arm trial. *Lancet Oncol* 2015;**16**:257–65. https://doi.org/10.1016/S1470-2045(15)70054-9.

Rodrigues G, Hoshino A, Kenific CM, et al. Tumour exosomal CEMIP protein promotes cancer cell colonization in brain metastasis. *Nat Cell Biol* 2019;**21**:1403–12. https://doi.org/10.1038/s41556-019-0404-4.

Rolland Y, Demeule M, Fenart L, Béliveau R. Inhibition of melanoma brain metastasis by targeting melanotransferrin at the cell surface. *Pigment Cell Melanoma Res* 2009;**22**:86–98. https://doi.org/10.1111/j.1755-148X.2008.00525.x.

Salehi A, Paturu MR, Patel B, et al. Therapeutic enhancement of blood–brain and blood–tumor barriers permeability by laser interstitial thermal therapy. *Neurooncol Adv* 2020;**2**: vdaa071. https://doi.org/10.1093/noajnl/vdaa071.

Sampson JH, Gunn MD, Fecci PE, Ashley DM. Brain immunology and immunotherapy in brain tumours. *Nat Rev Cancer* 2020;**20**:12–25. https://doi.org/10.1038/s41568-019-0224-7.

Sartorius CA, Hanna CT, Gril B, et al. Estrogen promotes the brain metastatic colonization of triple negative breast cancer cells via an astrocyte-mediated paracrine mechanism. *Oncogene* 2016;**35**:2881–92. https://doi.org/10.1038/onc.2015.353.

Seike T, Fujita K, Yamakawa Y, et al. Interaction between lung cancer cells and astrocytes via specific inflammatory cytokines in the microenvironment of brain metastasis. *Clin Exp Metastasis* 2011;**28**:13–25. https://doi.org/10.1007/s10585-010-9354-8.

Sevenich L, Bowman RL, Mason SD, et al. Analysis of tumour- and stroma-supplied proteolytic networks reveals a brain-metastasis-promoting role for cathepsin S. *Nat Cell Biol* 2014;**16**:876–88. https://doi.org/10.1038/ncb3011.

Sharma M, Balasubramanian S, Silva D, Barnett GH, Mohammadi AM. Laser interstitial thermal therapy in the management of brain metastasis and radiation necrosis after radiosurgery: an overview. *Expert Rev Neurother* 2016;**16**:223–32. https://doi.org/10.1586/14737175.2016.1135736.

Silver IA, Erecińska M. Extracellular glucose concentration in mammalian brain: continuous monitoring of changes during increased neuronal activity and upon limitation in oxygen supply in normo-, hypo-, and hyperglycemic animals. *J Neurosci* 1994;**14**:5068–76. https://doi.org/10.1523/JNEUROSCI.14-08-05068.1994.

Sjøbakk TE, Johansen R, Bathen TF, et al. Metabolic profiling of human brain metastases using in vivo proton MR spectroscopy at 3 T. *BMC Cancer* 2007;**7**:141. https://doi.org/10.1186/1471-2407-7-141.

Sjøbakk TE, Vettukattil R, Gulati M, et al. Metabolic profiles of brain metastases. *Int J Mol Sci* 2013;**14**:2104–18. https://doi.org/10.3390/ijms14012104.

Soto MS, Serres S, Anthony DC, Sibson NR. Functional role of endothelial adhesion molecules in the early stages of brain metastasis. *Neuro Oncol* 2014;**16**:540–51. https://doi.org/10.1093/neuonc/not222.

Sperringer JE, Addington A, Hutson SM. Branched-chain amino acids and brain metabolism. *Neurochem Res* 2017;**42**:1697–709. https://doi.org/10.1007/s11064-017-2261-5.

Tabatabaei SN, Girouard H, Carret A-S, Martel S. Remote control of the permeability of the blood–brain barrier by magnetic heating of nanoparticles: a proof of concept for brain drug delivery. *J Control Release* 2015;**206**:49–57. https://doi.org/10.1016/j.jconrel.2015.02.027.

Tawbi HA, Forsyth PA, Algazi A, et al. Combined Nivolumab and Ipilimumab in melanoma metastatic to the brain. *N Engl J Med* 2018;**379**:722–30. https://doi.org/10.1056/NEJMoa1805453.

Théry C, Zitvogel L, Amigorena S. Exosomes: composition, biogenesis and function. *Nat Rev Immunol* 2002;**2**:569–79. https://doi.org/10.1038/nri855.

Tiwary S, Morales JE, Kwiatkowski SC, Lang FF, Rao G, McCarty JH. Metastatic brain tumors disrupt the blood–brain barrier and alter lipid metabolism by inhibiting expression of the endothelial cell fatty acid transporter Mfsd2a. *Sci Rep* 2018;**8**:8267. https://doi.org/10.1038/s41598-018-26636-6.

Tominaga N, Kosaka N, Ono M, et al. Brain metastatic cancer cells release microRNA-181c-containing extracellular vesicles capable of destructing blood–brain barrier. *Nat Commun* 2015;**6**:6716. https://doi.org/10.1038/ncomms7716.

Tyran M, Carbuccia N, Garnier S, et al. A comparison of DNA mutation and copy number profiles of primary breast cancers and paired brain metastases for identifying clinically relevant genetic alterations in brain metastases. *Cancers* 2019;**11**:665. https://doi.org/10.3390/cancers11050665.

Valiente M, Obenauf AC, Jin X, et al. Serpins promote cancer cell survival and vascular co-option in brain metastasis. *Cell* 2014;**156**:1002–16. https://doi.org/10.1016/j.cell.2014.01.040.

van Vulpen M, Kal HB, Taphoorn MJB, El Sharouni SY. Changes in blood–brain barrier permeability induced by radiotherapy: implications for timing of chemotherapy? *Oncol Rep* 2002;**9**:683–8. https://doi.org/10.3892/or.9.4.683.

Wagner S, Czub S, Greif M, et al. Microglial/macrophage expression of interleukin 10 in human glioblastomas. *Int J Cancer* 1999;**82**:12–6. https://doi.org/10.1002/(sici)1097-0215(19990702)82:1<12::aid-ijc3>3.0.co;2-o.

Wang H, Ou Q, Li D, et al. Genes associated with increased brain metastasis risk in non–small cell lung cancer: comprehensive genomic profiling of 61 resected brain metastases versus primary non–small cell lung cancer (Guangdong Association Study of Thoracic Oncology 1036). *Cancer* 2019;**125**:3535–44. https://doi.org/10.1002/cncr.32372.

Warburg O. The metabolism of carcinoma cells. *J Cancer Res* 1925;**9**:148–63. https://doi.org/10.1158/jcr.1925.148.

Wu YJ, Muldoon LL, Gahramanov S, Kraemer DF, Marshall DJ, Neuwelt EA. Targeting αV-integrins decreased metastasis and increased survival in a nude rat breast cancer brain metastasis model. *J Neurooncol* 2012;**110**:27–36. https://doi.org/10.1007/s11060-012-0942-0.

Xing F, Kobayashi A, Okuda H, et al. Reactive astrocytes promote the metastatic growth of breast cancer stem-like cells by activating Notch signalling in brain. *EMBO Mol Med* 2013;**5**:384–96. https://doi.org/10.1002/emmm.201201623.

Xing F, Liu Y, Sharma S, et al. Activation of the c-Met pathway mobilizes an inflammatory network in the brain microenvironment to promote brain metastasis of breast cancer. *Cancer Res* 2016;**76**:4970–80. https://doi.org/10.1158/0008-5472.CAN-15-3541.

Xing F, Liu Y, Wu S-Y, et al. Loss of XIST in breast cancer activates MSN-c-Met and reprograms microglia via exosomal microRNA to promote brain metastasis. *Cancer Res* 2018;**78**:4316–30. https://doi.org/10.1158/0008-5472.CAN-18-1102.

Yang J, Mani SA, Donaher JL, et al. Twist, a master regulator of morphogenesis, plays an essential role in tumor metastasis. *Cell* 2004;**117**:927–39. https://doi.org/10.1016/j.cell.2004.06.006.

Yang X, Di J, Zhang Y, et al. The Rho-kinase inhibitor inhibits proliferation and metastasis of small cell lung cancer. *Biomed Pharmacother* 2012;**66**:221–7. https://doi.org/10.1016/j.biopha.2011.11.011.

Yano S, Shinohara H, Herbst RS, et al. Expression of vascular endothelial growth factor is necessary but not sufficient for production and growth of brain metastasis. *Cancer Res* 2000;**60**:4959–67.

Yao H, Price TT, Cantelli G, et al. Leukaemia hijacks a neural mechanism to invade the central nervous system. *Nature* 2018;**560**:55–60. https://doi.org/10.1038/s41586-018-0342-5.

Yu M, Bardia A, Wittner BS, et al. Circulating breast tumor cells exhibit dynamic changes in epithelial and mesenchymal composition. *Science* 2013;**339**:580–4. https://doi.org/10.1126/science.1228522.

Yuan H, Gaber MW, Boyd K, Wilson CM, Kiani MF, Merchant TE. Effects of fractionated radiation on the brain vasculature in a murine model: blood–brain barrier permeability, astrocyte proliferation, and ultrastructural changes. *Int J Radiat Oncol Biol Phys* 2006;**66**:860–6. https://doi.org/10.1016/j.ijrobp.2006.06.043.

Zhang L, Zhang S, Yao J, et al. Microenvironment-induced PTEN loss by exosomal microRNA primes brain metastasis outgrowth. *Nature* 2015;**527**:100–04. https://doi.org/10.1038/nature15376.

14 Benign Adult Brain Tumors and Pediatric Brain Tumors

Shun Yao, Umar Raza, and Farhana Akter

14.1 Introduction

Brain tumors in adults and children range from devastating malignant tumors with a dire prognosis to benign tumors that can be totally resected with a favorable outcome. The incidence rate for primary brain tumors in adults in the United States is approximately 23.8 per 100,000 persons. Of those, approximately two thirds of tumors are benign or borderline in nature (Ostrom et al., 2020). In this chapter we discuss the most common benign brain tumors in adults followed by a discussion on pediatric brain tumors (benign and malignant).

14.2 Meningioma

Meningiomas are the most frequently occurring primary intracranial neoplasm in adults, however are rare in children.

Accounting for 38.3% of all central nervous system (CNS) tumors, meningioma has the highest number of all estimated new CNS tumor cases within the United States (Osteom et al., 2020). The majority of meningiomas (80.6%) are found in the cerebral meninges, and the remainder are found in the spinal, orbital, intraventricular, epidural, and rarely extradural regions (Ostrom et al., 2020; Bi et al., 2016a). Currently, known risk factors include race (higher incidence in black vs. caucasian), age (over 65 years), gender (females vs. males, 2.3:1), and exposure to ionizing radiation(Ostrom et al., 2020). Patients with World Health Organization (WHO) Grade 1 meningiomas usually have a 10-year overall survival of 80–90% and progression-free survival (PFS) of 75–90% (Bi et al., 2016a). Ten-year relative survival for Grade 2 (also known as atypical) meningiomas ranges from 53% to 79% and PFS of 23–78%. WHO Grade 3 anaplastic meningiomas are associated with a poor prognosis and a 10-year overall survival rate of 14–34% and (Bi et al, 2016a).

In 2021, the WHO updated the classification and grading system for brain tumors, categorizing meningio- mas as a single tumor type with 15 distinct subtypes. WHO Grade 1 (Figure 14.1) meningiomas, comprising of nine subtypes, include the meningothelial, fibroblastic, and transitional subtype (Louis et al., 2021, Torp et al., 2021). The diagnosis of WHO Grade 2 and 3 meningiomas are based on several essential histopathological characteristics, including the mitotic activity (count of four or more per 10 high-powered fields), the presence of brain invasion, and/or at least three of the following morphological features: sheeting (loss of whorling or fascicular architecture), macronuclei, small cells with a high nucleus -cytoplasm ratio, high cellularity, and spontaneous necrosis (Louis et al., 2021).

Additional insights regarding prognosis can also be obtained from the location of the tumor. Meningiomas tend to differ in histology and mutational signatures according to the location in which they are found and this can provide valuable information regarding prognosis (Figure 14.2).

14.3 Molecular Landscape

Recent advances in genetic sequencing have enabled us to better understand the molecular drivers of meningioma, and therefore provide an opportunity to incorporate the molecular features of the tumor during diagnosis and classification.

14.3.1 Chromosomal Alterations

In 1967, Zang and Singer performed the first cytogenetic study to uncover the chromosomal aberrations underlying meningiomas, providing an unprecedented insight into the genetic drivers of meningiomas. They found a G-group chromosome (either chromosome 21 or 22) to be missing in all eight tumor samples of their study (Zang and Singer, 1967). Later studies established accumulative evidence that approximately two thirds of sporadic meningiomas present somatic copy number alterations (CNAs) in the chromosome 22 monosomy which carries the neurofibromatosis type 2 (*NF2*) gene

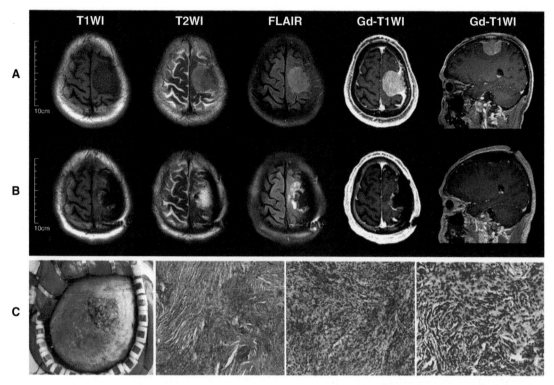

Figure 14.1 The illustration of a patient who achieved Simpson grade I resection and was diagnosed with a transitional meningioma (WHO Grade 1). Preoperative (A) and postoperative (B) magnetic resonance (MR) images include T_1-weighted image (T1WI), T2WI, fluid-attenuated inversion recovery (FLAIR), and gadolinium-enhanced (Gd)-T1WI. T1W1 is isointense gray and Gd-T1W1 shows intense and homogeneous enhancement with a dual tail. T2 and FLAIR is hyperintense gray. Edema is seen around the resected region in T2W1 and FLAIR images. (C) Meningioma invasion to the skull (left image). Histological images show spindle shaped tumor cells in a storiform pattern with a round nucleus, There are no signs of mitosis or tumor necrosis. Immunobiological stainings are positive for epithelial membrane antigen (+), somatostatin receptor2 (+), progesterone receptor (+), SOX10 (-), S-100 (+), CD34 (-), STAT-6 (-), and Ki 67.

(Bi et al., 2016b; Seizinger et al., 1987). Loss of heterozygosity on chromosome 1p is the second most common chromosomal abnormality in meningiomas and is observed as the most frequent cytogenetic abnormality in higher-grade tumors, such as anaplastic meningiomas (Cai et al., 2001). Studies show that loss of 1p is associated with tumor progression and poor outcomes (Cai et al., 2001). A recent 16-year follow-up case study also confirmed the loss of 1p as a reliable biomarker of meningioma progression (Hemmer et al., 2020). Along with 1p, alterations of chromosome 14 are also thought to be an important marker in meningioma progression and have been found in two thirds of WHO Grade 2 and all WHO Grade 3 meningiomas (Chukwueke and Wen, 2020). Loss of chromosomes 4p, 6q, 7p, 9p, 10q, 11p, 18q and gains in 17q and 20q have also been identified in meningiomas however at a low frequency (Chukwueke and Wen, 2020). The increased accumulation of these genomic alterations, including somatic CNAs,

rearrangements, and mutational burden, usually indicates a higher grade and aggressiveness of histopathological classification in meningiomas (Lee et al., 2010; Suppiah et al., 2019).

14.3.1.1 Neurofibromatosis Type 2 Mutation

The *NF2* gene is the first and most well-described oncogenic mutation in meningiomas, in which approximately 60% of patients will develop sporadic meningiomas in their lifetime (Bi et al., 2016). The *NF2* gene is a tumor suppressor gene, which contains 17 exons and is located on chromosome 22q12.2, encoding the protein Merlin (schwannoma) that serves as a membrane–cytoskeleton linker and prevents the process of cellular proliferation (James et al., 2009). Merlin has been identified as a negative moderator of a downstream target of mammalian target of rapamycin (mTOR) singling complex 1 but a positive moderator of mTOR singling complex 2 in *NF2*-deficient meningioma cells, resulting in tumor cell

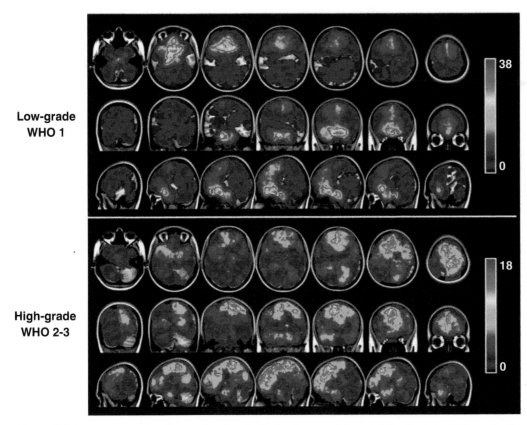

Figure 14.2 Frequency mapping of tumor location distribution in a population of 478 patients by WHO grade. The value of the color bar in the heatmaps represents the number of subjects that have the same tumor location in that brain area. The frequency map of WHO I meningiomas (*n* = 306, 63.3%) shows the preferred location in the middle and anterior cranial fossa. Tumors within the convexities of the central sulcus and sylvian fissure were typically of a higher grade.

proliferation and migration (James et al., 2009). Additionally, the loss of the *NF2* gene leads to a low level of Merlin product that subsequently causes a high-level expression of focal adhesion kinase (FAK), as a result of tumor cell growth and motility (Shapiro et al., 2014). An FAK inhibitor has been under investigation in meningiomas with *NF2* loss in a clinical trial (NCT02523014).

As an important early driver in the development of meningiomas, *NF2* mutation may be detected in both low-grade (~43%) and high-grade (~80%) meningiomas (Suppiah et al., 2019). Interestingly, a recent large cohort study investigating 3016 meningiomas revealed that *NF2* meningiomas are more frequently found in cerebral convexities and posterior skull base locations while non-*NF2* meningiomas are typically found within the anterior skull base structure (Youngblood et al., 2019).

14.3.1.2 Non-Neurofibromatosis Type 2 Mutations

Although substantial evidence has shown the significant role of *NF2* in the development of meningiomas, *NF2* mutations are only observed in half of all meningiomas (Suppiah et al., 2019). With the advances of next-generation sequencing technologies, additional gene mutations have been observed and investigated for therapeutic potential, including the pro-apoptotic E3 ubiquitin ligase tumor necrosis factor receptor-associated factor 7 (*TRAF7*), the pluripotency transcription factor Kruppel-like factor 4 (*KLF4*), the protooncogene v-Akt murine thymoma viral oncogene homolog 1 (*AKT1*), the Hedgehog pathway signaling member smoothened (*SMO*), telomerase reverse transcriptase (*TERT*), and cyclin-dependent kinase inhibitor 2A/B (*CDKN2A/B*). These non-NF2 mutated meningiomas are primarily non-malignant with intact chromosomes (Clark et al., 2013).

TRAF7, located on chromosome 16p13, is mutated in 12–25% of meningiomas and usually has a concomitant mutation with *AKT1* or *KLF4* (specifically K409Q; Clark et al., 2013). *KLF4* mutation is commonly located on chromosome 9q and is a critical regulator of cellular proliferation, resulting in the rapid growth of meningiomas (Clark et al., 2013). *TRAF7* and *KLF4* mutations are mutually exclusive with *NF2* mutation or chromosome 22 loss. *TRAF7/ KLF4* frequently occurs in the secretory variant of meningiomas and therefore is regarded as an important molecular biomarker for the histopathological diagnosis of secretory meningiomas (Clark et al., 2013; Reuss et al., 2013). *AKT1* mutation has been identified in approximately 10% of sporadic meningiomas and is known as a neoplasia-related recurrent mutation (Clark et al., 2013). All three above-mentioned mutations are almost exclusively identified in WHO Grade 1 meningiomas and more frequently located in anterior and midline skull base origins (Clark et al., 2013).

Smoothened (SMO) is a protein-coupled receptor and is a part of the Hedgehog signaling pathway. *SMO* mutation has been identified in 3–6% of non-*NF2* mutant meningiomas and involves the development of meningiomas via activating the Hedgehog signaling in meningiomas (Clark et al., 2013). *SMO*-mutant meningiomas are exclusively found in WHO Grade 1 meningiomas and more frequently originate from the anterior midline skull base. Additionally, the *SMO* mutations have been one of the few targetable genetic alterations for therapeutic potential in meningiomas, and several clinical trials with mTOR inhibitors have been under investigation, including Vismodegib (NCT02523014), Everolimus (NCT01880749), and AZD2014 (Vistusertib) (NCT03071874 and NCT02831257).

The loss of *CDKN2A/B* gene on chromosome 9p21, frequently found in grade 3 meningiomas are associated with a significantly shorter time to progression of the disease. Meningiomas with mutations in *TERT* promoter also show increased aggressiveness and reduced patient survival.

14.4 Preclinical Animal Models

In- vivo tumor models are invaluable in dissecting the mechanisms underlying tumorigenesis. These include xenografts, genetically engineered mice and chemically induced meninigioma models.

14.4.1 Xenograft Models

Patient-derived xenografts (PDX) can be engrafted heterotopically or orthotopically to induce meningiomas in animal models. The earliest successful attempt of PDX for meningiomas was reported in 1945 when Greene and Arnold injected human meningioma cells in the immune-privileged eyes of guinea pigs (Greene and Arnold, 1945) . The first heterotrophic mouse PDX model of meningiomas was reported in the 1970s when resected patient tumors were engrafted into flank of immunocompromised mice (Abedalthagafi et al., 2016). Both ortho- and heterotopic xenograft models using either PDX or established cell lines, such as Ben-Men-1 and IOMM-Lee, have greatly helped us in understanding the meningioma biology and in devising treatment strategies (Suppiah et al., 2019). Recent molecular characterization of xenografted tumors has revealed that PDX models of meningioma retain genetic, chromosomal, and histological features of parental tumors (Rath et al., 2011); however, lack of availability/accessibility of patient tumors and substantial heterogeneity between patients limit their use. In addition, the success rate of fresh engrafts is poor and PDX models often exhibit ventricular and leptomeningeal invasions, which are rare in human patients (McCutcheon et al., 2000). In order to overcome these obstacles, one strategy may be to use cryopreserved meningioma cells from human tumors, which results in tumor development with gene expression profiles comparable to the original tumor cells (Zhang et al., 2020).

14.4.2 Genetically Engineered Mouse Models

Genetically engineered mouse models (GEMMs) offer several advantages over xenograft models including intact immune systems and also the availability of tumor-stomal interactions in the microenvironment (Suppiah et al., 2019). Given the frequency of *NF2* inactivation in human meningioma, GEMMs for meningioma typically involve heterozygous germline deletion of *NF2*. Patients with these deletions develop neurofibromatosis type 2, a syndrome that is associated with growth of various tumors including multiple meningiomas(Choudhury and Raleigh, 2020). In mice, however, this leads to the formation of osteosarcomas instead of meningiomas (Petrilli and Fernández-Valle, 2016). To circumvent this problem, *NF2FL/FL* mice which contains genetic sequences (loxP) flanking the *NF2* gene have been created. The Cre recombination technique allows the injection of the adenovirus Cre recombinase into the cerebrospinal fluid (CSF). All loxP sites in cells that express Cre, which in *NF2FL/FL*, means the *NF2* gene, will be deleted. This leads to the formation of meningioma like tumors (McClatchey et al., 1998). Introducing heterozygous p53 mutation or Cre-mediated loss of *CDKN2AB* in *NF2FL/FL* mice can also result in high-grade meningiomas (Kalamarides et al., 2002). However, these double knockout mice also develop non-meningioma tumor-like sarcomas. Genetically engineered mouse models with *NF2* inactivation targeted to prostaglandin D2 synthase (*PDGF*) expressing arachnoid cells in meninges have been used successfully to create tumors (Peyre et al., 2015). Concurrent overexpression of platelet-derived growth factor (*PDGF*) in these mouse models results in more growth compared to *NF2* inactivation alone, but also the development of gliomas due to non-meningioma specific effects of genetic alterations (Peyre et al., 2015).

14.4.3 Chemically Induced Mouse Models

Chemical carcinogenesis through the use of e.g. Ethyl-nitrosourea (ENU) has been remarkably faithful in revealing underlying mechanisms of tumorigenesis (Russell et al., 1979). Their use has declined over the years with the development of alternative models. Mice heterozygous for p16 and p19 are susceptible to ENU- induced mutagenesis and can develop meningiomas (Morrison et al., 2007). However, the genetic landscape of these tumors is not well characterized, and therefore combining chemical carcinogens with GEMMs may be an invaluable approach to study the complex interaction between genotype and the environmental exposures that contributes to tumor development.

14.5 Pituitary Tumors

The pituitary gland is known as the "master gland" due to its important endocrine role of regulating vital hormone secretion (Figure 14.3). Pituitary tumors are frequently encountered intracranial neoplasms and are usually of the benign adenoma type. Prolactinomas and nonfunctioning adenomas are the most common types of pituitary adenomas. Histologically, this tumors are characterized by a granular cytoplasm and numerous round nuclei (Figure 14.4).

14.6 Animal models of pituitary tumors

Various animal models have been used to understand the biology of pituitary adenomas (PAs). These include xenograft and GEMMs.

14.6.1 Xenograft Models

The lack of commercially available cell lines derived from human PAs severely limits the feasibility of producing human cell line–based xenografts. To date, commercial murine cell lines such as AtT-20, GH3, and GH4-C1 as well as non-commercial human cell lines have been employed in-vitro and in-vivo studies. These xenograft models have greatly assisted in characterizing the function of various pathways, genes, and mutations in a variety of PAs. For instance, oncogenic fibroblast growth factor receptor 4 (*FFFR4*) expression (Ezzat et al., 2006; Jalali et al., 2016), overexpression of leucine Rich Repeats And Immunoglobulin Like Domains 1 (*LRIG1*) (Cheng et al., 2016), maternally Expressed 3 (*MEG3*) (Chunharojrith et al., 2015), inactivating mutations in pituitary transcription factor 1 (*PIT-1*) (Roche et al., 2012), tumor suppressive roles of miRNAs such as miR-524-5p (Zhen et al., 2017), persistent activation of the mitogen-activated protein kinase signal transduction pathway (MAPK) (Booth et al., 2014), and pituitary transforming gene (*PTTG*) protein stabilization (Fuertes et al., 2018) have been identified as key molecular mechanisms behind PAs. Murine cell line–based xenografts have also been extensively used to investigate the sensitivity of PAs toward existing chemo- and targeted therapies as well as against radiotherapy (Zhao et al., 2015), which has critically aided in identifying the anti-tumor roles for bafilomycin A1(McSheehy et al., 2003), bromocriptine and/or cabergoline (Lin et al., 2017), lanreotide (Ning et al., 2009), liquiritigenin (Wang et al., 2014), metformin (An et al., 2017), histone deacetylase inhibitor SAHA (Lu et al., 2017), thiazolidinediones (Mannelli et al., 2010), and Triptolide (Li et al., 2017) against PAs.

14.6.2 Genetically Engineered Mouse Models

Human familial disorder–associated tumor suppressor genes, have been modulated to develop animal models of PAs. Recent studies have shown that manipulation of *CDKN2B* and retinoblastoma (*RB*) genes, which have not been found associated with pituitary tumorigenesis in humans, also develop PAs in animal models (Gahete et al., 2019). Familial isolated pituitary adenoma (FIPA) patients harbor aryl hydrocarbon receptor interacting protein (AIP) mutations and predominantly develop growth hormone (GH)-secreting adenomas. In line with this, *AIP* +/– mice recapitulate the clinical scenario well and, despite their normal development, are predominantly prone to GH-secreting PAs. In addition, complete loss of *AIP* lesions, higher proliferation rates, and quicker penetrance

Posterior pituitary hormones

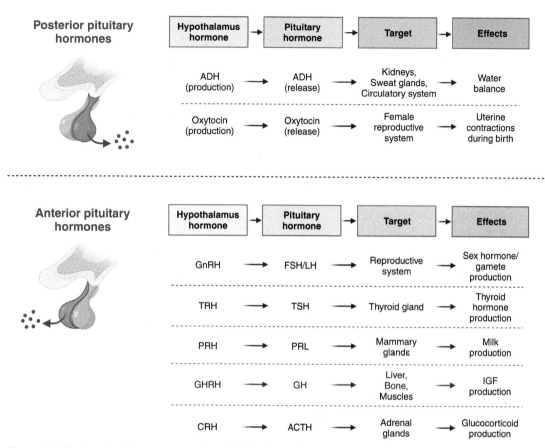

Hypothalamus hormone	Pituitary hormone	Target	Effects
ADH (production)	ADH (release)	Kidneys, Sweat glands, Circulatory system	Water balance
Oxytocin (production)	Oxytocin (release)	Female reproductive system	Uterine contractions during birth

Anterior pituitary hormones

Hypothalamus hormone	Pituitary hormone	Target	Effects
GnRH	FSH/LH	Reproductive system	Sex hormone/ gamete production
TRH	TSH	Thyroid gland	Thyroid hormone production
PRH	PRL	Mammary glands	Milk production
GHRH	GH	Liver, Bone, Muscles	IGF production
CRH	ACTH	Adrenal glands	Glucocorticoid production

Figure 14.3 Pituitary gland hormones and effects. ADH; Antidiuretic hormone, GnRH; Gonadotropin hormone-releasing hormone, FSH; Follicle-stimulating hormone, LH; Luteinizing hormone, TRH; Thyrotropin releasing hormone, TSH; thyroid stimulating hormone, PRH; Prolactin-releasing hormone, PRL; Prolactin, GHRH; Growth hormone-releasing hormone, GH; Growth hormone CRH; IGF; Insulin like growth factor; Corticotrophin-releasing hormone, ACTH; Adrenocorticotropic hormone

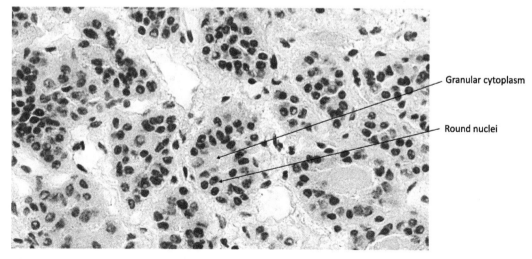

Granular cytoplasm

Round nuclei

Figure 14.4 Histological specimen of a pituitary adenoma.

of *AIP*-deficient tumors suggest close association between *AIP* loss and tumor aggressiveness in PAs. Of note, *AIP* knockout mice exhibit acromegaly like phenotype (Vierimaa et al., 2006). An *AIP*-deficient model has also aided in elucidating the molecular mechanisms underlying PAs as reduction in protein levels of aryl hydrocarbon receptor nuclear translocator 1 or 2 (ARNT or ARNT2) has been observed in these tumors which, in turn, have been shown to fluctuate the expression of key genes involved in tumorigenesis (Raitila et al., 2010). Like *AIP*, the *CDKN2C* knockout mice also develops acromegaly. However, *CDKN2C+/−* mice predominately develop somatotropinomas, exhibiting gigantism along with extensive organomegaly of the pituitary gland, spleen, and thymus (Franklin et al., 1998). *CDKN1B+/−* and *PRKAR1A+/−* models also develop other endocrine tumors such as adrenal tumors and follicular thyroid adenomas (Kiyokawa et al., 1996; Nakayama et al., 1996; Yin et al., 2008). Similarly, *MEN1*-knockout models develop PAs along with endocrine and neuroendocrine tumors (Bertolino et al., 2003; Biondi et al., 2004; Crabtree et al., 2003; Yin et al., 2008). *CDKN2B* knockout mouse models have revealed a tumor suppressor role for encoded protein, p19, in pituitary anterior lobe proliferation and these mice develop various tumors such as prolactinomas, GH and follicle-stimulating hormone (FSH) secreting adenomas (Bai et al., 2014). Germline heterozygous mutation in the Rb gene is associated with early/childhood retinoblastoma in humans, but mice harboring the same mutations develop pituitary carcinomas and can serve as in-vivo models for PAs (Jacks et al., 1992; Vooijs et al., 1998). *RB*-knockout based double-mutant models have also been developed in a quest to understand the interaction of *RB* with other PA-associated genes and to characterize the role of these combinations on tumorigenesis in the pituitary gland (Chesnokova et al., 2005; Guidi et al., 2006; Harvey et al., 1995; Loffler et al., 2007; Tsai et al., 2002). For instance, loss of ADP-ribosylation factor (*ARF*) deletion in *RB*-deficient mice ($RB^{+/−}/ARF^{+/−}$) accelerates pituitary gland tumorigenesis (Tsai et al., 2002). Mice heterozygous for both *RB* and Tp53 (tumor protein 53) developed endocrine tumors including pituitary tumors as well as lymphomas and sarcomas. In addition, tumor incidence was faster in these double-mutant mice compared to single-mutant ones (Harvey et al., 1995). In line with this, other double mutants ($CDK4^{R/R}/CDKN1B$; $CCNE1/P27^{−/−}$; $P18^{−/−}/P27^{−/−}$; $P18^{−/−}/ASU^{−/−}$; $INK4C/ARF$ and $MEN1^{+/−}/CDKN2^{−/−}$) involving cell-cycle regulators have also been shown to develop pituitary tumors, which aided in investigating

cyclin-dependent kinase (CDK) inhibitors (CKIs) as therapeutic options against pituitary adenomas (Franklin et al., 1998; Lloyd et al., 2002; Roussel-Gervais et al., 2010; Sotillo et al., 2005; Zindy et al., 2003).

Different animal models of PA have also been developed using gene knockin approach. For instance, growth hormone releasing hormone (*GHRH*) knockin model secretes excessive growth hormones and develops PA (Asa et al., 1992). A knockin model with corticotropin-releasing hormone (*CRH*) gene insertion develops Cushing's syndrome. *CRH*-transgenic animals, in particular, show endocrine abnormalities involving the hypothalamic–pituitary–adrenal axis, such as elevated plasma levels of adrenocorticotropic hormone (ACTH) and glucocorticoids, as well as physical changes associated with Cushing's syndrome, e.g., excessive fat accumulation, muscle atrophy, thin skin, and alopecia. These findings suggest that persistent corticotrophin-releasing hormone (CRF) production causes continuous stimulation of pituitary corticotrope cells, leading to high ACTH expression and subsequent glucocorticoid overproduction, thus resulting in Cushing's syndrome (Stenzel-Poore et al., 1992). Injection of mice harboring a *CRH* promoter mutation with *ENU* has shown to induce Cushing's disease, an approach which can serve as a chemical-induced in-vivo model for PA (Bentley et al., 2014). Overexpressing pituitary tumor-promoting genes such *PTTG* and the high-mobility group AT-hook (*HMGA*) has been shown to modulate the primary regulators of pituitary gland function. *PTTG* is a securing protein that plays a role in cell transformation, aneuploidy, apoptosis, and tumor microenvironment communication (Vlotides et al., 2007). It was initially discovered in rat pituitary tumor cells (Pei and Melmed, 1997), and later demonstrated to be overexpressed in human pituitary tumors as well (Sáez et al., 1999). Mice with pituitary gland-specific *PTTG* overexpression under the influence of pituitary specific alpha subunit glycoprotein promoter developed focal pituitary hyperplasia (Donangelo et al., 2006). On the other hand, pituitary gland-specific *PTTG* inactivation resulted in pituitary hypoplasia (Abbud et al., 2005) and knocking out *PTTG* in mice with heterozygous *Rb* background limits tumor growth (Chesnokova et al., 2005), confirming that *PTTG* plays a tumorigenic role in pituitary glands. In addition, mice with ubiquitous overexpression of *HMGA1* or *HMGA2* develop PAs characterized as mixed prolactinomas and somatotropinomas (Fedele et al., 2002, 2005). Of note, *HMGA2* promotes E2F Transcription Factor 1 (E2f1) transcriptional activity by interacting with RB, which in turn aids in the progression and development of PAs (Fedele et al., 2006).

In addition to mice gene knockin/knockout models, viral particle (oncovirus) induced GEMMs have also been established for PAs. The simian virus 40 (SV40) T antigen (SV40-Tag) has been shown to develop somatotropinomas when expressed under the control of bovine arginine vasopressin (AVP) promoter (Stefaneanu et al., 1992). On the other hand, mice with an SV40-Tag transgene under the control of the proopiomelanocortin promoter (POMC) have been shown to develop melanotroph tumors (Low et al., 1993). Similarly, a model of non-functioning adenomas has been established using SV40-Tag under the control of the Follicle Stimulating Hormone Subunit Beta (FSHB) promoter (Kumar et al., 1998). Finally, Cushing's disease has also been mimicked in animals by overexpressing the polyoma large T antigen under the control of polyoma early region promoter (Helseth et al., 1992).

14.7 Vestibular Schwannoma

Vestibular schwannomas (VS) are benign tumors (WHO grade 1) that typically arise from the distal neurilemmal portion of the inferior division of the vestibular nerve at or close to the neurilemmal–neuroglial junction. They represent approximately 90% of tumors arising in the cerebellopontine angle (CPA) and account for 8% all intracranial tumors. These tumors present with symptoms of tinnitus and hearing loss. However large tumors represent a threat to intracranial structures and can lead to the development of hydrocephalus, brainstem compression, herniation, and ultimately death. Although mostly benign, there is a small risk of malignant transformation (Chang and Welling, 2009).

The Koos grading is a classification system for VS designed to stratify tumors based on extrameatal extension and compression of the brainstem. Grade I represents small intracanalicular tumors; grade II are small tumors protruding to the CPA cistern; grade III tumors occupy the cerebellopontine cistern but do not displace the brainstem; grade IV tumors are large and displace the brainstem and cranial nerves.

Histologically, VS are well-circumscribed encapsulated masses, characterized by positive immunostaining for the S-100 protein with two distinct patterns of cellular architecture, these are known as Antoni regions. Antoni A regions refer to tightly organized fibrillary elongated tissue adjacent to loose microcytic tissue (Antoni B regions). Antoni A regions contain stacked nuclei known as palisades and elongated nuclei known as Verocay bodies (Figure 14.5).

Vestibular schwannomas can arise sporadically (95% cases) and are usually unilateral in nature or in the context of a familial syndrome such as neurofibromatosis type 2, an autosomal dominant disease representing 5% of all VSs, which is classically associated with bilateral tumors.

The *NF2* gene encodes for a tumor suppressor protein, which is located on chromosome 22q12.2. Mutations in the *NF2* gene causatively result in neurofibromatosis type 2, but are also found in unilateral sporadic schwannoma patients. There are over 200 mutations of *NF2* that have been identified; these include deletions, substitutions, insertions, and missense mutations. Sporadic VS differs from VS associated with *NF2* in that the mutational hit of the former involves somatic bi-allelic merlin gene inactivation, whereas in *NF2*-associated VS, one of the germline merlin alleles is already inactivated and therefore development of VS requires only an additional mutation or loss of the other allele. Loss of heterozygosity is also a frequent feature of sporadic VS.

Central to the pathogenesis of VS is loss of function of merlin, a product of the *NF2* gene, which belongs to the ERM (ezrin–radixin–moesin) family and is a putative tumor suppressor protein. Merlin interacts with many cellular proteins such as receptor tyrosine kinases and internalizes them, silencing their proliferation and thereby inducing contact-dependent growth inhibition.

Loss of merlin in the cytoplasm activates signal transduction of small G proteins Rac1 and Ras. Rac1 is a member of the Rho GTPase family and regulates signaling pathways such as MAPK and PI3K-Akt. Loss of merlin in the nucleus activates the E3 ubiquitin ligase CRL4DCAF1, which promotes oncogenesis by inhibiting the Hippo pathway.

Other molecular characteristics of VS include deregulation genes such as leucine zipper like post translational regulator 1 (*LZTR1*), SWI/SNF related, matrix associated, actin dependent regulator of chromatin, subfamily b, member 1 (*SMARCB1*), and Coenzyme Q6, Monooxygenase (*COQ6*). Among genes that are upregulated in VS are mediators of angiogenesis such as endoglin and osteonectin. Downregulated genes include tumor-suppressor genes such as RNA-binding motif protein 5 (*LUCA-15/RBM5*). A number of growth factors have also been implicated in VS progression and these include vascular endothelial growth factors (VEGFs), where increased expression may be correlated with rate of tumor growth (Chang and Welling, 2009; de Vries et al., 2015).

Animal models of VS include GEMMs such as Schwann cell *NF2* conditional knockouts. However they do not always develop intracranial schwannomas. This limitation can be overcome by crossing conditional *NF2* mutant mice with transgenic PostnCre mice in which the periostin promoter drives the expression of the Cre recombinase in the Schwann cell lineage.

Orthotopic transplantation models include the sciatic nerve model, the intracranial model and the hearing loss model. Mice models are limited by the small size of vestibular nerves and encasement in the internal auditory canal and therefore implantation can be technically challenging. The sciatic nerve model is a large nerve and therefore implantation is easier, however this does not reflect the symptoms induced by VS such as hearing loss. Similarly the intracranial model involves superficial injection through cranial windows and cannot simulate the neurological dysfunction seen in humans. Tumor cells injected into the auditory -vestibular nerve complex in mice via the internal auditory canal or into the cochleo-vestibular nerve of rats have been shown to induce hearing loss, however real-time imaging cannot be performed.

14.8 Pediatric Brain Tumors

Primary tumors of the CNS are one of the most common malignancies found in children and are associated with significant mortality and morbidity. Pediatric brain tumors are categorized into cell type/location. Gliomas are the most common brain tumors found in all age groups (Table 14.1).

14.9 Gliomas

Pediatric diffuse gliomas can be categorized according to their severity (diffuse low grade (LGG), high grade (HGG), circumscribed), location, or cellular architecture (Table 14.2).

Although pediatric gliomas are histologically indistinguishable from the adult type, there are a number of molecular differences. Two notable differences are the low prevalence of isocytrate dehydrogenase (*IDH*) mutations in LGGs and higher prevalence of histone gene mutations. The most common gene amplifications seen in the pediatric type are those of receptor tyrosine kinases including platelet-derived growth factor receptor A (*PDGFRA*), Epidermal Growth Factor Receptor (*EGFR*), KIT proto-oncogene (*KIT*), insulin like growth factor1 receptor (*IGF1R*), and MET Proto-Oncogene (*MET*). *PDGFRA* amplification is found more commonly in children, whereas *EGFR* is more commonly amplified in adults. *PDGFRA* amplification is found more commonly in children than adults, whereas *EGFR* is more commonly amplified in adults (Fangusaro, 2012).

Low-grade glionas include pilocytic astrocytoma (PA), subependymal giant cell astrocytoma (SEGA), pilomyxoid astrocytoma (PMA), pleomorphic xanthoastrocytoma

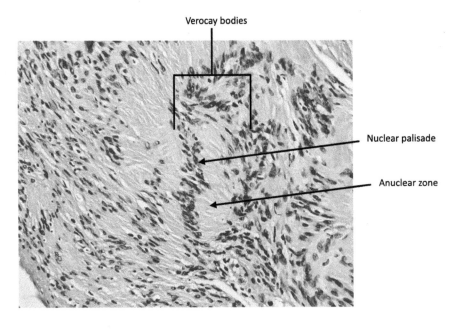

Figure 14.5 Verocay bodies are a component of "Antoni A," which are the dense areas of schwannomas located between palisading spindle cells in schwannomas. Distinct loose microcystic tissue adjacent to the Antoni A regions are known as Antoni B.

Verocay bodies

Nuclear palisade

Anuclear zone

(PXA,) and low-grade fibrillary astrocytoma or diffuse astrocytoma. Pilocytic astrocytoma is the most common type of glioma in children and accounts for approximately 20% of all pediatric brain tumors. They are characterized histologically by tightly packed cells surrounded by astrocytes. There may be numerous cytoplasmic extensions, Rosenthal fibers, eosinophilic granular bodies, and mitotic bodies. The most common genetic alteration in PA is aberration of the MAPK signaling pathway. One common mutation is the formation of fusion proteins such as those between *BRAF* (v-Raf murine sarcoma viral oncogene homolog B) protein and the protein KIAA1549, resulting in loss of BRAF regulation and activation of the MAPK kinase pathway, or that of BRAFV600E, where valine is substituted for glutamic acid leading to BRAF activation, resulting in high levels of the MYB transcription factor, *HIST1H3B* mutations, and gene deletions of *CDKN2A*, *TP53*, and *ADAM3*. Pilocytic astrocytomas are also seen in patients with neurofibromatosis; here, inactivation of the RAS-GTPase activating protein neurofibromin leads to constitutive activation of RAS resulting in tumors of the optic pathway. Other diseases associated with LGGs include tuberous sclerosis, which is often seen in patients with SEGA. These patients usually have mutations of *TSC1* (encoding the Hamartin protein) or the *TSC2* gene (encoding Tuberin protein), which are negative regulators of mTOR and cell growth. Inactivation of these genes leads to increased mTOR activity, enabling cell growth and proliferation (Fangusaro, 2012; Plant-Fox et al., 2021).

High-grade gliomas account for approximately 8–12% of primary CNS tumors in children. Both grade 2 tumors (anaplastic astrocytoma) and grade 4 tumors (glioblastoma) are categorized as HGG. In adults, they are much more common and often arise from malignant transformation of low-grade tumors. As with adults, HGGs are very aggressive and are associated with significant morbidity and mortality. They are histologically characterized by atypical nuclei, high mitotic activity, hypercellularity, microvascular proliferation, and pseudopalisading necrosis (Fangusaro, 2012; Plant-Fox et al., 2021).

In adults the most common genetic abnormality in HGG is *EGFR* amplification. In children, mutations in the p53 pathway are much more common. Other molecular aberrations in pediatric HGG include that of VEGF PDGFRA Abnormalities that are more commonly seen in adults but less so in children include mutations of the *RB* gene and the Phosphatase and tensin homolog (*PTEN*); amplifications of *MYC* Proto-oncogene (*MYC*), cell division protein kinase 6 (CDK6) and cyclin D2 (CCND2), and deletion of *CDKN2C*. Chromosomal

abnormalities in pediatric HGG include gains at 1p, 2q, and 21q as well as losses noted at 6q, 4q, 11q, and 16q. Approximately 10% of pediatric HGGs also have a V600E point mutation in *BRAF*. Molecular aberrations in the PI3 kinase (PI3K/mTOR) pathway are seen in both HGG and LGG (Fangusaro, 2012; Plant-Fox et al., 2021).

14.9.1 Diffuse Intrinsic Pontine Glioma

Although brainstem tumors are rare in adults, they are much more common in children. Diffuse intrinsic pontine glioma is the most common type of brainstem tumor in children. It has a dismal prognosis, with a 5-year survival rate of less than 1%. The cells of origin involved in DIPG are thought to be stem cell–like cells found in the subventricular zone and this hypothesis is supported by postmortem studies, magnetic resonance imaging (MRI) morphometric imaging, and histological analysis. Diffuse intrinsic pontine gliomas are usually classified as fibrillary astrocytomas on histopathological analysis (Johung and Monje, 2017).

The most common mutations include point mutations in *H3F3A* (encoding histone 3.3) and *HIST1H3B* (encoding histone 3.1) genes, leading to the substitution of a lysine by a methionine at position 27 (K27M). There is evidence of impaired function of polycomb repressive complex 2 (*PRC2*) methyltransferase leading to reduction in trimethylation of *H3K27*. There may be residual *PRC2* activity in DIPG cells and therefore this may be an additional therapeutic target to consider. *H3F3A* mutations confer a worse prognosis than *HIST1H3B* mutations. Mutations in *TP53* are commonly found in DIPGs, as are amplifications of the tyrosine kinase/Ras/phosphatidylinositol-3 pathway (Aziz-Bose and Monje, 2019; Johung and Monje, 2017).

Diffuse intrinsic pontine gliomas may also be classified into three molecular subgroups: MYCN, Silent, and H3K27M. The MYCN subgroup is high grade, with evidence of DNA hypermethylation and chromothripsis. The Silent subgroup has a lower genetic mutation burden. The H3K27M subgroup, is the most prevalent in DIPG, and is characterized by histone mutation, global DNA hypomethylation and multiple concurrent mutations (*TP53*, *PAX3*, *PGFRA*, *EGFR*, ATP-dependent helicase (*ATRX*), *NF1*, Protein Phosphatase, Mg2+/Mn2+ Dependent 1D (*PPM1D*), *PIK3CA*, *TERT*, neurotrophic tyrosine receptor kinase (*NTRK*), IL-13RA2, poly(ADP-ribose) polymerase 1 (*PARP*1), *PTEN*, Cyclin D1 (*CCND1/2/3*), cyclin dependent kinase (*CDK4/6*), and *MET* (Aziz-Bose and Monje, 2019; Johung and Monje, 2017).

Table 14.1 Pediatric brain tumors

Cell type	Name of tumor	Description
Glial cells	Glioma	Umbrella term to describe all glial tumors
Glial cells: astrocytes	Circumscribed astrocytic gliomas	Examples Grade 1 Pilocytic astrocytoma Pilomyxoid astrocytoma Grade 2/3 Pleomorphic xanthoastrocytomas (PXAs)
	Pediatric-type diffuse low-grade gliomas	- Diffuse astrocytoma, MYB- or MYBL1-altered - Angiocentric glioma - Polymorphous low-grade neuroepithelial tumor of the young - Diffuse low-grade glioma, MAPK pathway-altered
	Pediatric-type diffuse high-grade gliomas	- Diffuse midline glioma, H3 K27-altered - Diffuse hemispheric glioma, H3 G34-mutant
		- Diffuse Pediatric-type high-grade glioma, H3-wildtype and IDH-wildtype - Infant-type hemispheric glioma
Glial cells: oligodendrocytes	Oligodendroglioma	Most are grade 2 tumors Grade 2 tumors: Slow growing, can invade and become aggressive Grade 3: Very aggressive Anaplastic oligodendrogliomas
Ependymal cells	Ependymoma	Location: ventricles (spinal cord in adults) Can become anaplastic
Embryonal		Up to 20% of brain tumors in children are of this type More common in young children Rare in adults
Embryonal: neuroectodermal	Medulloblastoma	Location: cerebellum More common in children than adults
	Primitive neuroectodermal tumors (PNETs)	
Embryonal: teratoid/rhabdoid cells	Atypical teratoid rhabdoid tumor (ATRT)	Location: cerebellum/brainstem (50%) Rare Fast growing
Embryonal: germ cells	Germ cell tumors	Types: Germinomas: Most common type Choriocarcinomas Embryonal carcinomas Teratomas Yolk sac tumors
Mixed neuronal and glial cells	Gangliogliomas	Slow growing (grade 1)
Mixed	Dysembryoplastic neuroepithelial tumors (DNETs)	Slow growing (grade 2)
	Gangliogliomas	They are typically slow growing (grade 1) tumors
Schwann cells	Vestibular schwannoma	Rare in children. Vestibular schwannomas, more commonly known as acoustic neuromas, are benign brain tumors that develop on the balance (vestibular) and hearing or auditory nerves leading from the inner ear to the brain
Lymphocytes	Lymphomas	Rare in children Most lymphomas start in other parts of the body. Rarely found as primary tumors of the brain

Table 14.1 (cont.)

Cell type	Name of tumor	Description
Brainstem gliomas		Up to 20% of brain tumors in children are gliomas of the brainstem.
	Focal brainstem gliomas	Have distinct edges Less common
	Diffuse midline gliomas	Diffuse throughout brain stem When they start in the pons they care called diffuse intrinsic pontine gliomas (DIPGs)
Suprasellar/sellar	Craniopharyngioma	Rare Two types: Adamantinomatous (more common in children) Papillary (more common in adults)
Pituitary	Pituitary tumor	More common in young adolescents than young children Benign
Pineal gland	Pineal tumor	Difficult to treat Most common type: pineoblastoma
Ventricles	Choroid plexus tumors	Choroid plexus papillomas (benign) Choroid plexus carcinoma (malignant)
	Central neurocytomas	Benign
Meninges (arachnoid)	Meningioma	Rare in children Mostly benign Grade 1: Cells look mostly normal Grade 2: Atypical Grade 3: Anaplastic
Spinal cord	Ependymomas	5% of brain tumors in children are of this type Line ventricles or central canal of the spinal cord
	Chordoma	Location: Base of the skull or at the lower end of the spine. Can cause compression of spinal cord More common in adults than in children
Outside CNS	Neuroblastoma	Develop in nerve cells in abdomen/chest Most common in infants
Brain metastases		Less common than primary tumors in children

Diffuse intrinsic pontine gliomas can disseminate and invade nearby brainstem structures and extend to the leptomeninges, the supratentorial region, and to the subventricular zone. This is one of the significant barriers to optimal DIPG management, as surgery in these eloquent areas is very difficult.

14.10 Embryonal Tumors

Embryonal tumors are rare but highly malignant tumors with a propensity for dissemination.

14.10.1 Medulloblastoma

Medulloblastomas (MBs) are tumors found in the posterior fossa, usually the cerebellar vermis with potential for spread into the leptomeninges and the fourth ventricle. They are the most common primitive embryonal tumors of the CNS. Medulloblastomas can be histologically categorized into five subtypes: classic, desmoplastic, MB with extensive nodularity (MBEN), anaplastic, and large cell. In the updated 2021 WHO classification, these are classified into a a single tumor type: medulloblastoma, histologically defined. Genetic classification takes into the molecular background of the tumor and includes the Wingless (WNT) and Sonic Hedgehog (SHH) subgroups, and two groups with less well-defined molecular alterations, Group 3 (G3) and Group 4 (G4), which are also known as medulloblastoma, non-WNT/non-SHH(and De Braganca, 2016; Northcott et al., 2019).

Classic MBs are the most common type of MBs and are characterized by small cells with round nuclei and the presence of Homer Wright rosettes. The desmoplastic subgroup is characterized by nodules of neurocytic differentiations surrounded by primitive internodular regions. These

Table 14.2 Categorization of glioma according to cellular architecture

Histology	Low-grade glioma	Grade 1 – pilocytic astrocytoma
		Grade 2 – fibrillary astrocytoma
	High-grade glioma	Grade 3 – anaplastic astrocytoma
		Grade 4 – glioblastoma astrocytoma
Location/growth pattern		
Diffuse, pons	Diffuse intrinsic pontine gliomas	
Blood vessels	Angiocentric glioma	Rare, grade 1 LGG, elongated spindle-shaped bipolar cells, form pseudorosettes. Typically presents with seizures
Diffuse, multiple lobes	Gliomatosis cerebri	
Cell type		
Astrocytes	Pilocytic astrocytoma	
Astrocytes	Fibrillary astrocytoma	
Astrocytes	Anaplastic astrocytoma	
Astrocytes	Pleomorphic xanthoastrocytoma	Rare, benign, LGG Location: cerebral hemisphere, leptomeninges, rarely spinal cord
Ependymal cells	Ependymoma	Location: ventricles
Glial and sarcomatous cells	Gliosarcoma	
Glial and neuronal cells	Dysembryoplastic neuroepithelial tumor (DNET)	Location: cerebrum Low grade
	Ganglioglioma	Location: temporal lobe, sometimes cerebellum, spinal cord, brainstem
Oligodendrocytes	Oligodendroglioma	LGG Location: frontal lobe Spontaneous or associated with NF1/tuberous sclerosis
Optic nerve	Optic nerve gliomas	Slow growing Associated with NF1
Tectum	Tectal glioma	LGG
Thalamic/hypothalamic	Thalamic astrocytoma and hypothalamic astrocytoma	

tumors tend to have pericellular collagen deposition surrounding the nodules. Medulloblastoma with extensive nodularity is characterized by extensive areas of differentiated elements. The anaplastic group is characterized by cytologic pleomorphism, frequent mitiotic activity, and increased cell size. The large-cell subgroup has large cells with prominent nucleoli. The large-cell and anaplastic variant have been grouped together in the most recent WHO classification as they frequently coexist Torp et al., 2021

The WNT subgroup is associated with a prognosis and survival rates of approximately 90%. They are usually seen in older children and comprise approximately 15% of adults MB. These tumors usually have classic morphology. Common mutations found in the WNT subgroup occur in *CTNNB1* encoding β-catenin and loss of chromosome 6. Other mutations include that of adenomatous polyposis coli (APC), TP53, Transcription activator BRG1 (SMARCA4), Histone-lysine N-methyltransferase 2D (*KMT2D*), and DEAD-Box Helicase 3 X-Linked (*DDX3X*) (Millard and De Braganca, 2016; Northcott et al., 2019).

The SHH subgroup occurs more frequently in infants and young adolescents over the age of 16 and is also the most common molecular group in adults. The most common histological morphologies seen in SHH MB are the DN variants followed by classic and large-cell–anaplastic group. This subgroup is commonly associated with mutations in the SHH pathway genes including Patched1 (*PTCH1*) receptor, (*SMO*) activity, and suppressor of fused homolog (*SUFU*) and *SMO*. Amplifications of downstream mediators of this pathway such as GLI Family Zinc Finger 2 (*GLI2*) are also seen. SHH tumors with coexisting *TP53* abnormalities are associated with a very poor prognosis and are characterized by amplification of oncogenes including *MYC*, *MYCN*, and *GLI2* (Millard and De Braganca, 2016).

Group 3 are associated with the worst prognosis and patients often have metastatic disease. They are usually found in children and very rarely in adults. Mutations include loss of chromosome 17p, gain of 17q, identified recurrent translocations of *PVT1*, and high levels of *MYC* amplification and OTX2 amplification. Group 4 is typically present in older children. Mutations include loss of chromosome 17p, gain of 17q, identified recurrent translocations of plasmacytoma Variant Translocation (*PVT1*), and high levels of *MYC* amplification and orthodenticle homeobox 2 (*OTX2*) amplification. Group 4 is typically present in older children. Mutations include loss of chromosome 17p and gain of 17q. Other mutations include amplification of *MYCN*, *MLL2*, and *MLL3* and Lysine Demethylase 6A (*KDM6A*), and the presence of a tandem duplication of the Parkinson's gene synuclein alpha (*SNCA*)(Millard and De Braganca, 2016; Northcott et al., 2019).

14.11 Ependymoma

Ependymomas are tumors originating from epithelioid glial cells found lining the ventricles and the central canal within the spinal cord. They are the third most common malignant brain cancer in children and are typically found in the posterior fossa. In adults, they are rare and are typically intraspinal. Therefore, while these tumors arising from different regions are histologically similar, their clinical course often varies. They are often classified by genetic aberrations as follows: Posterior fossa (PF-EPN-SE (subependymoma), PF-EPN-B (group B), PF-EPN-A (group A)), Supratentorial (ST-EPN-SE (subependymoma, ST-EPN-YAP1 (YAP1 fusions), ST-EPN-RELA (RELA fusions)) and spinal ependymomas (SP-EPN-MPE (myxopapillary), SP-EPN-SE (subependymoma) and SP-EPN). They can also be categorized according to the WHO classification, which recognizes classic (Grade 2) tumors with characteristic perivascular pseudorosettes and can be further classified as cellular, clear cell or papillary or tanycytic. Myxopapillary ependymomas are also now considered grade 2 and have classic cuboidal tumor cells with vascular cores (Figure 14.6). Grade 3 has anaplastic features including cellular pleomorphism and frequent mitoses. Grade 1 tumors are benign and include subependymomas (Reni et al., 2007; Wu et al., 2016). Cytogenetic studies reveal loss of 22q as the commonest genetic abnormality. Gain of 1q is also frequently found. Ependymomas of the supratentorial region are characterized by a number of molecular aberrations such as activation of *EPHB2* (ephrin-type B receptor 2) and loss of *CDKN2*. Other aberrations include overexpression of the C11orf95 -RELA fusion pro- tein driving abnormal NF-κB transcription. The *NF2* gene may be an important driver of spinal ependymomas, however is less important for intracranial tumors (Reni et al., 2007). Despite advances in our understanding of the molecular aberrations of this tumor, the prognosis is still poor. The paucity of in vitro and in vivo model systems for ependymoma compound the difficulties in development of targeted therapies.

14.12 Craniopharyngiomas

Craniopharyngiomas are rare epithelial tumors that arise along the path of the craniopharyngeal duct. They are embryonic malformations of the sellar/parasellar region and are usually grade I (Müller, 2014; Müller et al., 2019). Histologically, they can be characterized by basaloid-appearing cells, inflammatory cells, and giant cells (Figure 14.7). Adamantinomatous craniopharyngiomas have 'wet' keratin, basal pallisading of tumor cell nuclei and stellate reticulum. These are typically absent in the papillary variant, which is characterized by stratified squamous epithelium surrounding fibrovascular tissue cores. Adamantinomatous craniopharyngiomas have a bimodal peak of incidence (5–15 years and 45–60 years). The most common mutations in this type are those of *CTNNB1* effecting β-catenin stability. The papillary variant is seen more commonly in adults. The most common mutation seen is that of *BRAFV600E*. Although craniopharyngiomas have a favorable prognosis; they frequently recur and can be associated with significant morbidity, e.g., due to endocrine deficits and resulting metabolic disturbances (Müller, 2014; Müller et al., 2019). Several animal models have been employed to study this tumor in mice. The two most successful approaches are xenograft models and GEMMs. Two GEMMs of the adamantinomatous type have been developed, however currently there are no models of the papillary type, limiting our ability to refine the role of BRAF inhibitors in the disease. In the embryonic GEMM model of the adamantinomatous type, exon 3 deletion from the *CTNNB1* locus of cells in the pituitary of a Hesx1–Cre mouse leads to tumor formation. In the inducible GEMM model, oncogenic beta–catenin is expressed in SRY–related HMG–box (SOX2) positive adult pituitary stem cells using tamoxifen–induced activation of the WNT pathway. However, both methods are limited due to only partial recapitulation of the human disease. A better understanding

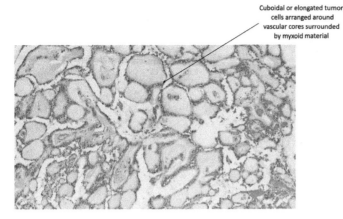

Cuboidal or elongated tumor cells arranged around vascular cores surrounded by myxoid material

Figure 14.6 Histology of a myxopapillary ependymoma.

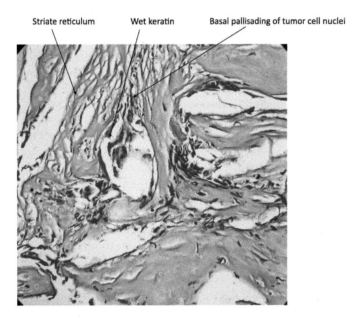

Striate reticulum   Wet keratin   Basal pallisading of tumor cell nuclei

Figure 14.7 Histology specimen of craniopharyngioma.

of the genetic landscapes in human disease will enable the development of new generation of GEMMs (Apps et al., 2017, Müller, 2014; Müller et al., 2019).

14.13 Pineal Tumor

Pineal tumors account for approximately 8% of intracranial tumors in children and approximately 1% in adults. The pineal gland is found above and posterior to the tectum of the midbrain. It contains pinealocytes, which synthesize and secrete N-acetyl-5methoxy-tryptamine, also known as melatonin. This hormone is rhythmically produced in response to changes in light and peaks in the middle of the night. It binds to G-protein-coupled receptors (MT1 and MT2) found in various places including the hypothalamus, pars tuberalis, and suprachiasmatic nucleus of the brain. It acts to establish the circadian rhythm and induction of sleep. It also has other effects including neuroprotection via stimulation of the antioxidant enzyme glutathione peroxidase, in the brain. Tumors found in the pineal gland include germ cell tumors, which account for approximately 50% of intracranial germ cell tumors. They are classified into six types: germinomas, choriocarcinomas, teratomas, embryonal carcinomas, yolk sac tumors and mixed germ cell tumors. Germinomas are the most common pineal tumors and are malignant in nature. Choriocarcinomas are uncommon but have a dismal

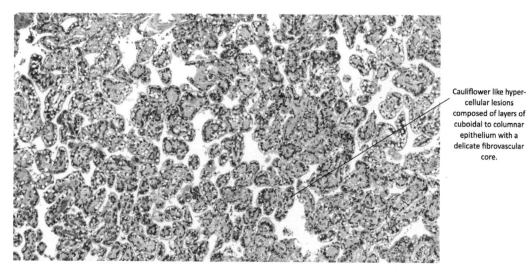

Cauliflower like hypercellular lesions composed of layers of cuboidal to columnar epithelium with a delicate fibrovascular core.

Figure 14.8 Histology of a choroid plexus papilloma.

prognosis. Other tumors include parenchymal tumors, include the slow growing pineocytomas, aggressive grade IV pineoblastomas, papillary tumors and pineal parenchymal tumors of intermediate differentiation. Pineal cysts are benign non-tumor lesions but are frequently observed during both MRI scans and autopsy studies. The two most common germline mutations found in the aggressive pineoblastomas are that of the tumor suppressors *RB1* and *DICER1* (Dicer 1, Ribonuclease III), and have been used to model the disease in mice. Inactivation of *RB* plus p53 via a whey acidic protein (WAP) promoter Cre deleter line, found in the pineal gland of mice can lead to the development of tumors that resemble the human disease with short latency and 100% penetrance. Disruption of *DICER1* plus p53 can also induce tumors, however usually with longer latency and reduced penetrance (Chung et al, 2020). Both benign and malignant tumors can present with hydrocephalus, Parinaud's syndrome (upward-gaze paresis, poor pupillary reaction to light and convergence-retraction nystagmus), bitemporal hemianopsia, and signs of endocrine deficiency (Favero et al., 2021; Hirato and Nakazato, 2001).

14.14 Choroid Plexus Tumor

The choroid plexus is a complex epithelial -endothelial convolute composed of an epithelium, stroma, and vascular supply and is responsible for the production of CSF. Choroid plexus tumors are rare neoplasms of neuroectodermal origin. Most cases present in children under 2 years of age. The most reported locations are the ventricles and

the most common presentation as a result is severe hydrocephalus and symptoms of overt intracranial hypertension. In the adult population, headaches are the most encountered symptom. They can be categorized according to their grade: Type 1 (benign choroid plexus papillomas), type 2 (atypical choroid plexus papillomas) and type 3 (malignant choroid plexus carcinomas (CPCs)). Choroid plexus carcinomas are highly malignant and characterized by numerous chromosomal aberrations. Histologically, they appear as lobulated masses with necrotic regions. The mechanisms underlying the tumor formation remain largely unknown, mostly due to the paucity of animal models reproducing the genetic alterations associated with this tumor. They were initially found in transgenic mice expressing SV40 T antigen. The most common underlying genetic mechanism is aberration of p53 and in humans there is an association with Li-Fraumeni syndrome. *RB* inactivation is also required for tumor initiation. Dysregulation of DNA maintenance and repair lead to tumor formation and are regulated by the oncogenes TATA-Box Binding Protein Associated Factor 12 (*TAF12*), Nuclear Transcription Factor Y Subunit C (*NFYC*) and RAD54 Like (*RAD54L*). Choroid plexus papillomas are indolent lesions that can often be cured with total resection. They are the most common type of choroid plexus tumors. They are often found in the lateral ventricle, followed by the fourth and third ventricles and, rarely, in the cerebellopontine angle. In adults, however they are more common in the fourth ventricle. There is an association with conditions such as Aicardi syndrome, von Hippel-Lindau disease and haemangioblastomas. On histology, they appear as cauliflower-like masses (Figure 14.8) (Thomas et al., 2021; Wolff et al., 2002).

Figure acknowledgements

The following images obtained with consent are credited to the authors of this chapter: Figures 14.1-14.2
The following image was created using a Biorender industrial license: Figure 14.3
The following images were created using a Shutterstock license: Figures 14.4-14.8

References

Abbud RA, Takumi I, Barker EM, et al. Early multipotential pituitary focal hyperplasia in the alpha-subunit of glycoprotein hormone-driven pituitary tumor-transforming gene transgenic mice. *Mol Endocrinol* 2005;**19**(5):1383–91. https://doi.org/10.1210/me.2004-0403.

Abedalthagafi M, Bi WL, Aizer AA, et al. Oncogenic PI3K mutations are as common as AKT1 and SMO mutations in meningioma. *Neuro Oncol* 2016;**18**(5):649–55. https://doi.org/10.1093/neuonc/nov316.

An J, Pei X, Zang Z, et al., Metformin inhibits proliferation and growth hormone secretion of GH3 pituitary adenoma cells. *Oncotarget* 2017;**8**(23):37538–49. https://doi.org/10.18632/oncotarget.16556.

Apps JR, Martinez-Barbera JP. Genetically engineered mouse models of craniopharyngioma: an opportunity for therapy development and understanding of tumor biology. Brain Pathol. 2017 May;**27**(3):364–369. doi: 10.1111/bpa.12501.

Asa SL, Kovacs K, Stefaneanu L, et al., Pituitary adenomas in mice transgenic for growth hormone-releasing hormone. *Endocrinology* 1992;**131**(5):2083–9. https://doi.org/10.1210/endo.131.5.1425411.

Aziz-Bose R, Monje M. Diffuse intrinsic pontine glioma: molecular landscape and emerging therapeutic targets. *Curr Opin Oncol* 2019;**31**(6):522–30. https://doi.org/10.1097/CCO.0000000000000577.

Bai F, Chan HL, Smith MD, Kiyokawa H, Pei X-H. $p19^{Ink4d}$ is a tumor suppressor and controls pituitary anterior lobe cell proliferation. *Mol Cell Biol* 2014;**34**(12):2121–34. https://doi.org/10.1128/MCB.01363-13.

Bentley L, Esapa CT, Nesbit MA, et al. An *N*-ethyl-*N*-nitrosourea induced corticotropin-releasing hormone promoter mutation provides a mouse model for endogenous glucocorticoid excess. *Endocrinology* 2014;**155**(3):908–22. https://doi.org/0.1210/en.2013-1247.

Bertolino P, Tong W-M, Herrera PL, et al. Pancreatic beta-cell-specific ablation of the multiple endocrine neoplasia type 1 (MEN1) gene causes full penetrance of insulinoma development in mice. *Cancer Res* 2003;**63**(16):4836–41.

Bi WL, Abedalthagafi M, Horowitz P, et al. Genomic landscape of intracranial meningiomas. *J Neurosurg* 2016a;**125**(3):525–35. https://doi.org/10.3171/2015.6.JNS15591.

Bi WL, Mei Y, Agarwalla PK, Beroukhim R, Dunn IF. Genomic and epigenomic landscape in meningioma. *Neurosurg Clinics* 2016b;**27**(2):167–79. https://doi.org/10.1016/j.nec.2015.11.009.

Biondi CA, Gartside MG, Waring P, et al. Conditional inactivation of the MEN1 gene leads to pancreatic and pituitary tumorigenesis but does not affect normal development of these tissues. *Mol Cell Biol* 2004;**24**(8):3125–31. https://doi.org/10.1128/MCB.24.8.3125-3131.2004.

Booth A, Trudeau T, Gomez C, Lucia MS, Gutierrez-Hartmann A. Persistent ERK/MAPK activation promotes lactotrope differentiation and diminishes tumorigenic phenotype. *Mol Endocrinol* 2014;**28**(12):1999–2011. https://doi.ord/10.1210/me.2014-1168.

Cai DX, Banerjee R, Scheithauer BW, Lohse CM, Kleinschmidt-Demasters BK, Perry A. Chromosome 1p and 14q FISH analysis in clinicopathologic subsets of meningioma: diagnostic and prognostic implications. *J Neuropathol Exp Neurol* 2001;**60**(6):628–36. https://doi.org/10.1093/jnen/60.6.628.

Chang LS, Welling DB. Molecular biology of vestibular schwannomas. *Methods Mol Biol* 2009;**493**:163–77. https://doi.org/10.1007/978-1-59745-523-7_10.

Cheng SQ, Fan H-Y, Xu X, et al, Over-expression of LRIG1 suppresses biological function of pituitary adenoma via attenuation of PI3K/AKT and Ras/Raf/ERK pathways in vivo and in vitro. *J Huazhong Univ Sci Technolog Med Sci* 2016;**36**(4):558–63. https://doi.org/10.1007/s11596-016-1625-4.

Chesnokova V, Kovacs K, Castro A-V, Zonis S, Melmed S. Pituitary hypoplasia in Pttg–/– mice is protective for Rb+/– pituitary tumorigenesis. *Mol Endocrinol* 2005;**19**(9):2371–9. https://doi.org/10.1210/me.2005-0137.

Choudhury A, Raleigh DR. Preclinical models of meningioma: cell culture and animal systems. *Handb Clin Neurol* 2020;**169**:131–6. https://doi.org/10.1016/B978-0-12-804280-9.00008-1.

Chukwueke UN, Wen PY. Medical management of meningiomas. In McDermott MW (Ed.), *Handbook of Clinical Neurology*. Elsevier, 2020: pp. 291–302.

Chung PED, Gendoo DMA, Ghanbari-Azarnier R, Liu JC, Jiang Z, Tsui J, Wang DY, Xiao X, Li B, Dubuc A, Shih D, Remke M, Ho B, Garzia L, Ben-David Y, Kang SG, Croul S, Haibe-Kains B, Huang A, Taylor MD, Zacksenhaus E. Modeling germline mutations in pineoblastoma uncovers lysosome disruption-based therapy. Nat Commun. 2020 Apr 14;**11**(1):1825. doi: 10.1038/s41467-020-15585-2.

Chunharojrith P, Nakayama Y, Jiang X, et al., Tumor suppression by MEG3 lncRNA in a human pituitary tumor derived cell line. *Mol Cell Endocrinol* 2015;**416**:27–35. https://doi.org/10.1016/j.mce.2015.08.018.

Clark VE, Erson-Omay EZ, Serin A, et al. Genomic analysis of non-NF2 meningiomas reveals mutations in TRAF7, KLF4,

AKT1, and SMO. *Science* 2013;**339**(6123):1077–80. https://doi.org/10.1126/science.1233009.

Crabtree JS, Scacheri PC, Ward JM, et al. Of mice and MEN1: insulinomas in a conditional mouse knockout. *Mol Cell Biol* 2003;**23**(17):6075–85. https://doi.org/10.1128/MCB.23.17.6075-6085.2003.

de Vries M, van der Mey AG, Hogendoorn PC. Tumor biology of vestibular Schwannoma: a review of experimental data on the determinants of tumor genesis and growth characteristics. *Otol Neurotol* 2015;**36**(7):1128–36. https://doi.org/10.1097/MAO.0000000000000788.

Donangelo I, Gutman S, Horvath E, et al. Pituitary tumor transforming gene overexpression facilitates pituitary tumor development. *Endocrinology* 2006;**147**(10):4781–91. https://doi.org/10.1210/en.2006-0544.

Ezzat S, Zheng L, Winer D, Asa SL. Targeting *N*-cadherin through fibroblast growth factor receptor-4: distinct pathogenetic and therapeutic implications. *Mol Endocrinol* 2006;**20**(11):2965–75. https//doi.org/10.1210/me.2006-0223.

Fangusaro J. Pediatric high grade glioma: a review and update on tumor clinical characteristics and biology. *Front Oncol* 2012;**2**:105. https://doi.org/10.3389/fonc.2012.00105.

Favero G, Bonomini F, Rezzani R. Pineal gland tumors: a review. *Cancers (Basel)* 2021;**13**(7):1547. https://doi.org/10.3390/cancers13071547.

Fedele M, Battista S, Kenyon L, et al. Overexpression of the HMGA2 gene in transgenic mice leads to the onset of pituitary adenomas. *Oncogene* 2002;**21**(20):3190–8. https://doi.org/10.1038/sj.onc.1205428.

Fedele M, Pentimalli F, Baldassarre G, et al. Transgenic mice overexpressing the wild-type form of the HMGA1 gene develop mixed growth hormone/prolactin cell pituitary adenomas and natural killer cell lymphomas. *Oncogene* 2005;**24**(21):3427–35. https://doi.org/10.1038/sj.onc.1208501.

Fedele M, Visone R, De Martino I, et al. HMGA2 induces pituitary tumorigenesis by enhancing E2F1 activity. *Cancer Cell* 2006;**9**(6):459–71. https://doi.org/10.1016/j.ccr.2006.04.024

Franklin DS, Godfrey VL, Lee H, et al. CDK inhibitors p18 (INK4c) and p27(Kip1) mediate two separate pathways to collaboratively suppress pituitary tumorigenesis. *Genes Dev* 1998;**12**(18):2899–911. https://doi.org/10.1101/gad.12.18.2899.

Fuertes M, Sapochnik M, Tedesco L, et al. Protein stabilization by RSUME accounts for PTTG pituitary tumor abundance and oncogenicity. *Endocr Relat Cancer* 2018;**25**(6):665–76. https://doi.org/10.1530/ERC-18-0028.

Gahete MD, Jiménez-Vacas JM, Alors-Pérez E, et al. Mouse models in endocrine tumors. *J Endocrinol* 2019;**240**(3):R73–93. https://doi.org/10.1530/JOE-18-0571

Greene HSN, Arnold H. The homologous and heterologous transplantation of brain and brain tumors. *J Neurosurg* 1945;**2**(4):315–31. https://doi.org/10.3171/jns.1945.2.4.0315.

Guidi CJ, Mudhasani R, Hoover K, et al. Functional interaction of the retinoblastoma and Ini1/Snf5 tumor suppressors in cell growth and pituitary tumorigenesis. *Cancer Res* 2006;**66**(16):8076–82. https://doi.org/10.1158/0008-5472.CAN-06-1451.

Harvey M, Vogel H, Lee EY, Bradley A, Donehower LA. Mice deficient in both p53 and Rb develop tumors primarily of endocrine origin. *Cancer Res* 1995;**55**(5):1146–51.

Helseth A, Siegel GP, Haug E, Bautch VL. Transgenic mice that develop pituitary tumors. A model for Cushing's disease. *Am J Pathol* 1992;**140**(5):1071–80.

Hemmer S, Sippl C, Sahm F, Oertel J, Urbschat S, Ketter R. The loss of 1p as a reliable marker of progression in a child with aggressive meningioma: a 16-year follow-up case report. *Ped Neurosurg* 2020;**55**(6):418–25. https://doi.org/10.1159/000512001.

Hirato J, Nakazato Y. Pathology of pineal region tumors. *J Neurooncol* 2001;**54**(3):239–49. https://doi.org/10.1023/a:1012721723387.

Jacks T, Fazeli A, Schmitt EM, Bronson RT, Goodell MA, Weinberg RA. Effects of an Rb mutation in the mouse. *Nature* 1992;**359**(6393):295–300. https://doi.org/10.1038/359295a0.

Jalali S, Monsalves E, Tateno T, Zadeh G. Role of mTOR inhibitors in growth hormone-producing pituitary adenomas harboring different FGFR4 genotypes. *Endocrinology* 2016;**157**(9):3577–87. https://doi.org/10.1210/en.2016-1028.

James MF, Han S, Polizzano C, et al. NF2/merlin is a novel negative regulator of mTOR complex 1, and activation of mTORC1 is associated with meningioma and schwannoma growth. *Mol Cell Biol* 2009;**29**(15):4250–61. https://doi.org/10.1128/MCB.01581-08.

Johung TB, Monje M. Diffuse intrinsic pontine glioma: new pathophysiological insights and emerging therapeutic targets. *Curr Neuropharmacol* 2017;**15**(1):88–97. https://doi.org/10.2174/1570159x14666160509123229.

Kalamarides M, Niwa-Kawakita M, Leblois H, et al. Nf2 gene inactivation in arachnoidal cells is rate-limiting for meningioma development in the mouse. *Genes Dev* 2002;**16**(9):1060–5. https://doi.org/10.1101/gad.226302.

Kiyokawa H, Kineman RD, Manova-Todorova KO, et al., Enhanced growth of mice lacking the cyclin-dependent kinase inhibitor function of p27(Kip1). *Cell* 1996;**85**(5):721–32. https://doi.org/10.1016/s0092-8674(00)81238-6.

Kumar TR, Graham KE, Asa SL, Low MJ. Simian virus 40 T antigen-induced gonadotroph adenomas: a model of human null cell adenomas. *Endocrinology* 1998:**139**(7):3342–51. https://doi.org/10.1210/endo.139.7.6100.

Lee Y, Liu J, Patel S, et al. Genomic landscape of meningiomas. *Brain Pathol* 2010;**20**(4):751–62. https://doi.org/10.1111/j.1750-3639.2009.00356.x.

Li R, Zhang Z, Wang J, et al. Triptolide suppresses growth and hormone secretion in murine pituitary corticotroph tumor cells via NF-kappaB signaling pathway. *Biomed Pharmacother* 2017;**95**:771–9. https://doi.org/10.1016/j.biopha.2017.08.127.

Lin SJ, Wu ZR, Cao L, et al. Pituitary tumor suppression by combination of cabergoline and chloroquine. *J Clin Endocrinol Metab* 2017;**102**(10):3692–703. https://doi.org/10.1210/jc .2017-00627.

Lloyd RV, Ruebel KH, Zhang S, Jin L. Pituitary hyperplasia in glycoprotein hormone alpha subunit-, p18(INK4C)-, and p27 (kip-1)-null mice: analysis of proteins influencing p27(kip-1) ubiquitin degradation. *Am J Pathol* 2002;**160**(3): 1171–9. https://doi.org/10.1016/S0002-9440(10)64936-X.

Loffler KA, Biondi CA, Gartside MG, et al. Lack of augmentation of tumor spectrum or severity in dual heterozygous Men1 and Rb1 knockout mice. *Oncogene* 2007;**26** (27):4009–17. https://doi.org/10.1038/sj.onc.1210163.

Louis DN, Perry A, Wesseling P, et al. The 2021 WHO Classi cation of Tumors of the Central Nervous System: a summary. Neuro-Oncology. 2021;**23**(8):1231–1251. https://doi.org/10.10 93/neuonc/noab106.

Low MJ, Liu B, Hammer GD, Rubinstein M, Allen RG. Post-translational processing of proopiomelanocortin (POMC) in mouse pituitary melanotroph tumors induced by a POMC-simian virus 40 large T antigen transgene. *J Biol Chem* 1993;**268**(33):24967–75.

Lu J, Chatain GP, Bugarini A, et al. Histone deacetylase inhibitor SAHA is a promising treatment of cushing disease. *J Clin Endocrinol Metab* 2017;**102**(8):2825–35. 10.1210/jc.2017-00464.

Mannelli M, Cantini G, Poli G, et al. Role of the PPAR-γ system in normal and tumoral pituitary corticotropic cells and adrenal cells. *Neuroendocrinology* 2010;**92**(Suppl 1):23–7. https://doi .org/10.1159/000314312.

Manoranjan B, Mahendram S, Almenawer SA, et al. The identification of human pituitary adenoma-initiating cells. *Acta Neuropathol Commun* 2016;**4**(1):125. https://doi.org/10.1186/s 40478-016-0394-4.

McClatchey AI, Saotome I, Mercer K, et al. Mice heterozygous for a mutation at the Nf2 tumor suppressor locus develop a range of highly metastatic tumors. *Genes Dev* 1998;**12** (8):1121–33. https://doi.org/10.1101/gad.12.8.1121.

McCutcheon IE, Friend KE, Gerdes TM, Zhang BM, Wildrick DM, Fuller GN. Intracranial injection of human meningioma cells in athymic mice: an orthotopic model for meningioma growth. *J Neurosurg* 2000;**92**(2):306–14. https:// doi.org/10.3171/jns.2000.92.2.0306.

McSheehy PM, Troy H, Kelland LR, Judson IR, Leach MO, Griffiths JR. Increased tumour extracellular pH induced by Bafilomycin A1 inhibits tumour growth and mitosis in vivo and alters 5-fluorouracil pharmacokinetics. *Eur J Cancer* 2003;**39**(4):532–40. 10.1016/s0959-8049(02)00671-8.

Millard NE, De Braganca KC. Medulloblastoma. *J Child Neurol* 2016;**31**(12):1341–53. https://doi.org/10.1177/08830738156008 66. Erratum in *J Child Neurol*, 2016.

Morrison JP, Satoh H, Foley J, et al. *N*-ethyl-*N*-nitrosourea (ENU)-induced meningiomatosis and meningioma in p16

(INK4a)/p19(ARF) tumor suppressor gene-deficient mice. *Toxicol Pathol* 2007;**35**(6):780–7. https://doi.org/10.1080 /01926230701584130.

Müller HL. Craniopharyngioma. *Endocr Rev* 2014;**35**(3):513–43. https://doi.org/10.1210/er.2013-1115.

Müller HL, Merchant TE, Warmuth-Metz M, Martinez-Barbera JP, Puget S. Craniopharyngioma. *Nat Rev Dis Primers* 2019;**5**(1):75. https://doi.org/10.1038/s41572-019-0125-9.

Nakayama K, Ishida N, Shirane M, et al. Mice lacking p27(Kip1) display increased body size, multiple organ hyperplasia, retinal dysplasia, and pituitary tumors. *Cell* 1996;**85**(5):707–20. https:// doi.org/10.1016/s0092-8674(00)81237-4.

Ning S, Knox SJ, Harsh GR, Culler MD, Katznelson L. Lanreotide promotes apoptosis and is not radioprotective in GH3 cells. *Endocr Relat Cancer* 2009;**16**(3):1045–55. https//doi .org/10.1677/ERC-09-0003.

Northcott PA, Robinson GW, Kratz CP, et al. Medulloblastoma. *Nat Rev Dis Primers* 2019;**5**(1):11. https://doi.org/10.1038/s415 72-019-0063-6.

Ostrom QT, Patil N, Cioffi G, Waite K, Kruchko C, Barnholtz-Sloan JS. CBTRUS statistical report: primary brain and other central nervous system tumors diagnosed in the United States in 2013–2017. *Neuro-Oncology* 2020;**22**(Suppl_1):iv1–96. https:// doi.org/10.1093/neuonc/noaa200.

Pei L, Melmed S. Isolation and characterization of a pituitary tumor-transforming gene (PTTG). *Mol Endocrinol* 1997;**11** (4):433–41. https://doi.org/10.1210/mend.11.4.9911.

Petrilli AM, Fernández-Valle C. Role of Merlin/NF2 inactivation in tumor biology. *Oncogene* 2016;**35**(5):537–48. https://doi.org/10.1038/onc.2015.125.

Peyre M, Salaud C, Clermont-Taranchon E, et al. PDGF activation in PGDS-positive arachnoid cells induces meningioma formation in mice promoting tumor progression in combination with Nf2 and Cdkn2ab loss. *Oncotarget* 2015;**6** (32):32713–22. https://doi.org/10.18632/oncotarget.5296.

Plant-Fox AS, O'Halloran K, Goldman S. Pediatric brain tumors: the era of molecular diagnostics, targeted and immune-based therapeutics, and a focus on long term neurologic sequelae. *Curr Probl Cancer* 2021;**45**(4):100777. https://doi.org/10.1016/j.currproblcancer.2021.100777.

Raitila A, Lehtonen HJ, Arola J, et al. Mice with inactivation of aryl hydrocarbon receptor-interacting protein (Aip) display complete penetrance of pituitary adenomas with aberrant ARNT expression. *Am J Pathol* 2010;**177**(4):1969–76. https:// doi.org/10.2353/ajpath.2010.100138.

Rath P, Miller DC, Litofsky NS, et al. Isolation and characterization of a population of stem-like progenitor cells from an atypical meningioma. *Exp Mol Pathol* 2011;**90** (2):179–88. https://doi.org/10.1016/j.yexmp.2010.12.003.

Reni M, Gatta G, Mazza E, Vecht C. Ependymoma. *Crit Rev Oncol Hematol* 2007;**63**(1):81–9. https://doi.org/10.1016/j .critrevonc.2007.03.004.

Reuss DE, Piro RM, Jones DTW, et al. Secretory meningiomas are defined by combined KLF4 K409Q and TRAF7 mutations. *Acta Neuropathol* 2013;**125**(3):351–8. https://doi.org/10.1007/s00401-013-1093-x.

Roche C, Rasolonjanahary R, Thirion S, et al. Inactivation of transcription factor pit-1 to target tumoral somatolactotroph cells. *Hum Gene Ther* 2012;**23**(1):104–14. https://doi.org/10.1089/hum.2011.105.

Roussel-Gervais A, Bilodeau S, Vallette S, et al. Cooperation between cyclin E and p27(Kip1) in pituitary tumorigenesis. *Mol Endocrinol* 2010;**24**(9):1835–45. https://doi.org/10.1210/me.2010-0091.

Russell WL, Kelly EM, Hunsicker PR, Bangham JW, Maddux SC, Phipps EL. Specific-locus test shows ethylnitrosourea to be the most potent mutagen in the mouse. *PNAS* 1979;**76**(11):5818–9. https://doi.org/10.1073/pnas.76.11.5818.

Sáez C, Japón MA, Ramos-Morales F, et al. hpttg is over-expressed in pituitary adenomas and other primary epithelial neoplasias. *Oncogene* 1999;**18**(39):5473–6. https://doi.org/10.1038/sj.onc.1202914.

Seizinger BR, de la Monte S, Atkins L, Gusella JF, Martuza RL. Molecular genetic approach to human meningioma: loss of genes on chromosome 22. *PNAS* 1987;**84**(15):5419–23. https://doi.org/10.1073/pnas.84.15.5419.

Shapiro IM, Kolev VN, Vidal CM, et al. Merlin deficiency predicts FAK inhibitor sensitivity: a synthetic lethal relationship. *Sci Transl Med* 2014;**6**(237):237ra68–237ra68. https://doi.org/10.1126/scitranslmed.3008639.

Sotillo R, Renner O, Dubus P, et al., Cooperation between Cdk4 and p27kip1 in tumor development: a preclinical model to evaluate cell cycle inhibitors with therapeutic activity. Cancer Res, 2005. **65**(9): p. 3846-52. https://doi.org/10.1158/0008-5472.CAN-04-4195.

Stefaneanu L, Rindi G, Horvath E, Murphy D, Polak JM, Kovacs K. Morphology of adenohypophysial tumors in mice transgenic for vasopressin-SV40 hybrid oncogene. *Endocrinology* 1992;**130**(4):1789–95. https://doi.org/10.1210/endo.130.4.1312426.

Stenzel-Poore MP, Cameron VA, Vaughan J, Sawchenko PE, Vale W. Development of Cushing's syndrome in corticotropin-releasing factor transgenic mice. *Endocrinology* 1992;**130**(6):3378–86. https://doi.org/10.1210/endo.130.6.1597149.

Suppiah S, Nassiri F, Bi WL, et al. Molecular and translational advances in meningiomas. *Neuro Oncol* 2019;**21**(Suppl_1):i4–17. https://doi.org/10.1093/neuonc/noy178.

Thomas C, Soschinski P, Zwaig M, et al. The genetic landscape of choroid plexus tumors in children and adults. *Neuro Oncol* 2021;**23**(4):650–60. 10.1093/neuonc/noaa267.

Torp SH, Solheim O, Skjulsvik AJ. The WHO 2021 Classification of Central Nervous System tumours: a practical update on what neurosurgeons need to know-a minireview. Acta Neurochir (Wien). 2022 Sep;164(9):2453-2464. doi: 10.1007/s00701-022-05301-y.

Tsai KY, MacPherson D, Rubinson DA, et al., ARF mutation accelerates pituitary tumor development in Rb+/− mice. *PNAS* 2002;**99**(26):16865–70. https://doi.org/10.1073/pnas.262499599.

Vierimaa O, Georgitsi M, Lehtonen R, et al. Pituitary adenoma predisposition caused by germline mutations in the AIP gene. *Science* 2006;**312**(5777):1228–30. https://doi.org/10.1126/science.1126100.

Vlotides G, Eigler T, Melmed S. Pituitary tumor-transforming gene: physiology and implications for tumorigenesis. *Endocr Rev* 2007;**28**(2):165–86. https://doi.org/

Vooijs M, van der Valk M, te Riele H, Berns A. Flp-mediated tissue-specific inactivation of the retinoblastoma tumor suppressor gene in the mouse. *Oncogene* 1998;**17**(1):1–12. https://doi.org/10.1038/sj.onc.1202169.

Wang D, Wong H-K, Feng Y-B, Zhang Z-J. Liquiritigenin exhibits antitumour action in pituitary adenoma cells via Ras/ERKs and ROS-dependent mitochondrial signalling pathways. *J Pharm Pharmacol* 2014;**66**(3):408–17. https://doi.org/10.1111/jphp.12170.

Wolff JE, Sajedi M, Brant R, Coppes MJ, Egeler RM. Choroid plexus tumours. *Br J Cancer* 2002;**87**(10):1086–91. https://doi.org/10.1038/sj.bjc.6600609.

Wu J, Armstrong TS, Gilbert MR. Biology and management of ependymomas. *Neuro Oncol* 2016;**18**(7):902–13. https://doi.org/10.1093/neuonc/now016.

Yin Z, Williams-Simons L, Parlow AF, Asa S, Kirschner LS. Pituitary-specific knockout of the Carney complex gene Prkar1a leads to pituitary tumorigenesis. *Mol Endocrinol* 2008;**22**(2):380–7. https://doi.org/10.1210/me.2006-0428.

Youngblood MW, Duran D, Montejo JD, et al. Correlations between genomic subgroup and clinical features in a cohort of more than 3000 meningiomas. *J Neurosurg* 2019;**133**(5):1345–54. https://doi.org/10.3171/2019.8.JNS191266.

Zang KD, Singer H. Chromosomal constitution of meningiomas. *Nature* 1967;**216**(5110):84–5. https://doi.org/10.1038/216084a0.

Zhang H, Qi L, Du Y, et al. Patient-derived orthotopic xenograft (PDOX) mouse models of primary and recurrent meningioma. *Cancers (Basel)* 2020;**12**(6):E1478. https://doi.org/10.3390/cancers12061478.

Zhao Y, Xiao Z, Chen W, Yang J, Li T, Fan B. Disulfiram sensitizes pituitary adenoma cells to temozolomide by regulating O6-methylguanine-DNA methyltransferase expression. *Mol Med Rep* 2015;**12**(2):2313–22. https://doi.org/10.3892/mmr.2015.3664.

Zhen W, Qiu D, Zhiyong C, et al. MicroRNA-524-5p functions as a tumor suppressor in a human pituitary tumor-derived cell line. *Horm Metab Res* 2017;**49**(7):550–7. https://doi.org/10.1055/s-0043-106437.

Zindy F, Nilsson LM, Nguyen L, et al. Hemangiosarcomas, medulloblastomas, and other tumors in Ink4c/p53-null mice. *Cancer Res* 2003;**63**(17):5420–7.

Chapter 15

Biomechanics of the Spine

Gaetano De Biase and Kingsley Abode-Iyamah

15.1 Introduction

The human spine consists of 33 vertebrae grouped into five different regions. From superior to inferior there are seven cervical vertebrae, 12 thoracic vertebrae, five lumbar vertebrae, five fused sacral vertebrae, and four small fused coccygeal vertebrae (Figure 15.1). The spine is a functionally complex and significant component of the human body that not only provides bony protection to the spinal cord but also provides an incredible amount of flexibility to the trunk and serves as the mechanical linkage between the upper and lower extremities, allowing movement in all three planes. Biomechanics, the application of mechanical principles to living organisms, is crucial in understanding how the bony and soft spinal components interact to ensure spinal stability, and how this is affected by degenerative disorders, trauma, and tumors. Understanding spine biomechanics may provide important insights to clinicians on the etiology of spine diseases, such as adverse mechanical loading conditions or unfavorable biochemical environments

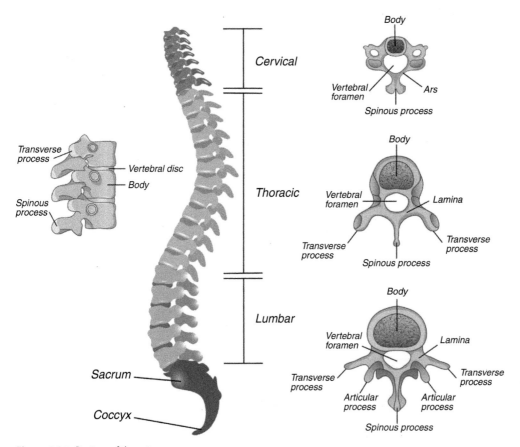

Figure 15.1 Regions of the spine.

which can trigger intervertebral disc degeneration. The occipital cervical junction has a complex network of ligamentous connection and movement that goes beyond the scope of this review.

15.2 The Motion Segment

The motion segment, considered the functional unit of the spine, is composed of two adjacent vertebrae, the intervertebral disc, the facet joints, and the spinal ligaments. Each motion segment includes three joints: the vertebral bodies separated by the intervertebral discs; a symphysis; and the right and left facet joints between the superior and inferior articular processes, diarthroses of the gliding type lined with articular cartilage.

15.3 Definition of Stability

White et al. (1975) have defined spine stability as the ability of the spine under physiologic loads to limit patterns of displacement so as not to damage or irritate the spinal cord or nerve roots and, in addition, to prevent incapacitating deformity or pain caused by structural changes. The loss of stability – instability – is an important cause of axial back pain, especially at the lumbar level. White and Panjabi (1978) characterized instability as the loss of the ability of the spine under physiologic loads to maintain its patterns of displacement so there is no initial or additional neurologic deficit, no major deformity, and no incapacitating pain. Instability leads to increased and abnormal movements in the motion segment. These abnormal movements of the spine can result from degenerative changes or from congenital malformation of the spinal column. Additionally, trauma can lead to injury in the spine, resulting in instability.

15.4 Normal Spine Motion

Within each motion segment the vertebral body can execute three translational movements along and three rotational movements around each of the x-, y-, and z-Cartesian axes of the space and various combinations of those movements. The axis around which a vertebral body rotates at a definite point in time is called the instantaneous axis of rotation (IAR). Normally functioning motion units have an IAR confined to a relatively limited area somewhere within the motion unit; if instability develops, the IAR can noticeably enlarge and even shift outside of the physical space of the unit. The physiologic range of motion (ROM) is characterized by a neutral zone (NZ) and an elastic zone (EZ). When applying a force to a motion segment, the functional unit will be displaced from a resting neutral position to a position in which a resistance in experienced. The initial motion on either side of the neutral position, the NZ, is characterized by low resistance and high flexibility, thus allowing large motions with minimal effort. If the NZ increases in size it may allow excessive motion, thus leading to instability. The NZ is followed by the EZ, in which tissues follow Hooke's law; thus, the degree of deformation is proportional to the deforming force. This represents a zone of high stiffness, in which the resistance to movement increases linearly and more load is required per unit displacement (Panjabi, 1992). This biphasic behavior allows movements near the neutral posture with minimal muscle effort, while ensuring stability toward the end of joint range.

15.5 The Three-Column Model

To better explain the impact of fractures on spinal stability, Denis (1983) developed the widely used three-column model, in which disruption of two columns is required to cause instability. The anterior column is formed by the anterior longitudinal ligament, the anterior annulus fibrosus and intervertebral disc, and the anterior half of the vertebral body. The middle column consists of the posterior longitudinal ligament, the posterior annulus fibrosus and the posterior half of the vertebral body. The posterior column contains the posterior bony complex (posterior arch) and the posterior ligamentous complex (supraspinous ligament, interspinous ligament, capsule, and ligamentum flavum). This model thus considers compression fractures to be stable, and chance fractures, burst fractures and fracture–dislocations unstable (Panjabi et al., 1995). To simplify and standardize the process of classifying spinal injuries the now widely adopted AO Spine injury classification system was developed. For every fracture three distinct components are taken into consideration: morphology of the fracture, presence of neurological signs, and presence of ligamentous injuries or comorbid conditions (modifiers); injuries are broadly classified into: type A, compression injuries; type B, failure of the posterior or anterior tension band without evidence of either gross translation or the potential for gross translation; type C, failure of all elements leading to dislocation or displacement. Another commonly used scale used for scoring fractures is the thoracolumbar injury classification and severity score (TLICS), which is based on three parameters: injury morphology, posterior ligamentous complex integrity, and patient neurology.

15.6 Regional Biomechanics of the Spine

Each vertebral region is characterized by unique anatomic and biomechanic features that predispose them to specific injuries. Normally, the spine is characterized by a curvilinear sagittal conformation with a thoracic kyphotic curve and lordotic cervical and lumbar curves. Any alterations in the physiologic curvatures lead to changes in the momentum, the perpendicular distance from the IAR to the gravitational force vector, which results in modifications to the normal weight distribution. Due to the abrupt differences in stiffness and biomechanical properties that occur at the cervicothoracic, thoracolumbar, and lumbosacral junctions these areas are more prone to injury and degeneration.

15.6.1 The Cervical Spine

The cervical region is the most mobile of the spine, with a range of motion of 80–90° of flexion, 70° of extension, 20–45° of lateral flexion, and up to 90° of rotation to both sides (Miele et al., 2012). Lysell (1969) studied on autopsy specimens the relationship between motion and disc degeneration in the cervical spine. He graded the intervertebral discs for degeneration and did not find an association between range of motion of a specific level and the extent of its disc degeneration.

15.6.2 The Thoracic Spine

Due to the costochondral reinforcement the thoracic spine is relatively stiff and is characterized by a kyphotic curvature. Gregersen and Lucas (1967) measured the axial rotation (rotation in the transverse plane) in young male subjects by inserting Steinmann pins in the spinous processes and measuring the angular displacement of the pins. They found an average of 6° of rotation at each thoracic level, with the maximal rotation identified in the middle portion of the thoracic spine. Due to the stiffness provided by the rib cage in this region it is thought to constitute a fourth column to the thoracic spine.

15.6.3 The Lumbar Spine

While the lumbar vertebrae are larger, thus providing more axial strength, this region is significantly more mobile than the thoracic spine and also lacks the stability provided by the ribs, and all these factors lead to an increase in susceptibility to injury. The high incidence of clinically relevant disc disease at L4–L5 and L5–S1 is related to the fact that these segments undergo the most motion and are under the highest loads.

15.7 The Intervertebral Disc

The intervertebral disc is made primarily of proteoglycans and collagen, and is composed of the centrally located nucleus pulposus and its outer boundaries are defined by the annulus fibrosus. The disc is subject to many different types of load and is a very resilient structure. Several studies have found that even when subjected to high compressive loads that lead to permanent deformation, upon cessation of the load, no herniation of the nucleus pulposus had occurred (Hirsch, 1955; Markolf and Morris, 1974; Virgin, 1951). Under compression loading of a vertebra–disc–vertebra, no disc herniation was reported, and the first component to fail was the vertebra secondary to fracture of the end plate (Brown et al., 1957). Studies looking at tensile properties of intervertebral discs have revealed the anterior and posterior regions to be stronger than the lateral and central ones. Experiments have also been performed to study the behavior of lumbar disc under direct shear. Markolf (1972) found the horizontal shear stiffness to be 260 N/nm, indicating that clinical annular disruption implies that the disc has been exposed to a combination of torsion bending and tension, and not just pure shear. When subjected to compression load, the pressure in the nucleus pulposus increases. Nachemson (1966) and Nachemson and Morris (1964) measured the disc pressure *in vivo* using a needle with a pressure transducer located on its tip. Interestingly, although the portion of body above the L3 disc accounts only for 60% of total body weight, the load on the L3 disc in the sitting position and while standing with a 20° of flexion is about 200% total body weight, and simply adding 20 kg of weight in the hands leads to a 300% body weight load. It has been suggested that after a fusion the increased range of motion and intradiscal pressure (IDP) adjacent to instrumentation may play a role in adjacent segment disease. Cadaveric studies have found that instrumentation with either PEEK or Ti rods results in decreased motion at the instrumented levels while increasing IDP at the adjacent level (Abode-Iyamah et al., 2014).

15.8 Spine Ligaments

Ligaments are structures that resist tensile forces, but buckle when compressed and transfer tensile loads from one bone to another. There are seven spine ligaments: the anterior and posterior longitudinal ligaments, the intertransverse and capsular ligament, the interspinous and supraspinous ligaments, and the ligamentum flavum. They allow adequate and low-resistance physiologic motion between the vertebrae while restricting movements within physiologic limits in order to protect the spinal cord; they are also effective at absorbing and dissipating suddenly applied external energy, thus offering a level of protection in traumatic situations. The shock-absorbing properties of the spine ligaments tend to deteriorate with age and with disc degeneration, as their large amount of elastic fibers gets replaced by fibrous tissue (Tkaczuk, 1968). Noyes et al. (1974a, 1974b) studied ligament failure under traumatic loads and found that at low speeds of load application the failure was more often in the bone at the points of attachment, while at higher speeds failure was most likely to occur within the ligament itself. The intra- and supraspinous ligament also acts as a tensile posterior tension band of the spine preventing excessive flexion.

15.9 The Vertebra

Despite the structure of the vertebrae being similar in the different portions of the spine, the vertebral size increases from C1 to L5, thus providing mechanical support to the progressively increasing loads to which they are subjected, as shown by several studies that have found the compression strength of the vertebrae to increase from C3 to L3 (from 1500 N to 7000 N; Bell et al., 1967). Interestingly, Weaver and Chalmers (1966) found that the strength properties of vertebral cancellous bone cubes of the L3, L4, and L5 vertebrae are comparable, thus concluding that differences in vertebral strength with spine level is likely due to the different vertebral size. Vertebral strength decreases with age, and a small (25%) decrease in osseous tissue leads to significant (50%) loss of vertebral strength. Furthermore, in the elderly, due to degenerative disc collapse, forces are no longer evenly distributed on the endplates and the posterior facets bear much more of the load.

15.10 Conclusions

Spine biomechanics is a complex field routed in the principles of physics. Understanding spine biomechanics may provide important insights to clinicians on the etiology of spine diseases, such as adverse mechanical loading conditions or unfavorable biochemical environments which can trigger intervertebral disc degeneration.

Figure acknowledgements

The following image was created using a Shutterstock license: Figure 15.1

References

Abode-Iyamah K, Kim SB, Grosland N, et al. Spinal motion and intradiscal pressure measurements before and after lumbar spine instrumentation with titanium or PEEK rods. *J Clin Neurosci* 2014;21:651–5. https://doi.org/10.1016/j.jocn.2013.08.010.

Bell GH, Dunbar O, Beck JS, Gibb A. Variations in strength of vertebrae with age and their relation to osteoporosis. *Calcif Tissue Res* 1967;1(1):75–86. https//doi.org/10.1007/BF02008077.

Brown T, Hansen RJ, Yorra AJ Some mechanical tests on the lumbosacral spine with particular reference to the intervertebral discs; a preliminary report. *J Bone Joint Surg Am* 1957;39-A (5):1135–64.

Denis F. The three column spine and its significance in the classification of acute thoracolumbar spinal injuries. *Spine* 1983;8:817–31. https://doi.org/10.1097/00007632-198311000-00003.

Gregersen GG, Lucas DB. An in vivo study of the axial rotation of the human thoracolumbar spine. *J Bone Joint Surg Am* 1967;49:247–62.

Hirsch C. The reaction of intervertebral discs to compression forces. *J Bone Joint Surg Am* 1955;37-A:1188–96.

Lysell E. Motion in the cervical spine. An experimental study on autopsy specimens. *Acta Orthop Scand Suppl* 1969;123:1+. https//doi.org/10.3109/ort.1969.40.suppl-123.01.

Markolf KL. Deformation of the thoracolumbar intervertebral joints in response to external loads: a biomechanical study using autopsy material. *J Bone Joint Surg Am* 1972;54:511–33.

Markolf KL, Morris JM. The structural components of the intervertebral disc. A study of their contributions to the ability of the disc to withstand compressive forces. *J Bone Joint Surg Am* 1974;56:675–87.

Miele VJ, Panjabi MM, Benzel EC. Anatomy and biomechanics of the spinal column and cord. *Handb Clin Neurol* 2012;109:31–43. https://doi.org/10.1016/B978-0-444-52137-8.00002-4.

Nachemson A. The load on lumbar disks in different positions of the body. *Clin Orthop* 1966;45:107–22.

Nachemson A, Morris JM. In vivo measurements of intradiscal pressure. Discometry, a method for the determination of pressure in the lower lumbar discs. *J Bone Joint Surg Am* 1964;46:1077–92.

Noyes FR, DeLucas JL, Torvik PJ. Biomechanics of anterior cruciate ligament failure: an analysis of strain-rate sensitivity and mechanisms of failure in primates. *J Bone Joint Surg Am* 1974a;56:236–53.

Noyes FR, Torvik PJ, Hyde WB, DeLucas JL. Biomechanics of ligament failure. II. An analysis of immobilization, exercise, and reconditioning effects in primates. *J Bone Joint Surg Am* 1974b;56:1406–18.

Panjabi MM. The stabilizing system of the spine. Part II. Neutral zone and instability hypothesis. *J Spinal Disord* 1992;5:390–6; discussion 397. https://doi.org/10.1097/00002517-199212000-00002.

Panjabi MM, Oxland TR, Kifune M, Arand M, Wen L, Chen A. Validity of the three-column theory of thoracolumbar fractures. A biomechanic investigation. *Spine* 1995;20:1122–7. https://doi.org/10.1097/00007632-199505150-00003.

Tkaczuk H. Tensile properties of human lumbar longitudinal ligaments. *Acta Orthop Scand Suppl* 1968;115:1+. https://doi.org/10.3109/ort.1968.39.suppl-115.01.

Virgin WJ. Experimental investigations into the physical properties of the intervertebral disc. *J Bone Joint Surg Br* 1951;33-B:607–11. https://doi.org/10.1302/0301-620X.33B4.607.

Weaver JK, Chalmers J. Cancellous bone: its strength and changes with aging and an evaluation of some methods for measuring its mineral content. *J Bone Joint Surg Am* 1966;48(2):289–98.

White AA, Johnson RM, Panjabi MM, Southwick WO. Biomechanical analysis of clinical stability in the cervical spine. *Clin Orthop* 1975;109:85–96. https://doi.org/10.1097/00003086-197506000-00011.

White AA, Panjabi MM. The basic kinematics of the human spine. A review of past and current knowledge. *Spine* 1978;3:12–20. https://doi.org/10.1097/00007632-197803000-00003.

Degenerative Cervical Myelopathy

T.J. Florence, Joel S. Beckett, and Langston T. Holly

16.1 Introduction

Key traits distinguish humans from other species. Beyond language, two of these most prominent traits include manual dexterity and bipedal locomotion. Our hands enable an array of feats at a multitude of scales – from microsurgical clipping of a ruptured aneurysm, to hewing the stone needed to build the pyramids. Likewise, our two legs afford some the ability to pirouette, tap dance, or high jump. Even comparatively simple actions, such as buttoning shirt buttons or ambulating, rely on a complex interaction between the neural circuitry of the brain and spinal cord (Kandel et al., 2000). Descending commands are conditioned and modified by local circuits; these same impulses are modified in real time by ascending sensory and proprioceptive information.

Degenerative cervical myelopathy (DCM, also known as cervical spondylotic myelopathy) is a clinical syndrome characterized by clumsiness of the upper extremities, gait difficulty, hyperreflexia, and spasticity of the lower extremities (Clarke and Robinson, 1956; Stookey, 1928). The most common cause of non-traumatic myelopathy (Moore and Blumhardt, 1997), it is caused by compression of the cervical spinal cord secondary to degeneration of extradural elements (Baron and Young, 2007). While many of the fundamental pathologic processes remain to be elucidated (Karadimas et al., 2015), DCM can be thought of as a pathologic alteration in the relationship between sensorimotor and reflexive circuitry of the brain and spinal cord. In this chapter we will consider the neurobiology of spinal motor control and its anatomical substrates. We will demonstrate how compression alters afferent, efferent, and local circuitry in the context of these behaviors, informed in part from work on spinal cord injury. Finally, we will discuss how the brain attempts to compensate for this pathological state via plastic changes in sensorimotor network.

16.2 Neurobiology of the Cervical Cord

In DCM, spinal cord injury leads to aberrant motor control. A significant body of research has elucidated the role spinal neural circuits play in shaping movement. Understanding the neurobiology of movement and the pathophysiology of DCM relies on a firm understanding of cervical cord anatomy, which will be briefly reviewed here.

16.2.1 Anatomy of the Cervical Cord

Consider an axial hemi-section of the cervical spinal cord as positions on a clock face. Along the circumference of the spinal cord are organized distinct white matter tracts (Figure 16.1). At the noon position are the dorsal columns, a pair of white matter tracts which convey proprioceptive, fine-touch, and vibratory information. At one o'clock, axons from sensory dorsal root ganglion neurons enter the spinal cord en route to organized nuclear synapses within the central gray matter. From two to three o'clock is the lateral corticospinal tract, carrying upper motor neuron fibers directly from the contralateral cortex and critical for fine motor control; just inferior to it is the rubrospinal tract, which plays a role in coordinating movement between body segments. Along the extreme edge of the cord between two and six o'clock are the spinocerebellar tracts, which convey additional proprioceptive information from Golgi tendon organs and spindles of muscle fibers. Between three and five o'clock exists the spinothalamic tract, conveying pain, temperature, and pressure information from the extremities to sensory thalamus. Just deep to this is the reticulospinal tract, important for unconscious motor control of antigravity movement. Finally, at six o'clock resides a cluster of white matter tracts: the ventral corticospinal tract, containing uncrossed upper motor neurons; the tectospinal tract, involved in visual orientation; and the vestibulospinal tract, modulating head and body orientation and upright posture (Martin, 2003).

Within the core of the spinal cord is the butterfly-shaped central gray matter. The dorsal horns contain the cell bodies of neurons receiving sensory information

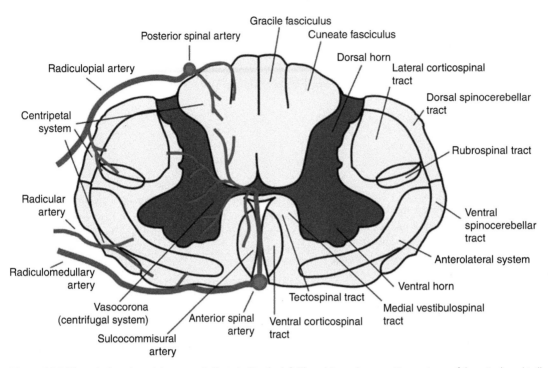

Figure 16.1 The spinal cord arterial anatomy is illustrated to the left. The white and gray matter anatomy of the spinal cord is illustrated to the right.

from dorsal root ganglia synapses; this information is conveyed to appropriate white matter tracts or local neurons controlling spinal reflexes. The ventral horns contain the cell bodies of lower motor neurons receiving information from primarily corticospinal tracts, in turn directly activating muscles.

From a vascular perspective, the spinal cord is supplied by two arterial systems: the centrifugal ("radiating out") system and the centripetal ("radiating in") system (Figure 16.1). The centrifugal system originates with the anterior spinal artery, which dives into the cord itself along the ventral commissure, as it becomes the sulco-commisural artery. It branches radially deep within the cord. The centripetal system originates with radiculopial arteries laterally and the paired posterior spinal arteries dorsally. It forms an anastomotic, mesh-like pial network around the cord, which perforates from the periphery. Venous drainage occurs via an anterior median vein and variable posterior veins, which are widely anastomotic (Santillan et al., 1910).

16.2.2 Neurobiology of Movement

Motor control in the human nervous system is hierarchically organized (Kandel et al., 2000). Initiation of voluntary movement, high-level control, and motor planning

begin in the premotor and motor cortex. Motor signals exit layer V of the cortex, and are conditioned by subcortical structures in the striatum, cerebellum, and brainstem. The majority of descending corticospinal fibers decussate at the medullary pyramids and become the lateral corticospinal tracts; additional fibers descend via the so-called "extra-pyramidal" tracts (Martin, 2003).

The local circuits of the spinal cord are the final effectors of descending motor commands. However, like infantry battalions receiving orders from a general, spinal circuits exhibit significant moment-to-moment autonomy in carrying out commands. This model was dramatically demonstrated in a series of experiments at the beginning of the twentieth century using a decerebrate feline preparation. The pioneering neuroscientist Charles Sherrington demonstrated that cats in which the brain was surgically disconnected from the spinal cord retained the ability to walk on a moving treadmill (Sherrington, 1906, 1910). Subsequent experiments would show that these experimental animals stumble, but recover, over obstacles placed on the treadmill; moreover, they retained the ability to transition from running to walking gait as the treadmill cycled through different speeds (Whelan,

1996). These experiments powerfully demonstrate that normal behavior depends to a significant degree on relatively independent local spinal circuitry.

16.2.3 Proprioceptive Feedback Enables Closed-Loop Control

Just as descending commands direct spinal circuits to execute motor commands, spinal circuits send afferent information toward the cerebrum to inform motor commands. The primary afferent source of proprioceptive information in the spinal cord travels via the dorsal columns (Kandel et al., 2000). In the cervical spine, the dorsal columns are divided into two fasciculi: the gracile fasciculus carries proprioceptive information from the lower extremities; the more lateral cuneate fasciculus carries analogous information from the upper extremities. Each delivers information to its respective nucleus in the medial lemniscus of the medulla, en route to the ventral thalamus and sensory cortex (Martin, 2003).

The nervous system uses ascending proprioceptive information to influence motor planning via a process termed closed-loop control. With respect to movement, the nervous system is limited to altering the force of muscle contraction and thus the acceleration of limbs or grasped objects. In closed-loop control, the expected outcome of an action is compared to the actual outcome; if these differ, an error signal is generated and minimized via online correction (Madhav and Cowan, 2020). The value of closed-loop control is evident to anyone who has picked up an unexpectedly empty jug of milk. At finer scales, it is critical for enabling fine digit control necessary for tying sutures or buttoning buttons.

Closed-loop proprioceptive further enables us to walk on two legs. Bipedal walking is a dynamically unstable process: the swing phase of one leg is dependent on carrying forward momentum of the body via pendulous movement about the stance phase of the opposite leg (Chao, 1986). Flexor and extensor contractions must be coordinated across the body axis, both laterally and along the neuraxis (Dietz, 2003). As no surface is perfectly flat, numerous unconscious corrections continuously occur to prevent falling.

16.2.4 Fine Motor Control

As mentioned above, to effect motor action, the nervous system must activate muscle sarcomeres through activation of motor neurons. Yet clearly, the force required for common tasks vary widely: grabbing an egg from the refrigerator requires significantly less force than giving a firm handshake. The nervous system solves this problem through something known as the size principle (Henneman and Olson, 1965; Mendell, 2005). Motor neurons vary in size; small motor neurons activate relatively few sarcomeres, and large motor neurons recruit significantly more. Differences in membrane properties ensure that small motor neurons are activated prior to activation of large motor neurons. This allows the firing rate of descending upper motor neurons to linearly encode the force exerted by a muscle. In sum, the size principle allows the nervous system to direct a given muscle to exert a wide range of forces.

The organization of descending corticospinal tracts interfaces with spinal motor neurons via this size principle. Some corticospinal neurons interface monosynaptically with individual motor neurons; others synapse on to local interneurons, which in turn synapse on a larger motor pool. Evidence from lesioning experiments in primates suggest that the lateral corticospinal tracts in particular are necessary for individual digit control required for the manipulation of small objects (Lemon, 1993; Zaaimi et al., 2012). Taken together, these suggest that fine manual motor control depends on cortical signals conveyed via the lateral corticospinal tracts and the regulated recruitment of motor pools at the appropriate spinal level.

16.3 Degenerative Cervical Myelopathy

Degenerative cervical myelopathy describes both a syndrome and its underlying cause (Fehlings and Skaf, 1998; Karadimas et al., 2015). It refers generally to a constellation of symptoms, including upper- and lower-motor neuron signs, resulting from insult to the spinal cord. Specifically, these include weakness with hyperreflexia, sensory or proprioceptive deficits, and, in late stages, bowel or bladder dysfunction. In DCM, the critical insult is compression arising from degenerative changes ("spondylosis") of cervical intervertebral disks, vertebrae, and ligamentous structures. Patients relate non-specific difficulties with walking, generally with insidious onset (Nurick, 1972). Common chief complaints on presentation include upper-extremity weakness and numbness, and lack of functional use of the hands, particularly with fine-motor tasks like handwriting or buttoning shirt buttons (Crandall and Batzdorf, 1966). Bladder and bowel dysfunction may be seen in patients with severe disease. Patients may complain of Lhermitte's sign, an electric-shock like sensation, on neck flexion. Cervical and upper-extremity radiculopathy and occipital headache can also be present, although these are not classical features of the myelopathic syndrome (Rao, 2002).

16.4 Pathophysiology of Degenerative Cervical Myelopathy

The pathophysiology of DCM can be considered on the basis of extradural and intradural processes. Outside the cervical cord, degenerative changes of the bony and ligamentous spine lead to stenosis of the spinal canal and compression of the cervical cord (Baron and Young, 2007). Anteriorly, this process begins with disc degeneration. As vertebral discs age, they dehydrate in an eccentric pattern, causing inward buckling of the central annular lamellae and outward bucking of the annulus fibrosis (Rao, 2002). Disc degeneration leads to two primary issues. First, joints lose their restricted degrees of freedom and become hypermobile (Mihara et al., 2000). Second, with decreased buffering of weight-bearing forces, adjacent vertebral bodies must accommodate greater extremes of mechanical stress. Uncinate hypertrophy and formation of osteophytic bars may constitute an adaptive response to these two stressors by increasing the surface area of axial weight-bearing elements and reducing joint mobility (Carette and Fehlins, 2005; McCormack and Weinstein, 1996). Posterior narrowing may result from age-related hypertrophy of the ligamentum flavum and facet hypertrophy (Muthukumar, 2005). In addition to the aforementioned degenerative causes of cord compression, other

progressive entities such as ossification of the posterior longitudinal ligament (OPLL) can lead to clinically significant stenosis, particularly in patients of Asian descent (Choi et al., 2011; Figure 16.2). Degenerative stenosis is exacerbated if patients have a congenitally narrow spinal canal (<13 mm) or anatomical listheses (Hayashi et al., 1987).

Beyond static compression, dynamic forces also imperil cord function. In cervical flexion, the cord moves anteriorly, and may become draped and stretched over retropulsed discs or osteophytes. In extension, laminar shingling leads to posterior buckling of the ligamentum flavum. Cadaveric studies suggest that neck flexion can decrease canal diameter by 10%, while extension in the presence of flaval buckling can decrease canal diameter by 24% (Chen et al., 1994). In addition to transient increases in compression, these introduce shear forces that directly alter neuronal excitability and lead to axonal injury (Shi and Pryor, 2002).

16.4.1 Intradural Processes

Multifactorial processes contribute to intraspinal pathology in DCM. Much of our understanding of ultrastructural change comes from a landmark paper in which autopsies were performed on nine patients suffering from uncorrected DCM who expired from unrelated causes (Ogino et al., 1983). Findings were stratified based on degree of spinal compression as measured by the anterior–posterior (AP) ratio, measured along all vertebral segments of the cervical spine. In cases displaying mild

(a)

(b)

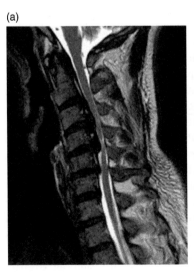
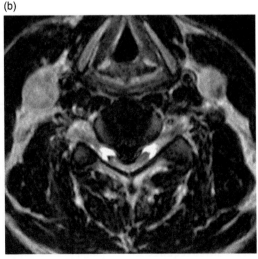

Figure 16.2 Forty-five-year-old gentleman with OPLL and progressive difficulty in ambulation and hand function. Sagittal (a) and axial MRI (b) demonstrate severe spinal cord compression

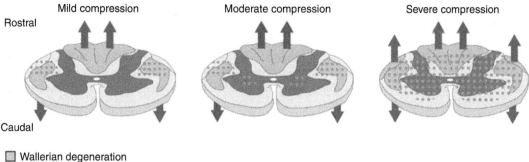

Rostral

Mild compression   Moderate compression   Severe compression

Caudal

☐ Wallerian degeneration
∴ Intrasegmental damage

Figure 16.3 Increasing compression leads to progressive damage to the white and gray matter of the cervical spine accompanied by Wallerian degeneration caudal and cephalad to the primary injury.

compression (defined as AP ratio in the neighborhood of 40%), ascending Wallerian degeneration and demyelination was observed throughout the dorsal columns above the site of maximal compression; descending degeneration was observed in the lateral corticospinal tracts (Figure 16.3). At maximally compressive levels, local infarction was observed in lateral white matter tracts. With more pronounced progression (20–40% AP ratio), local demyelination of the lateral corticospinal tracts worsened; this was accompanied by cavitation and neuronal loss in central gray matter. Even more significant compression (AP ratio < 20%) was associated with extensive necrosis and cavitation within central gray matter, as well as gliosis and necrosis of lateral and dorsal columns. Remarkably, anterior white matter tracts remained relatively well preserved across all degrees of compression.

16.4.2 Lessons From Diffusion Tensor Imaging

A strong prediction from these data is that in symptomatic patients, degree of compression would correlate not just with anatomic disruption, but with symptom severity as well. This has since been investigated using diffusion tensor imaging (DTI) in the cervical spine. Briefly, DTI visualizes white matter tracts by detecting the fractional anisotropy (FA), or asymmetric movement, of water molecules within them. In the stenotic degenerative spine, compression reduces the relative linearity of spinal white matter, lowering FA. In a longitudinal study of 66 patients with varying levels of spinal stenosis, the modified Japanese Orthopeadic Association (mJOA) score, a standardized assessment of myelopathic severity, was linearly correlated with FA to a remarkable extent (Ellingson et al., 2018). Moreover, unlike standard MRI, the microstructural pathological

alterations captured by DTI were sensitive to changes in neurological status for individual patients over time.

These ultrastructural and microstructural changes suggest a neuroanatomical basis for the symptomatology of degenerative cervical myelopathy. Spasticity likely occurs as a result of the diminished influence of lateral corticospinal tracts, and may lead to disordered recruitment of motor pools necessary for fine motor control (Adams and Hicks, 2005). This loss of descending control, as well as the dysregulation of gray matter reflexive circuits, lead to hyperreflexia (Little et al., 1999). Degradation of the dorsal columns reduces proprioceptive information sent to the central brain, disrupting closed-loop control of movement (Dietz, 2002).

16.4.3 Ischemia and Hypoxia

Spinal cord ischemia has long been proposed to play a significant pathogenic role in DCM (Brain et al., 1948), beginning in the middle of the twentieth century, with the observation of vessel wall thickening and hyalinization within the anterior spinal artery and its branching arterioles (Mair and Druckman, 1953). Further, foraminal stenosis has been shown to decrease radiculomedullary arterial diameter (Taylor, 1953); autopsy studies have demonstrated terminal branches of the anterior superior alveolar nerve and the penetrating pial plexus curved and stretched around osteophytes (Breig et al., 1966). In a canine model, the dual insults of arterial ligation and cord compression recapitulate parenchymal cavitation seen in human autopsy (Gooding et al., 2009). A working pathophysiological model (Karadimas et al., 2015) suggests that increased vascular resistance from stenosis, together with increased parenchymal pressure from direct compression, decreases cord perfusion.

Similar findings have been elucidated in humans that demonstrate a link between spinal cord ischemia and DCM. Using dynamic susceptibility contrast perfusion MRI before and after intravenous contrast administration, Ellingson et al. (2019) independently assessed both cord perfusion and hypoxia/ischemia in patients with DCM. We found that spinal cord blood volume and spinal cord relative oxygen extraction fraction (rOEF) was correlated with degree of compression as assessed by AP diameter. However, spinal cord hypoxia was not statistically correlated with the degree of spinal cord compression. Therefore, although spinal cord diameter was associated with decreased blood flow, the degree of spinal cord hypoxia is in large part dependent on the ability of the spinal cord to extract oxygen. As the spinal cord becomes more compressed and the blood flow becomes more impaired, there is an apparent stimulus to extract more oxygen form the compromised vasculature, likely a compensatory mechanism to minimize hypoxia in the face of ischemia. The spinal cord rOEF is tightly correlated with the mJOA score, with higher oxygen extraction being associated with a worse neurological status. This suggests that while stenosis may reduce blood flow, relative spinal cord deoxygenation may play an even more direct role in pathophysiology.

16.4.4 Molecular Spinal Cord Changes

Cellular biochemical changes accompany cord dysfunction. Commonly utilized to investigate the biochemistry of pathological conditions within the brain, magnetic resonance spectroscopy (MRS) provides the ability to non-invasively sample the molecular makeup within defined tissue voxels. MRS research in DCM has focused on the diagnostic and prognostic utility of metabolites with distinct signal peaks, such as N-acetyl-asparatate (NAA), choline (Cho), and lactate. N-acetyl-asparatate is found almost exclusively in neurons and axons, and a reduction of this metabolite is associated with neuronal damage commonly seen in pathological processes that damage CNS tissue. Choline is a common component of many phospholipids, and fluctuations of this marker are an indication of cellular turnover related to both membrane synthesis and degradation. A lactate peak generally indicates substantial anaerobic metabolism and a derangement in the normal cellular biochemical oxidative process.

In DCM patients, a higher spinal cord Cho/NAA ratio is significantly correlated with a poorer neurological function (Salamon et al., 2013). This cellular biomarker Cho/NAA ratio assays both the integrity of axons and neurons as well as the amount of cellular injury and turnover, and indicates that patients with either elevated choline (increased cellular injury and turnover), decreased NAA (axonal or neuronal injury), or both had more severe myelopathy. In contrast, patients with a lower Cho/NAA ratio have been found to have a greater neurological improvement following surgery (Holly et al., 2017), suggesting that this biomarker can be used to assess preoperative spinal cord viability in patients undergoing surgical intervention. The finding that DCM patients commonly have lactate peaks in their MRS spectra further implicates ischemia in the pathogenesis of this disorder (Holly et al., 2009).

16.4.5 Lessons From Spinal Cord Injury

Although DCM represents a distinct entity from traumatic spinal cord injury (SCI), parallel pathologic mechanisms are likely at play. Among these include mechanical stretch-induced axonal injury, which almost certainly occurs as part of the dynamic cord insult cascade discussed above. Electrophysiologic studies have shown stepwise aberrations in membrane properties of spinal cord white matter during stretch injury (Shi and Pryor, 2002). These include a transient increase in membrane permeability directly caused by stretch. This is followed by transient conductive failure secondary to demyelination, followed by permanent conductive failure, likely the result of direct axonal injury.

As in SCI, excitotoxicity likely plays a significant role. The cells of the central nervous system expend significant energy to maintain hyperpolarizing ionic gradients via the Na–K ATPase and other ionic channels (Stys, 1998). Disrupted energy metabolism and direct cell lysis promote an excitatory milieu. This becomes a feedforward process as more cells depolarize to excitatory thresholds, in turn releasing excitatory neurotransmitters like glutamate (Park et al., 2004). Beyond the resulting osmotic injury, there is evidence for direct ionic injury to tissue both via cations and free radicals (Stys, 1998).

There is scant evidence for necrosis as a contributing factor in DCM, except at the severe range of spinal compression. Instead, neuronal and oligodendrocytic loss likely occur via apoptosis, or programmed cell death. Oligodendrocytes are known to be particularly sensitive to ischemic changes (Karadimas et al., 2010), potentially explaining white matter demyelination observed in autopsy specimens. Experimental models demonstrate delayed apoptosis can continue to occur in the spinal cord weeks after insertion of a compressive implant (Karadimas et al., 2013). Given that apoptosis is an active process, cell loss in DCM may represent a paradoxically adaptive process to accommodate the decreased metabolic reserve of chronically hypoperfused tissue (Ellingson et al., 2019).

16.4.6 Compensatory Plasticity in the Cerebrum

The human cortex is famously plastic. Functional changes in the cortex after spinal cord injury are well established; compensatory plasticity in the setting of degenerative cervical myelopathy remains understudied. In one pioneering study, patients with clinically and radiographically confirmed DCM underwent functional magnetic resonance imaging both prior to decompressive surgery and at delayed intervals after surgical intervention (Holly et al., 2007). Compared to healthy controls, these patients displayed expanded cortical representation for motor tasks (wrist or ankle dorsiflexion) in the maximally affected extremity. Remarkably, this expanded representation regressed to resemble those of healthy controls after decompression.

This functional adaptation occurs in concert with structural changes to the brain. Utilizing DTI, synchronous microstructural cerebral white matter changes have been captured in the corticospinal tract within the internal capsule and corona radiata in DCM patients with evidence of microstructural spinal cord injury (Figure 16.4). Both spinal and cerebral DTI demonstrated proportionally similar decreases in FA that were significantly associated with a lower mJOA score and poorer neurological function. Woodworth et al. (2019) examined the relationship between myelopathic symptom severity and cortical thickness in patients with DCM compared to healthy controls. Significant atrophy was observed in brain areas critical for sensorimotor physiology. In particular, primary sensory cortex, sensorimotor precuneus, and the putaminal nucleus of the basal ganglia all displayed atrophy, the degree of which significantly was significantly correlated with mJOA score. These aforementioned studies suggest a fascinating hypothesis: although the primary pathology of DCM is localized to the spine, the capacity for functional recovery after decompressive surgery may at least depend in part on the reversibility of DCM-induced upstream micro- and microstructural cerebral alterations.

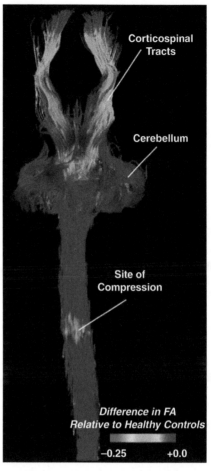

Figure 16.4 DTI tractography in a DCM patient demonstrating significant synchronous alterations in FA at the site of spinal cord compression and in the cerebral white matter

16.5 Conclusion

Movements directed by the central nervous system rely on a complex interplay between brain and spinal circuits. While the brain directs high-level features of movement, the final executor of motor commands resides at the local spinal level. Local circuits play a critical role in shaping movement and informing the brain of unforeseen error. This relationship is disrupted in DCM, in a manner predicted by ultrastructural changes to the predicted cord itself. The pathophysiology is multifactorial, initiated by bony and ligamentous processes, and propagated by compression, ischemia, biochemistry, and a host of cellular processes. The finding that DCM induces plastic changes in motor cortex that regress after decompressive surgery highlights that significant work remains in describing a complete picture of the circuit pathology inherent to degenerative cervical myelopathy. Identifying prognostic indicators of postoperative recovery remains one of the most important questions in the field.

Figure acknowledgements

The following images are credited to the authors of this chapter: Figures 16.1–16.2, 16.4
The following image has been adapted from Ogino et al., 1983: Figure 16.3

References

Adams MM, Hicks AL. Spasticity after spinal cord injury. *Spinal Cord* 2005;**43**(10):577–86. https://doi.org/10.1038/sj.sc.3101757.

Baron EM, Young WF. Cervical spondylotic myelopathy: a brief review of its pathophysiology, clinical course, and diagnosis. *Neurosurgery* 2007;**60**(1_Suppl.):35–42. https://doi.org/10.1227/01.NEU.0000215383.64386.82.

Brain R, Knight GC, Bull JWD. Discussion on rupture of the intervertebral disc in the cervical region. *J R Soc Med* 1948;**41**(8):509–16.

Breig A, Turnbull I, Hassler O. Effects of mechanical stresses on the spinal cord in cervical spondylosis. A study on fresh cadaver material. *J Neurosurg* 1966;**25**(1):45–56. https://doi.org/10.3171/jns.1966.25.1.0045.

Carette S, Fehlings MG. Cervical radiculopathy. *N Engl J Med* 2005;**353**(4):392–9. www.nejm.org/doi/abs/10.1056/NEJMcp043887

Chao EYS. Biomechanics of the human gait. In *Frontiers in Biomechanics*. Springer, 1986: 225–44. https://doi.org/10.1007/978-1-4612-4866-8_17

Chen I-H, Vasavada A, Panjabi MM. Kinematics of the cervical spine canal. *J Spinal Disord* 1994;**7**(2):93–101. http://journals.lww.com/00002517-199407020-00001

Choi BW, Song KJ, Chang H. Ossification of the posterior longitudinal ligament: a review of literature. *Asian Spine J* 2011;**5**(4):267–76. https://doi.org/10.4184/asj.2011.5.4.267.

Clarke E, Robinson PK. Cervical myelopathy: a complication of cervical spondylosis. Brain 1956;**79**(3):483–510. https://doi.org/10.1093/brain/79.3.483.

Crandall PH, Batzdorf U. Cervical spondylotic myelopathy. *J Neurosurg* 1966;**25**(1):57–66. https://doi.org/10.3171/jns.1966.25.1.0057.

Dietz V. Proprioception and locomotor disorders. *Nat Rev Neurosci* 2002;**3**(10):781–90. https://doi.org/10.1038/nrn939.

Dietz V. Spinal cord pattern generators for locomotion. *Clin Neurophysiol* 2003;**114**(8):1379–89. https://doi.org/10.1016/s1388-2457(03)00120-2.

Ellingson BM, Salamon N, Woodworth DC, Yokota H, Holly LT. Reproducibility, temporal stability, and functional correlation of diffusion MR measurements within the spinal cord in patients with asymptomatic cervical stenosis or cervical myelopathy. *J Neurosurg Spine* 2018;**28**(5):472–80. https://doi.org/10.3171/2017.7.SPINE176.

Ellingson BM, Woodworth DC, Leu K, Salamon N, Holly LT. Spinal cord perfusion MR imaging implicates both ischemia and hypoxia in the pathogenesis of cervical spondylosis. *World Neurosurg* 2019;**128**:e773–81. https://doi.org/10.1016/j.wneu.2019.04.253

Fehlings MG, Skaf G. A review of the pathophysiology of cervical spondylotic myelopathy with insights for potential novel mechanisms drawn from traumatic spinal cord injury. *Spine (Phila Pa 1976)* 1998;**23**(24):2730–7. https://doi.org/10.1097/00007632-199812150-00012.

Gooding MR, Wilson CB, Hoff JT. Experimental cervical myelopathy. Effects of ischemia and compression of the canine cervical spinal cord. *J Neurosurg* 2009;**43**(1):9–17. https://doi.org/10.3171/jns.1975.43.1.0009.

Hayashi H, Okada K, Hamada M, Tada K, Ueno R. Etiologic factors of myelopathy. A radiographic evaluation of the aging changes in the cervical spine. *Clin Orthop Relat Res* 1987;**214**:200–09. www.ncbi.nlm.nih.gov/pubmed/3791744

Henneman E, Olson CB. Relations between structure and function in the design of skeletal muscles. *J Neurophysiol* 1965;**28**:581–98. https://doi.org/10.1152/jn.1965.28.3.581.

Holly LT, Dong Y, Albistegui-Dubois R, Marehbian J, Dobkin B. Cortical reorganization in patients with cervical spondylotic myelopathy. *J Neurosurg Spine* 2007;**6**(6):544–51. https://thejns.org/view/journals/j-neurosurg-spine/6/6/article-p544.xml

Holly LT, Ellingson BM, Salamon N. Metabolic imaging using proton magnetic spectroscopy as a predictor of outcome after surgery for cervical spondylotic myelopathy. *Clin Spine Surg* 2017;**30**(5):E615–9. https://doi.org/10.1097/BSD.0000000000000248.

Holly LT, Freitas B, McArthur D, Salamon N. Proton magnetic resonance spectroscopy to evaluate spinal cord axonal injury in cervical spondylotic myelopathy. *J Neurosurg Spine* 2009;**10**:194–200. https://doi.org/10.3171/2008.12.SPINE08367.

Kandel E, Schwartz J, Jessell TM. *Principles of Neural Science.* 4th ed. New York: McGraw-Hill; 2000.

Karadimas S, Gialeli C, Klironomos G, et al. The role of oligodendrocytes in the molecular pathobiology and potential molecular treatment of cervical spondylotic myelopathy. *Curr Med Chem* 2010;**17**(11):1048–58. https://doi.org/10.2174/092986710790820598.

Karadimas SK, Gatzounis G, Fehlings MG. Pathobiology of cervical spondylotic myelopathy. *Eur Spine J* 2015;**24**(2):132–8. https://doi.org/10.1007/s00586-014-3264-4.

Karadimas SK, Moon ES, Yu WR, et al. A novel experimental model of cervical spondylotic myelopathy (CSM) to facilitate translational research. *Neurobiol Dis* 2013;54:43–58. http://dx.doi.org/10.1016/j.nbd.2013.02.013

Lemon R. Cortical control of the primate hand. *Exp Physiol* 1993;78(3):263–263. https://doi.org/10.1113/expphysiol.1993.sp003686.

Little JW, Ditunno JF, Stiens SA, Harris RM. Incomplete spinal cord injury: neuronal mechanisms of motor recovery and hyperreflexia. *Arch Phys Med Rehabil* 1999;80(5):587–99. https://doi.org/10.1016/s0003-9993(99)90204-6.

Madhav MS, Cowan NJ. The synergy between neuroscience and control theory: the nervous system as inspiration for hard control challenges. *Annu Rev Control Robot Auton Syst* 2020;3(1):243–67. https://doi.org/10.1146/annurev-control-060117-104856.

Mair WGP, Druckman R. The pathology of spinal cord lesions and their relation to the clinical features. *Brain* 1953;76(1):70–91. https://doi.org/10.1093/brain/76.1.70.

Martin J. *Neuroanatomy (Text and Atlas)*. 3rd ed. McGraw-Hill Medical; 2003.

McCormack BM, Weinstein PR. Cervical spondylosis – an update. *West J Med* 1996;165(1–2):43–51.

Mendell LM. The size principle: a rule describing the recruitment of motoneurons. *J Neurophysiol* 2005;93(6):3024–6. https://doi.org/10.1152/classicessays.00025.2005.

Mihara H, Ohnari K, Hachiya M, Kondo S, Yamada K. Cervical myelopathy caused by C3–C4 spondylosis in elderly patients: a radiographic analysis of pathogenesis. *Spine (Phila Pa 1976)* 2000;25(7):796–800. https://doi.org/10.1097/00007632-200004010-00006.

Moore AP, Blumhardt LD. A prospective survey of the causes of non-traumatic spastic paraparesis and tetraparesis in 585 patients. *Spinal Cord* 1997;35(6):361–7. https://doi.org/10.1038/sj.sc.3100422.

Muthukumar N. Ossification of the ligamentum flavum as a result of fluorosis causing myelopathy: report of two cases. *Neurosurgery* 2005;56(3):E622. https://doi.org/10.1227/01.NEU.0000154062.14313.6D.

Nurick S. The pathogenesis of the spinal cord disorder associated with cervical spondylosis. *Brain* 1972;95(1):87–100. https://doi.org/10.1093/brain/95.1.87.

Ogino H, Tada K, Okada K, et al. Canal diameter, anteroposterior compression ratio, and spondylotic myelopathy of the cervical spine. *Spine (Phila Pa 1976)* 1983;8(1):1–15. https://doi.org/10.1097/00007632-198301000-00001.

Park E, Velumian AA, Fehlings MG. The role of excitotoxicity in secondary mechanisms of spinal cord injury: a review with an emphasis on the implications for white matter degeneration. *J Neurotrauma* 2004;21(6):754–74. https://doi.org/10.1089/0897715041269641.

Rao R. Neck pain, cervical radiculopathy, and cervical myelopathy. *J Bone Jt Surg Am* 2002;84(10):1872–81. https://doi.org/10.2106/00004623-200210000-00021.

Salamon N, Ellingson BM, Nagarajan R, Gebara N, Thomas A, Holly LT. Proton magnetic resonance spectroscopy of human cervical spondylosis at 3T. *Spinal Cord* 2013;51(7):558–63. https://doi.org/10.1038/sc.2013.31.

Santillan A, Nacarino V, Greenberg E, Riina HA, Gobin YP, Patsalides A. Vascular anatomy of the spinal cord. *J Neurointerv Surg* 2012;4(1):67–74.

Sherrington CS. *The Integrative Action of the Nervous System.* Yale University Press, 1906.

Sherrington CS. Flexion–reflex of the limb, crossed extension–reflex, and reflex stepping and standing. *J Physiol* 1910;40(1–2):28–121. https://doi.org/10.1113/jphysiol.1910.sp001362.

Shi R, Pryor JD. Pathological changes of isolated spinal cord axons in response to mechanical stretch. *Neuroscience* 2002;110(4):765–77. https://doi.org/10.1016/s0306-4522(01)00596-6.

Stookey B. Compression of the spinal cord due to ventral extradural cervical chondromas: diagnosis and surgical treatment. *Arch Neurol Psychiatry* 1928;20(2):275–91. https://doi.org/10.1001/archneurpsyc.1928.02210140043003.

Stys PK. Anoxic and ischemic injury of myelinated axons in CNS white matter: from mechanistic concepts to therapeutics. *J Cereb Blood Flow Metab* 1998;18(1):2–25. https://doi.org/10.1097/00004647-199801000-00002.

Taylor AR. Mechanism and treatment of spinal-cord disorders associated with cervical spondylosis. *Lancet* 1953;261(6763):717–20. https://linkinghub.elsevier.com/retrieve/pii/S0140673653918479

Whelan PJ. Control of locomotion in the decerebrate cat. *Prog Neurobiol* 1996;49(5):481–515. https://doi.org/10.1016/0301-0082(96)00028-7.

Woodworth DC, Holly LT, Mayer EA, Salamon N, Ellingson BM. Alterations in cortical thickness and subcortical volume are associated with neurological symptoms and neck pain in patients with cervical spondylosis. *Clin Neurosurg* 2019;84(3):588–97. https://doi.org/10.1093/neuros/nyy066.

Zaaimi B, Edgley SA, Soteropoulos DS, Baker SN. Changes in descending motor pathway connectivity after corticospinal tract lesion in macaque monkey. *Brain* 2012;135(7):2277–89. https://doi.org/10.1093/brain/aws115.

Spondylolisthesis

Yike Jin, Ann Liu, Ravi Medikonda, and Timothy F. Witham

17.1 Introduction

First described in 1782 by the Belgian obstetrician Herbiniaux, spondylolisthesis is defined as the slippage of one vertebra over another. The century after Herbiniaux's description saw multiple reports on spondylolisthesis and several theories regarding its etiology. In 1963, Newman and Stone reported five types of spondylolisthesis based on a 15-year study of over 300 cases: dysplastic, isthmic, degenerative, traumatic, and pathological (Figures 17.1 and 17.2). The Wiltse classification (Table 17.1), still used today, built upon Newman and Stone's initial work (Wiltse and Winter, 1983).

17.2 Pathobiology

The spine can be simplified into three longitudinal columns of stability (the anterior, middle, and posterior spinal columns; Denis, 1983) and the three-joint complex consisting of the intervertebral disc and posterior facets (Yong-Hing and Kirkaldy-Willis, 1983). The lumbosacral

Table 17.1 Wiltse classification of spondylolisthesis (Wiltse and Winter, 1983)

Type I	Dysplastic (congenital)	Congenital dysplasia of the neural arch
Type II	Isthmic	Lesions in the pars interarticularis
A	Lytic	Separation of the pars due to a fatigue fracture
B	Elongated but intact pars	Microfractures of the pars with healing leading to elongation
C	Acute	Acute fracture secondary to severe trauma
Type III	Degenerative	Longstanding intersegmental instability
Type IV	Post traumatic	Severe injury/trauma to bones other than the pars
Type V	Pathologic	Local or general bone disease

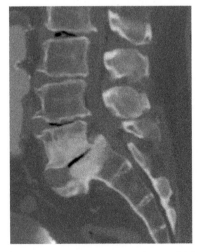

Figure 17.1 Degenerative L5–S1 spondylolisthesis.

(a) (b)

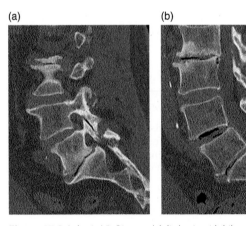

Figure 17.2 Isthmic L5–S1 spondylolisthesis with bilateral pars fractures.

spine provides stability of the axial skeleton by supporting physiological loads, preventing non-physiological motion, and protecting neural elements (Hammerberg, 2005). Static stability relies on the overall coronal and sagittal balance of the spinal column and integrity of the osteo-discal-ligamentous complex, while stability during dynamic functioning is dependent on the neuromuscular system as well as the osteo-discal-ligamentous complex (Hammerberg, 2005).

Abnormalities in these complex components can lead to pathology by altering the spine's normal biomechanics and ability to distribute force and stress. In general with spondylolisthesis, when the posterior bony elements are dissociated from the anterior column, high shear forces on the disc can lead to slippage of the vertebral bodies on one another (Hammerberg, 2005). Each subtype of spondylolisthesis has a different pathobiology. In dysplastic spondylolisthesis, dysplasia of both the lumbar and upper sacral facets predisposes L5 to slip anteriorly on the sacrum (Cunningham et al., 2020). In degenerative spondylolisthesis, the inciting pathology is disc degeneration, leading to increased stress on the facet joints and ligaments. This ultimately results in instability of the segment, which in turn promotes facet degeneration, laxity of ligaments, and osteophyte formation in an attempt to restabilize the mobile segment (Cunningham et al., 2020). In isthmic spondylolisthesis with a pars interarticular defect, the shear forces placed on the pars fracture prevent normal healing, resulting in an ineffectual lamina and pars and forward displacement of one vertebra on another (Cunningham et al., 2020).

17.3 Biomechanical Models

A limited number of biomechanical models have been developed for lumbar spondylolisthesis, primarily for degenerative and isthmic spondylolisthesis.

17.3.1 Degenerative Spondylolisthesis

To date, very few models of degenerative lumbar spondylolisthesis have been developed. In 1999, Suzuki et al. described a porcine model utilizing five lumbosacral spine specimens to assess the biomechanical properties of a posterior stabilization device. To prepare the functional L4–L5 complex, the surrounding adipose and paraspinal musculature were dissected from the complex, maintaining the ligaments, intervertebral discs, and facet joint capsules. To create the degenerative spondylolisthesis model, the posterior half of the L4–L5 intervertebral disc, the posterior longitudinal ligament (PLL), and the ligamentum were transected in the horizontal plane of the intact motion segment. The anterior longitudinal ligament (ALL), interspinous, and supraspinous ligaments were maintained. The anterior aspect of the superior articular process and the posterior aspect of the inferior articular process were also partially resected. This preparation allowed for anterior instability and migration of the L4 vertebra when flexed. Biomechanical testing was performed using an electric oil pressure servo-controlled fatigue-testing machine (Saginomiya Co., Tokyo, Japan) and allowed the motion segment to move in flexion and extension, with limited lateral bending and axial rotation. Each specimen was loaded to a combined flexion and extension bending moment of 1.9 Nm, and during this first loading cycle, the degenerative spondylolisthesis group of spines had a significantly greater mean range of motion and anterior translation, and a significantly decreased mean flexural initial stiffness (Suzuki et al., 1999).

In 2001, Crawford et al. recreated instability in human cadaveric lumbar spines by resecting tissue incrementally as follows: (1) Facets were resected using standard Kerrison rongeurs; (2) nucleus pulposus and annulus fibrosis were removed using pituitary rongeurs and curettes (a small wall of approximately 2 mm of the lateral annulus fibrosis was maintained bilaterally); and (3) ALL and PLL were separated from the vertebral body using a periosteal elevator (Crawford et al., 2001). Biomechanical testing was conducted with a standard servohydraulic test system (MTS, Minneapolis, MN) with a system of cables and pulleys. A non-contacting stereophotogrammetric optical system (Optotrak 3020, Northern Digital, Waterloo, ON, Canada) was used to monitor the 3D motion of the specimen (Crawford et al., 2001). There are several criticisms of this model compared to *in vivo* degenerative spondylolisthesis. First, the complete facetectomy used as one of the major steps of destabilization does not exist *in vivo* (Melnyk et al., 2013). Additionally, the maximal shear force of 50 N that was applied is less than what is predicted *in vivo*. Finally, no compressive force (representing body weight and muscles) was applied (Melnyk et al., 2013).

To address these criticisms, Melnyk et al. (2013) used eight human cadaveric lumbar spines, which each underwent shear and flexibility testing in five conditions:

1. Intact.
2. Both facet capsules were incised on the posterior aspect of the joint, and a 2 mm gap was created between the articular processes with a surgical burr.
3. A 4 mm gap was created between both facet joints with a surgical burr.

4. Nucleotomy was performed by resecting 2–3 mm of the inferior edge of the lamina with a Kerrison rongeur, removing ligamentum flavum, making a stab incision in the middle of the posterior annulus and PLL, and removal of the nucleus pulposus with pituitary and discectomy rongeurs.

5. The posterior annulus, PLL, and inner annular fibers were excised while the outermost anterior and lateral annular fibers were preserved.

Biomechanical testing was performed on a custom apparatus and compressive forces were applied from –50 N (posterior shear) to 250 N (anterior shear). Flexibility testing was performed on a spine motion stimulator, and a motion capture system (Optotrak 3020, Northern Digital, Waterloo, ON, Canada) was used to record the 3D motion. Under physiological shear loads, this model was able to achieve anterolisthesis of 3.1 mm (Melnyk et al., 2013).

17.3.2 Isthmic Spondylolisthesis

Ex vivo models of isthmic spondylolisthesis have been created in both immature and mature spines in an attempt to understand the patho-mechanism from spondylolysis to spondylolisthesis. Sairyo et al. used immature calf spines harvested between age 6 and 8 months (Sairyo et al., 1998). Each specimen was freed of all soft tissues except the interconnecting ligaments, intervertebral discs, and facet joints. Bilateral pars defects were created to the rostral vertebra. The specimens were then assigned to two groups: Group 1 where the disc was left intact, and Group 2 where 75% of the anterior-to-posterior depth of the disc and the ALL was dissected along the mid-disc plane, but not removed (a significant region of the nucleus was also incised). Biomechanical testing was completed with a uniaxial MTS machine (445 controller, MTS system, Minneapolis, MN). Both groups had displacement through the superior growth plate and osseous endplate of the caudal vertebra at around 980 N of anterior-posterior shearing force (Sairyo et al., 2001). A major limitation of this study is the histologic and radiologic differences between calf and human spines, and thus the study was also replicated using immature Chacma baboon spinal segments (Konz et al., 2001). Failure through the growth plate was also seen by Kajiura et al. (2001), who used immature (neonates, 2 months old, and 24 months old) calf spines and created bilateral pars defects with a drill and chisel. Biomechanical testing was completed with a uniaxial MTS machine (Test Star IIS;

MTS Systems, Minneapolis, MN) with anteroposterior shearing forces applied at a rate of 25 mm/min (Kajiura et al., 2001).

For mature spine models, Patwardhan et al. (2002) used five adult lumbar spine specimens by creating bilateral pars fractures at L5 and excising a portion of the L5–S1 nucleus. The specimens were then tested with: (1) a pure compressive load up to 1200 N, (2) a combined compressive-shear load up to 1200 N, and (3) flexion–extension moments without a compressive preload. Anterior slip of L5 was seen after a combined compressive shear load across L5–S1 (Patwardhan et al., 2002). Beadon et al. (2008) used five functional porcine spinal units with manually created defects in the disc and pars. The anterior 25% of the disc was sectioned with a scalpel at 30° to the horizontal axis. Rongeurs were used to create defects in the pars and inferior facets. A static cranial–caudal compressive load was applied via an actuator (Instron 591, Instron, Canton, MS), and a dynamic pure shear load was applied cyclically using a materials testing device (Instron 8874, Instron, Canton, MS). All specimens had bilateral fracture of the pars; continued cyclic testing lead to grade 2 isthmic spondylolisthesis (Beadon et al., 2008).

A few *in vivo* models have been described. Österman et al. (1996) operated on 31 rabbits at the age of 4 weeks and divided into three groups. In Group A, the L7–S1 level was exposed and the L7 inferior articular processes were resected bilaterally with disruption of the facet joint capsules (referred to as posterior element disruption). In Group B, posterior element disruption as well as L6–L7 fusion with wiring and polymethylmethacrylate application were performed. In Group C, posterior element disruption with an L7–S1 disc herniation was performed. The rabbits were followed up to 6 months until adulthood. All groups had statistically significant ventral slipping of L7, despite the lack of compressive loading and extension/ flexion stress associated with an upright spine (Österman et al., 1996). Sakamaki et al. (2003) used 4- and 26-week-old Wistar rats who underwent L5 laminectomy and bilateral L5–L6 facetectomy. Both L5 vertebral slippage and deformities of the L6 vertebral body were seen in young rats not adult rats, mimicking those seen in pediatric patients with spondylolysis (Sakamaki et al., 2003).

17.4 Clinical Research

17.4.1 Degenerative Spondylolisthesis

The Spine Patient Outcomes Research Trial (SPORT) was a large multicenter prospective trial which was designed to compare the effectiveness of surgery and non-surgical management of spinal stenosis, intervertebral disc herniation, and degenerative spondylolisthesis whose results were first published in 2006 (Weinstein et al., 2006). Of the patients enrolled in SPORT, 607 had degenerative spondylolisthesis and were split between a randomization cohort ($n = 304$) who were randomized to either surgical treatment (of either decompression and fusion or decompression alone) or non-operative management and an observational cohort who were not randomized. The as-treated analysis demonstrated significant advantage for surgery at 3 months, 1 year, and 2 year follow-up when considering the primary outcomes of Short Form Health Survey (SF-36) and Oswestry Disability Index (ODI).

Given this demonstrated advantage of surgery, one of the next points of debate in the treatment of degenerative spondylolisthesis is the role of instrumented fusion. The North American Spine Society (NASS) guidelines updated in 2014 gave Grade B recommendations that suggested that surgical decompression and fusion, with or without instrumentation, for patients with symptomatic lumbar stenosis and degenerative lumbar spondylolisthesis lead to better clinic outcomes than decompression alone (Matz et al., 2016). The guidelines also suggested that instrumentation increases the chance of overall fusion in these surgeries.

Shortly after this update, in 2016, two randomized control studies published in the *New England Journal of Medicine* (NEJM) had conflicting conclusions on this topic. Ghogawala and colleagues conducted a randomized control trial (SLIP trial) with 66 patients with symptomatic lumbar stenosis and stable lumbar spondylolisthesis to either decompression only or decompression and posterolateral fusion with SF-36 and ODI at 2 years after surgery being the primary and secondary outcomes (Ghogawala et al., 2016). SLIP reported a statistically significant 5.7 point average increase in change of SF-36 scores with the fusion group compared to the decompression only group at 2-year follow-up which was increased to 6.7 points at 4-year follow-up. At 4-year follow-up there was also noted to be an average 9-point improvement in ODI when comparing patients who underwent fusion compared to decompression alone. The cumulative reoperative rate was also noted to be significantly higher in the decompression only group (34% versus 15%, $p < 0.05$), which taken in context with the other findings suggests a clinically significant advantage to instrumented fusion compared to decompression alone.

Försth and colleagues conducted a similar trial with conflicting results. Their study was a randomized control study design that included 247 patients with lumbar stenosis (cross-section of dural sac <75 mm), of which 135 were determined to have degenerative spondylolisthesis (>3 mm displacement; Försth et al., 2016). Patients were enrolled from seven Swedish hospitals, and after being stratified by the presence of spondylolisthesis were randomized to either decompression only or decompression with fusion with the primary outcome being ODI scores at 2 years and 5 years after surgery. Secondary outcomes included scores from European Quality of Life–5 Dimensions (EQ-5D), visual-analogue scales (VAS) for back and leg pain, and the Zurich Claudication Questionnaire (ZCQ), which is another measurement of disability. At 2 years after surgery, Försth and colleagues reported no significant difference in ODI scores between spondylolisthesis patients who underwent decompression versus decompression and fusion (21 ± 18 versus 25 ± 19, $p = 0.11$), and differences in the secondary outcomes such as EQ-5D (0.63 ± 0.31 versus 0.69 ± 0.28, $p = 0.20$), ZCQ and VASs were similarly not significant. Although only 144 of the total 247 patients were enrolled early enough for 5-year follow-up, the trend of insignificance between ODIs from the two treatment groups persisted. Försth and colleagues also accentuated the differences in terms of resource use between the two arms with significant increases in length of hospital stay (7.4 ± 8.4 versus 4.1 ± 6.1, $p < 0.001$) and average operation costs ($\$12,200$ versus $\$5,400$) when comparing fusion with decompression only. At 2 years after surgery it was also noted that there was no significant difference between the use of auxiliary health services/benefits such as number of outpatient visits, sick leave benefits, or chronic opioid use.

Systematic reviews and meta-analyses have sought to try to reconcile these seemingly conflicting conclusions. Liang and colleagues published a meta-analysis in 2017 which reviewed four randomized control trials and 13 observational studies comparing decompression and fusion with decompression alone and demonstrated that patient satisfaction rates were significantly higher among patients who underwent decompression and fusion (risk ratio (RR) 0.87; 95% confidence interval (CI) 0.76, 0.99; $I^2 = 49\%$; $p = 0.04$) and leg pain scores were significantly more improved when compared to decompression alone (standardized mean differences (SMD) 0.11; 95% CI 0.03, 0.19; $I^2 = 0\%$; $p = 0.005$) (Liang et al., 2017). It is important to note that no significant differences were found in ODI, back pain score, reoperation rate, or complication rates.

17.4.2 Isthmic Spondylolisthesis

The literature for isthmic spondylolisthesis focuses primarily on exploring the relative efficacy of various surgical procedures for fusion (Noorian et al., 2018). Several studies have demonstrated that surgical reduction, while conferring better radiographic outcomes, does not significantly affect clinical outcomes when compared to *in situ* fusion. Lian and colleagues demonstrated that in 88 patients with isthmic spondylolisthesis, those who had *in situ* fusions had non-inferior VAS, ODI, and Japanese Orthopedic Association (JOA) scores, and had a similar incidence of surgical complications (Lian et al., 2014). When considering various types of fusion surgery, studies have suggested the that use of an interbody may improve overall outcomes. Cunningham and Robertson (2011) demonstrated in a prospective cohort observational study with mean follow-up of 94 months that patients who underwent posterior lumbar interbody fusion (PLIF) had significantly improved pain and function scores as measured by Low Back Outcome Score (LBOS) and (SF)-12v2. To date, the literature remains relatively heterogeneous in reporting outcomes with regard to different surgical approaches such as ALIF, PLIF, and TLIF (Kim et al., 2009, 2010; Yang et al., 2016), and there are insufficient data to support relative superiority of any one approach.

17.5 Challenges and Future Work

Given the heterogeneity of its pathobiology, spondylolisthesis has been a difficult disease pathology to model in the laboratory. One major criticism of the use of animal models is the subtle differences between animal spine and human spine anatomy. Additionally, most of the models described are done *ex vivo*, relying on machines to simulate the variety of forces exerted on the spine. Degenerative spondylolisthesis is also particularly challenging to replicate as it is due to years of degeneration and tissue adaptation. Further work is needed to develop better models to accurately replicate the various types of spondylolisthesis in order to better study this spine pathology.

From a clinical research standpoint, further large randomized control studies are needed to assess not only the efficacy of more modern techniques of treatments of spondylolisthesis but also the longitudinal socioeconomic impact of various treatments options. While existing trials have touched upon the potential cost of medical management and various surgical approaches, further work is needed to better quantify the effect of recovery time, lost work efficiency/days, complications and need for reoperation, and need for long-term follow-up into the overall calculus of impact on healthcare and the workforce.

17.6 Treatment

Despite the utility of non-operative treatments in symptomatic management, the mainstay treatment for refractory spondylolisthesis remains surgical. While there is still a lack of overwhelming consensus on the optimal surgical approach, studies have suggested that decompression and fusion procedures seem to be correlated with increased patient satisfaction and possibly improved clinical function scores on validated questionnaires. *In situ* fusions have been shown to be non-inferior to fusion with reduction, but data do suggest that fusions with use of an interbody are associated with better long-term pain and function outcomes.

Figure acknowledgements

The following images obtained with consent are credited to the authors of this chapter: Figures 17.1-17.2

References

Beadon K, Johnston JD, Siggers K, et al. A repeatable *ex vivo* model of spondylolysis and spondylolisthesis. *Spine* 2008;33:2387–93. https://doi.org/10.1097/BRS.0b013e318184e775.

Crawford NR, Cagli S, Sonntag VK, Dickman CA. Biomechanics of grade I degenerative lumbar spondylolisthesis. Part 1: *in vitro* model. *J Neurosurg* 2001;94:45–50. https://doi.org/10.3171/spi.2001.94.1.0045.

Cunningham, B, Mueller K, Hawken J. Biomechanical considerations and mechanisms of injury in spondylolisthesis. *Semin Spine Surg* 2020;32:100803.

Cunningham J, Robertson P. Long-term outcomes following lumbar spine fusion for adult isthmic spondylolisthesis: a comparison of PLIF versus PLF. *Spine J* 2011;11:S135. https://doi.org/10.1016/j.spinee.2011.08.327.

Denis F. The three column spine and its significance in the classification of acute thoracolumbar spinal injuries. *Spine* 1983;8:817–31. https://doi.org/10.1097/00007632-198311000-00003.

Försth P, Ólafsson G, Carlsson T, et al. A randomized, controlled trial of fusion surgery for lumbar spinal stenosis. N Engl J Med 2016;374(15):1413–23. https://doi.org/10.1056/NEJMoa1513721.

Ghogawala Z, Dziura J, Butler WE, et al. Laminectomy plus fusion versus laminectomy alone for lumbar spondylolisthesis. *N Engl J Med* 2016;374(15):1424–34. https://doi.org/10.1056/NEJMoa1508788.

Hammerberg KW. New concepts on the pathogenesis and classification of spondylolisthesis. *Spine* 2005;**30**:S4–11. https://doi.org/10.1097/01.brs.0000155576.62159.1c.

Herbiniaux G. *Traite sur Divers Accouchements Laborieux, et sur les Polypes de la Matrice.* JL DeBoubers, 1782.

Kajiura K, Katoh S, Sairyo K, Ikata T, Goel VK, Murakami RI. Slippage mechanism of pediatric spondylolysis: biomechanical study using immature calf spines. *Spine* 2001;**26**:2208–13. https://doi.org/10.1097/00007632-200110150-00010.

Kim JS, Kim DH, Lee SH. Comparison between instrumented Mini-TLIF and instrumented circumferential fusion in adult low-grade lytic spondylolisthesis: can mini-TLIF with PPF replace circumferential fusion? *J Korean Neurosurg Soc* 2009;**45** (2):74–80. https://doi.org/10.3340/jkns.2009.45.2.74.

Kim JS, Lee KY, Lee SH, Lee HY. Which lumbar interbody fusion technique is better in terms of level for the treatment of unstable isthmic spondylolisthesis? J Neurosurg Spine 2010;**12** (2):171–7. https://doi.org/10.3171/2009.9.SPINE09272.

Konz RJ, Goel VK, Grobler LJ, et al. The pathomechanism of spondylolytic spondylolisthesis in immature primate lumbar spines *in vitro* and finite element assessments. *Spine* 2001;**26**: E38–49. https://doi.org/10.1097/00007632-200102150-00003.

Lian XF, Hou TS, Xu JG, et al. Single segment of posterior lumbar interbody fusion for adult isthmic spondylolisthesis: reduction or fusion in situ. *Eur Spine J* 2014;**23**(1):172–9. https://doi.org/10.1007/s00586-013-2858-6.

Liang HF, Liu SH, Chen ZX, Fei QM. Decompression plus fusion versus decompression alone for degenerative lumbar spondylolisthesis: a systematic review and meta-analysis. *Eur Spine J* 2017;**26**(12):3084–95. https://doi.org/10.1007/s00586-017-5200-x.

Matz PG, Meagher RJ, Lamer T, et al. Guideline summary review: an evidence-based clinical guideline for the diagnosis and treatment of degenerative lumbar spondylolisthesis. *Spine J* 2016;**16**:439–48. https://doi.org/10.1016/j.spinee.2015.11.055.

Melnyk AD, Kingwell SP, Zhu Q, et al. An *in vitro* model of degenerative lumbar spondylolisthesis. *Spine* 2013;**38**:E870–E877. https://doi.org/10.1097/BRS.0b013e3182945897.

Newman PH, Stone KH. The etiology of spondylolisthesis with a special investigation. *J Bone Joint Surg* 1963;**45**:39–59. https://doi.org/10.1302/0301-620X.45B1.39.

Noorian S, Sorensen K, Cho W. A systematic review of clinical outcomes in surgical treatment of adult isthmic spondylolistesis. *Spine J* 2018;**18**(8):1441–54. https://doi.org/10.1016/j.spinee.2018.04.022.

Österman K, Österman H. Experimental lumbar spondylolisthesis in growing rabbits. *Clin Orthop Relat Res* 1996;**332**:274–80.

Patwardhan A, Ghanayem A, Simonds J, et al. An experimental model of adult-onset slip progression in isthmic spondylolistesis. *Stud Health Technol Inform* 2002;**91**:322–4.

Sairyo K, Goel VK, Grobler LJ, et al. The pathomechanism of isthmic lumbar spondylolisthesis. A biomechanical study in immature calf spines. *Spine* 1998;**23**:1442–6. https://doi.org/10.1097/00007632-199807010-00002.

Sakamaki T, Sairyo K, Katoh S, et al. The pathogenesis of slippage and deformity in the pediatric lumbar spine: a radiographic and histologic study using a new rat *in vivo* model. *Spine* 2003;**28**:645–51. https://doi.org/10.1097/01.BRS.0000051915.35828.17.

Suzuki K, Mochida J, Chiba M, Kikugawa H. Posterior stabilization of degenerative lumbar spondylolisthesis with a Leeds–Keio artificial ligament. A biomechanical analysis in a porcine vertebral model. *Spine* 1999;**24**:26–31. https://doi.org/10.1097/00007632-199901010-00007.

Weinstein JN, Tosteson TD, Lurie JD, et al. Surgical vs nonoperative treatment for lumbar disk herniation: the Spine Patient Outcomes Research Trial (SPORT): a randomized trial. *JAMA* 2006;**296**:2441–50. https://doi.org/ 10.1001/jama.296.20.2451.

Wiltse LL, Winter RB. Terminology and measurement of spondylolisthesis. *J Bone Joint Surg Am* 1983;**65**:768–72.

Yang EZ, Xu JG, Liu XK, et al. An RCT study comparing the clinical and radiological outcomes with the use of PLIF or TLIF after instrumented reduction in adult isthmic spondylolisthesis. *Eur Spine J* 2016;**25**(5):1587–94. https://doi.org/10.1007/s00586-015-4341-z.

Yong-Hing K, Kirkaldy-Willis WH. The pathophysiology of degenerative disease of the lumbar spine. *Orthop Clin North Am* 1983;**14**:491–504.

Chapter 18

Radiculopathy

Yingda Li and Michael Y. Wang

18.1 Introduction

Radiculopathy refers to pathology at the nerve root level, manifest as positive symptoms such as pain, paresthesias and dysesthesias, and negative symptoms such as numbness and weakness. While a number of causes for radiculopathy exist (Table 18.1), the archetypal etiology is lumbar disc herniation, leading to compression of the traversing or, less commonly, exiting nerve root. Such mechanical bases for radiculopathy were first recognized nearly a century ago, initially in the lumbar region by Mixter and Barr (1934), followed by the cervical spine by Semmes and Murphey in 1943.

As experience increased and matured, however, it became clear that a purely mechanical basis for radiculopathy was insufficient to explain a number of common clinical observations. First, the natural history of acute radiculopathy related to disc herniation remained favorable in the majority of patients (in the order of 80%), and that symptomatic improvement occurred despite non-surgical measures, i.e., without directly addressing the presumed offending compression (Weinstein et al., 2006). While spontaneous disc resorption was sometimes observed, clinical improvement usually preceded radiographic resolution (Komori et al., 1996). Furthermore, the predilection for certain types of disc herniations to

resorb, including sequestered fragments (Komori et al., 1996) and those that contrast enhanced (Komori et al., 1998), pointed to a peculiar, vascularized local microenvironment. In response, an additional chemical theory was proposed in the 1970s (Marshall and Trethewie, 1973).

Other apparently counterintuitive observations included a bi-directional discord between clinical and radiological severity, such as why some patients with significant stenosis on imaging remained asymptomatic (Brinjikji et al., 2015), yet others with seemingly innocuous findings such as annular fissures presented, on occasion, with debilitating radicular pain (Peng et al., 2007). In addition, the propensity for foraminal and extra-foraminal disc herniations to cause exquisite pain (Lejeune et al., 1994), as well as relatively high rates of dysesthesia following intraoperative manipulation (Yeung and Tsou, 2002; Figure 18.1), cultivated interest in the dorsal root ganglion (DRG), housed within the intervertebral foramen, as a key pathogenic structure, particularly in chronic neuropathic pain (Krames, 2014).

In this chapter, we begin by addressing the mechanical and chemical theories of radiculopathy and the animal models that led to them. This is followed by a discussion of potential mechanisms leading to chronic neuropathic pain and central sensitization, specifically in the context of radiculopathy. The unique features of the DRG are highlighted, as well as its potential role in sensitization and symptom maintenance. Specific clinical corollaries of pathophysiologic data are illuminated as they arise. We conclude by highlighting some of the knowledge gaps that currently exist, and suggest areas for future research.

18.2 Mechanical Basis for Radiculopathy

A mechanical basis remains the oldest and perhaps most intuitive and widely accepted of radiculopathy theories; the often observed immediate relief of radicular pain following discectomy attests to its cogency. The earliest animal experiments on mechanical radiculopathy came in the

Table 18.1 Select causes of radiculopathy

Cause	Subtype
Disc herniation	Paracentral
Stenosis	Foraminal
Tumor	Extra-foraminal
Trauma	Lateral recess
Infection	Foraminal
Miscellaneous, including	Dynamic, e.g., spondylolisthesis
non-compressive causes	Benign, e.g., Schwannoma
	Malignant, e.g., metastasis
	Iatrogenic
	Epidural scar
	Chemical radiculitis including bone morphogenetic protein

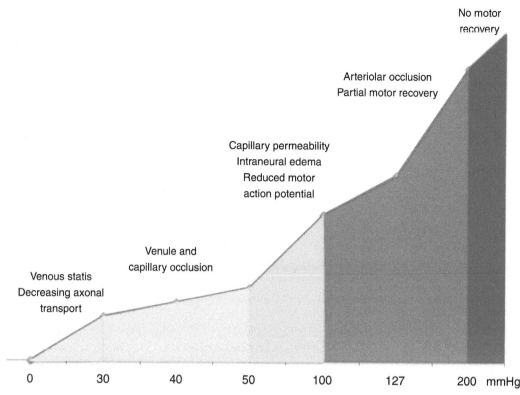

No motor
recovery

Arteriolar occlusion
Partial motor recovery

Capillary permeability
Intraneural edema
Reduced motor
action potential

Venule and
capillary occlusion

Venous statis
Decreasing axonal
transport

| 0 | 30 | 40 | 50 | 100 | 127 | 200 | mmHg |

Figure 18.1 Summary of findings of the Swedish balloon compression experiments, correlating graded mechanical compression (measured in mmHg) with vascular compromise, edema, and electrophysiologic decrement. While not illustrated here, the acuity of compression played an equally, if not more important, role.

form of a canine model, correlating neural deformation with reversible conduction block, conducted by Gelfan and Tarlov in the 1950s (Gelfan and Tarlov, 1956). However, the first sham-controlled studies systematically addressing the various end-organ effects of nerve root compression were not conducted until the late 1980s at the University of Gothenburg in Sweden (Olmarker, 1991).

18.2.1 Balloon Compression Model

In their porcine model, employing an inflatable balloon secured to the coccygeal epidural space, Olmarker and Rydivek et al. systematically assessed the effects of graded cauda equina compression on local hemodynamics, electrophysiology, and histopathology (Olmarker et al., 1989a, 1989b, 1990b). Several vital observations were made. First, susceptibility to compression varied between different components of the local vasculature, with cessation of flow occurring much earlier in venules and capillaries than their arteriolar counterparts (Olmarker et al., 1989b). Second, reductions in nutritional delivery,

assessed using a tagged analog for glucose and oxygen, appeared to correlate with both degree as well as, and perhaps more importantly, acuity of compression (Olmarker et al., 1990b). This latter finding was replicated when intraneural edema was assessed using Evans blue dye, with extravasation more pronounced following rapid and sustained compression (Olmarker et al., 1989a). Furthermore, while reductions in motor action potentials correlated with both acuity and magnitude, irreversibility was only observed in the rapid compression group (Olmarker et al., 1990a). Taken together, these findings supported a time-sensitive compression effect, and were the first to shed scientific light on certain clinical conundrums, including why some patients with severe, albeit chronic radiological stenosis remained clinically indolent, while others with acute disc herniations suffered debilitating pain and, on occasion, significant neurological deficit that never completely recovered. Figure 18.2 summarizes the key findings from this seminal series of experiments.

255

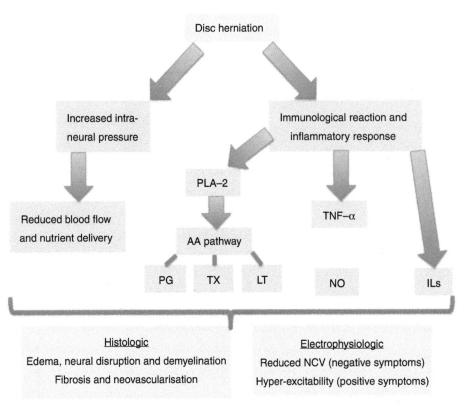

Figure 18.2 Summary of the mechanical (green) and chemical (red) bases of radiculopathy. Abbreviations: AA, arachidonic acid; IL, interleukin; LT, leukotriene; NCV, nerve conduction velocity; nitric oxide; PG, prostaglandin; PLA-2, phospholipase A2, TNF-a, tumor necrosis factor alpha; TX, thromboxane.

18.2.2 Other Mechanical Models

In addition to the balloon compression paradigm, other mechanical models were developed over time. Using ameroid constrictors, the same research group demonstrated early and late histologic changes following compression, with nerve fiber disruption, hyperemia, and hemorrhage by 1 week, and demyelination, fibrosis, and neovascularization by 4 weeks (Cornefjord et al., 1997). Rat studies using silk ligation were some of the first to study the behavioral effects of compression, correlating degree of neural deformation with severity of mechanical allodynia (Winkelstein et al., 2002), while others employing a stainless steel rod inserted into the intervertebral foramen led to thermal hyperalgesia as well as a hyperexcitable and aberrantly firing DRG (Hu and Xing, 1998). This unique electrosensitivity of the DRG will be expanded upon later in its dedicated section.

18.2.3 Structural Susceptibility of Nerve Roots to Compression

These extrinsic compression models, however, only formed one part of the equation, another crucial component being the unique microstructural vulnerabilities of the nerve root and the macroscopic stressors placed upon it in disease states. First, in contrast to their peripheral nerve counterparts (compression of which led more commonly to sensory disturbance than pain per se), nerve roots lack well-developed peri- and epineuria, potentially rendering them more susceptible to mechanical injury (Rydevik et al., 1984). Second, vascular supply to nerve roots is inherently more tenuous, including a hypovascular "watershed zone" irrigated internally from the vasa corona of the spinal cord and externally via radicular arteries coursing through the intervertebral foramina (Olmarker, 1991). In a porcine model, clip ligation of the root as it exited its foramen led to nearly twice the reduction in blood flow than when applied as it entered more proximally (Naito et al., 1990).

Furthermore, nerve roots (and DRG) are held within a relatively rigid nerve root sheath, analogous to the denticulate ligaments of the spinal cord of pial origin, while studies of intraoperative nerve tension in patients with compressive pathology demonstrated nerve "flattening" and loss of physiological "glide" (Smith et al., 1993),

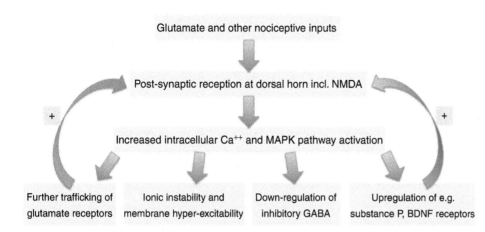

Figure 18.3 Mechanisms involved in the initial phases of central sensitization. BDNF, brain-derived neurotrophic factor; Ca++, calcium; GABA, γ-amino-butyric acid; MAPK, mitogen-activated protein kinase; NMDA, N-methyl-D-aspartate.

often "tethered" by periradicular adhesive tissue, with concomitant reductions in intraradicular blood flow (Kobayashi et al., 2003) and nerve conduction (Kobayashi et al., 2010). The contribution of the ventral dural ligaments (of Hofmann; Wadhwani et al., 2004) may further impede nerve root movement.

Despite this growing body of evidence supporting a mechanical basis for radiculopathy, the need for an additional trigger has long been recognized, dating back to human studies conducted in the 1950s, in which postoperative tension exerted on normal lumbar roots via intraoperatively placed nylon threads failed to elicit symptoms (Smyth and Wright, 1958), while more recently manipulation of normal roots during lumbar surgery performed under local anesthesia produced paresthesias but seldom pain (Kuslich et al., 1991). All of these pointed to an alternative non-mechanical pathway by which radicular symptoms developed.

18.3 Chemical Basis for Radiculopathy

Despite inflammatory reactions at laminectomy being first detected in the 1950s and use of epidural steroid injections in the treatment of radicular pain being mainstream for over half a century (Stafford et al., 2007), rigorous scientific evidence supporting a chemical basis for radiculopathy (Figure 18.3) has only been established over the last two decades or so (Olmarker et al., 1993).

18.3.1 Nucleus Pulposus as Chemically Active

In landmark studies conducted by the same Swedish group that drove the mechanical theory, small volumes of non-compressive nucleus pulposus were harvested from porcine disc and placed epidurally, and its effects

compared to autologous fat (Olmarker et al., 1993). Nerve conduction velocities, along with blood flow, were significantly reduced in the disc group, while endoneurial pressures were significantly increased. Systemic administration of the anti-inflammatory methylprednisolone seemingly restored nerve conduction (Olmarker et al., 1994), while also reducing vascular permeability (Byröd et al., 2000). These electrophysiologic derangements were replicated in canine models in which the annulus was simply incised, along with axonal disruption and vascular stasis (Kayama et al., 1996), supporting potential cytokine "leak" as a possible source for the radicular pain occasionally witnessed in patients with annular tears. Studies that followed suggested a potentially synergistic effect when nerve roots were exposed to both disc material as well as mechanical compression, manifesting as reduced conduction velocities (Takahashi et al., 2003), more pronounced spontaneous pain behaviors (Olmarker et al., 2002), allodynia and hyperalgesia, and increased expression of nerve growth factor (NGF; Onda et al., 2005), which, as we shall later see, may be an important chemical mediator in sensitization. In further support of the nucleus pulposus being chemically active, studies deploying cultured cells continued to show dampened nerve conduction (Kayama et al., 1998), while those using disc material subjected to freezing (leading to cell lysis) did not (Olmarker et al., 1997).

18.3.2 Possible Immunologic Response

Two conclusions could be drawn from these data: that the disc itself contains pro-inflammatory cytokines, or that the disc provokes an immunologic response and activation of the inflammatory cascade occurs secondarily. While the latter hypothesis seems counterintuitive given the autologous source of disc material, one must remember the relatively avascular and potentially immunologically "privileged" environment in which it normally resides, i.e., within the confines of the annulus. Possible autoantibodies to disc material have been found in both humans (Marshall et al., 1977) and rabbits (Bobechko and Hirsch, 1965) dating back to the 1960s. More recently, antibodies to glycosphingolipids, ubiquitous in cell membranes and detected in autoimmune conditions such as Guillain–Barre syndrome, were detected in the serum of patients undergoing lumbar discectomy (Brisby et al., 2002).

18.3.3 Tumor Necrosis Factor Alpha

A number of chemical mediators have been implicated in radiculopathy, although it remains unclear as to their exact position within the inflammatory "chain of events," including whether they originate from the disc itself. One of the key cytokines appears to be tumor necrosis factors (TNF-α), initially put forth due to the striking similarity between its effects on neural tissue and those aforementioned of the nucleus pulposus, including increased vascular permeability, demyelination, hypercoagulability, and hyperalgesia, as well as their responsiveness to anti-inflammatory and immuno-modulatory therapies (Mulleman et al., 2006). TNF-α has, in fact, been detected in the nucleus pulposus of pigs, and its antagonism by doxycycline led to reversal of disc-induced reductions in nerve conduction (Olmarker and Larsson, 1998), although it must be conceded that this drug non-selectively inhibits a number of other cytokines. Furthermore, nitric oxide (NO), which is upregulated by TNF-α and mediates a significant proportion of its inflammatory effects, has been identified in human disc herniations (Kang et al., 1996), while recent trials evaluating the epidural administration of etanercept, a potent TNF-α inhibitor, have shown promising results in patients with radicular pain when compared to corticosteroids, which form the current standard of care (Ohtori et al., 2012).

18.3.4 Phospholipase A2

Evidence also supports phospholipase A2 (PLA-2) being an important chemical mediator of radiculopathy. Phospholipase A2, which has been detected in high concentrations in human disc herniations (Saal et al., 1990), liberates arachidonic acid (AA), the precursor to prostaglandins (PG), leukotrienes (LT) and thromboxane (TX),

which have all been found in disc specimens, namely PGE2, LT-B4 and TX-B2 (Kang et al., 1996; Nygaard et al., 1997). Inhibition of cyclooxygenase (COX), which catalyzes the AA pathway, restored nerve conduction and reduced hyperalgesia in porcine, canine, and rodent nucleus pulposus models using diclofenac (Cornefjord et al., 2002), indomethacin (Arai et al., 2004) and an epidural COX-2 inhibitor (Kawakami et al., 2002), respectively. Furthermore, PLA-2 applied to the rat epidural space produced significant electrical hyperexcitability, sensorimotor deficit as well as demyelination (Chen et al., 1997), while chymopapain, a now largely obsolete agent previously used in chemonucleolysis, reduced PLA-2 activity in rat sciatic nerves subject to the inflammatory effects of chromic gut (Sawin et al., 1997), offering a possible explanation as to why clinical response to chymopapain often preceded reduction in disc size. Furthermore, the hyperalgesic effects of chromic gut loosely placed around lumbar roots were attenuated by epidural injection of betamethasone, corresponding with reductions in PLA-2 activity (Lee et al., 1998). Importantly, this identification of PLA-2 in non-discogenic models suggests that the chemical theory is more broadly applicable to other causes of radiculopathy.

18.3.5 Other Candidate Cytokines

A number of other cytokines have been detected in human disc herniations, both lumbar and cervical, including inter-leukins (IL) 1α, 1β, 6, and 8, and matrix metalloproteinases (MMPs; Kang et al., 1995; Kang et al., 1996; Takahashi et al., 1996). Matrix metalloproteinases have been implicated in disc resorption (Haro et al., 2000), while IL-6 has been detected in the cerebrospinal fluid of patients with lumbar stenosis (Ohtori et al., 2011). Similar cytokine profiles have been found in the epidural lavage of rats subjected to chemical irritation by nucleus pulposus (Cuéllar et al., 2013), although replicating this result in humans has thus far proved elusive (Scuderi et al., 2006). The inflammatory cell most commonly isolated in disc herniations and implicated in cytokine production has been the macrophage (Mulleman et al., 2006).

Crucially, a difference in cytokine expression between contained and non-contained discs has been demonstrated (Nygaard et al., 1997), including in comparisons with "healthy" discs removed as part of surgery for cervical burst fractures (Kang et al., 1995). These findings lend further support to exposure of previously insulated disc material to the vascularized epidural environment being a necessary inciting event in the chemical theory.

18.4 Chronic Neuropathic Pain and Central Sensitization

While mechanical and chemical theories may sufficiently account for some of the acute manifestations of radiculopathy, the mechanisms underlying the transition from an acute to chronic neuropathic state have received significantly less attention, despite chronic spine-related pain being the most disabling condition worldwide (Driscoll et al., 2014). Experimental evidence on this subject has largely been borrowed and extrapolated from models of peripheral nerve injury, i.e., distal to the DRG. Before proceeding further, however, it is prudent to offer some definitions of relevant terminology.

18.4.1 Definition of Chronic Neuropathic Pain and Central Sensitization

Chronic neuropathic pain, as defined by the International Association for the Study of Pain (IASP), refers to pain caused by any condition involving the somatosensory system lasting for more than 3 months (Scholz et al., 2019), of which chronic painful radiculopathy is a subtype. Central sensitization refers to a state of hyperresponsiveness of nociceptive neurons in the central nervous system (CNS) to normal or subthreshold afferent input, hallmarked by hyperalgesia (heightened response to normally painful stimuli, usually assessed using thermal means) and allodynia (pain in response to customarily non-painful stimuli, usually assessed using mechanical stressors) (IASP, n.d.). While hyperalgesia and allodynia are often cited in chronic neuropathic pain, which may be driven by central sensitization, they are neither necessary nor sufficient for its diagnosis. Furthermore, in the context of chronic radiculopathy, the unique mechanical and chemical effects of persistent compressive pathology, such as disc herniation, remain unclear. Despite this, an understanding of central sensitization, and the resultant "uncoupling" between stimulus intensity (or even presence) and symptom severity, may be key to explaining the dreaded (but thankfully uncommon) observation of certain patients never improving following onset of radiculopathy, even in spite of surgery (which is a "peripheral" intervention).

18.4.2 Secondary Hyperalgesia Versus Deviations From Foerster and Keegan–Garrett Maps

Fundamentally, central sensitization represents activity-dependent plasticity following neural injury, usually localized to the dorsal horn in the literature, recruiting previously subthreshold synaptic inputs to nociceptive neurons, generating augmented action potentials (Woolf, 2011). In addition to hyperalgesia and allodynia, central sensitization may manifest as secondary hyperalgesia, that is, painful response to stimulus outside of the zone supplied by the initially injured neural pathway (IASP, n.d.). This must be differentiated from radicular pain patterns that deviate from classical Foerster (1933) and Keegan and Garrett (1948) maps (derived from dorsal root sectioning and disc herniation studies, respectively), which may be explained by variations in plexus organization and intradural connections between rootlets (McAnany et al., 2019). Furthermore, pain specifically in the scapular region often occurs as part of cervical radiculopathy, likely owing to the distribution of the corresponding dorsal rami (Tanaka et al., 2006).

18.4.3 Mechanisms of Central Sensitization

Molecular mechanisms for central sensitization have been established (Figure 18.4), with perhaps the glutamate-NMDA receptor (N-methyl-D-aspartate) stream the most well-known, leading to increased intracellular calcium and converging on mitogen-activated protein kinase (MAPK) pathways that effect trafficking of further glutamate receptors to the cell membrane, including AMPA (α-amino-3-hydroxy-5-methyl-4-isoxazolepropionic acid), as well as transcriptional upregulation of nociceptive and growth factor receptors, deprivation of the stabilizing potassium, and downregulation of the inhibitory GABA (γ-amino-butyric acid) (Woolf, 2011). (Interestingly, the gabapentinoids commonly used to treat neuropathic pain, while initially designed to be analogs of GABA, appear to exact their action via inactivation of voltage-gated calcium channels; Rose and Kam, 2002.) Other implicated receptors and mediators include metabotropic glutamate receptors (mGluR), substance P, calcitonin gene-related peptide (CGRP) and brain-derived neurotrophic factor (BDNF) (Latremoliere and Woolf, 2009). A positive feedback loop is thus created and maintenance of postsynaptic hyperexcitability ensues. Over time, potentiation, both homo- (leading to "windup" pain) and heterosynaptic, with the more deeply seated Aβ fibers (usually associated with touch) sprouting into more superficial cord laminae normally occupied by nociceptive c-fiber terminals, resulting in a phenotypic "switch" (Woolf, 2011).

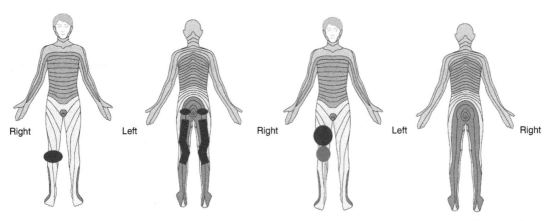

Figure 18.4 Pre- (left) and postoperative (right) patient-driven pain drawings demonstrating new right-sided pain (blue), dysesthesias (red), and numbness (yellow) following right L3 -4 transforaminal surgery, likely reflective of DRG irritation

18.4.4 Central Sensitization in Radiculopathy

Direct evidence connecting central sensitization to radiculopathy is limited when compared to the peripheral nerve injury literature. Significantly higher concentrations of glutamate have, however, been detected in the herniated portions of a disc when compared to contained parts harvested during discectomy, while injection of the same glutamate into the rat epidural space resulted in radiolabelling of the DRG (Harrington et al., 2000). More recently, epidural infusion of glutamate in rats led to hyperalgesia and allodynia, as well as increased expression of NDMA receptors within the dorsal horn (Osgood et al., 2010). Further evidence supporting central responses following root injury came from a rat ligation model, using both chemical (chromic gut) and mechanical (silk) insults, with both astrocytic and microglial (the CNS equivalent of the macrophages previously alluded to) activation in the corresponding cord segment over a 6-week period, starting at day 3 (Hashizume et al., 2000). Furthermore, IL-1α and β, 6 and 10, as well as TNF-α were expressed in the same cord segments at day 7, and appeared to correlate with both degree of root deformation and severity of allodynia (Winkelstein et al., 2001). Finally, in patients with isolated C6 radiculopathy lasting at least 30 days, increased somatosensory evoked potentials (SSEPs) were observed following stimulation of the ipsilateral C6 dermatome, but not the contralateral side or the C7 distribution (Tinazzi et al., 2000).

18.5 Dorsal Root Ganglion in Neuropathic Pain

18.5.1 Structural Features and Functional Implications

The DRG, long dismissed as a "passive" storage organ, has garnered growing interest recently as both a pathophysiologic substrate and therapeutic target in radiculopathy, based on clinical observations of its susceptibility to intraoperative manipulation (Figure 18.4), as well as promising pain responses to DRG lesioning (Van Zundert et al., 2007) and stimulation (Harrison et al., 2018). In fact, C2 ganglionectomy is a well-established treatment option for recalcitrant occipital neuralgia (Wang and Levi, 2002). The unique ultrastructural properties of the DRG rendering it more liable to mechanical and vascular compromise were discussed earlier, while its ability to generate autonomous or "ectopic" impulses (akin to a pacemaker), in both anti- and orthodromic directions, despite being proximal to the site of initial injury, was first described by Wall and Devor in rats in the 1980s (Wall and Devor, 1983). Moreover, as a bipolar (or, more strictly, pseudo-unipolar) neuron, DRGs comprise the richest collection of sensory nerves in the body, as well as constituting some of the longest, reaching up to 1.5 meters in length (Krames, 2014). Furthermore, it has long been established that DRGs lack a blood–neural barrier (Arvidson, 1979), making them naturally a chemical target.

18.5.2 Kambin's Triangle Versus "Prism'"

Classical anatomical teaching posits the DRG within the intervertebral foramen, lying near the apex of the hypotenuse of Kambin's triangle (the other two limbs of this triangle being formed by the traversing root and the intervertebral disc) (Tumalán et al., 2019). More recent data, however, point to significant variation in its position (Fanous et al., 2019), while the triangle concept may be overly simplistic and ignores its bony boundaries, especially the superior articular process (which also serves as a principal point of compression in degenerative conditions), leading some to suggest that it be more aptly depicted as a "prism" (Fanous et al., 2019).

Taken together, these findings suggest a pivotal role for the DRG in both the generation and perpetuation of radicular pain and sensory alteration, perhaps as the "missing link" unifying the mechanical and chemical theories with central sensitization, being a potential target for both spondylotic compression and acute pro-inflammatory cytokines, and a source of molecules mediating central sensitization, as well as being its principal effector or modulatory organ (or even an accessory site for its genesis).

18.5.3 Electrochemical Environment

The aforementioned unique electrical properties of the DRG have also been demonstrated in feline models, with the DRG exhibiting repetitive and sustained firing in response to minimal acute compression, while preexisting injury was a necessary precondition to hyperexcitability at the nerve root and spinal nerve levels (Howe et al., 1977). This hyperexcitability, mediated in part by TNF-α via tetrodoxin-resistant (TTX-R) sodium channels (mechanical hypersensitivity) and transient receptor potential vallinoid (TRPV-1) channels (thermal hypersensitivity) (Jin and Gerau, 2006), may account for the acute allodynia and hyperalgesia occasionally seen in radiculopathy, earlier than might have been anticipated for central sensitization.

Chemically, its cell bodies are surrounded by satellite glial cells, which carry receptors for many of the cytokines implicated in inflammatory radiculopathy, while the neurons themselves harbor several substances implicated in both nociception and central sensitization, including ILs, substance P, and CGRP (Krames, 2014). Its modulation of information relayed to the dorsal horn has been evidenced by the detection of labeled TNF-α injected into the DRG of rats subject to sciatic nerve injury, but not in uninjured specimens (Shubayev and Myers, 2002).

Furthermore, a new family of purinergic ligand-gated ion channels (activated by adenosine triphosphate, ATP) specific to sensory ganglia, the P2X receptors, have been identified in both DRG (Chen et al., 1995) and dorsal horn, and, in the latter instance, contribute to upregulation of BDNF (Coull et al., 2005), identified earlier as an important ingredient in central sensitization, including in silencing GABA. P2X expression was also increased in rat DRG exposed to nuclear material, but not in response to mild mechanical displacement (Sato et al., 2012).

18.5.4 Growth Factors and Dorsal Root Ganglion "Sensitization"

In addition, both BDNF and NGF have been detected locally in the lumbar roots and DRG of rats exposed to nucleus pulposus, correlating with signs of sensitization, as well as sympathetic "sprouting" in the case of NGF (Ramer et al., 1998), while endoneurial injection of NGF into normal roots produced dose-dependent mechanical allodynia and BDNF upregulation (Obata et al., 2002). Finally, upregulation of both growth factors was witnessed in the superjacent L4 DRG 2 weeks following ligation of the rat L5 spinal nerve, while corresponding thermal hyperalgesia was attenuated by local administration of antibodies to each (Fukuoka et al., 2001). This seemingly independent, growth factor-driven secondary hyperalgesic effect supports the novel hypothesis that the DRG itself may serve as a sensitization station.

18.6 Conclusions and Future Directions

In this chapter, we have presented the mechanical, chemical, central, and ganglionic mechanisms underlying radiculopathy, and, in doing so, attempted to shed light upon some of the common clinical conundrums faced by neurosurgeons in daily practice. However, a number of knowledge gaps persist, giving rise to several areas for future research.

Firstly, animal models, which currently dominate the radiculopathy literature, are clearly different to humans, especially given the subjectivity of pain, and findings from experimental research are not necessarily translatable to clinical practice. Secondly, it is difficult to capture the impact of the spectrum of spondylotic changes incurred upon the upright human spine using quadruped animal models; there have been only isolated reports of more pronounced and prolonged allodynia following epidural placement of disc material harvested from the tails of rats previously subjected to compression (Kawakami et al., 2003), suggesting potential chemical modulation by degeneration. Thirdly, while the use of static stressors such as disc herniation and suture ligation have proved fruitful, the cumulative effects of repetitive, dynamic, and potentially progressive insults, including conditions such as spondylolisthesis and spinal settling, remain unknown.

Furthermore, the majority of experimental studies have focused on the acute phase of radiculopathy (and mostly limited to the lumbar spine), while evidence for chronic neuropathic pain has largely been borrowed from non-radicular animal models. Better understanding of the evolution of mechanical and chemical derangements, including transition into established central sensitization, may lead to more temporally specific treatments, while also providing a pathophysiologic explanation for this intermediary "therapeutic window" that is currently largely driven by clinical gestalt, and in doing so unlocking the relationship between symptom duration and recoverability (Takenaka and Aono, 2017). Very little experimental evidence supports the 6-week trial of conservative treatment customarily afforded patients, with the few that do largely focusing on the histologic aftermath, such as progressive axonal loss, particularly of large-diameter myelinated fibers, after 8 weeks of compression following an initial period of regeneration in in rats (Jancalek and Dubovy, 2007). Equally, a paucity of data exists on the effects of surgery on the chemical milieu and central sensitization.

To date, most models of radiculopathy have treated mechanical and chemical contributions separately; such a binary approach is unlikely to reflect reality. In fact, certain studies have demonstrated a synergistic effect on hyperalgesia, both in severity and duration, when nucleus pulposus has been used both to chemically irritate as well as mechanically compress lumbar nerve roots in rats (Hou et al., 2003; Kawakami et al., 2003). In addition, the majority of studies have treated radiculopathy as a single entity, while clinical observations, including sensorimotor recovery that often lags behind pain relief, and dysesthesias being relatively unique to the DRG, suggest otherwise. In a human discectomy model, contact pressure between disc and nerve root, measured via a transducer placed between the two, correlated with severity of motor deficit but not limitation to straight leg raise (Takahashi et al., 1999). Furthermore, the outcome metrics used in the majority of animal studies, i.e., mechanical allodynia and thermal hyperalgesia, more closely mirror symptoms seen in chronic neuropathic pain and central sensitization, and may be relatively uncommon in human radiculopathy, at least during the acute phase (Mahn et al., 2011).

In addition, an increased appreciation for the pathophysiology underlying radiculopathy, particularly chemical bases and central sensitization, may improve our clinical acumen, including reducing nihilism toward patients in the emergency room with severe pain or neurological deficit without significant radiological compression, and those in clinic with generalized non-dermatomal symptomatology that may in fact reflect secondary hyperalgesia. Finally, in situations where both spinal and non-spinal pathology, such as hip osteoarthropathy and peripheral neuropathy, coexist, a biomarker pointing to a radicular origin, potentially derived from chemical studies, may become the ultimate diagnostic panacea. Moving forward, collaboration between clinicians and scientists will be critical to bridging these knowledge and translational voids.

Figure acknowledgements

The following images are credited to the authors of this chapter: Figures 18.1-18.4

References

Arai I, Mao GP, Otani K, Konno S, Kikuchi S, Olmarker K. Indomethacin blocks the nucleus pulposus-induced effects on nerve root function. An experimental study in dogs with assessment of nerve conduction and blood flow following experimental disc herniation. *Eur Spine J* 2004;**13**(8):691–4. https://doi.org/10.1007/s005860100268.

Arvidson B. Distribution of intravenously injected protein tracers in peripheral ganglia of adult mice. *Exp Neurol* 1979;**63**(2):388–410. https://doi.org/10.1016/0014-4886(79)90134-1.

Bobechko WP, Hirsch C. Auto-immune response to nucleus pulposus in the rabbit. *J Bone Joint Surg Br* 1965;**47**:574–80.

Brinjikji W, Luetmer PH, Comstock B, et al. Systematic literature review of imaging features of spinal degeneration in asymptomatic populations. *Am J Neuroradiol* 2015;**36**(4):811–6. https://doi.org/10.3174/ajnr.A4173.

Brisby H, Balague F, Schafer D, et al. Glycosphingolipid antibodies in serum in patients with sciatica. *Spine* 2002;**27** (4):380–6. https://doi.org/10.1097/00007632-200202150-00011.

Byröd G, Otani K, Brisby H, Rydevik B, Olmarker K. Methylprednisolone reduces the early vascular permeability increase in spinal nerve roots induced by epidural nucleus pulposus application. *J Orthop Res* 2000;**18**(6):983–7. https://doi.org/10.1002/jor.1100180619.

Chen C, Cavanaugh JM, Ozaktay AC, Kallakuri S, King AI. Effects of phospholipase A2 on lumbar nerve root structure and function. *Spine* 1997;**22**(10):1057–64. https://doi.org/10.1097/00007632-199705150-00002.

Chen CC, Akopian AN, Sivilotti L, Colquhoun D, Burnstock G, Wood JN. A P2X purinoceptor expressed by a subset of sensory neurons. *Nature* 1995;**377**(6548):428–31. https://doi.org/10.1038/377428a0.

Cornefjord M, Olmarker K, Otani K, Rydevik B. Nucleus pulposus-induced nerve root injury: effects of diclofenac and ketoprofen. *Eur Spine J* 2002;**11**(1):57–61. https://doi.org/10.1007/s005860100299.

Cornefjord M, Sato K, Olmarker K, Rydevik B, Nordborg C. A model for chronic nerve root compression studies. Presentation of a porcine model for controlled, slow-onset compression with analyses of anatomic aspects, compression onset rate, and morphologic and neurophysiologic effects. *Spine* 1997;**22**(9):946–57. https://doi.org/10.1097/00007632-199705010-00003.

Coull JA, Beggs S, Boudreau D, et al. BDNF from microglia causes the shift in neuronal anion gradient underlying neuropathic pain. *Nature* 2005;**438**(7070):1017–21. https://doi.org/10.1038/nature04223.

Cuéllar JM, Borges PM, Cuéllar VG, Yoo A, Scuderi GJ, Yeomans DC. Cytokine expression in the epidural space: a model of noncompressive disc herniation-induced inflammation. *Spine* 2013;**38**(1):17–23. https://doi.org/10.1097/BRS.0b013e3182604baa.

Driscoll T, Jacklyn G, Orchard J, et al. The global burden of occupationally related low back pain: estimates from the Global Burden of Disease 2010 study. *Ann Rheum Dis* 2014;**73**(6):975–81. https://doi.org/10.1136/annrheumdis-2013-204631.

Fanous AA, Tumialán LM, Wang MY. Kambin's triangle: definition and new classification schema. *J Neurosurg Spine* [published online ahead of print Nov 29, 2019]. https://doi.org/10.3171/2019.8.SPINE181475.

Foerster O. The dermatomes in man. *Brain* 1933;**56**:1–39.

Fukuoka T, Kondo E, Dai Y, Hashimoto N, Noguchi K. Brain-derived neurotrophic factor increases in the uninjured dorsal root ganglion neurons in selective spinal nerve ligation model. *J Neurosci* 2001;**21**(13):4891–900. https://doi.org/10.1523/JNEUROSCI.21-13-04891.

Gelfan S, Tarlov IM. Physiology of spinal cord, nerve root and peripheral nerve compression. *Am J Physiol* 1956;**185**:217–29. https://doi.org/10.1152/ajplegacy.1956.185.1.217.

Haro H, Crawford HC, Fingleton B, et al. Matrix metalloproteinase-3-dependent generation of a macrophage chemoattractant in a model of herniated disc resorption. *J Clin Invest* 2000;**105**(2):133–41. https://doi.org/10.1172/JCI7090.

Harrington JF, Messier AA, Bereiter D, Barnes B, Epstein MH. Herniated lumbar disc material as a source of free glutamate available to affect pain signals through the dorsal root ganglion. *Spine* 2000;**25**(8):929–36. https://doi.org/10.1097/00007632-200004150-00006.

Harrison C, Epton S, Bojanic S, Green AL, Fitzgerald JJ. The efficacy and safety of dorsal root ganglion stimulation as a treatment for neuropathic pain: a literature review. *Neuromodulation* 2018;**21**(3):225–33. https://doi.org/10.1111/ner.12685.

Hashizume H, Deleo JA, Colburn RW, Weinstein JN. Spinal glial activation and cytokine expression after lumbar root injury in the rat. *Spine* 2000;**25**(10):1206–17. https://doi.org/10.1097/00007632-200005150-00003.

Hou SX, Tang JG, Chen HS, Chen J. Chronic inflammation and compression of the dorsal root contribute to sciatica induced by the intervertebral disc herniation in rats. *Pain* 2003;**105**(1–2):255–64. https://doi.org/10.1016/s0304-3959(03)00222-7.

Howe JF, Loeser JD, Calvin WH. Mechanosensitivity of dorsal root ganglia and chronically injured axons: a physiological basis for the radicular pain of nerve root compression. *Pain* 1977;**3**(1):25–41. https://doi.org/10.1016/0304-3959(77)90033-1.

Hu SJ, Xing JL. An experimental model for chronic compression of dorsal root ganglion produced by intervertebral foramen stenosis in the rat. *Pain* 1998;**77**(1):15–23. https://doi.org/10.1016/S0304-3959(98)00067-0.

International Association for the Study of Pain (IASP). Pain terminology. www.iasp-pain.org/Education/Content.aspx?ItemNumber=1698#Centralsensitization.

Jancalek R, Dubovy P. An experimental animal model of spinal root compression syndrome: an analysis of morphological changes of myelinated axons during compression radiculopathy and after decompression. *Exp Brain Res* 2007;**179**(1):111–9. https://doi.org/10.1007/s00221-006-0771-5.

Jin X, Gereau RW. Acute p38-mediated modulation of tetrodotoxin-resistant sodium channels in mouse sensory neurons by tumor necrosis factor-alpha. *J Neurosci* 2006;**26**(1):246–55. https://doi.org/10.1523/JNEUROSCI.3858-05.2006.

Kang JD, Georgescu HI, McIntyre-Larkin L, Stefanovic-Racic M, Donaldson WF, Evans CH. Herniated lumbar intervertebral discs spontaneously produce matrix metalloproteinases, nitric oxide, interleukin-6, and prostaglandin E2. *Spine* 1996;**21**(3):271–7. https://doi.org/10.1097/00007632-199602010-00003.

Kang JD, Georgescu HI, McIntyre-Larkin L, Stefanovic-Racic M, Evans CH. Herniated cervical intervertebral discs spontaneously produce matrix metalloproteinases, nitric oxide, interleukin-6, and prostaglandin E2. *Spine* 1995;**20**(22):2373–8. https://doi.org/10.1097/00007632-199511001-00001.

Kawakami M, Hashizume H, Nishi H, Matsumoto T, Tamaki T, Kuribayashi K. Comparison of neuropathic pain induced by the application of normal and mechanically compressed nucleus pulposus to lumbar nerve roots in the rat. *J Orthop Res* 2003;**21**(3):535–9. https://doi.org/10.1016/S0736-0266(02)00192-4.

Kawakami M, Matsumoto T, Hashizume H, Kuribayashi K, Tamaki T. Epidural injection of cyclooxygenase-2 inhibitor attenuates pain-related behavior following application of nucleus pulposus to the nerve root in the rat. *J Orthop Res* 2002;**20**(2):376–81. https://doi.org/10.1016/S0736-0266(01)00114-0.

Kayama S, Konno S, Olmarker K, Yabuki S, Kikuchi S. Incision of the anulus fibrosus induces nerve root morphologic, vascular, and functional changes. An experimental study. *Spine* 1996;**21** (22):2539–43. https://doi.org/10.1097/00007632-199611150-00002.

Kayama S, Olmarker K, Larsson K, Sjögren-jansson E, Lindahl A, Rydevik B. Cultured, autologous nucleus pulposus cells induce functional changes in spinal nerve roots. *Spine* 1998;**23**(20):2155–8. https://doi.org/10.1097/00007632-199810150-00002.

Keegan JJ, Garrett FD. The segmental distribution of the cutaneous nerves in the limbs of man. *Anat Rec* 1948;**102** (4):409–37. https://doi.org/10.1002/ar.1091020403.

Kobayashi S, Shizu N, Suzuki Y, Asai T, Yoshizawa H. Changes in nerve root motion and intraradicular blood flow during an intraoperative straight-leg-raising test. *Spine* 2003;**28**(13):1427–34. https://doi.org/10.1097/01.BRS.0000067087.94398.35

Kobayashi S, Takeno K, Yayama T, et al. Pathomechanisms of sciatica in lumbar disc herniation: effect of periradicular adhesive tissue on electrophysiological values by an intraoperative straight leg raising test. *Spine* 2010;**35**(22):2004–14. https://doi.org/10.1097/BRS.0b013e3181d4164d.

Komori H, Okawa A, Haro H, Muneta T, Yamamoto H, Shinomiya K. Contrast-enhanced magnetic resonance imaging in conservative management of lumbar disc herniation. *Spine* 1998;**23**(1):67–73. https://doi.org/10.1097/00007632-199801010-00015.

Komori H, Shinomiya K, Nakai O, Yamaura I, Takeda S, Furuya K. The natural history of herniated nucleus pulposus with radiculopathy. *Spine* 1996;**21**(2):225–9. https://doi.org/10.1097/00007632-199601150-00013.

Krames ES. The role of the dorsal root ganglion in the development of neuropathic pain. *Pain Med* 2014;**15**(10):1669–85. https://doi.org/10.1111/pme.12413.

Kuslich SD, Ulstrom CL, Michael CJ. The tissue origin of low back pain and sciatica: a report of pain response to tissue stimulation during operations on the lumbar spine using local anesthesia. *Orthop Clin North Am* 1991;**22**(2):181–7.

Latremoliere A, Woolf CJ. Central sensitization: a generator of pain hypersensitivity by central neural plasticity. *J Pain* 2009;**10** (9):895–926. https://doi.org/10.1016/j.jpain.2009.06.012.

Lee HM, Weinstein JN, Meller ST, Hayashi N, Spratt KF, Gebhart GF. The role of steroids and their effects on phospholipase A2. An animal model of radiculopathy. *Spine* 1998;**23**(11):1191–6. https://doi.org/10.1097/00007632-199806010-00001.

Lejeune JP, Hladky JP, Cotten A, Vinchon M, Christiaens JL. Foraminal lumbar disc herniation. Experience with 83 patients. *Spine* 1994;**19**(17):1905–08. https://doi.org/10.1097/00007632-199409000-00007.

Lindahl O, Rexed B. Histologic changes in spinal nerve roots of operated cases of sciatica. *Acta Orthop Scand* 1951;**20**(3):215–25. https://doi.org

Mahn F, Hüllemann P, Gockel U, et al. Sensory symptom profiles and co-morbidities in painful radiculopathy. *PLoS One* 2011;**6**(5):e18018. https://doi.org/10.1371/journal.pone.0018018.

Marshall LL, Trethewie ER. Chemical irritation of nerve-root in disc prolapse. *Lancet* 1973;**2**(7824):320. https://doi.org/10.1016/s0140-6736(73)90818-0.

Marshall LL, Trethewie ER, Curtain CC. Chemical radiculitis. A clinical, physiological and immunological study. *Clin Orthop Relat Res* 1977;**129**:61–7.

McAnany SJ, Rhee JM, Baird EO, et al. Observed patterns of cervical radiculopathy: how often do they differ from a standard, "Netter diagram" distribution? *Spine J* 2019;**19** (7):1137–42. https://doi.org/10.1016/j.spinee.2018.08.002

Mixter WJ, Barr JS. Rupture of the intervertebral disc with involvement of the spinal canal. *N Engl J Med* 1934;**211**:210–4. https://doi.org/10.1056/NEJM193408022110506.

Mulleman D, Mammou S, Griffoul I, Watier H, Goupille P. Pathophysiology of disk-related sciatica. I – Evidence supporting a chemical component. *Joint Bone Spine* 2006;**73** (2):151–8. https://doi.org/10.1016/j.jbspin.2005.03.003.

Naito M, Owen JH, Bridwell KH, Oakley DM. Blood flow direction in the lumbar nerve root. *Spine* 1990;**15**(9):966–8. https://doi.org/10.1097/00007632-199009000-00023.

Nygaard OP, Mellgren SI, Osterud B. The inflammatory properties of contained and noncontained lumbar disc herniation. *Spine* 1997;**22**(21):2484–8. https://doi.org/10.1097/00007632-199711010-00004.

Obata K, Tsujino H, Yamanaka H, et al. Expression of neurotrophic factors in the dorsal root ganglion in a rat model of lumbar disc herniation. *Pain* 2002;**99**(1–2):121–32. https://doi.org/10.1016/s0304-3959(02)00068-4.

Ohtori S, Miyagi M, Eguchi Y, et al. Epidural administration of spinal nerves with the tumor necrosis factor-alpha inhibitor, etanercept, compared with dexamethasone for treatment of sciatica in patients with lumbar spinal stenosis: a prospective randomized study. *Spine* 2012;**37**(6):439–44. https://doi.org/10.1097/BRS.0b013e318238af83.

Ohtori S, Suzuki M, Koshi T, et al. Proinflammatory cytokines in the cerebrospinal fluid of patients with lumbar radiculopathy. *Eur Spine J* 2011;**20**(6):942–6. https://doi.org/10.1007/s00586-010-1595-3.

Olmarker K. Spinal nerve root compression. Nutrition and function of the porcine cauda equina compressed in vivo. *Acta Orthop Scand Suppl* 1991;**242**:1–27.

Olmarker K, Brisby H, Yabuki S, Nordborg C, Rydevik B. The effects of normal, frozen, and hyaluronidase-digested nucleus pulposus on nerve root structure and function. *Spine.* 1997;**22** (5):471–5. https://doi.org/10.1097/00007632-199703010-00001.

Olmarker K, Byröd G, Cornefjord M, Nordborg C, Rydevik B. Effects of methylprednisolone on nucleus pulposus-induced nerve root injury. *Spine* 1994;**19**(16):1803–8. https://doi.org/10.1097/00007632-199408150-00003.

Olmarker K, Holm S, Rydevik B. Importance of compression onset rate for the degree of impairment of impulse propagation in experimental compression injury of the porcine cauda equina. *Spine* 1990a;**15**(5):416–9. https://doi.org/10.1097/00007632-199005000-00013.

Olmarker K, Larsson K. Tumor necrosis factor alpha and nucleus-pulposus-induced nerve root injury. *Spine* 1998;**23**(23):2538–44. https://doi.org/10.1097/00007632-199812010-00008.

Olmarker K, Rydevik B, Hansson T, Holm S. Compression-induced changes of the nutritional supply to the porcine cauda equina. *J Spinal Disord* 1990b;**3**(1):25–9.

Olmarker K, Rydevik B, Holm S. Edema formation in spinal nerve roots induced by experimental, graded compression. An experimental study on the pig cauda equina with special reference to differences in effects between rapid and slow onset of compression. *Spine* 1989a;**14**(6):569–73.

Olmarker K, Rydevik B, Holm S, Bagge U. Effects of experimental graded compression on blood flow in spinal nerve roots. A vital microscopic study on the porcine cauda equina. *J Orthop Res* 1989b;**7**(6):817–23. https://doi.org/10.1002/jor.1100070607.

Olmarker K, Rydevik B, Nordborg C. Autologous nucleus pulposus induces neurophysiologic and histologic changes in porcine cauda equina nerve roots. *Spine* 1993;**18**(11):1425–32.

Olmarker K, Størkson R, Berge OG. Pathogenesis of sciatic pain: a study of spontaneous behavior in rats exposed to experimental disc herniation. *Spine* 2002;**27**(12):1312–7. https://doi.org/10.1097/00007632-200206150-00013.

Onda A, Murata Y, Rydevik B, Larsson K, Kikuchi S, Olmarker K. Nerve growth factor content in dorsal root ganglion as related to changes in pain behavior in a rat model of experimental lumbar disc herniation. *Spine* 2005;**30**(2):188–93. https://doi.org/10.1097/01.brs.0000150830.12518.26.

Osgood DP, Kenney EV, Harrington WF, Harrington JF. Excrescence of neurotransmitter glutamate from disc material has nociceptive qualities: evidence from a rat model. *Spine J* 2010;**10**(11):999–1006. https://doi.org/10.1016/j.spinee.2010.07.390.

Peng B, Wu W, Li Z, Guo J, Wang X. Chemical radiculitis. *Pain* 2007;**127**(1–2):11–6. https://doi.org/10.1016/j.pain.2006.06.034.

Ramer MS, Kawaja MD, Henderson JT, Roder JC, Bisby MA. Glial overexpression of NGF enhances neuropathic pain and adrenergic sprouting into DRG following chronic sciatic constriction in mice. *Neurosci Lett* 1998;**251**(1):53–6. https://doi.org/10.1016/s0304-3940(98)00493-5.

Rose MA, Kam PC. Gabapentin: pharmacology and its use in pain management. *Anaesthesia* 2002;**57**(5):451–62. https://doi.org/10.1046/j.0003-2409.2001.02399.x.

Rydevik B, Brown MD, Lundborg G. Pathoanatomy and pathophysiology of nerve root compression. *Spine* 1984;**9**(1).7–15. https://doi.org/10.1097/00007632-198401000-00004.

Saal JS, Franson RC, Dobrow R, Saal JA, White AH, Goldthwaite N. High levels of inflammatory phospholipase A2 activity in lumbar disc herniations. *Spine* 1990;**15**(7):674–8. https://doi.org/10.1097/00007632-199007000-00011.

Sato KT, Satoh K, Sekiguchi M, et al. Local application of nucleus pulposus induces expression of P2X3 in rat dorsal root ganglion cells. *Fukushima J Med Sci* 2012;**58**(1):17–21. https://doi.org/10.5387/fms.58.17.

Sawin PD, Traynelis VC, Rich G, et al. Chymopapain-induced reduction of proinflammatory phospholipase A2 activity and amelioration of neuropathic behavioral changes in an *in vivo* model of acute sciatica. *J Neurosurg* 1997;**86**(6):998–1006. https://doi.org/10.3171/jns.1997.86.6.0998.

Scholz J, Finnerup NB, Attal N, et al. The IASP classification of chronic pain for ICD-11: chronic neuropathic pain. *Pain* 2019;**160**(1):53–59. https://doi.org/10.1097/j.pain.0000000000001365.

Scuderi GJ, Brusovanik GV, Brusovamik v G, et al. Cytokine assay of the epidural space lavage in patients with lumbar intervertebral disk herniation and radiculopathy. *J Spinal Disord Tech* 2006;**19**(4):266–9. https://doi.org/10.1097/01.bsd.0000204501.22343.99.

Semmes RE, Murphey MF. The syndrome of unilateral rupture of the sixth cervical intervertebral disk with compression of the seventh cervical nerve root: a report of four cases with symptoms simulating coronary disease. *JAMA* 1943;**121**:1209–14. https://doi.org/10.1001/jama.1943.02840150023006.

Shubayev VI, Myers RR. Anterograde TNF alpha transport from rat dorsal root ganglion to spinal cord and injured sciatic nerve. *Neurosci Lett* 2002;**320**(1–2):99–101. https://doi.org/10.1016/s0304-3940(02)00010-1.

Smith SA, Massie JB, Chesnut R, Garfin SR. Straight leg raising. Anatomical effects on the spinal nerve root without and with fusion. *Spine* 1993;**18**(8):992–9.

Smyth MJ, Wright V. Sciatica and the intervertebral disc; an experimental study. *J Bone Joint Surg Am* 1958;**40**-A(6):1401–18.

Stafford MA, Peng P, Hill DA. Sciatica: a review of history, epidemiology, pathogenesis, and the role of epidural steroid injection in management. *Br J Anaesth* 2007;**99**(4):461–73. https://doi.org/10.1093/bja/aem238.

Takahashi H, Suguro T, Okazima Y, Motegi M, Okada Y, Kakiuchi T. Inflammatory cytokines in the herniated disc of the lumbar spine. *Spine* 1996;**21**(2):218–24. https://doi.org/10.1097/00007632-199601150-00011.

Takahashi K, Shima I, Porter RW. Nerve root pressure in lumbar disc herniation. *Spine* 1999;**24**(19):2003–06. https://doi.org/10.1097/00007632-199910010-00007.

Takahashi N, Yabuki S, Aoki Y, Kikuchi S. Pathomechanisms of nerve root injury caused by disc herniation: an experimental study of mechanical compression and chemical irritation. *Spine* 2003;**28**(5):435–41. https://doi.org/10.1097/01.BRS.0000048645.33118.02.

Takenaka S, Aono H. Prediction of postoperative clinical recovery of drop foot attributable to lumbar degenerative diseases, via a Bayesian network. *Clin Orthop Relat Res* 2017;**475**(3):872–80. https://doi.org/10.1007/s11999-016-5180.

Tanaka Y, Kokubun S, Sato T, Ozawa H. Cervical roots as origin of pain in the neck or scapular regions. *Spine* 2006;**31**(17):E568–73. https://doi.org/10.1097/01.brs.0000229261.02816.48.

Tinazzi M, Fiaschi A, Rosso T, Faccioli F, Grosslercher J, Aglioti SM. Neuroplastic changes related to pain occur at multiple levels of the human somatosensory system: a somatosensory-evoked potentials study in patients with cervical radicular pain. *J Neurosci* 2000;**20**(24):9277–83. https://doi.org/10.1523/JNEUROSCI.20-24-09277.2000.

Tumialán LM, Madhavan K, Godzik J, Wang MY. The history of and controversy over Kambin's triangle: a historical analysis of the lumbar transforaminal corridor for endoscopic and surgical approaches. *World Neurosurg* 2019;**123**:402–08. https://doi.org/10.1016/j.wneu.2018.10.221.

Van Zundert J, Patijn J, Kessels A, Lamé I, Van Suijlekom H, Van Kleef M. Pulsed radiofrequency adjacent to the cervical dorsal root ganglion in chronic cervical radicular pain: a double blind sham controlled randomized clinical trial. *Pain* 2007;**127**(1–2):173–82. https://doi.org/10.1016/j.pain.2006.09.002.

Wadhwani S, Loughenbury P, Soames R. The anterior dural (Hofmann) ligaments. *Spine* 2004;**29**(6):623–7. https://doi.org/10.1097/01.brs.0000115129.59484.24.

Wall PD, Devor M. Sensory afferent impulses originate from dorsal root ganglia as well as from the periphery in normal and nerve injured rats. *Pain* 1983;**17**(4):321–39. https://doi.org/10.1016/0304-3959(83)90164-1.

Wang MY, Levi AD. Ganglionectomy of C-2 for the treatment of medically refractory occipital neuralgia. *Neurosurg Focus* 2002;**12**(1):E14. https://doi.org/10.3171/foc.2002.12.1.15.

Weinstein JN, Tosteson TD, Lurie JD, et al. Surgical vs nonoperative treatment for lumbar disk herniation: the Spine Patient Outcomes Research Trial (SPORT): a randomized trial. *JAMA* 2006;**296**(20):2441–50. https://doi.org/10.1001/jama.296.20.2441.

Winkelstein BA, Rutkowski MD, Weinstein JN, Deleo JA. Quantification of neural tissue injury in a rat radiculopathy model: comparison of local deformation, behavioral outcomes, and spinal cytokine mRNA for two surgeons. *J Neurosci Methds* 2001;**111**(1):49–57. https://doi.org/10.1016/s0165-0270(01)00445-9.

Winkelstein BA, Weinstein JN, Deleo JA. The role of mechanical deformation in lumbar radiculopathy: an *in vivo* model. *Spine* 2002;**27**(1):27–33. https://doi.org/10.1097/00007632-200201010-00009.

Woolf CJ. Central sensitization: implications for the diagnosis and treatment of pain. *Pain* 2011;**152**(3 Suppl):S2–15. https://doi.org/10.1016/j.pain.2010.09.030.

Yeung AT, Tsou PM. Posterolateral endoscopic excision for lumbar disc herniation: Surgical technique, outcome, and complications in 307 consecutive cases. *Spine* 2002;**27**(7):722–31. https://doi.org/10.1097/00007632-200204010-00009.

Spinal Tumors

Ziev B. Moses, Matthew Trawczynski, and John E. O'Toole

19.1 Introduction

Tumors of the spine are a heterogeneous group of neoplasms involving the spinal column and spinal cord. They can be distinguished based on their location within the spine into three groups: intradural–intramedullary, intradural–extramedullary, and extradural (see Figure 19.1). Another classification seeks to separate out these tumors based on their cell of origin, with primary spine tumors arising from either the spinal cord itself, its surrounding coverings including the leptomeninges, bone, cartilage, and soft tissue, or as secondary tumors arising from spinal involvement of a systemic neoplasm such as myeloma or as a metastasis from a distant site. This chapter seeks to discuss current evidence on the genetic, epigenetic, and cellular underpinnings of spine tumors with emphasis on the pathobiology and mechanisms underlying these neoplasms.

19.2 Intramedullary Spinal Cord Tumors

19.2.1 Astrocytomas

Intramedullary spinal cord astrocytomas are recognized as glial neoplasms similar to their primary brain analogues. Astrocytomas and ependymomas comprise the majority of all intramedullary spine tumors (Grimm and Chamberlain, 2009). Pilocytic astrocytomas (WHO grade I) are rare in the spine, and the majority of spinal cord astrocytomas are infiltrative (WHO grade II or higher). In grade I astrocytomas, BRAF, a member of the mitogen-activated protein kinase (MAPK) pathway, is altered and results in abnormal cell division. Two major mutations involved in *BRAF* include a fusion oncogene involving *BRAF* and *KIAA1549*, and a valine to glutamate mutation known as BRAF V600E (Horbinski, 2013). Both mutations result in constitutive activation of the MAPK pathway. The fusion oncogene variant is found to be

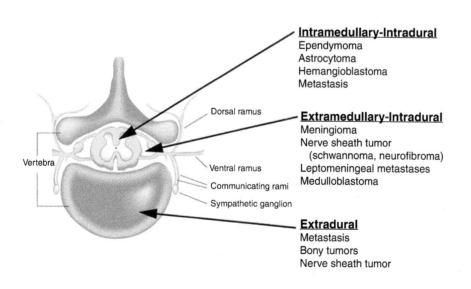

Intramedullary-Intradural
Ependymoma
Astrocytoma
Hemangioblastoma
Metastasis

Dorsal ramus

Extramedullary-Intradural
Meningioma
Nerve sheath tumor
    (schwannoma, neurofibroma)
Leptomeningeal metastases
Medulloblastoma

Vertebra

Ventral ramus

Communicating rami

Sympathetic ganglion

Extradural
Metastasis
Bony tumors
Nerve sheath tumor

Figure 19.1 Distribution of primary spinal cord tumors by location.

more common among spinal cord pilocytic astrocytomas, with one recent study discovering that of 17 spinal cord astrocytomas, 80% of grade I astrocytomas had *BRAF* mutations (Shankar et al., 2016). Of these, 30% involved the *BRAF–KIAA1549* fusion protein and 50% had a *BRAF* copy number gain. None of the 17 specimens was found to have the *BRAF V600E* mutation. Cyclin-dependent kinase inhibitor 2A (*CDKN2A*) encodes the tumor suppressor protein p16 and has been found to be mutated in grade I astrocytomas. In one study of 147 pilocytic astrocytomas in a pediatric cohort, p16 loss of heterozygosity was more common in midbrain, brainstem, and spinal cord locations (Horbinski et al., 2010). Grade II astrocytomas have been found to have similar alterations as grade I, including the *BRAF–KIAA1549* translocation and *BRAF* amplification (Shankar et al., 2016). Grades III and IV astrocytomas have been shown to harbor a mutation in histone 3 variant H3.3 (H3F3A). In the cohort above of 17 astrocytomas, all four grades III and IV astrocytomas shared *H3F3A K27M* mutations (Shankar et al., 2016). In addition, studies have shown

that *TP53* mutations are common in high-grade spinal cord astrocytomas but not *IDH1*, which is more common in their brain analog (Nagaishi et al., 2016; Shankar et al., 2016; Yanamadala et al., 2016). See Figure 19.2 for a depiction of the most commonly found mutations in a cohort of spinal cord astrocytomas.

19.2.2 Ependymomas

Ependymomas are divided into three grades including subependymoma and myxopapillary ependymoma (WHO grade I), classic ependymoma (WHO grade II), and anaplastic ependymoma (grade III) (DeWitt et al., 2017). While the majority of pediatric ependymomas are intracranial, spinal cord ependymomas are most common in adults aged 20–40 (Hasselblatt, 2009). Ependymomas are thought to arise from radial glia-like stem cells, contrary to prior hypotheses that they originate from ependymal cells lining the central canal (Johnson et al., 2010). New research on the genetics of ependymoma have found important differences between

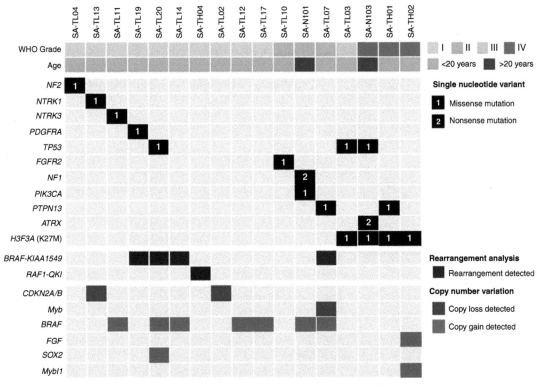

Figure 19.2 Genomic characterization of spinal cord astrocytomas.

spinal and cranial types (Nagasawa et al., 2013). With regard to ependymoma initiation, CDKN2A has been implicated in pediatric spinal ependymomas but not their intracranial analogs (Korshuhnov et al., 2003). It appears spinal ependymomas have higher rates of *NF2* mutations (Bettegowda et al., 2013; Singh et al., 2002). In another study including 10 spinal ependymomas, mRNA expression levels were found to be higher in the following proteins in the spinal type compared with the supratentorial and posterior fossa groups: homeoboxB5 (HOXB5), phospholipase A2 group 5 (PLA2G5), and inter-a-trypsin inhibitor heavy chain 2 (ITIH2) (Korshuhnov et al., 2003). Myxopapillary ependymomas, which are most often limited to the distal spinal cord, tend to express the highest levels of *HOX* genes, which are associated with normal development of the lumbosacral zone (Barton et al., 2010; Wellik, 2007). Specifically, the genes *HOXC10, HOXD10, HOXA13,* and *HOXB13* are the most highly expressed *HOX* genes and may serve as therapeutic targets (Barton et al., 2010).

19.2.3 Hemangioblastomas

Hemangioblastomas account for 2–8% of intramedullary tumors, with approximately 25% of hemangioblastoma patients having evidence of von Hippel–Lindau (VHL) disease (Glasker, 2005; Ostrom et al., 2014). The *VHL* gene regulates vascular proliferation by encoding E3 ubiquitin ligase, which acts on hypoxia-inducible factor 1α (HIF-1α). VHL disease is transmitted in an autosomal dominant fashion with 90% penetrance and affects multiple organ systems including the kidneys, pancreas, and adrenal glands (Glasker, 2005). While 80% of hemangioblastomas occur in the posterior fossa, approximately 20% affect the spine, most commonly in the cervical or lumbar regions (Ostrom et al., 2014). At least one study has shown that spinal hemangioblastomas are more strongly associated with VHL syndrome (88% of cases) and have significant VHL expression in comparison with those found in sporadic cases (21%) (Takai et al., 2010). While surgery is the mainstay for symptomatic spinal hemangioblastomas, anti-HIF-1α and anti-VEGF drugs remain promising avenues of treatment for hemangioblastoma despite limited clinical studies.

19.2.4 Germ Cell Tumors

Germ cell tumors typically arise in the pineal or suprasellar region, whereas primary germ cell tumors of the spine are infrequent. While spinal seeding of germ cell tumors has been described, primary tumors within the spinal cord are exceedingly rare, with germinoma being the most common. In at least one literature review, primary spinal germ cell tumors were most commonly found in the thoracolumbar region (70%), with B-HCG overproduction found in 40% of patients (Biswas et al., 2009). Findings of syncytiotrophoblastic giant cells (STGCs) are associated with higher rates of recurrence (Uematsu et al., 1992). Currently, the pathobiology and treatment plan mirror those in the intracranial space (Loya et al., 2013; Mehta et al., 2011).

19.2.5 Gangliogliomas

A ganglioglioma is a slow-growing neoplasm of the central nervous system (CNS) associated with seizures and often found in the temporal lobes, while its presence in the spinal cord is exceedingly rare. Reported spinal cases number less than 100 and have largely been seen in young adults and children (Hamburger et al., 1997). Histopathological analysis reveals both ganglion cells and neoplastic glial cells similar to their intracranial counterparts, and the majority are considered benign WHO grade I tumors (Louis et al., 2007). In a screen of 1320 CNS tumors, BRAF V600E mutations were found in approximately 20% of gangliogliomas (Schindler et al., 2011). Indeed, one case report details the successful treatment of a recurrent spinal ganglioglioma with Vemurafenib, a small molecule inhibitor of mutated BRAF (Garnier et al., 2019). Surgical excision remains the mainstay of treatment, but as the pathobiology is better understood additional treatments may become available.

19.2.6 Primary Melanoma

Primary malignant melanoma of the CNS represents approximately 1% of all melanomas and is rarely reported on in the literature (Brat et al., 1999; Farrokh et al., 2001; Schneider et al., 1987; Skarli et al., 1994). It is considered primary in the absence of lesions outside the CNS and the diagnosis is confirmed by histology. Originating from the neural crest cell-derived melanocytes, these neoplasms can behave aggressively. Given its infrequent incidence, its unique pathobiology is uncertain compared with metastatic melanoma.

19.2.7 Central Nervous System Lymphoma

Extranodal lymphoma of the CNS is often a manifestation of advanced systemic disease. In the spine, it often presents with spinal cord compression due to extradural disease, either as an isolated seeding

269

or an enlarging adjacent nodal mass (Eeles et al., 1991). However, primary CNS lymphoma, particularly isolated primary spinal lymphoma, is rare and often presents subdurally or within the spinal cord. In one literature review of 37 cases of isolated primary spinal lymphoma, histology revealed the majority of these to be diffuse large B-cell lymphomas (Zheng et al., 2010). Treatment is often surgical with decompression followed by chemoradiation based on the pathological findings (Hashi et al., 2018).

19.2.8 Other Tumors

The neoplasm types discussed thus far are not unique to the spine. They originate in a variety of primary sites including bone, nervous tissue, or soft tissue. This highlights the incredible complexity and heterogeneity of spinal tumors, as most are driven by underlying (e.g., early in tumor cell lineage) epigenetic, genetic, or protein-level changes rather than tissue-specific alterations. Many of these have undergone in-depth basic science investigation, but the extreme rarity of others has resulted in less research attention given to several tumor classes. One of these, known as a primitive neuroectodermal tumor (PNET), presents extremely rarely as a primary intramedullary or extramedullary spinal tumor (Ma et al., 2020). Some studies have demonstrated significant histologic and genetic overlap between PNET neoplasms and Ewing sarcoma (Desai et al., 2010). These tumors are known to be at least partially driven by chromosomal translocations, notably fusions of the *EWSR1* gene with ETS-transcription factor family members or zinc-finger family genes (Sumegi et al., 2011). One study also identified a unique EWSR1–SMARCA5 translocation in the lumbosacral spine of a 5-year old female, where SMARCA5 belongs to the WSTF–SNF2h chromatin-remodeling gene family (Sumegi et al., 2011). These findings suggest a heterogeneous and often co-dependent interplay of chromosomal, epigenetic, and genetic factors at play in spinal lesion tumorigenesis.

Other diverse tumor types – including lipomas and hamartomas – have also previously been found to occur as primary spinal lesions. Lipomas may also present as intramedullary lesions, compressing critical neural tracts and resulting in various neuropathic symptoms. These may be classified into transitional, dorsal, or chaotic lipomas, among other subcategories (Pang et al., 2010). Dorsal dysraphic lipomas, which are congenital, present more commonly than subpial lipomas (Pasalic et al., 2018). Challenges remain, however, to accurate and efficient lipoma classification. One recent study of 64 patients with lumbosacral lipomas investigated the histological patterns of lipoma subcategories, finding abundant connective tissue, peripheral nerve fibers, thickened blood vessels, and occasionally CNS glial tissue across different lipoma types that was not consistent with current standards in nomenclature (Jones et al., 2018). Future basic research is needed before spinal lipomas may be potentially reclassified to more accurately reflect their pathophysiology. Notably, similar to lipomas, intramedullary hamartomas may also be composed of varying cell types and histological landmarks. Some reports have described hamartomas composed of two germ cell lines (e.g., ectodermal and mesodermal tissue), but others have reported at least three germ cell lines co-occurring with stratified squamous epithelium and adnexal sebaceous glands (Samak et al., 2016). These studies suggest that future work is needed before lipomas and hamartomas may be reclassified or segregated into subcategories based on molecular profiling, gene sequencing, or chromosomal alterations.

19.3 Intradural Extramedullary Spinal Cord Tumors

19.3.1 Meningioma

Meningiomas are intradural extramedullary lesions arising from arachnoid cap cells within arachnoid villi. These neoplasms bear attachment to dura, and it is estimated that up to 25% of all primary spinal tumors are meningiomas (Chamberlain and Tredway, 2011). Over 80% of spinal meningiomas are diagnosed in females, which is likely due to differences in endogenous sex hormones (Buerki et al., 2018). A wide variety of genetic and epigenetic alterations have been described in meningiomas, but a tumor classification system rooted in molecular diagnostics (versus histologic markers of malignancy) has not yet been established. The most commonly reported genetic alterations in spinal meningiomas include chromosome 22q deletion and altered NF2 expression (Karsy et al., 2015; Sayagues et al., 2006). Researchers using microarray studies and interphase fluorescence in-situ hybridization techniques have found spinal meningiomas to more commonly represent a single tumor cell clone than intracranial meningiomas, suggesting that spinal lesions could have a lower degree of intratumor heterogeneity than cranial lesions (Sayagues et al., 2006). They found that spinal meningiomas were also more likely to be of a psammomatous or transitional subtype, uniquely expressing a number of genes not associated with intracranial meningiomas: *HOXA5, HOXA7, HOXB6, KLF4,*

FOSL2, RGS16, and *SOCS3*, among others. See Figure 19.3 for a schematic depicting differences in clonal evolution of spinal meningiomas and intracranial meningiomas. Recent reports have confirmed key differences between genetic alterations in cranial and spinal meningiomas, notably that spinal meningiomas more commonly have a decreased expression of E-cadherin, an adhesive protein whose deletion can induce epithelial to mesenchymal (EMT) cell migration (Foda et al., 2019). See Figure 19.4 for an illustration summarizing EMT. As is seen, spinal meningiomas carry unique gene expression signatures that differentiate these lesions from intracranial meningiomas, possibly suggesting differences in early tumor clonal evolution.

19.3.2 Nerve Sheath Tumors

Schwannomas and neurofibromas are nerve sheath tumors originating from the dorsal root or peripheral nerves, respectively. They are mostly benign, with schwannomas generally causing mass effect that displaces nerves and neurofibromas encircling them (Chamberlain and Tredway, 2011). Mutations in *NF1* (17q11) and *NF2* (22q12) are most commonly associated with these neoplasms, as they are often found in familial neurofibromatosis (Jett and Friedman, 2010; Karsy et al., 2015). *NF1* codes for neurofibromin, which is decreased in neurofibromatosis. This decreased expression leads to increased cell proliferation and decreased apoptosis via the Ras-GTP, MAPK, and mTOR signal transduction pathways (Gottfried et al., 2010). *NF2* codes for merlin, a tumor suppressor protein. When dephosphorylated, merlin is active via a closed configuration in association with 4.1–ezrin–radixin–moesin domain and carboxy-terminal domains. Absent merlin function results in cytoskeletal and cell adhesion disruption (Asthagiri et al., 2009).

19.4 Spinal Column Tumors

19.4.1 Chordoma

Chordomas are notochord-derived locally aggressive tumors that make up approximately 1–4% of all primary bone tumors (Healey and Lane, 1989). Histopathologically, they are defined by their physaliphorous cells, which are pathognomonic of the disease and have a homolog in the evolution of notochordal tissue. In a familial chordoma study, duplications of 6q27 were found, which contains the *brachyury* gene,

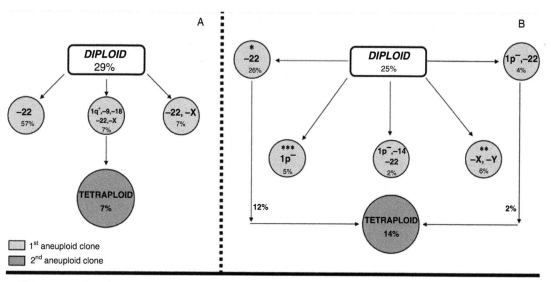

* 1/36 cases corresponded to a grade II tumor
** 2/8 cases corresponded to a grade II tumor
*** 1/7 cases corresponded to a grade II tumor

Figure 19.3 Schematic depicting differences in intratumor clonal evolution between spinal (A) and cranial (B) meningiomas. Per cent values indicate the percent of cases having the listed cytogenetic profile. Source: Sayagues JM, Tabernero MD, Maillo A, et al. Microarray-based analysis of spinal versus intracranial meningiomas: different clinical, biological, and genetic characteristics associated with distinct patterns of gene expression.

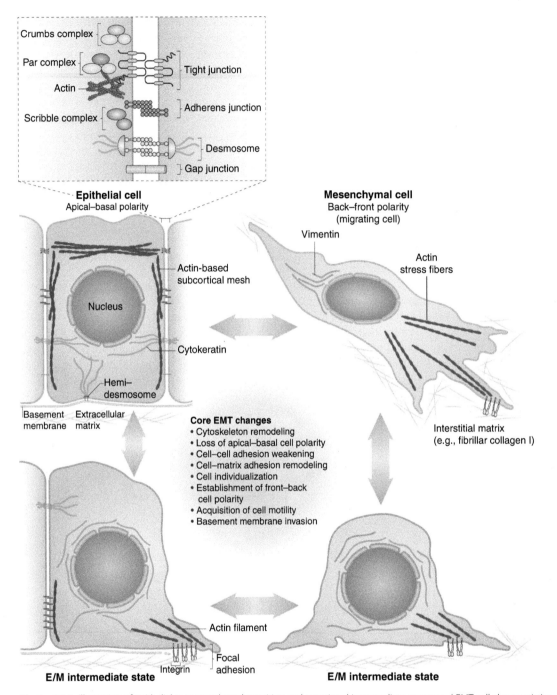

Figure 19.4 Illustration of epithelial to mesenchymal transition and associated intermediate stages and EMT cell characteristics.

further supporting its notochordal origin and genetic susceptibility to chordoma (Yang et al., 2009). In another study of 104 sporadic chordomas, PI3K signaling mutations were found in up to 16% of tumors (Tarpey et al., 2017). Building on evidence of tyrosine kinase receptor activation and downstream signaling, a number of agents targeting this pathway have been studied in chordoma with some clinical benefit, including imatinib, lapatinib, and sorafenib (Bompas et al., 2015; Magnaghi et al., 2018; Stacchiotti et al., 2013).

19.4.2 Sarcoma

Spinal sarcomas are primary tumors originating from bone or connective tissue. These include Ewing's sarcoma, osteosarcoma, chondrosarcoma, and fibrosarcoma. When Ewing's sarcoma presents as a primary lesion in the spine it usually affects the sacral ala and frequently invades the spinal canal (91% of cases) (Ilaslan et al., 2004). Due to its rarity, few basic studies have investigated primary spinal Ewing's sarcoma. One report found positive staining for neuronal enolase, synaptophysin, and chromogranin in this tumor type, which was identified via its expression of CD99 (Saeedinia et al., 2012). Basic studies of primary spinal osteosarcomas are also few, but some studies have identified differential gene expression between different osteosarcoma subtypes, including changes in angiopoietin 1, IGFBP3, ferredoxin 1, BMP, decorin, and fibulin 1 expression (Katonis et al., 2013; Kubista et al., 2011). Chondrosarcomas may be differentiated by differences in gene involvement in primary versus secondary lesions. Exostosin genes, responsible for heparan sulfate biosynthesis, are inactive in secondary chondrosarcomas but active in primary tumors (Katonis et al., 2011). In fibrosarcoma, neurotrophic tyrosine receptor kinase gene fusions are frequently reported (>90%), especially in the infantile form (Bourgeois et al., 2000; Forschner et al., 2020). In addition, these tumors stain positive for vimentin, smooth muscle actin, desmin, S-100, and potentially CD34 (Bourgeois et al., 2000). As is seen, each of these tumors has unique gene hallmarks.

19.4.3 Plasmacytoma

Solitary bone plasmacytoma (SBP) represents a condition along a continuum of hematopoietic disorders ranging from monoclonal gammopathy of unknown significance to multiple myeloma. Of plasmacytomas, there are SBPs, extramedullary plasmacytomas, and multiple solitary plasmactyomas (MSPs). Criteria for SBP include a solitary lesion, less than 10% bone marrow plasmacytosis, a biopsy of the lesion containing a plasma cell neoplasm, and negative imaging for other lesions (Soutar et al., 2004). Given the low incidence of spinal plasmacytoma, prognostic factors associated with genetic abnormalities have not been discovered as in multiple myeloma (Kitamura et al., 2018). However, at least one case report describes a difficult to treat relapsed CD138-

low MSP with a 17p deletion (Kitamura et al., 2018). The patient was successfully treated with an autologous hematopoietic stem cell transplantation followed by Bortezomib maintenance therapy.

19.5 Metastatic Tumors of the Spine

19.5.1 Mechanisms of Metastasis

Tumors occupying the extradural space are most commonly metastases originating from primary tumors outside of the spine. The spine itself is the most frequent location of metastasis to bone (Maccauro et al., 2011). A wide variety of mechanisms drive spinal metastases, many of which are currently poorly understood. Neoplastic dissemination is classically divided into three routes of spread: hematogenous, contiguous, or lymphatic. In addition to the route of metastasis, a wide variety of factors are necessary for a primary tumor to seed bony or nervous tissue around the spine. First, it is theorized that tumor cells undergo EMT (Yang et al., 2020), which is a process of de-differentiation by which cells gain migratory "stem-like" characteristics and decrease the expression of adhesive proteins such as E-cadherin with an increased expression of CD44 (Gdowski et al., 2017; Maccauro et al., 2011; Thiery et al., 2009). See Figure 19.4 for a summary of EMT. Cells also begin to secrete proteinases that destroy the extracellular matrix, rendering escape from the tumor stroma possible (DeClerck, 2000). Tumor cells begin to spread through the vasculature; they often favor seeding in regions with the highest red bone marrow, such as the vertebral bodies or ribs, because these are highly vascular (Maccauro et al., 2011). This in combination with relatively slow blood-flow velocity results in ideal conditions for tumor seeding through microthrombi formation, adhesion, migration, and infiltration into those extravascular spaces with the most favorable tumor microenvironment. Tumor cells are then able to begin secreting a variety of cytokines and chemokines to cause osteoclastic or osteoblastic lesions. As can be seen, a wide variety of factors contribute to spinal metastases.

Some studies have also demonstrated that dural tissue itself could promote a favorable microenvironment for nearby bone metastasis, particularly to the posterior third of the vertebral body. Researchers examined dural conditioned media (DCM), performing RNA-sequencing studies of dural fibroblasts (Szerlip et al., 2018). They found that DCM promoted the proliferation and survival of some prostate and breast cancer cell lines by inducing signaling proteins involved in several receptor tyrosine kinase pathways including pAKT, pERk1/2, and pSTAT3. They also found that DCM promotes the proliferation of bone marrow myeloid cells, which represent a significant subpopulation of cells within the spine. These results suggest that dural tissue itself may be a driving force in creating a favorable microenvironment for spinal metastases.

It is well known that certain primary tumors have a preference for metastasizing to the spine. The pathophysiology behind why specific tumor types metastasize more commonly to certain regions is also multifactorial. For example, breast cancer often spreads to the thoracic spine because of both favorable anatomy and unique changes in gene expression signatures. The venous drainage system of the breast is routed through the azygous vein, which communicates with the thoracic spine through Batson's plexus (Gdowski et al., 2017; Maccauro et al., 2011). Basic studies have also demonstrated spine-specific ligand receptor interactions, namely that of CX3CL1 and CX3CR1 operating through the Src/FAK pathway in breast cancer metastasis to the spine (Liang et al., 2018). This pathway has previously been identified as a central signaling pathway responsible for cell migration, actin regulation, and anchorage-independent growth by the Src-induced phosphorylation of FAK (Westhoff et al., 2004). Similarly, the metastasis of lung adenocarcinoma to spine has been found to be associated with CXCL17 expression, which contributes to upregulating the Src/FAK pathway (Liu et al., 2020). COL5A1 has also been identified as a driver in lung adenocarcinoma (Liu et al., 2018). As is seen, microenvironmental, anatomic, and gene expression signatures all contribute to tumorigenesis and metastasis in the spine.

19.5.2 Drop Metastases

"Drop metastasis" refers to the process of intracranial tumors spreading to the spine via cerebrospinal fluid pathways. Metastasis of a variety of tumors occurs by this mechanism, including medulloblastoma and rarely glioblastomas or ependymomas and even solid-organ metastases to the brain among others. The precise mechanisms of drop metastases are poorly understood, but it is hypothesized they occur via myelinated tract infiltration, tumor cell exfoliation into cerebrospinal fluid, or mechanical transfer during surgery (Wright et al., 2019). In one study, researchers conducted whole exome sequencing and epigenetic analysis comparing an H3K27M-mutant pineal parenchymal tumor with its spinal drop metastases, finding that the metastasis had additional mutations and chromosomal amplifications (Fomchenko et al., 2019). Future studies are needed to further characterize genetic and epigenetic differences between primary intracranial lesions and spinal drop metastases.

19.6 Conclusion and Future Directions

In this chapter we reviewed common trends in basic science in the field of spinal oncology. We discussed genetic and epigenetic features of intramedullary, intradural–extramedullary, and extradural metastatic tumors of the spine. We highlighted important principles of tumor classification schemes, epithelial to mesenchymal transition, cell migration, and the wide interplay of factors involved in tumorigenesis. As we have shown, future studies are needed to more precisely understand the mechanisms behind spinal tumorigenesis and metastasis. In particular, tumor stratification is a critical area of future research in spinal oncology. Molecular diagnostics are needed in combination with novel grading schemes for many primary tumors of the spine, similar to the current WHO grading guidelines for malignant gliomas which incorporate epigenetic and chromosomal molecular markers. This is especially relevant for current grading schemes involving lipomas, hamartomas, and other tumors, which largely have been shown to be inconsistent. Overall, the field of spinal oncology is an exciting and rapidly developing field where future basic science studies are needed to develop novel treatment strategies for many of the tumors discussed here.

Figure acknowledgements

The following image is credited to Karsy et al., 2015: Figure 19.1
The following image is credited to Shankar et al., 2016: Figure 19.2
The following image is credited to Sayagues et al., 2006: Figure 19.3
The following image is credited to Yang et al., 2020: Figure 19.4

References

Asthagiri AR, Parry DM, Butman JA, et al. Neurofibromatosis type 2. *Lancet* 2009;**373**(9679):1974–86. https://doi.org/10.1016/S0140-6736(09)60259-2.

Barton VN, Donson AM, Kleinschmidt-DeMasters BK, Birks DK, Handler MH, Foreman NK. Unique molecular characteristics of pediatric myxopapillary ependymoma. *Brain Pathol* 2010;**20**(3):560–70. https://doi.org/10.1111/j.1750-3639.2009.00333.x

Bettegowda C, Agrawal N, Jiao Y, et al. Exomic sequencing of four rare central nervous system tumor types. *Oncotarget* 2013;**4**(4):572–83. https://doi.org/10.18632/oncotarget.964.

Biswas A, Puri T, Goyal S, et al. Spinal intradural primary germ cell tumour–review of literature and case report. *Acta Neurochir (Wien)* 2009;**151**(3):277–84. https://doi.org/10.1007/s00701-009-0200-1.

Bompas E, Le Cesne A, Tresch-Bruneel E, et al. Sorafenib in patients with locally advanced and metastatic chordomas: a phase II trial of the French Sarcoma Group (GSF/GETO). *Ann Oncol* 2015;**26**(10):2168–173. https://doi.org/10.1093/annonc/mdv300.

Bourgeois JM, Knezevich SR, Mathers JA, Sorensen PH. Molecular detection of the *ETV6–NTRK3* gene fusion differentiates congenital fibrosarcoma from other childhood spindle cell tumors. *Am J Surg Pathol* 2000;**24**(7):937–46. https://doi.org/10.1097/00000478-200007000-00005.

Brat DJ, Giannini C, Scheithauer BW, Burger PC. Primary melanocytic neoplasms of the central nervous systems. *Am J Surg Pathol* 1999;**23**(7):745–54. https://doi.org/10.1097/00000478-199907000-00001.

Buerki RA, Horbinski CM, Kruser T, Horowitz PM, James CD, Lukas RV. An overview of meningiomas. *Future Oncol* 2018;**14**(21):2161–77. https://doi.org/10.2217/fon-2018-0006.

Chamberlain MC, Tredway TL. Adult primary intradural spinal cord tumors: a review. *Curr Neurol Neurosci Rep* 2011;**11**(3):320–8. https://doi.org/10.1007/s11910-011-0190-2.

DeClerck YA. Interactions between tumour cells and stromal cells and proteolytic modification of the extracellular matrix by metalloproteinases in cancer. *Eur J Cancer* 2000;**36**(10):1258–68. https://doi.org/10.1007/s11910-011-0190-2.

Desai SS, Jambhekar NA. Pathology of Ewing's sarcoma/PNET: current opinion and emerging concepts. *Indian J Orthop* 2010;**44**(4):363–8. https://doi.org/10.4103/0019-5413.69304.

DeWitt JC, Mock A, Louis DN. The 2016 WHO classification of central nervous system tumors: what neurologists need to know. *Curr Opin Neurol* 2017;**30**(6):643–9. https://doi.org/10.1097/WCO.0000000000000490.

Eeles RA, O'Brien P, Horwich A, Brada M. Non-Hodgkin's lymphoma presenting with extradural spinal cord compression: functional outcome and survival. *Br J Cancer* 1991;**63**(1):126–9. https://doi.org/10.1038/bjc.1991.25.

Farrokh D, Fransen P, Faverly D. MR findings of a primary intramedullary malignant melanoma: case report and literature review. *Am J Neuroradiol* 2001;**22**(10):1864–6.

Foda AAM, Alam MS, Ikram N, Rafi S, Elnaghi K. Spinal versus intracranial meningioma: expression of E-cadherin and Fascin with relation to clinicopathological features. *Cancer Biomark* 2019;**25**(4):333–9. https://doi.org/10.3233/CBM-190164.

Fomchenko EI, Erson-Omay EZ, Kundishora AJ, et al. Genomic alterations underlying spinal metastases in pediatric H3K27M-mutant pineal parenchymal tumor of intermediate differentiation: case report. *J Neurosurg Pediatr* 2019. Online ahead of print. https://doi.org/10.3171/2019.8.PEDS18664.

Forschner A, Forchhammer S, Bonzheim I. *NTRK* gene fusions in melanoma: detection, prevalence and potential therapeutic implications. *J Dtsch Dermatol Ges* 2020;**18**(12):1387–92. https://doi.org/10.1111/ddg.14160.

Garnier L, Ducray F, Verlut C, et al. Prolonged response induced by single agent vemurafenib in a BRAF V600E spinal ganglioglioma: a case report and review of the literature. *Front Oncol* 2019;**9**:177. https://doi.org/10.3389/fonc.2019.00177.

Gdowski AS, Ranjan A, Vishwanatha JK. Current concepts in bone metastasis, contemporary therapeutic strategies and ongoing clinical trials. *J Exp Clin Cancer Res* 2017;**36**(1):108. https://doi.org/10.1186/s13046-017-0578-1.

Glasker S. Central nervous system manifestations in VHL: genetics, pathology and clinical phenotypic features. *Fam Cancer* 2005;**4**(1):37–42. https://doi.org/10.1007/s10689-004-5347-6.

Gottfried ON, Viskochil DH, Couldwell WT. Neurofibromatosis Type 1 and tumorigenesis: molecular mechanisms and therapeutic implications. *Neurosurg Focus* 2010;**28**(1):E8. https://doi.org/10.3171/2009.11.FOCUS09221.

Grimm S, Chamberlain MC. Adult primary spinal cord tumors. *Expert Rev Neurother* 2009;**9**(10):1487–95. https://doi.org/10.1586/ern.09.101.

Hamburger C, Buttner A, Weis S. Ganglioglioma of the spinal cord: report of two rare cases and review of the literature. *Neurosurgery* 1997;**41**(6):1410–15; discussion 1415–6. https://doi.org/10.1097/00006123-199712000-00038.

Hashi S, Goodwin CR, Ahmed AK, Sciubba DM. Management of extranodal lymphoma of the spine: a study of 30 patients. *CNS Oncol* 2018;**7**(2):CNS11. https://doi.org/10.2217/cns-2017-0033.

Hasselblatt M. Ependymal tumors. *Recent Results Cancer Res* 2009;**171**:51–66. https://doi.org/10.1007/978-3-540-31206-2_3.

Healey JH, Lane JM. Chordoma: a critical review of diagnosis and treatment. *Orthop Clin North Am* 1989;**20**(3):417–26.

Horbinski C. To *BRAF* or not to *BRAF*: is that even a question anymore? *J Neuropathol Exp Neurol* 2013;**72**(1):2–7. https://doi.org/10.1097/NEN.0b013e318279f3db.

Horbinski C, Hamilton RL, Nikiforov Y, Pollack IF. Association of molecular alterations, including *BRAF*, with biology and outcome in pilocytic astrocytomas. *Acta Neuropathol* 2010;**119**(5):641–9. https://doi.org/10.1007/s00401-009-0634-9.

Ilaslan H, Sundaram M, Unni KK, Dekutoski MB. Primary Ewing's sarcoma of the vertebral column. *Skeletal Radiol* 2004;**33**(9):506–13. https://doi.org/10.1007/s00256-004-0810-x

Jett K, Friedman JM. Clinical and genetic aspects of neurofibromatosis 1. *Genet Med.* 2010;**12**(1):1–11. https://doi.org/10.1097/GIM.0b013e3181bf15e3.

Johnson RA, Wright KD, Poppleton H, et al. Cross-species genomics matches driver mutations and cell compartments to

model ependymoma. *Nature* 2010;**466**(7306):632–6. https://doi
.org/10.1038/nature09173.

Jones V, Wykes V, Cohen N, Thompson D, Jacques TS. The
pathology of lumbosacral lipomas: macroscopic and
microscopic disparity have implications for embryogenesis and
mode of clinical deterioration. *Histopathology* 2018;**72**(7):1136–
44. https://doi.org/10.1111/his.13469.

Karsy M, Guan J, Sivakumar W, Neil JA, Schmidt MH,
Mahan MA. The genetic basis of intradural spinal tumors and
its impact on clinical treatment. *Neurosurg Focus* 2015;**39**(2):E3.
https://doi.org/10.3171/2015.5.FOCUS15143.

Katonis P, Alpantaki K, Michail K, et al. Spinal
chondrosarcoma: a review. *Sarcoma* 2011;**2011**:378957. https://
doi.org/10.1155/2011/378957.

Katonis P, Datsis G, Karantanas A, et al. Spinal osteosarcoma.
Clin Med Insights Oncol 2013;**7**:199–208. https://doi.org/10
.4137/CMO.S10099.

Kitamura H, Kubota Y, Yamaguchi K, et al. Successful
autologous hematopoietic stem cell transplantation followed by
bortezomib maintenance in a patient with relapsed CD138-low
multiple solitary plasmacytomas harboring a 17p deletion.
Intern Med 2018;**57**(6):855–60. https://doi.org/10.2169/internal
medicine.9446-17.

Korshunov A, Neben K, Wrobel G, et al. Gene expression
patterns in ependymomas correlate with tumor location, grade,
and patient age. *Am J Pathol* 2003;**163**(5):1721–7. https://doi
.org/10.1016/S0002-9440(10)63530-4.

Kubista B, Klinglmueller F, Bilban M, et al. Microarray analysis
identifies distinct gene expression profiles associated with
histological subtype in human osteosarcoma. *Int Orthop* 2011;**35**
(3):401–11. https://doi.org/10.1007/s00264-010-0996-6.

Liang Y, Yi L, Liu P, et al. CX3CL1 involves in breast cancer
metastasizing to the spine via the Src/FAK signaling pathway.
J Cancer 2018;**9**(19):3603–12. https://doi.org/10.7150/jca.26497.

Liu W, Wei H, Gao Z, et al. *COL5A1* may contribute the
metastasis of lung adenocarcinoma. *Gene* 2018;**665**:57–66.
https://doi.org/10.1016/j.gene.2018.04.066.

Liu W, Xie X, Wu J. Mechanism of lung adenocarcinoma spine
metastasis induced by CXCL17. *Cell Oncol (Dordr)* 2020;**43**
(2):311–20. https://doi.org/10.1007/s13402-019-00491-7.

Louis DN, Ohgaki H, Wiestler OD, et al. The 2007 WHO
classification of tumours of the central nervous system. *Acta
Neuropathol* 2007;**114**(2):97–109. https://doi.org/10.1007/s00401-
007-0243-4.

Loya JJ, Jung H, Temmins C, Cho N, Singh H. Primary spinal
germ cell tumors: a case analysis and review of treatment
paradigms. *Case Rep Med* 2013;**2013**:798358. https://doi.org/10
.1155/2013/798358.

Ma J, Ma S, Yang J, Jia G, Jia W. Primary spinal primitive
neuroectodermal tumor: a single center series with literature
review. *J Spinal Cord Med* 2020;**43**(6):895–903. https://doi.org/
10.1080/10790268.2018.1547862.

Maccauro G, Spinelli MS, Mauro S, Perisano C, Graci C,
Rosa MA. Physiopathology of spine metastasis. *Int J Surg Oncol*
2011;**2011**:107969. https://doi.org/10.1155/2011/107969.

Magnaghi P, Salom B, Cozzi L, et al. Afatinib is a new
therapeutic approach in chordoma with a unique ability to
target EGFR and brachyury. *Mol Cancer Ther* 2018;**17**(3):603–
13. https://doi.org/10.1158/1535-7163.MCT-17-0324.

Mehta VA, Kretzer RM, Orr B, Jallo GI. Primary intramedullary
spinal germ cell tumors. *World Neurosurg* 2011;**76**(5):478 e471–
6. https://doi.org/10.1016/j.wneu.2011.01.024.

Nagaishi M, Nobusawa S, Yokoo H, et al. Genetic mutations in
high grade gliomas of the adult spinal cord. *Brain Tumor Pathol*
2016;**33**(4):267–9. https://doi.org/10.1007/s10014-016-0263-7.

Nagasawa DT, Trang A, Choy W, et al. Genetic expression
profiles of adult and pediatric ependymomas: molecular
pathways, prognostic indicators, and therapeutic targets. *Clin
Neurol Neurosurg* 2013;**115**(4):388–99. https://doi.org/10.1016/j
.clineuro.2012.12.006.

Ostrom QT, Gittleman H, Liao P, et al. CBTRUS statistical
report: primary brain and central nervous system tumors
diagnosed in the United States in 2007–2011. *Neuro Oncol*
2014;**16**(Suppl 4):iv1–63. https://doi.org/10.1093/neuonc/
nou223.

Pang D, Zovickian J, Oviedo A. Long-term outcome of total and
near-total resection of spinal cord lipomas and radical
reconstruction of the neural placode, part II: outcome analysis
and preoperative profiling. *Neurosurgery* 2010;**66**(2):253–72;
discussion 272–3. https://doi.org/10.1227/01
.NEU.0000363598.81101.7B.

Pasalic I, Brgic K, Nemir J, Kolenc D, Njiric N, Mrak G.
Intramedullary spinal cord lipoma mimicking a late subacute
hematoma. *Asian J Neurosurg* 2018;**13**(4):1282–4. https://doi
.org/10.4103/ajns.AJNS_112_18.

Saeedinia S, Nouri M, Alimohammadi M, Moradi H,
Amirjamshidi A. Primary spinal extradural Ewing's sarcoma
(primitive neuroectodermal tumor): report of a case and meta-
analysis of the reported cases in the literature. *Surg Neurol Int*
2012;**3**:55. https://doi.org/10.4103/2152-7806.96154.

Samak EM, Abdel Latif AM, Ghany WA, Hewedi IH, Amer A,
Moharram H. Spinal intramedullary hamartoma with acute
presentation in a 13-month old infant: case report. *J Neurosurg
Pediatr* 2016;**18**(2):177–82. https://doi.org/10.3171/2016
.2.PEDS15561.

Sayagues JM, Tabernero MD, Maillo A, et al. Microarray-based
analysis of spinal versus intracranial meningiomas: different
clinical, biological, and genetic characteristics associated with
distinct patterns of gene expression. *J Neuropathol Exp Neurol*
2006;**65**(5):445–54. https://doi.org/10.1097/01
.jnen.0000229234.13372.d8.

Schindler G, Capper D, Meyer J, et al. Analysis of *BRAF* V600E
mutation in 1,320 nervous system tumors reveals high mutation
frequencies in pleomorphic xanthoastrocytoma, ganglioglioma

and extra-cerebellar pilocytic astrocytoma. *Acta Neuropathol* 2011;**121**(3):397–405. https://doi.org/10.1007/s00401-011-0802-6.

Schneider SJ, Blacklock JB, Bruner JM. Melanoma arising in a spinal nerve root. Case report. *J Neurosurg* 1987;**67**(6):923–7. https://doi.org/10.3171/jns.1987.67.6.0923.

Shankar GM, Lelic N, Gill CM, et al. *BRAF* alteration status and the histone *H3F3A* gene K27M mutation segregate spinal cord astrocytoma histology. *Acta Neuropathol* 2016;**131**(1):147–50. https://doi.org/10.1007/s00401-015-1492-2.

Singh PK, Gutmann DH, Fuller CE, Newsham IF, Perry A. Differential involvement of protein 4.1 family members DAL-1 and NF2 in intracranial and intraspinal ependymomas. *Mod Pathol* 2002;**15**(5):526–31. https://doi.org/10.1038/modpathol.3880558.

Skarli SO, Wolf AL, Kristt DA, Numaguchi Y. Melanoma arising in a cervical spinal nerve root: report of a case with a benign course and malignant features. *Neurosurgery* 1994;**34**(3):533–7; discussion 637. https://doi.org/10.1227/00006123-199403000-00023.

Soutar R, Lucraft H, Jackson G, et al. Guidelines on the diagnosis and management of solitary plasmacytoma of bone and solitary extramedullary plasmacytoma. *Clin Oncol (R Coll Radiol)* 2004;**16**(6):405–13. https://doi.org/10.1016/j.clon.2004.02.007.

Stacchiotti S, Tamborini E, Lo Vullo S, et al. Phase II study on lapatinib in advanced EGFR-positive chordoma. *Ann Oncol* 2013;**24**(7):1931–6. https://doi.org/10.1093/annonc/mdt117.

Sumegi J, Nishio J, Nelson M, Frayer RW, Perry D, Bridge JA. A novel t(4;22)(q31;q12) produces an *EWSR1–SMARCA5* fusion in extraskeletal Ewing sarcoma/primitive neuroectodermal tumor. *Mod Pathol* 2011;**24**(3):333–42. https://doi.org/10.1038/modpathol.2010.201.

Szerlip NJ, Calinescu A, Smith E, et al. Dural cells release factors which promote cancer cell malignancy and induce immunosuppressive markers in bone marrow myeloid cells. *Neurosurgery* 2018;**83**(6):1306–16. https://doi.org/10.1093/neuros/nyx626.

Takai K, Taniguchi M, Takahashi H, Usui M, Saito N. Comparative analysis of spinal hemangioblastomas in sporadic disease and Von Hippel–Lindau syndrome. *Neurol Med Chir (Tokyo)* 2010;**50**(7):560–7. https://doi.org/10.2176/nmc.50.560.

Tarpey PS, Behjati S, Young MD, et al. The driver landscape of sporadic chordoma. *Nat Commun* 2017;**8**(1):890. https://doi.org/10.1038/s41467-017-01026-0.

Thiery JP, Acloque H, Huang RY, Nieto MA. Epithelial–mesenchymal transitions in development and disease. *Cell* 2009;**139**(5):871–90. https://doi.org/10.1016/j.cell.2009.11.007.

Uematsu Y, Tsuura Y, Miyamoto K, Itakura T, Hayashi S, Komai N. The recurrence of primary intracranial germinomas. Special reference to germinoma with STGC (syncytiotrophoblastic giant cell). *J Neurooncol* 1992;**13**(3):247–56. https://doi.org/10.1007/BF00172477.

Wellik DM. Hox patterning of the vertebrate axial skeleton. *Dev Dyn.* 2007;**236**(9):2454–63. https://doi.org/10.1002/dvdy.21286.

Westhoff MA, Serrels B, Fincham VJ, Frame MC, Carragher NO. SRC-mediated phosphorylation of focal adhesion kinase couples actin and adhesion dynamics to survival signaling. *Mol Cell Biol* 2004;**24**(18):8113–33. https://doi.org/10.1128/MCB.24.18.8113-8133.2004.

Wright CH, Wright J, Onyewadume L, et al. Diagnosis, treatment, and survival in spinal dissemination of primary intracranial glioblastoma: systematic literature review. *J Neurosurg Spine* 2019:1–10. Online ahead of print. https://doi.org/10.3171/2019.5.SPINE19164.

Yanamadala V, Koffie RM, Shankar GM, et al. Spinal cord glioblastoma: 25 years of experience from a single institution. *J Clin Neurosci* 2016;**27**:138–41. https://doi.org/10.1016/j.jocn.2015.11.011.

Yang J, Antin P, Berx G, et al. Guidelines and definitions for research on epithelial–mesenchymal transition. *Nat Rev Mol Cell Biol* 2020;**21**(6):341–52. https://doi.org/10.1038/s41580-020-0237-9.

Yang XR, Ng D, Alcorta DA, et al. T (brachyury) gene duplication confers major susceptibility to familial chordoma. *Nat Genet* 2009;**41**(11):1176–8. https://doi.org/10.1038/ng.454

Zheng JS, Wang M, Wan S, et al. Isolated primary non-Hodgkin's lymphoma of the thoracic spine: a case report with a review of the literature. *J Int Med Res* 2010;**38**(4):1553–60. https://doi.org/10.1177/147323001003800440.

Acute Spinal Cord Injury and Spinal Trauma

Dominique M. O. Higgins, Pavan S. Upadhyayula, Michael Argenziano, and Paul McCormick

20.1 Introduction

Spinal cord injury (SCI) is a debilitating problem with a global incidence of 8 to 246 cases per million (Furlan et al., 2013) and an associated significant increase in healthcare cost. Spinal cord injury research generally focuses on two broad categories: minimizing initial insult via modulation of primary and secondary injury cascades, or on novel therapeutic strategies aimed at recovering function. To this end, numerous SCI preclinical models have been developed, and promising clinical trials have arisen as a result, highlighting the importance of choosing the optimal model in relation to one's scientific question. In this chapter we will highlight relevant spinal cord anatomy, embryology, and the pathophysiology of SCI with a focus on how these factors relate to preclinical models of SCI and spinal cord trauma. We hope to highlight important factors necessary for future research.

20.2 Spinal Cord Anatomy

20.2.1 Basic Organization

The spinal cord is organized in vertical columns that span the junction between the central and peripheral nervous systems. Cross-sections of the spinal cord show gray matter organized in a butterfly pattern, surrounded by white matter tracts peripherally. The spinal cord has an anterior median fissure and a posterior median septum or raphe that helps signify the midline. The central gray matter includes neuronal cell bodies, dendrites, interneurons, glial cells, and axons. The gray matter is organized into 10 distinct regions, Rexed 1–10, named for Bror Rexed's anatomical study of cats (Rexed, 1952, 1954). Rexed 1–9 are organized dorsal to ventral while Rexed 10 is located around the central canal. A full description of the Rexed nuclei can be found in Table 20.1 (Bennett et al., 1980, 1981; Honda and Lee, 1985; Mannen and Sugiura, 1976; Schoenen, 1982a, 1982b).

The white matter columns of the spinal cord surround the gray matter and can broadly be categorized as either ascending tracts or descending tracts. The ascending tracts of the spinal cord are sensory, which include: the dorsal column–medial lemnisci, the anterior and lateral spinothalamic tracts, and the spinocerebellar tracts (Rothwell, 1994). Descending white matter tracts are generally motor tracts (Lemon, 2008; Rothwell, 1994). Descending motor tracts are broadly grouped based on whether they travel through the medullary pyramids. The anterior and lateral corticospinal tracts carry voluntary motor movement from the motor cortex or supplementary motor area directly to lower motor neurons synapsing in the anterior horn cells. The extrapyramidal tracts generally maintain posture, muscle tone, and reflexes; the largest extrapyramidal tracts are the rubrospinal tract, the vestibulospinal tract, and the reticulospinal tract. The rubrospinal tract is broadly responsible for flexor movements of the upper limbs, while the reticulospinal tract is essential for postural coordination. The vestibulospinal tract integrates sensory information from the vestibular nuclei to maintain posture and muscle tone in extensor or antigravity muscles. A complete cross-section of the gray matter nuclei and white matter tracts can be found in Figure 20.1.

20.2.2 Embryology

Spinal cord development is made possible by the notochord, a craniocaudal collection of mesenchymal and endodermal cells that form a notochordal process by day 19 with complete closure of the notochord by day 25 of embryonic development (Ramesh et al., 2017). Although the notochord itself is fated to become the intervertebral discs of the spinal cord, it secretes the factors necessary for patterning of the neural tube that arises from neuroepithelial cells on the dorsal side of the notochord (Ramesh et al., 2017). The process of creating the neural plate and subsequent neural tube from ectodermal cells is known as

Table 20.1 Spinal cord gray matter summary – Rexed nuclei summary

Rexed nuclei	Cytoarchitecture	Description
Laminae 1	Waldeyer cells (medium/small neurons); Nissl-positive large neurons	Entry point for the dorsal roots (sensory)
Laminae II	Smallest cells in the dorsal horn with abundant dendrites	Substantia gelatinosa, synapse point for axons carrying noxious and temperature impulse (lateral spinothalamic tract)
Laminae III	Large pale cells with light nucleus and prominent nucleolus	Nucleus proprius: along with laminae IV, synapse point for axons carrying vibration/pressure sensation and proprioceptive impulses to the dorsal columns/medial lemniscus
Laminae IV	Large and small cells juxtaposed	Nucleus proprius: along with laminae III, synapse point for axons carrying vibration/pressure sensation and proprioceptive impulses to the dorsal columns/medial lemniscus
Laminae V	10 neuronal types with greatest number of dendritic connections. Lightly staining medial zone and darkly staining lateral reticulated zone	Sensory afferents received from skin and visceral nociceptors
Laminae VI	Medial zone with compact small cells, lateral zone with loose large star-shaped cells	Corresponds with the nuclei of Cajal, implicated in reflex withdrawal from painful stimuli and with synapses to lamina VIII coordinating spinal reflexes
Laminae VII	Intermediolateral gray horn: medial zone of interneurons/propriospinal neurons, lateral zone of posture and movement	From C8 to L3 origin of ipsilateral spinocerebellar tract. From T1 to L2 preganglionic sympathetic neurons
Laminae VIII	Triangular/star-shaped heavy staining nerve cells	Interneurons and proprioceptive neurons coordinating spinal reflexes and the synapse point for vestibulospinal and reticulospinal tracts
Laminae IX	Abundant Nissl staining	Medial motor column innervates proximal muscles while lateral motor column present in cervical/lumbar regions innervates distal muscles of shoulder/pelvic girdle
Laminae X	Centrally located around the central canal	Axons that cross to opposite side of cord

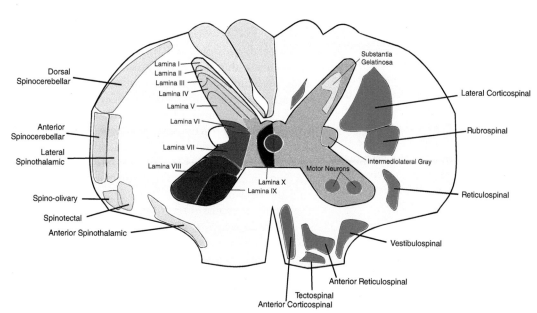

Figure 20.1 Cross-section of spinal cord demonstrating ascending and descending tracts. Ascending tracts are depicted in blue and descending tracts are depicted in red. Author's artwork

neuralation (O'Rahilly and Müller, 2006). The first neurons to appear are motor neurons in the anterior horn of the cervical spine (28 days post conception) and the first synapses to appear are also in the cervical spinal cord (44 days post conception; O'Rahilly and Müller, 2006). Although beyond the scope of this chapter, the patterning of the spinal cord, both in rostrocaudal and ventrodorsal axes, is strictly regulated by transcription factors and cytoskeletal elements (Ferretti et al., 2006). Two intermediate filament markers, nestin and vimentin, are associated with embryonic development of the neural tube and formation of the early spinal cord. Interestingly, animals such as salamanders that are able to regenerate their spinal cord are shown to have dedicated ependymoglial cells with inducible nestin and vimentin expression following injury (Ferretti et al., 2006). Numerous studies have shown that differential regulation of master regulator genes during neurulation and embryological development play a key role in pathophysiologic differences between species (Fougerousse et al., 2000; Semple et al., 2013). This becomes important in understanding mechanisms of neurogenesis and potential mechanisms of repair in different animal models.

20.3 Pathophysiology of Spinal Cord Injury

Spinal cord injury is thought to occur primarily in two phases, an acute primary phase, and a subacute to chronic secondary phase. Primary injury in SCI relates to the immediate, mostly mechanical trauma, that the spinal cord suffers. This primary injury event usually comprises disruption, dislocation, compression, transection, and/or distraction of the spinal cord. These insults directly stress neurons, oligodendrocytes, and endothelial cells/vasculature. The primary injury leads to ischemia and edema, both of which can trigger a variety of cell cascades that amplify SCI. The downstream cascades during the secondary phase broadly fall into three main categories: inflammatory or immune-mediated injury, reactive oxygen species and lipid peroxidation, and neuronal cell death and demyelination (Ahuja et al., 2017).

20.3.1 Mechanisms of Secondary Injury

20.3.1.1 Inflammatory and Immune-Mediated Injury

The inflammatory cascade involves a host of second messengers, typically released from the recruitment of immune cells. Initial studies in animal and human models have

shown therapeutic effects of immune depletion, either through high-dose steroid use or through direct inhibition of macrophages, neutrophils, or other immune compartments (Bracken and Holford, 2002; Rossignol et al., 2007). However, similar to cancer-associated immune cells, it is now well recognized that there are both positive and negative immune mediators. As such, complete immune response inhibition can have negative effects on recovery. Macrophages, for example, can either create devastating inflammation and scar formation or be critical in debris clearance and wound healing. The exact markers underlying these differences are not yet known, but classic macrophage expression markers including CX3CR1 and MAC-2 have been implicated (Orr and Gensel, 2018; Wang et al., 2015). Microglia are key inducers of central nervous system (CNS) inflammation, but also secrete growth factors necessary for neuron survival (Badimon et al., 2020; Werneburg et al., 2017). Beyond macrophages, neutrophils have been linked to propagation of the SCI injury through release of enzymes, cytokines, and free radicals (Kubota et al., 2012; Kumar et al., 2018; Neirinckx et al., 2014; Nguyen et al., 2007; Saiwai et al., 2010). T lymphocytes can be primed against myelin due to release of myelin auto-antigens creating further demyelination. In sum, although immune cells are important for debris clearance and eventual wound healing, it is often found that both innate and adaptive immune cells can propagate worsening of the SCI through the release of cytokines and free radicals.

20.3.1.2 Reactive Oxygen Species and Lipid Peroxidation

The secondary cascade in SCI causes a host of metabolic alterations within spinal cord cells. Changes to local vasculature, immune microenvironment, and a secondary cascade of inflammatory cells all shift cells toward generation of large quantities of reactive oxygen species (ROS), which are highly reactive and capable of propagating and damaging lipid membranes, proteins, and DNA (Müller and Gürster, 1993; Su et al., 2019). While oxygen's role as an electron acceptor is critical to normal cell metabolism and the electron transport chain, dysregulated metabolism in the presence of transition metals can create ROS.

Multiple animal studies have shown this process of ROS generation and membrane lipid peroxidation occurs in the secondary cascade of spinal cord injury. As with the normal ROS cascade, the three steps of initiation, propagation, and termination can occur with radicalization of free-floating oxygen molecules or with the radicalization of carboxylic end chains of polyunsaturated fatty acids.

The high fat content in the spinal cord has highlighted the importance of lipid peroxidation and the associated regulated cell death cascade, ferroptosis, in spinal cord injury. Initial studies have demonstrated that induction of ferroptosis through infusion of iron (Fe^{2+}) and peroxide can create histologic lesions similar to SCI (Anderson et al., 1985; Liu et al., 1998). Moreover, other studies have shown that SCI-induced lipid peroxidation occurs as quickly as one hour following insult and is associated with depletion of native antioxidants (i.e., vitamin E, ascorbic acid, glutathione) (Hall et al., 1992; Lemke et al., 1990; Lucas et al., 2002; Pietronigro et al., 1983).

This ROS cascade and associated lipid peroxidation triggers the loss of membrane integrity and functioning ion channels, leading to dysregulation of microvasculature, glutamate excitotoxicity, and mitochondrial dysfunction, creating a vicious feedback cycle (Carrico et al., 2009; Hall and Wolf, 1986; Monyer et al., 1990). Loss of membrane integrity and unregulated ionic flux is associated with spontaneous activation of proteases, leading to apoptosis and necrosis of surrounding tissue (Whalen et al., 2008). Animal studies have shown lipid peroxidation breakdown products accumulate within minutes of an SCI and that they may peak as early as 3 h following injury (Barut et al., 1993; J.-B. Liu et al., 2004).

Studies examining antioxidants and specific lipid peroxidation blockers have also had promise in preclinical SCI models (Anderson et al., 1985; Demopoulos et al., 1982; Hall and Braughler, 1982; Hall et al., 1992; Kamencic et al., 2001; D. Liu et al., 2004; Stockwell et al., 2017; Yune et al., 2008). Importantly, studies examining ROS antioxidants have been correlated with improved clinical outcomes following SCI. A small study ($n = 30$) by Heller et al. (2019) showed that levels of selenium, a trace element key for selenoproteins that comprise the rate-limiting step in lipid peroxide detoxification, is inversely correlated with outcomes following traumatic SCI.

20.3.1.3 Neuronal Cell Death and Demyelination

Demyelination occurs both in the acute and chronic phases following SCI. Initial insult with the inflammatory cascade, vascular dysregulation, and membrane permeabilization leads to death of oligodendrocytes, leading to rapid early demyelination around the injury focus (Rowland et al., 2008). While most injury and neuronal cell death occurs through a dual process of edema and necrosis, oligodendrocytes have been shown to undergo apoptosis through a Fas-mediated microglial activation

(Casha et al., 2001, 2005). Fas, also known as CD95, is a transmembrane protein that when bound to its ligand initiates a cascade of events that ultimately lead to cleavage of caspase-3 and initiation of apoptosis (Volpe et al., 2016). Although rodent studies have highlighted the importance of spared demyelinated neurons in functional recovery, no human studies have shown similar findings (Kakulas, 2004; Nashmi and Fehlings, 2001; Norenberg et al., 2004; Totoiu et al., 2004). This may be due to the fact that human neurons are more likely to undergo cell death following demyelination. This loss of white matter due to oligodendrocyte apoptosis can continue for weeks, leading to profound and persistent demyelination along white matter tracts spreading beyond the lesion focus (Beattie et al., 2000). In this subacute to chronic period following SCI, oligodendrocyte progenitor cells – a CNS oligodendrocyte precursor cell capable of differentiation into neurons, astrocytes, or oligodendrocytes – regenerate the lost oligodendrocyte population. The myelin generated from this new population of oligodendrocytes is unable to cover all demyelinated axons leading to a myelin deficit with uncovered neurons prone to dysfunction or degeneration (Alizadeh et al., 2015; Hackett et al., 2016).

20.4 Mechanisms of Spinal Cord Injury Repair

After the primary and secondary injury cascades, recovery and repair of the spinal cord occurs. These lesions, once they reach a steady state, generally have three components: a non-neural core, an astroglial scar, and a surrounding region of viable neural tissue (O'Shea et al., 2017). The non-neural core contains pericytes and fibroblasts along with diverse immune cells that aid in the clearance of cellular debris. This inflammatory process is blocked off by astrocytes as early as 24 h after SCI. The formation of a complete scar generally occurs by 3 weeks following SCI. Although astrocytes are the predominant cell type, oligodendrocyte progenitor cells are also intermixed within scar formation. The viable neural tissue surrounding these two areas can often undergo circuit reorganization. In some instances this is pathologic, leading to neuropathic pain, muscle spasms, or dysautonomia. In some cases, most notably after cord hemi-section such as in Brown–Sequard syndrome, spontaneous recovery of function can occur. Although the astrocytosis is necessary for edema resolution and restoration of the blood–brain barrier (BBB) (Rowland et al., 2008), the astroglial scar often is an impediment to many types of regenerative therapies as it acts as a mechanical blockade from neuronal regeneration or remyelination.

20.4.1 Clinical Trials Targeted at Improving Spinal Cord Injury Outcomes

Management of SCI has made numerous improvements in the recent years. These improvements can be directly traced to an understanding of the pathophysiologic mechanisms of SCI. As described, the initial insult often involves vascular compromise. For this reason numerous clinical trials aimed at mean arterial pressure (MAP) support have demonstrated improvement in clinical outcomes (Levi et al., 1993; Vale et al., 1997). Perhaps the clearest demonstration of the importance of MAP support was by Hawryluk et al., who used q1 minute MAP data showing that MAP support for 2–3 days following injury was associated with improved neurological outcome in acute SCI (Hawryluk et al., 2015; Readdy and Dhall, 2016). Early steroid use demonstrated improvement in outcomes, such as in the National Acute SCI Study (NASCIS) I–III, which were large multicenter clinical trials (Anderson et al., 1985; Bracken and Holford, 2002). More recently, however, high-dose steroid use has fallen out of favor, due to the potential for harmful side effects outweighing marginal benefit (Bracken et al., 1997; Ohtani et al., 1994; Pointillart et al., 2000). Management of intrathecal spinal cord pressure is another active area of research, as emerging data suggest that spinal fluid drainage may help to improve cord perfusion and recovery (Martirosyan et al., 2015). Finally, numerous preclinical and clinical studies have evaluated use of growth factors or stem cell–based treatments aimed at preventing neuronal degradation or at the creation of new neurons and synaptic connections (Curtis et al., 2018; Kucher et al., 2018; Levi et al., 2019; Tabakow et al., 2013; Xiao et al., 2018). These clinical trials have demonstrated safety and sporadic improvements in function, but numerous questions remain. Mechanisms of delivery, location of delivery (i.e., intramedullary, intrathecal), chronicity of treatment, and even the necessity for surgical excision of local scar are all important areas of future study for optimization of these treatment paradigms. Another area of clinical investigation includes the use of brain–machine interfaces or exoskeleton devices (Chaudhary et al., 2016; Guger et al., 2003). These devices aim to produce functional recovery without neurological recovery (Ajiboye et al., 2017; Rohm

et al., 2013). An important outstanding question for therapeutic applications of brain–computer interfaces is the optimization of training methods that can be applied universally to different patients with different pathologies (Kawase et al., 2017; Tidoni et al., 2017).

20.4.2 Importance of Species in Animal Models of Spinal Cord Injury

Animal models of SCI span the gamut between small rodents and larger animals including cats, dogs, pigs, and non-human primates. In general, small rodents such as rats and mice are most commonly used in SCI research due to low cost and ease of handling. No animal perfectly mimics the anatomy of the human spinal cord or the pathology of human SCI. There exist advantages and disadvantages with each model and it is important to know how animal models recapitulate human pathology.

Of rodents, rats are known to have pathophysiology post-SCI that more closely mimics human pathology, and are the most common species in animal models of SCI. In both rats and humans, a syrinx encased in white matter is often formed following traumatic SCI (Noble and Wrathall, 1985; Zhang et al., 2018). This syrinx generally forms both cranially and caudally to the site of injury (Bunge et al., 1993; Josephson et al., 2001). Magnetic resonance imaging studies of rat SCI show findings that are consistent with human SCI; namely, that lesion size and spinal cord atrophy are strongly correlated with functional outcome (Metz et al., 2000).

These similarities, however, are not universal. Locomotion, an extensively studied topic in the SCI field, appears to be differentially modulated by descending tracts. In humans, the corticospinal tract is essential to walking as evidenced by the inability for normal locomotion following bilateral lesions to the corticospinal tract. Electroencephalographic studies have shown that all muscle activity involved in normal uncomplicated locomotion seems to have a cortical source (Nathan, 1994; Nielsen, 2003; Petersen et al., 2012). On the contrary, in rats corticospinal lesions are permissive of gait; gait is more dependent on descending pathways such as the rubrospinal and reticulospinal tract (Schucht et al., 2002). Importantly, rats are also able to functionally bridge across spinal cord lesions to regain function. The ability for descending redundant motor tracts like the rubrospinal or reticulospinal tracts to arborize with propriospinal neurons and bridge spinal cord lesions is a key factor explaining how rats have higher degree of functional recovery following SCI than humans (Filli et al.,

2014; Ghosh et al., 2010; Kennedy, 1990; Zörner et al., 2014). It is important to note that arborization between rubrospinal or reticulospinal tracts and propriospinal neurons are also implicated in human and primate recovery following SCI (Baker and Perez, 2017; Tohyama et al., 2017).

The mouse has numerous additional features that diverge from human SCI. First, the mouse does not form a syrinx post-traumatic SCI (Göritz et al., 2011; Ma et al., 2001). Following acute injury such as transection, proliferation of cells is able to keep the spinal cord in contact preventing the formation of a syrinx (Göritz et al., 2011). A study by Inman and Steward (2003) showed extension of ascending sensory axons into connective tissue scar that formed following acute crush injury in c57/B6J mice. Both these findings highlight the increased potential for functional recovery in mice compared to humans and other animal models.

Many initial SCI studies were undertaken in the feline species. The use of feline models of SCI has been instrumental in understanding mechanisms of recovery of hindlimb locomotion following various spinal lesions (Frigon, 2013). Like humans, cats have a higher center of gravity during locomotion compared to other models such as rodents. Furthermore, cats can be trained to freely walk on a treadmill at various speeds and inclines. Spinal anatomy of cats is also more similar to humans – the major component of the feline corticospinal tract lies in the dorsolateral spinal cord, as in humans (Frigon, 2013). Due to its larger physical size, the cat has been used to develop several experimental techniques that were then translated to smaller models such as rodents. This includes a model of fictive locomotion, where a decerebrate paralyzed animal undergoes the neural processes of locomotion without any physical motion (Gerasimenko et al., 2003; Grillner and Zangger et al., 1979; Jordan et al., 2008; Whelan, 1996). Thus, feline models have allowed for the detailed identification of the neuronal subtypes within the mammalian spinal cord (Domínguez-Rodríguez et al., 2020; Eccles et al., 1957; Jankowska et al., 2007).

Canines, while comprising only 2.3% of all animal models of SCI (Sharif-Alhoseini et al., 2017), have been integral in the translational understanding of SCI in humans. Canines undergo spontaneous SCI through intervertebral disc herniation. Canines also demonstrate similar comorbidities to humans, such as obesity and cardiovascular disease (Moore et al., 2018; van der Scheer et al., 2017). Thus, studies in canines with spontaneous non-traumatic SCI requiring euthanasia present a unique opportunity for translational study of therapies (Jeffery et al., 2006, 2011; Levine et al., 2011; Moore et al., 2017).

The pig is thought to be the best non-primate model of SCI as it has similar structural, neuronal, and vascular anatomy along with similar secondary responses to SCI as humans. The vascular anatomy of the pig is similar to that of a human with similar ventral and dorsal spinal arteries along with arteries of similar caliber. Even though there exist key differences between pig and human spinal cords, such as the significant arterial supply provided by the median sacral artery – an artery that is redundant in humans – the pig is still optimal for the study of spinal cord ischemia and reperfusion due to the similar vascular anatomy and ability to use similar surgical equipment (Mazensky et al., 2017; Simon and Oberhuber, 2016). There exists marked similarity between the contribution of segmental thoracic and lumbar arteries in the pig and human spinal cords. The formation of post-traumatic syrinx in both animals also shows similar pathophysiologic responses to SCI (Navarro et al., 2012; Strauch et al., 2007). Moreover, the organization and location of various tracts including the corticospinal tract and the spinothalamic tract – both located ventrolaterally – is similar between humans and pigs (Breazile and Kitchell, 1968). Multiple metrics demonstrate similar immune and inflammatory profiles of pigs to humans. Perhaps most telling is the fact that the number of orthologous gene families between pigs and humans is 10 times as many as the number of orthologous gene families between mice and humans (Amit et al., 2009; Schomberg et al., 2017; Zakaryan et al., 2015).

20.4.3 Mechanisms of Injury in Animal Models of Spinal Cord Injury

Human SCI predominantly occurs through either direct impact with compression, distraction, or laceration and transection (Alizadeh et al., 2019). Although animal models are generally limited to a single mechanism of injury, human SCI usually comprises multiple injury mechanisms. In general, animal models have been created to replicate these mechanisms of injury. These animal models fall into four broad categories: contusion, transection, compression, and distraction/dislocation models (Cheriyan et al., 2014). Most studies use contusion models (43.4%) followed by transection (34.3%) and compression (20.5%). There is a paucity of distraction/dislocation studies (1.1%) likely due to the lack of standardized models for this type of injury (Sharif-Alhoseini et al., 2017).

20.4.3.1 Contusion Model

The most widely used contusion model is the Multicenter Animal Spinal Cord Injury Study (MASCIS) impactor model (Basso et al., 1996). This involves the dropping of a specific weight from a specific height onto a laminectomized portion of a rat spinal cord. Recent studies have broadened this to studies into a variety of animal models (Hu et al., 2010; Jones et al., 2012). Concerns with the MASCIS impactor include the possibility for a double impact due to a bounce of the weight dropping mechanism as well as an issue with exact reproducibility (Cheriyan et al., 2014). Two other contusion models aimed at addressing this problem are the Infinite Horizon Impactor and the Ohio State University Impactor, both of which use computer-based systems to create reproducible contusions. The contusion mechanism of SCI is associated with numerous pathologic findings. Choo et al. (2008) describe these findings in a rat contusion model and show prominent neuronal loss of mitochondrial cytochrome c in the contusion epicenter. The authors show relative preservation of axonal integrity and white matter tracts with levels that are similar to sham controls. These findings point to a gray-matter dominant, white-matter sparing phenotype that is important to consider when evaluating outcomes.

20.4.3.2 Compression Models

Compression models were first explored to create more reproducible SCI. The most common type of compression model uses an aneurysm clip applied to laminectomized spine. Although there is a level of compressive injury, it is generally believed the mechanism of injury is due to vascular compromise and ischemia (Zivin and DeGirolami, 1980). Another such method was the use of balloon compression that compresses the spinal cord through inflation in the epidural or subdural space (Aslan et al., 2009; Fukuda et al., 2005; Nesathurai et al., 2006). Two other methods for compressive injury include the calibrated forceps model and spinal cord strapping. The calibrated forceps uses mechanical forceps to compress the spinal cord to a given depth. Spinal cord strapping is the one method that does not require a laminectomy and involves threading a suture around the spinal cord in a blind fashion and then using weights to deliver compressive force to the cord. All these methods have been shown to induce graded functional and histologic responses along with the characteristics of secondary injury including edema, hemorrhage, and cavitation (Abdullahi et al., 2017). Recent microdialysis studies have shown increased elevation of lactate to pyruvate ratio following compressive versus contusive injury, further indicating an ischemic mechanism following spinal cord compression (Okon et al., 2013). Therefore, it is believed this model of SCI may reproduce surgical SCI more accurately than traumatic SCI (Cheriyan et al., 2014).

20.4.3.3 Transection Models

Transection models are commonly used in preclinical studies even though transection is an infrequent mechanism of clinical SCI. Currently, many studies aimed at functional neuronal recovery through stem cell therapies use transection models. Numerous animal models have demonstrated spontaneous recovery of function following transection, demonstrating a major caveat to preclinical studies using transection models. For example, rat hind-limb movement was found to spontaneously occur following thoracic level transection as soon as 1 week following insult (Basso et al., 2006). Cats were similarly able to support weight following spinal cord hemi-section and these changes facilitated increased capacity for recovery following subsequent SCI (Martinez et al., 2011). Multiple mechanisms may explain this functional recovery phenomenon. In rats, the increased plasticity through the reticulospinal tract or propriospinal neurons is thought to bypass the hemi-sected descending corticospinal tract (Ballermann and Fouad, 2006; Courtine et al., 2008). In cats, a spinal pattern generating neurons below the injury level maintains and primes neurons for functional recovery (Ballermann and Fouad, 2006; Barrière et al., 2008). Some argue that the increased interaction with the environment experienced by quadrupedal animals may make them more prone to this increased plasticity (Onifer et al., 2011).

20.4.3.4 Dislocation/Distraction Models

Dislocation or distraction models are the least commonly used in preclinical studies. It is important to note that the study by Choo and colleagues. in rats showed that there existed prominent differences between the dislocation and distraction models. Dislocation models showed increased axonal permeability, high levels of beta amyloid precursor accumulation (a marker of neurofilament degradation and axonal damage), and large amounts of reactive changes including reactive astrocytes and microglia activation (Choo et al., 2008). In histologic areas, distraction injury showed much fewer changes to both gray and white matter. Multiple distraction models have been reported (Cheriyan et al., 2014). In general, these models, including the Harrington distractor and the University of Texas Arlington distractor, have used slow-velocity distraction (Dabney et al., 2004; Zhang et al., 2014). This mechanism is dissimilar from human SCI, which generally occurs at high velocity. The University of British Columbia distractor is capable of high-velocity distraction but has yet to be validated with concrete pathophysiologic endpoints (Choo et al., 2009).

20.5 Final Considerations

A 2017 meta-analysis of SCI studies shows that a majority of animal studies in SCI use either rat (72.4%) or mouse (16%) animal models (Sharif-Alhoseini et al., 2017). Any project examining SCI in a preclinical model should be able to identify the correlation between the model in use and relevant human pathology. Moreover, the intervention of choice should specifically target a mechanism of secondary injury in SCI, or be aimed at aiding a mechanism of regeneration or recovery. Thorough analysis of the accuracy and precision of different SCI models and an understanding of the trade-offs that are inherent when moving from large animal to small animal SCI models is imperative.

Moreover, bowel and bladder function, autonomic function, breathing, and fine motor coordination are some of the most important factors contributing to patient outcomes following SCI. In contrast, animal models of SCI generally focus on thoracic-level injuries and examine locomotion (55.9% of all studies) and sensation (10.2% of studies), with only 4% of studies examining bowel or bladder function or autonomic responses (Sharif-Alhoseini et al., 2017). The general discordance between promising preclinical studies and their clinical impact highlights the importance of using the appropriate preclinical models along with examining the appropriate outcomes that can most impact patient care.

Figure acknowledgements

The following image is credited to the authors of this chapter: Figure 20.1

References

Abdullahi D, Annuar AA, Mohamad M, Aziz I, Sanusi J. Experimental spinal cord trauma: a review of mechanically induced spinal cord injury in rat models. *Rev Neurosci* 2017:28:15–20. https://doi.org/10.1515/revneuro-2016-0050.

Ahuja CS, Wilson JR, Novi S, et al. Traumatic spinal cord injury. *Nat Rev Dis Primers* (2017;3:17018. https://doi.org/10.1038/nrdp.2017.18.

Ajiboye AB, Willett FR, Young DR, et al. Restoration of reaching and grasping movements through brain-controlled muscle stimulation in a person with tetraplegia: a proof-of-concept demonstration. *Lancet* 2017;389:1821–30. https://doi.org/10.1016/S0140-6736(17)30601-3.

Alizadeh A, Dyck SM, Karimi-Abdolrezaee S. Myelin damage and repair in pathologic CNS: challenges and prospects. *Front Mol Neurosci* 2015;8:35. https://doi.org/10.3389/fnmol.2015.00035.

Alizadeh A, Dyck SM, Karimi-Abdolrezaee S. Traumatic spinal cord injury: an overview of pathophysiology, models and acute injury mechanisms. *Front Neurol* 2019:10:282. https://doi.org/10.3389/fneur.2019.00282

Amit I, Garber M, Chevrier N, et al. Unbiased reconstruction of a mammalian transcriptional network mediating pathogen responses. *Science* 2009;326:257–63. https://doi.org/10.1126/science.1179050.

Anderson DK, Means ED. Iron-induced lipid peroxidation in spinal cord: protection with mannitol and methylprednisolone. *J Free Radic Biol Med* 1985;1:59–64. https://doi.org/10.1016/0748-5514(85)90030-3.

Anderson DK, Saunders RD, Demediuk P, et al. Lipid hydrolysis and peroxidation in injured spinal cord: partial protection with methylprednisolone or vitamin E and selenium. *Cent Nerv Syst Trauma* 1985;2:257–67. https://doi.org/10.1089/cns.1985.2.257.

Aslan A, Cemek M, Eser, O, et al. Does dexmedetomidine reduce secondary damage after spinal cord injury? An experimental study. *Eur Spine J* 2009;18:336–44. https://doi.org/10.1007/s00586-008-0872-x.

Badimon A, Strasburger HJ, Ayata P, et al. Negative feedback control of neuronal activity by microglia. *Nature* 2020;586:417–23. https://doi.org/10.1038/s41586-020-2777-8.

Baker SN, Perez MA. Reticulospinal contributions to gross hand function after human spinal cord injury. *J Neurosci* 2017;37:9778–84. https://doi.org/10.1523/JNEUROSCI.3368-16.2017.

Ballermann M, Fouad K. Spontaneous locomotor recovery in spinal cord injured rats is accompanied by anatomical plasticity of reticulospinal fibers. *Eur J Neurosci* 2006;23:1988–96. https://doi.org/10.1111/j.1460-9568.2006.04726.x.

Barrière G, Leblond H, Provencher J, Rossignol S. Prominent role of the spinal central pattern generator in the recovery of locomotion after partial spinal cord injuries. *J Neurosci* 2008;28:3976–87. https://doi.org/10.1523/JNEUROSCI.5692-07.2008.

Barut S, Canbolat A, Bilge T, Aydin Y, Cokneşeli B, Kaya U. Lipid peroxidation in experimental spinal cord injury: time-level relationship. *Neurosurg Rev* 1993;16:53–9. https://doi.org/10.1007/BF00308614.

Basso DM, Beattie MS, Bresnahan, JC, et al. MASCIS evaluation of open field locomotor scores: effects of experience and teamwork on reliability. Multicenter animal spinal cord injury study. *J Neurotrauma* 1996;**13**:343–59. https://doi.org/10.1089/neu.1996.13.343.

Basso DM, Fisher LC, Anderson AJ, Jakeman LB, McTigue DM, Popovich PG. Basso Mouse Scale for locomotion detects differences in recovery after spinal cord injury in five common mouse strains. *J. Neurotrauma* 2006;**23**:635–59. https://doi.org/10.1089/neu.2006.23.635.

Beattie MS, Farooqui AA, Bresnahan JC. Review of current evidence for apoptosis after spinal cord injury. *J Neurotrauma* 2000;**17**:915–25. https://doi.org/10.1089/neu.2000.17.915.

Bennett GJ, Abdelmoumene M, Hayashi H, Dubner R. Physiology and morphology of substantia gelatinosa neurons intracellularly stained with horseradish peroxidase. *J Comp Neurol* 1980;**194**:809–27. https://doi.org/10.1002/cne.901940407.

Bennett GJ, Abdelmoumene M, Hayashi H, Hoffert MJ, Dubner R. Spinal cord layer I neurons with axon collaterals that generate local arbors. *Brain Res* 1981;**209**:421–6. https://doi.org/10.1016/0006-8993(81)90164-5.

Bracken MB, Holford TR. Neurological and functional status 1 year after acute spinal cord injury: estimates of functional recovery in National Acute Spinal Cord Injury Study II from results modeled in National Acute Spinal Cord Injury Study III. *J Neurosurg* 2002;**96**:259–66. https://doi.org/10.3171/spi.2002.96.3.0259.

Bracken MB, Shepard MJ, Holford TR, et al. Administration of methylprednisolone for 24 or 48 hours or tirilazad mesylate for 48 hours in the treatment of acute spinal cord injury. Results of the Third National Acute Spinal Cord Injury Randomized Controlled Trial. National Acute Spinal Cord Injury Study. *JAMA* 1997;**277**:1597–604.

Breazile JE, Kitchell RL. A study of fiber systems within the spinal cord of the domestic pig that subserve pain. *J Comp Neurol* 1968;**133**:373–82. https://doi.org/10.1002/cne.901330307.

Bunge RP, Puckett WR, Becerra JL, Marcillo A, Quencer RM. Observations on the pathology of human spinal cord injury. A review and classification of 22 new cases with details from a case of chronic cord compression with extensive focal demyelination. *Adv Neurol* 1993;**59**:75–89.

Carrico KM, Vaishnav R, Hall ED. Temporal and spatial dynamics of peroxynitrite-induced oxidative damage after spinal cord contusion injury. *J Neurotrauma* 2009;**26**:1369–78. https://doi.org/10.1089/neu.2008-0870.

Casha S, Yu WR, Fehlings MG. Oligodendroglial apoptosis occurs along degenerating axons and is associated with FAS and p75 expression following spinal cord injury in the rat. *Neuroscience* 2001;**103**:203–18. https://doi.org/10.1016/s0306-4522(00)00538-8.

Casha S, Yu WR, Fehlings MG. FAS deficiency reduces apoptosis, spares axons and improves function after spinal cord

injury. *Exp Neurol* 2005;**196**:390–400. https://doi.org/10.1016/j.expneurol.2005.08.020.

Chaudhary U, Birbaumer N, Ramos-Murguialday A. Brain–computer interfaces for communication and rehabilitation. *Nat Rev Neurol* 2016;**12**:513–25. https://doi.org/10.1038/nrneurol.2016.113.

Cheriyan T, Ryan DJ, Weinreb JH, et al. Spinal cord injury models: a review. *Spinal Cord* 2014;**52**:588–95. https://doi.org/10.1038/sc.2014.91.

Choo AM, Liu J, Dvorak M, Tetzlaff W, Oxland TR. Secondary pathology following contusion, dislocation, and distraction spinal cord injuries. *Exp Neurol* 2008;**212**: 490–506. https://doi.org/10.1016/j.expneurol.2008.04.038.

Choo AM-T, Liu J, Liu Z, Dvorak M, Tetzlaff W, Oxland TR. Modeling spinal cord contusion, dislocation, and distraction: characterization of vertebral clamps, injury severities, and node of Ranvier deformations. *J Neurosci Methods* 2009;**181**:6–17. https://doi.org/10.1016/j.jneumeth.2009.04.007.

Courtine G, Song B, Hoy RR, et al. Recovery of supraspinal control of stepping via indirect propriospinal relay connections after spinal cord injury. *Nat Med* 2008;**14**:69–74. https://doi.org/10.1038/nm1682.

Curtis E, Martin JR, Gabel B, et al. A first-in-human, Phase I study of neural stem cell transplantation for chronic spinal cord injury. *Cell Stem Cell* 2018;**22**:941–50. https://doi.org/10.1016/j.stem.2018.05.014.

Dabney KW, Ehrenshteyn M, Agresta CA, et al. A model of experimental spinal cord trauma based on computer-controlled intervertebral distraction: characterization of graded injury. *Spine* 2004;**29**:2357–64. https://doi.org/10.1097/01.brs.0000143108.65385.74.

Demopoulos HB, Flamm ES, Seligman ML, Pietronigro DD, Tomasula J, DeCrescito V. Further studies on free-radical pathology in the major central nervous system disorders: effect of very high doses of methylprednisolone on the functional outcome, morphology, and chemistry of experimental spinal cord impact injury. *Can J Physiol Pharmacol* 1982;**60**:1415–24. https://doi.org/10.1139/y82-210.

Domínguez-Rodríguez LE, Stecina K, García-Ramírez DL, et al. Candidate interneurons mediating the resetting of the locomotor rhythm by extensor group I afferents in the cat. *Neuroscience* 2020;**450**:96–112. https://doi.org/10.1016/j.neuroscience.2020.09.017.

Eccles JC, Eccles RM, Lundberg A. The convergence of monosynaptic excitatory afferents on to many different species of alpha motoneurones. *J Physiol* 1957;**137**:22–50. https://doi.org/10.1113/jphysiol.1957.sp005794.

Ferretti P, Mackay M, Walder S. The developing human spinal cord contains distinct populations of neural precursors. *Neurodegener Dis* 2006;**3**:38–44. https://doi.org/10.1159/000092091.

Filli L, Engmann AK, Zörner B, et al. Bridging the gap: a reticulo-propriospinal detour bypassing an incomplete spinal cord injury. *J Neurosci* 2014;**34**:13399–410. https://doi.org/10.1523/JNEUROSCI.0701-14.2014.

Fougerousse F, Bullen P, Herasse M, et al. Human–mouse differences in the embryonic expression patterns of developmental control genes and disease genes. *Hum Mol Genet* 2000;**9**:165–73. https://doi.org/10.1093/hmg/9.2.165.

Frigon A. The cat model of spinal cord injury. In Aldskogius H. (Ed.), *Animal Models of Spinal Cord Repair.* Humana Press, 2013; 159–83.

Fukuda S, Nakamura T, Kishigami Y, et al. New canine spinal cord injury model free from laminectomy. *Brain Res Brain Res Protoc* 2005;**14**:171–80. https://doi.org/10.1016/j.brainresprot.2005.01.001.

Furlan JC, Sakakibara BM, Miller WC, Krassioukov AV. Global incidence and prevalence of traumatic spinal cord injury. *Can J Neurol Sci* 2013;**40**:456–64. https://doi.org/10.1017/s0317167100014530.

Gerasimenko YP, Avelev VD, Nikitin OA, Lavrov IA. Initiation of locomotor activity in spinal cats by epidural stimulation of the spinal cord. *Neurosci Behav Physiol* 2003;**33**:247–54. https://doi.org/10.1023/a:1022199214515.

Ghosh A, Fleiss F, Sydekum E, et al. Rewiring of hindlimb corticospinal neurons after spinal cord injury. *Nat Neurosci* 2010;**13**:97–104. https://doi.org/10.1038/nn.2448.

Göritz C, Dias DO, Tomilin N, Barbacid M, Shupliakov O, Frisén J. A pericyte origin of spinal cord scar tissue. *Science* 2011; **333**:238–42 https://doi.org/10.1126/science.1203165.

Grillner S, Zangger P. On the central generation of locomotion in the low spinal cat. *Exp Brain Res* 1979;**34**:241–61. https://doi.org/10.1007/BF00235671.

Guger C, Edlinger G, Harkam W, Niedermayer I, Pfurtscheller G. How many people are able to operate an EEG-based brain-computer interface (BCI)? *IEEE Trans Neural Syst Rehabil Eng* 2003;**11**:145–7. https://doi.org/10.1109/TNSRE.2003.814481.

Hackett AR, Lee D-H, Dawood A, et al. STAT3 and SOCS3 regulate NG2 cell proliferation and differentiation after contusive spinal cord injury. *Neurobiol Dis* 2016;**89**:10–22. https://doi.org/10.1016/j.nbd.2016.01.017

Hall ED, Braughler JM. Effects of intravenous methylprednisolone on spinal cord lipid peroxidation and Na$^+$ + K$^+$)-ATPase activity. Dose–response analysis during 1st hour after contusion injury in the cat. *J Neurosurg* 1982;**57**:247–53. https://doi.org/10.3171/jns.1982.57.2.0247.

Hall ED, Wolf DL. A pharmacological analysis of the pathophysiological mechanisms of posttraumatic spinal cord ischemia. *J Neurosurg* 1986;**64**:951–61. https://doi.org/10.3171/jns.1986.64.6.0951.

Hall ED, Yonkers PA, Andrus PK, Cox JW, Anderson DK. Biochemistry and pharmacology of lipid antioxidants in acute brain and spinal cord injury. *J Neurotrauma* 1992;**9**(Suppl 2):S425–42.

Hawryluk G, Whetstone W, Saigal R, et al. Mean arterial blood pressure correlates with neurological recovery after human spinal cord injury: analysis of high frequency physiologic data. *J Neurotrauma* 2015;**32**:1958–67. https://doi.org/10.1089/neu.2014.3778.

Heller RA, Seelig J, Bock T, et al. Relation of selenium status to neuro-regeneration after traumatic spinal cord injury. *J Trace Elem Med Biol* 2019;**51**:141–9. https://doi.org/10.1016/j.jtemb.2018.10.006.

Honda CN, Lee CL. Immunohistochemistry of synaptic input and functional characterizations of neurons near the spinal central canal. *Brain Res* 1985;**343**:120–8. https://doi.org/10.1016/0006-8993(85)91165-5.

Hu R., Zhou J, Luo C, et al. Glial scar and neuroregeneration: histological, functional, and magnetic resonance imaging analysis in chronic spinal cord injury. *J Neurosurg Spine* 2010;**13**:169–80. https://doi.org/10.3171/2010.3.SPINE09190.

Inman DM, Steward O. Ascending sensory, but not other long-tract axons, regenerate into the connective tissue matrix that forms at the site of a spinal cord injury in mice. *J Comp Neurol* 2003;**462**:431–49. https://doi.org/10.1002/cne.10768.

Jankowska E, Maxwell DJ, Bannatyne BA. On coupling and decoupling of spinal interneuronal networks. *Arch Ital Biol* 2007;**145**:235–50.

Jeffery ND, Hamilton L, Granger N. Designing clinical trials in canine spinal cord injury as a model to translate successful laboratory interventions into clinical practice. *Vet Rec* 2011;**168**:102–07. https://doi.org/10.1136/vr.d475.

Jeffery ND, Smith PM, Lakatos A, Ibanez C, Ito D, Franklin RJM. Clinical canine spinal cord injury provides an opportunity to examine the issues in translating laboratory techniques into practical therapy. *Spinal Cord* 2006;**44**:584–93. https://doi.org/10.1038/sj.sc.3101912.

Jones CF, Lee JHT, Kwon BK, Cripton PA. Development of a large-animal model to measure dynamic cerebrospinal fluid pressure during spinal cord injury: laboratory investigation. *J Neurosurg Spine* 2012;**16**:624–35. https://doi.org/10.3171/2012.3.SPINE11970.

Jordan LM, Liu J, Hedlund PB, Akay T, Pearson KG. Descending command systems for the initiation of locomotion in mammals. *Brain Res Rev* 2008;**57**:183–91. https://doi.org/10.1016/j.brainresrev.2007.07.019.

Josephson A, Greitz D, Klason T, Olson L, Spenger C. A spinal thecal sac constriction model supports the theory that induced pressure gradients in the cord cause edema and cyst formation. *Neurosurgery* 2001;**48**:636–45; discussion 645–6. https://doi.org/10.1097/00006123-200103000-00039.

Kakulas BA. Neuropathology: the foundation for new treatments in spinal cord injury. *Spinal Cord* 2004;**42**:549–63. https://doi.org/10.1038/sj.sc.3101670.

Kamencic H, Griebel RW, Lyon AW, Paterson PG, Juurlink BH. Promoting glutathione synthesis after spinal cord trauma decreases secondary damage and promotes retention of function. *FASEB J* 2001;**15**:243–50. https://doi.org/10.1096/fj.00-0228com.

Kawase T, Sakurada T, Koike Y, Kansaku K. A hybrid BMI-based exoskeleton for paresis: EMG control for assisting arm movements. *J Neural Eng* 2017;**14**:016015. https://doi.org/10.1088/1741-2552/aa525f.

Kennedy PR. Corticospinal, rubrospinal and rubro-olivary projections: a unifying hypothesis. *Trends Neurosci* 1990;**13**:474–9. https://doi.org/10.1016/0166-2236(90)90079-p.

Kubota K, Saiwai H, Kumamaru H, et al. Myeloperoxidase exacerbates secondary injury by generating highly reactive oxygen species and mediating neutrophil recruitment in experimental spinal cord injury. *Spine* 2012;**37**:1363–9. https://doi.org/10.1097/BRS.0b013e31824b9e77.

Kucher K, Johns D, Maier D, et al. First-in-man intrathecal application of neurite growth-promoting anti-Nogo-A antibodies in acute spinal cord injury. *Neurorehabil Neural Repair* 2018;**32**:578–89. https://doi.org/10.1177/1545968318776371.

Kumar H, Choi H, Jo M-J, et al. Neutrophil elastase inhibition effectively rescued angiopoietin-1 decrease and inhibits glial scar after spinal cord injury. *Acta Neuropathol Commun* 2018;**6**:73. https://doi.org/10.1186/s40478-018-0576-3.

Lemke M, Frei B, Ames BN, Faden AI. Decreases in tissue levels of ubiquinol-9 and -10, ascorbate and alpha-tocopherol following spinal cord impact trauma in rats. *Neurosci Lett* 1990;**108**:201–06. https://doi.org/10.1016/0304-3940(90)90731-n.

Lemon RN. Descending pathways in motor control. *Annu Rev Neurosci* 2008;**31**:195–218. https://doi.org/10.1146/annurev.neuro.31.060407.125547.

Levi AD, Anderson KD, Okonkwo DO, et al. Clinical outcomes from a multi-center study of human neural stem cell transplantation in chronic cervical spinal cord injury. *J Neurotrauma* 2019;**36**:891–902. https://doi.org/10.1089/neu.2018.5843.

Levi L, Wolf A, Belzberg H. Hemodynamic parameters in patients with acute cervical cord trauma: description, intervention, and prediction of outcome. *Neurosurgery* 1993;**33**:1007–16; discussion 1016–7.

Levine JM, Levine GJ, Porter BF, Topp K, Noble-Haeusslein LJ. Naturally occurring disk herniation in dogs: an opportunity for pre-clinical spinal cord injury research. *J Neurotrauma* 2011;**28**:675–88. https://doi.org/10.1089/neu.2010.1645.

Liu D, Liu J, Sun D, Wen J. The time course of hydroxyl radical formation following spinal cord injury: the possible role of the iron-catalyzed Haber–Weiss reaction. *J Neurotrauma* 2004;**21**:805–16. https://doi.org/10.1089/0897715041269650.

Liu D, Sybert TE, Qian H, Liu J. Superoxide production after spinal injury detected by microperfusion of cytochrome c. *Free Radic Biol Med* 1998;**25**:298–304. https://doi.org/10.1016/s0891-5849(98)00055-0.

Liu J-B, Tang T-S, Xiao D-S. Changes of free iron contents and its correlation with lipid peroxidation after experimental spinal cord injury. *Chin J Traumatol* 2004:**7**:229–32.

Lucas JH, Wheeler DG, Guan Z, Suntres Z, Stokes BT. Effect of glutathione augmentation on lipid peroxidation after spinal cord injury. *J Neurotrauma* 2002;**19**:763–75. https://doi.org/10.1089/08977150260139138.

Ma M, Basso DM, Walters P, Stokes BT, Jakeman LB. Behavioral and histological outcomes following graded spinal cord contusion injury in the C57Bl/6 mouse. *Exp Neurol* 2001;**169**:239–54. https://doi.org/10.1006/exnr.2001.7679.

Mannen H, Sugiura Y. Reconstruction of neurons of dorsal horn proper using Golgi-stained serial sections. *J Comp Neurol* 1976;**168**:303–12. https://doi.org/10.1002/cne.901680205.

Martinez M, Delivet-Mongrain H, Leblond H, Rossignol S. Recovery of hindlimb locomotion after incomplete spinal cord injury in the cat involves spontaneous compensatory changes within the spinal locomotor circuitry. *J Neurophysiol* 2011;**106**:1969–84. https://doi.org/10.1152/jn.00368.2011.

Martirosyan N L, Kalani MYS, Bichard WD, et al. Cerebrospinal fluid drainage and induced hypertension improve spinal cord perfusion after acute spinal cord injury in pigs. *Neurosurgery* 2015;**76**:461–8; discussion 468–9. https://doi.org/10.1227/NEU.0000000000000638.

Mazensky D, Flesarova S, Sulla I. Arterial blood supply to the spinal cord in animal models of spinal cord injury. A review. *Anat Rec* 2017;**300**:2091–106. https://doi.org/10.1002/ar.23694.

Metz GA, Curt A, van de Meent H, Klusman I, Schwab ME, Dietz V. Validation of the weight-drop contusion model in rats: a comparative study of human spinal cord injury. *J Neurotrauma* 2000;**17**:1–17. https://doi.org/10.1089/neu.2000.17.1.

Monyer H, Hartley DM, Choi D W. 21-Aminosteroids attenuate excitotoxic neuronal injury in cortical cell cultures. *Neuron* 1990;**5**:121–6. https://doi.org/10.1016/0896-6273(90)90302-v.

Moore SA, Granger N, Olby NJ, et al. Targeting translational successes through CANSORT-SCI: using pet dogs to identify effective treatments for spinal cord injury. *J Neurotrauma* 2017;**34**:2007–18. https://doi.org/10.1089/neu.2016.4745.

Moore SA, Zidan N, Spitzbarth I, et al. Development of an International Canine Spinal Cord Injury observational registry: a collaborative data-sharing network to optimize translational studies of SCI. *Spinal Cord* 2018;**56**:656–65. https://doi.org/10.1038/s41393-018-0145-4.

Müller K, Gürster D. Hydroxyl radical damage to DNA sugar and model membranes induced by anthralin (dithranol). *Biochem Pharmacol* 1993;**46**:1695–704. https://doi.org/10.1016/0006-2952(93)90573-f.

Nashmi R, Fehlings MG. Changes in axonal physiology and morphology after chronic compressive injury of the rat thoracic spinal cord. *Neuroscience* 2001;**104**:235–51. https://doi.org/10.1016/s0306-4522(01)00009-4.

Nathan PW. Effects on movement of surgical incisions into the human spinal cord. *Brain* 1994;**117**(Pt 2):337–46. https://doi.org/10.1093/brain/117.2.337.

Navarro R, Juhas S, Keshavarzi S, et al. Chronic spinal compression model in minipigs: a systematic behavioral, qualitative, and quantitative neuropathological study. *J Neurotrauma* 2012;**29**:499–513. https://doi.org/10.1089/neu.2011.2076.

Neirinckx V, Coste C, Franzen F, Gothot A, Rogister B, Wislet S. Neutrophil contribution to spinal cord injury and repair. *J Neuroinflammation* 2014;**11**:150. https://doi.org/10.1186/s12974-014-0150-2.

Nesathurai S, Graham WA, Mansfield K, et al. Model of traumatic spinal cord injury in *Macaca fascicularis*: similarity of experimental lesions created by epidural catheter to human spinal cord injury. *J Med Primatol* 2006;**35**:401–04. https://doi.org/10.1111/j.1600-0684.2006.00162.x.

Nguyen HX, O'Barr TJ, Anderson AJ. Polymorphonuclear leukocytes promote neurotoxicity through release of matrix metalloproteinases, reactive oxygen species, and TNF-alpha. *J Neurochem* 2007;**102**:900–12. https://doi.org/10.1111/j.1471-4159.2007.04643.x.

Nielsen JB. How we walk: central control of muscle activity during human walking. *Neuroscientist* 2003;**9**:195–204. https://doi.org/10.1177/1073858403009003012.

Noble LJ, Wrathall JR. Spinal cord contusion in the rat: morphometric analyses of alterations in the spinal cord. *Exp Neurol* 1985;**88**:135–49. https://doi.org/10.1016/0014-4886(85)90119-0.

Norenberg MD, Smith J, Marcillo A. The pathology of human spinal cord injury: defining the problems. *J Neurotrauma* 2004;**21**:429–40. https://doi.org/10.1089/089771504323004575.

O'Rahilly RR, Müller F. *The Embryonic Human Brain: An Atlas Of Developmental Stages*. John Wiley & Sons, 2006.

O'Shea TM, Burda JE, Sofroniew MV. Cell biology of spinal cord injury and repair. *J Clin Invest* 2017;**127**:3259–70. https://doi.org/10.1172/JCI90608.

Ohtani K, Abe H, Kadoya S. Beneficial effects of methylprednisolone sodium succinate in the treatment of acute spinal cord injury. *Sekitsui Sekizui* 1994;**7**:633–47.

Okon EB, Streijger F, Lee JHT, Anderson LM, Russell AK, Kwon BK. Intraparenchymal microdialysis after acute spinal cord injury reveals differential metabolic responses to contusive versus compressive mechanisms of injury. *J Neurotrauma* 2013;**30**:1564–76. https://doi.org/10.1089/neu.2013.2956.

Onifer SM, Smith GM, Fouad K. Plasticity after spinal cord injury: relevance to recovery and approaches to facilitate it. *Neurotherapeutics* 2011;**8**:283–93. https://doi.org/10.1007/s13311-011-0034-4.

Orr MB, Gensel JC. Spinal cord injury scarring and inflammation: therapies targeting glial and inflammatory responses. *Neurotherapeutics* 2018;**15**:541–53. https://doi.org/10.1007/s13311-018-0631-6.

Petersen TH, Willerslev-Olsen M, Conway BA, Nielsen JB. The motor cortex drives the muscles during walking in human subjects. *J Physiol* 2012;**590**:2443–52. https://doi.org/10.1113/jphysiol.2012.227397.

Pietronigro DD, Hovsepian M, Demopoulos HB, Flamm ES. Loss of ascorbic acid from injured feline spinal cord. *J Neurochem* 1983;**41**:1072–6. https://doi.org/10.1111/j.1471-4159.1983.tb09053.x.

Pointillart V, Petitjean ME, Wiart L, et al. Pharmacological therapy of spinal cord injury during the acute phase. *Spinal Cord* 2000;**38**:71–6. https://doi.org/10.1038/sj.sc.3100962.

Ramesh T, Nagula SV, Tardieu GG, et al. Update on the notochord including its embryology, molecular development, and pathology: a primer for the clinician. *Cureus* 2017;**9**:e1137. https://doi.org/10.7759/cureus.1137

Readdy WJ, Dhall SS. Vasopressor administration in spinal cord injury: should we apply a universal standard to all injury patterns? *Neural Regeneration Res* 2016);**11**:420–1. https://doi.org/10.4103/1673-5374.179051.

Rexed B. The cytoarchitectonic organization of the spinal cord in the cat. *J Comp Neurol* 1952;**96**:414–95. https://doi.org/10.1002/cne.900960303.

Rexed B. A cytoarchitectonic atlas of the spinal cord in the cat. *J Comp Neurol* 1954;**100**:297–379. https://doi.org/10.1002/cne.901000205.

Rohm M, Schneider M, Müller C, et al. Hybrid brain–computer interfaces and hybrid neuroprostheses for restoration of upper limb functions in individuals with high-level spinal cord injury. *Artif Intell Med* 2013;**59**:133–42. https://doi.org/10.1016/j.artmed.2013.07.004.

Rossignol S, Schwab M, Schwartz M, Fehlings MG. Spinal cord injury: time to move? *J Neurosci* 2007;**27**:11782–92. https://doi.org/10.1523/JNEUROSCI.3444-07.2007.

Rothwell J. Ascending and descending pathways of the spinal cord. In Rothwell J (Ed.), *Control of Human Voluntary Movement*. Springer Netherlands, 1994; 217–51.

Rowland JW, Hawryluk GWJ, Kwon B, Fehlings MG. Current status of acute spinal cord injury pathophysiology and emerging therapies: promise on the horizon. *Neurosurg. Focus* 2008;**25**:E2. https://doi.org/10.3171/FOC.2008.25.11.E2.

Saiwai H, Ohkawa Y, Yamada H, et al. The LTB4–BLT1 axis mediates neutrophil infiltration and secondary injury in experimental spinal cord injury. *Am J Pathol* 2010;**176**:2352–66. https://doi.org/10.2353/ajpath.2010.090839

Schoenen J. Dendritic organization of the human spinal cord: the motoneurons. *J Comp Neurol* 1982a;**211**:226–47. https://doi.org/10.1002/cne.902110303.

Schoenen J. The dendritic organization of the human spinal cord: the dorsal horn. *Neuroscience* 1982b;**7**:2057–87. https://doi.org/10.1016/0306-4522(82)90120-8.

Schomberg DT, Miranpuri GS, Chopra A, et al. Translational relevance of swine models of spinal cord injury. *J Neurotrauma* 2017;**34**:541–51. https://doi.org/10.1089/neu.2016.4567.

Schucht P, Raineteau O, Schwab ME, Fouad K. Anatomical correlates of locomotor recovery following dorsal and ventral lesions of the rat spinal cord. *Exp Neurol* 2002;**176**:143–53. https://doi.org/10.1006/exnr.2002.7909.

Semple BD, Blomgren K, Gimlin K, Ferriero DM, Noble-Haeusslein LJ. Brain development in rodents and humans: Identifying benchmarks of maturation and vulnerability to injury across species. *Prog Neurobiol* 2013;**106–107**:1–16. https://doi.org/10.1016/j.pneurobio.2013.04.001.

Sharif-Alhoseini M, Khormali M, Rezaei M, et al. Animal models of spinal cord injury: a systematic review. *Spinal Cord* 2017;**55**:714–21. https://doi.org/10.1038/sc.2016.187

Simon F, Oberhuber A. Ischemia and reperfusion injury of the spinal cord: experimental strategies to examine postischemic paraplegia. *Neural Regeneration Res* 2016;**11**:414–15. https://doi.org/10.4103/1673-5374.179050.

Stockwell BR, Freidmann Angeli JP, Bayir H, et al. Ferroptosis: a regulated cell death nexus linking metabolism, redox biology, and disease. *Cell* 2017;**171**:273–85. https://doi.org/10.1016/j.cell.2017.09.021.

Strauch JT, Lauten A, Zhang N, Wahlers T, Griepp RB. Anatomy of spinal cord blood supply in the pig. *Ann Thorac Surg* 2007);**83**:2130–4. https://doi.org/10.1016/j.athoracsur.2007.01.060.

Su L-J, Zhang J-H, Gomez H, et al. Reactive oxygen species-induced lipid peroxidation in apoptosis, autophagy, and ferroptosis. *Oxid Med Cell Longev* 2019;**2019**:5080843. https://doi.org/10.1155/2019/5080843.

Tabakow P, Jarmundowicz W, Czapiga B, et al. Transplantation of autologous olfactory ensheathing cells in complete human spinal cord injury. *Cell Transplant* 2013;**22**:1591–612. https://doi.org/10.3727/096368912X663532.

Tidoni E, Gergondet P, Fusco G, Kheddar A, Aglioti SM. The role of audio-visual feedback in a thought-based control of a humanoid robot: a BCI study in healthy and spinal cord injured people. *IEEE Trans Neural Syst Rehabil Eng* 2017;**25**:772–81. https://doi.org/10.1109/TNSRE.2016.2597863.

Tohyama T, Kinoshita M, Kobayashi K, et al. Contribution of propriospinal neurons to recovery of hand dexterity after corticospinal tract lesions in monkeys. *Proc Natl Acad Sci U S A* 2017;**114**:604–09. https://doi.org/10.1073/pnas.1610787114.

Totoiu MO, Nistor GI, Lane TE, Keirstead HS. Remyelination, axonal sparing, and locomotor recovery following transplantation of glial-committed progenitor cells into the MHV model of multiple sclerosis. *Exp Neurol* 2004;**187**:254–65. https://doi.org/10.1016/j.expneurol.2004.01.028.

Vale FL, Burns J, Jackson AB, Hadley MN. Combined medical and surgical treatment after acute spinal cord injury: results of a prospective pilot study to assess the merits of aggressive medical resuscitation and blood pressure management. *J Neurosurg* 1997;**87**:239–46. https://doi.org/10.3171/jns.1997.87.2.0239.

van der Scheer JW, Martin Ginis KA, Ditor DS, et al. Effects of exercise on fitness and health of adults with spinal cord injury: a systematic review. *Neurology* 2017;**89**:736–45. https://doi.org/10.1212/WNL.0000000000004224.

Volpe E, Sambucci M, Battistini L, Borsellino G. Fas–Fas ligand: checkpoint of T cell functions in multiple sclerosis. *Front Immunol* 2016l7:382. https://doi.org/10.3389/fimmu.2016.00382.

Wang X, Cao K, Sun X, et al. Macrophages in spinal cord injury: phenotypic and functional change from exposure to myelin debris. *Glia* 2015;**63**:635–51. https://doi.org/10.1002/glia.22774.

Werneburg S, Feinberg PA, Johnson KM, Schafer DP. A microglia–cytokine axis to modulate synaptic connectivity and function. *Curr Opin Neurobiol* 2017;**47**:138–45. https://doi.org/10.1016/j.conb.2017.10.002.

Whalen MJ, Dalkara T, You Z, et al. Acute plasmalemma permeability and protracted clearance of injured cells after controlled cortical impact in mice. *J Cereb Blood Flow Metab* 2008;**28**:490–505. https://doi.org/10.1038/sj.jcbfm.9600544.

Whelan PJ. Control of locomotion in the decerebrate cat. *Prog Neurobiol* 1996;**49**:481–515. https://doi.org/10.1016/0301-0082(96)00028-7.

Xiao Z, Tang F, Zhao Y, et al. Significant improvement of acute complete spinal cord injury patients diagnosed by a combined criteria implanted with NeuroRegen scaffolds and mesenchymal stem cells. *Cell Transplant* 2018;**27**:907–15. https://doi.org/10.1177/0963689718766279.

Yune TY, Lee JY, Jiang MH, Kim DW, Choi SY, Oh TH. Systemic administration of PEP-1–SOD1 fusion protein improves functional recovery by inhibition of neuronal cell death after spinal cord injury. *Free Radic Biol Med* 2008;**45**:1190–200. https://doi.org/10.1016/j.freeradbiomed.2008.07.016.

Zakaryan H, Cholakyans V, Simonyan L, et al. A study of lymphoid organs and serum proinflammatory cytokines in pigs infected with African swine fever virus genotype II. *Arch Virol* 2015;**160**:1407–14. https://doi.org/10.1007/s00705-015-2401-7.

Zhang C, Chen K, Han X, et al. Diffusion tensor imaging in diagnosis of post-traumatic syringomyelia in spinal cord injury in rats. *Med Sci Monit* 2018;**24**:177–82. https://doi.org/10.12659/MSM.907955.

Zhang N, Fang M, Chen H, Gou F, Ding M. Evaluation of spinal cord injury animal models. *Neural Regeneration Res* 2014;**9**:2008–12. https://doi.org/10.4103/1673-5374.143436.

Zivin JA, DeGirolami U. Spinal cord infarction: a highly reproducible stroke model. *Stroke* 1980;**11**:200–02. https://doi.org/10.1161/01.str.11.2.200.

Zörner B, Bachmann LC, Filli L, et al. Chasing central nervous system plasticity: the brainstem's contribution to locomotor recovery in rats with spinal cord injury. *Brain* 2014;**137**:1716–32. https://doi.org/10.1093/brain/awu078.

21 Traumatic Brain Injury

Kristin A. Keith and Jason H. Huang

21.1 Introduction

Traumatic brain injury (TBI) is one of the leading causes of morbidity and mortality worldwide, with an estimated annual incidence of 69 million individuals worldwide (Dewan et al., 2019). In 2014, the CDC documented 2.5 million TBI-related emergency department (ED) visits in the United States (US) with 288,000 TBI-related hospitalizations and 56,800 TBI-associated mortalities (CDC, 2014). Furthermore, TBI is the leading cause of long-term disability in children and young adults within the US population, with annual cost estimates in patients suffering from TBI varying from $56 billion to $221 billion (Capizzi et al., 2020).

21.2 Categories of Traumatic Brain Injury

Traumatic brain injury can be categorized based on the unique physical mechanisms associated with each type of primary insult, resulting in three categories: (1) closed head, (2) penetrating, and (3) explosive blast TBI, as described below (Ng and Lee, 2019).

Closed-head TBI typically results from blunt force trauma with a compression contact force causing disruption of the immediately underlying structures, consequently resulting in stretch and shear injuries of both the axons and blood vessels. Depending on the severity of the impact, brain displacement secondary to resulting shock may lead to compression of adjacent brain parenchyma and reduction of cerebral blood flow. Upon initial impact of the brain, focal disruption of the axon results in disruption of axonal transport leading to axonal swelling followed by Wallerian degeneration (Frati et al., 2017).

Penetrating TBI results from penetration of a foreign object through the skull, dura, and into the underlying brain parenchyma, and poses a significantly increased morbidity and mortality as compared to closed-head injuries. Laceration of the brain parenchyma results in localized damage, intracranial hemorrhage, cerebral edema, and ischemia secondary to reduced blood flow. The high pressure from the projectile directly results in crush injury and cell necrosis along the leading edge of the projectile, creating a permanent tract, while the extent of the resulting injury remains largely dependent upon the velocity of the object – i.e., invasion of a high-velocity projectile object can lead to additional tissue cavitation resulting in increased damage secondary to the associated shockwave (Vakil and Singh, 2017).

Explosives can be classified as either low explosives, such as gunpowder which is readily combustible, or high explosives, such as trinitrotoluene (TNT) or cyclonite (RDX), which produce a shattering effect when detonated due to the instability of the molecules resulting in the production of shock or pressure waves. Effects of blast-induced TBI can be categorized into five separate injury patterns: primary (shockwaves generated from the explosion/blast), secondary (blunt/penetrating injury secondary to a fragment of debris propelled by the explosion), tertiary (acceleration/deceleration characterized by the kinetic energy released during the explosion), quaternary (flash burns), and quinary (factors released during the detonation of the explosive charge) (Cernak, 2017). Studies have indicated that pressure-wave propagation following the blast-injury results in stimulation of systemic inflammation contributing to neurodegeneration (Cernak, 2010, 2017; Valiyaveettil et al., 2013). Furthermore, blast-induced neurotrauma (BINT)-specific neurodegeneration was reported by Shively and Perl (2017) and Shively et al. (2016) in both the acute and chronic phase. In the acute phase, early astroglial scarring was seen involving the subpial glial plate, penetrating cortical blood vessels, gray–white matter junctions, and structures lining the ventricles. In the chronic phase, prominent astroglial scarring involved the same brain regions and all patients with a history of chronic blast exposure were diagnosed with post-traumatic stress disorder (PTSD) prior to death. Additionally, patients with BINT demonstrated greater hypometabolism on positron emission tomography

(PET) scans as compared to blunt TBI patients – particularly in the right superior parietal lobe and posterior cingulate cortex (Mendez et al., 2013).

21.3 Pathophysiology

Traumatic brain injury is defined by two distinct phases: (1) acute, primary injury which occurs during the direct insult and is secondary to mechanical forces disrupting cell integrity, and (2) delayed, secondary injury that occurs hours to months following the initial trauma. The acute, primary injury can result in either focal brain injury or diffuse brain injury; however, studies have suggested that both focal and diffuse brain injuries frequently coexist in the setting of moderate-to-severe TBI (Ng and Lee, 2019; Skandsen et al., 2010).

Secondary brain injury occurs due to biochemical, cellular, and physiological events triggered by a primary insult leading to delayed, prolonged injury from a variety of underlying mechanisms including: edema, excitotoxicity, mitochondrial dysfunction, oxidative stress, lipid peroxidation, neuroinflammation, axon degeneration, and apoptotic cell death (Cernak, 2017; Ng and Lee, 2019; Ray et al., 2002) .

21.3.1 Excitotoxicity

Studies have demonstrated that blood–brain barrier (BBB) breakdown and primary neuronal cell death result in the release of excitatory amino acids, particularly glutamate. An acute increase in extracellular glutamate levels has been detected in both experimental models and patients secondary to damaged cellular membranes following TBI, and ultimately, have been shown to lead to overstimulation of glutamate receptors, which is further precipitated by a reduction in the overall presence of astrocytic sodium-dependent glutamate transporters GLAST and GLT-1 (Landeghem et al., 2006; Raghavendra Rao et al., 2002). Studies have suggested that release of glutamate is associated with age – such that, elderly TBI patient have increased levels of glutamate as compared to younger TBI patients (Kaur and Sharma, 2018).

Glutamate activates ionotropic glutamate receptors (iGluRs), N-methyl-D-aspartate (NMDA) receptor, and α-amino-3-hydroxy-5-methyl-4-isoxazole propionate (AMPA) receptor, allowing Na^+, K^+, and Ca^{2+} ionic flux, resulting in neuronal membrane depolarization, alteration of ion homeostasis, and activation of downstream signaling molecules including Ca^{2+}/calmodulin-dependent protein kinase II, mitogen-activated protein kinase (MAPK), and protein phosphatase 2B (calcineurin) (Bales et al., 2010; Faden et al., 1989; Folkerts et al., 2007; Landeghem et al., 2006; Lu et al., 2008; Meldrum, 2000; Ng and Lee, 2019). Additionally, activation of NMDA receptors promotes the production of reactive oxygen species (ROS) and nitric oxide (NO), further exacerbating cellular injury via protein oxidation, cleavage of DNA, and mitochondrial electron transport chain inhibition, leading to cell death (Kaur and Sharma, 2018). Glutamate has also been shown to activate metabotropic glutamate receptors (mGluRs), which regulate Ca^{2+} and downstream GTP-binding proteins, thereby triggering the activation of phospholipase C inositol-1,4,5-triphosphate leading to release of Ca^{2+} (Weber, 2012). Ultimately, disruption of Ca^{2+} homeostasis due to excess release of excitatory amino acids and neuronal mechanical damage results in activation of caspases and calpains, leading to activation of apoptosis and necrosis (Frati et al., 2017).

21.3.2 Oxidation

Traumatic brain injury results in the production of ROS and free radicals due to dysfunctional mitochondria, activated neutrophils, excitotoxic pathways, and increased accumulation of Ca^{2+}. Studies have demonstrated that oxidative stress causes damage to cellular structures and plays a significant role in post-traumatic secondary injury following TBI, particularly to neuronal structures such as axons (Ansari et al., 2008). Excitotoxicity and depletion of the endogenous antioxidant process lead to excessive production of ROS leading to protein oxidation, DNA cleavage, cellular peroxidation, and vascular peroxidation resulting in disruption of the mitochondrial electron transport chain (ETC). The development of ROS further perpetuates the viscous cycle – mechanical axonal damage results in an increase in intracellular Ca^{2+}, primarily resulting in mitochondrial Ca^{2+} sequestration leading to formation of ROS and oxidative stress. Production of ROS triggers lipid peroxidation–mediated oxidative damage to the mitochondrial membrane, causing loss of mitochondrial membrane potential and respiratory failure that leads to failure of ATP production and mitochondrial permeability transition (MPT). The resulting mitochondrial permeability leads to efflux of mitochondrial-sequestered Ca^{2+}, further exacerbating the activation of calpain and caspase 3 (biomarker reflective of apoptosis and neurodegeneration) leading to proteolysis of neuronal structures (Hill et al., 2017).

Studies have demonstrated increased oxidative markers, including 3-nitrotyrosine (3-NT) and 4-hydroxynonenal (4-HNE), both of which are produced by the formation of peroxynitrite (PN) due to excessive NO and free radicals (Hall et al., 2004; Ng and Lee, 2019), which play a role in activation of cytotoxic cascades. Additionally, Synapsin I, a major substrate for cyclic AMP-dependent protein kinase and Ca^{2+}-dependent protein kinase in the presynaptic terminal responsible for regulation of neurotransmitter release, and PSD-95, a core scaffolding protein of the post-synaptic terminal responsible for regulating synaptic strength via regulation of the abundance of AMPA receptors, demonstrated time-dependent decrease in the ipsilateral hippocampus in TBI patients associated with increased oxidative stress (Ansari et al., 2008; Hill et al., 2017). Furthermore, it has been shown that increased ROS may play a role in the facilitation of the MPT, ultimately leading to apoptosis (Kaur and Sharma, 2018).

21.3.3 Mitochondrial Dysfunction

Mitochondrial dysfunction remains prevalent in secondary injury associated with TBI, particularly with ROS production and the mitochondrial permeability transition pore (mPTP) production. The mPTP, an internal mitochondrial membrane protein that allows mitochondrial influx/efflux, is produced secondary to sequestration of Ca^{2+} leading to mitochondrial swelling due to disruption of cristae. Studies proposed that such mitochondrial dysfunction resulted in localized death of the axon via the proposed mechanism, which was further supported by the protection of mitochondria with the use of Cyclosporin-A, a known inhibitor of mPTP (Sullivan et al., 1999).

In summary, glutamate toxicity induces mitochondrial injury resulting in sequestration and mitochondrial overloading of Ca^{2+} leading to mitochondrial dysfunction, which further enhances energy failure leading to production of reactive nitrogen species (RNS) and ROS by the mitochondria. These processes combined lead to impaired oxidative phosphorylation, mitochondrial respiration, and transport of ions, ultimately resulting in generation of the mPTP. Production of the mPTP leads to mitochondrial collapse and depletion of cytoplasmic ATP, further amplifying cellular energy failure and calcium dysregulation, thereby initiating apoptosis and necrosis (Kaur and Sharma, 2018).

21.3.4 Inflammation

The primary insult of TBI results in cellular damage thereby activating and initiating neuroinflammatory cascades, which pose a complex interaction in TBI in that they facilitate neurorepair as well as resulting in secondary brain injury. There are two components of post-traumatic neuroinflammation – a cellular component composed of glial cells, microglia, astrocytes, and infiltrating leukocytes, and the immune mediators composed of pro-inflammatory cytokines, anti-inflammatory cytokines, and chemotactic cytokines.

Previous studies have attempted to associate inflammatory cytokines with post-TBI outcomes with conflicting results, although the most widely studied inflammatory cytokine, IL-6, has been shown to be significantly upregulated in CSF within as little as 1 h following TBI, with peak expression occurring between 2 and 5 h post-injury (Woodcock and Morganti-Kossmann, 2013). Furthermore, it has been suggested that increased serum concentration remains indicative of severe TBI and has been associated with BBB dysfunction (Hergenroeder et al., 2010; Woodroofe et al., 1991). Although studies have demonstrated that IL-6 is significantly elevated in cerebrospinal fluid (CSF) as compared to serum following TBI, a complex paradigm exists in that serum IL-6 has been shown to be upregulated following polytrauma including orthopedic injuries, burns, and multi-organ dysfunction system – all of which are commonly seen in TBI patients (Hergenroeder et al., 2010; Sapan et al., 2016; Woodroofe et al., 1991).

21.4 Animal Models

A wide variety of animal models exist in studying TBI with each offering benefits and trade-offs. For example, large-animal models recapitulate human physiology far better and share a gyrencephalic brain; however, they have higher costs and extended generational time frames.

21.4.1 Fluid Percussion Injury

Fluid percussion injury (FPI) remains the most established model that is extensively utilized in studying mixed focal and diffuse TBI, particularly due to the ease of reproducibility and standardized protocol (Figure 21.1). Furthermore, the FPI model recapitulates many of the injuries commonly seen in TBI in humans, thereby making the FPI model clinically relevant (Alder et al., 2011). Studies have been shown to successfully reproduce histopathology associated with TBI including focal contusion within the cerebral cortex with accompanying petechial or intraparenchymal hemorrhage, cerebral edema, and progressive gray matter damage (Thompson et al., 2005).

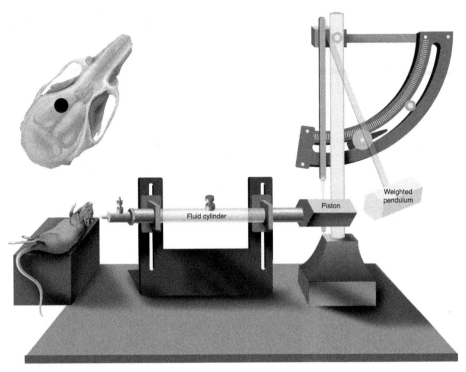

Figure 21.1 Schematic diagram showing experimental setup of the fluid percussion injury (FPI) animal model of traumatic brain injury (TBI) with anesthetized mouse. The FPI model is produced by applying a direct fluid pulse of approximately 20 ms directly to the surface of the dura following a craniotomy via a surgically implanted injury hub (i.e., a leur-lock syringe cap) to produce a brief deformation of the underlying brain parenchyma. The fluid pulse is generated when the weighted pendulum strikes the piston at the end of the fluid cylinder.

Protocol: Animals are anesthetized as per institutional protocol; then, the heads of the animals are shaved and inserted into a stereotaxic frame. Strict sterile technique is maintained throughout the course of the surgical procedure as detailed below. A 3-mm craniotomy was performed with dura intact over the right parietal cortex between the lambda and the bregma approximately 2 mm to the right of midline. A 3-mm injury cap (made from a female leur-lock cap) is positioned over the craniectomy site and secured with glue. A small amount of methyl-methacrylate dental acrylic solution is used to create a seal with cement around the injury hub to ensure the fluid bolus remains within the cranial cavity. The injury hub is filled with 0.9 per cent NaCl to keep the dura moist during the recovery phase. Injury pressure pulses are delivered ranging 0.9–2.1 atm in magnitude and lasting approximately 20 ms in duration over the exposed dura (Alder et al., 2011). The injury cap was removed, the scalp sutured, and animals returned to home cages for recovery.

21.4.2 Controlled Cortical Impact

Controlled cortical impact (CCI) produces brain injury using a pneumatic or electromagnetic impactor to compress exposed brain and produce varying severity of brain injury (Dixon et al., 1991). As with the FPI mode, the CCI model has been successfully shown to mimic injuries produced with TBI, including cortical tissue loss, acute subdural hematoma, axonal injury, concussion, and BBB dysfunction (Osier and Dixon, 2016). Initially thought to only produce focal gray matter injuries, studies have suggested the CCI model produces more widespread degeneration, including white matter, hippocampus, and thalamus (Yang et al., 2010). To date, CCI models have been successfully replicated in ferrets, rats, mice, swine, and monkeys (Xiong et al., 2013; Figure 21.2).

Protocol: Animals are anesthetized as per institutional protocol (as previously mentioned). Strict sterile technique is maintained throughout the course of the surgical procedure. A midline incision is made, the soft tissues are reflected, and a craniectomy performed as detailed.

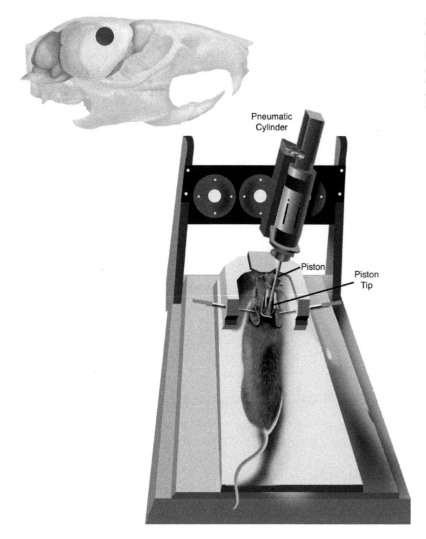

Figure 21.2 Schematic diagram showing experimental setup of the controlled cortical impact (CCI) animal model of traumatic brain injury (TBI) with anesthetized mouse in situ. Assembly of the controlled cortical impact device includes pneumatic cylinder with a piston mounted precisely along an adjustable horizontal crossbar.

Pneumatic Cylinder

Piston

Piston Tip

A 5-mm craniotomy is performed over the left parietotemporal cortex, while maintaining the dura mater intact. The controlled cortical impact is conducted using a beveled 3-mm flat-tip impounder at velocity 5.7–6 m/s with cortical deformation 1 mm (Hunt et al., 2012). Surgical site closed with suture.

21.4.3 Closed Head Impact Model of Engineered Rotational Acceleration

Closed Head Impact Model of Engineered Rotational Acceleration (CHIMERA) is a non-surgical, diffuse closed-head injury model characterized by direct impact as well as unconstrained head motion following impact. Furthermore, studies have shown that CHIMERA-induced TBI results in the reliable recapitulation of several key behavioral, biochemical, and neuropathological characteristics that remain the hallmark of TBI, including widespread microgliosis, widespread persistent diffuse axonal injury (DAI), activation of inflammatory reaction, and functional deficits (Namjoshi et al., 2014).

Protocol: The CHIMERA impactor consists of an aluminum frame that supports an animal holding platform, composed of a fixed head plate maintaining the animal in the supine position and a body plate that secures the animal's torso, above a pneumatic impactor system. The pneumatic impactor system delivers impact via a 50-g free-floating chrome steel piston with a surrounding steel barrel to maintain the appropriate trajectory.

Animals were anesthetized per institutional protocol and were placed supine such that the top of the animal's head lay flat over a hole in the head plate so that the piston strikes the vertex of the head covering a 5-mm area surrounding the bregma. Twenty four hours following the initial impact, a second identical impact was delivered. Of note, approximately 3 per cent of the CHIMERA TBI animal models did not regain consciousness for >45 min or displayed severe motor dysfunction following the impact and were therefore euthanized (Namjoshi et al., 2014).

21.4.4 modCHIMERA

Recently, in 2018, the CHIMERA model was further expanded to the modCHIMERA model, which was designed to establish a range of injury severities and specifically target the complicated mild-to-moderate TBI. The modCHIMERA model is characterized by a direct impact followed by a semi-restrained linear and rotational acceleration. It is hypothesized that models that include both impact and inertial elements (including both linear and rotational acceleration) maximize clinical validity as both are generally present in human TBI, which remains the basis for the modCHIMERA model. Development of the modCHIMERA model was similar to the CHIMERA model with two specific modifications: (1) the use of a semi-rigid helmet for protection of the skull from skull fractures, and (2) use of a foam-lined rigid cradle to partially restrict spine flexion.

Protocol: Animals were anesthetized per institutional protocol and a semi-rigid helmet was placed immediately posterior to the animal's eyes. The animal was subsequently placed in the supine position in a foam-lined cradle attached to the CHIMERA device with the stage set at a 10-degree angle with the head positioned over the impact site 4 mm posterior to the lateral canthus of the eye at midline. Two separate impact intensities were used (1.7 J using 8 psi air pressure and 2.1 J using 9.8–10 psi air pressure). Following impact, each animal model and cradle was allowed to freely rotate 180 degrees attached to the CHIMERA device. The animals were quickly removed from the cradle and assessed for any signs of ineffective respirations or apnea, and if observed, lateral fingertip chest percussion was performed at a rate of 350 percussions/min until effective breathing returned (Sauerbeck et al., 2018).

21.4.5 Impact–Acceleration Model

The Impact–Acceleration Model, also known as the Weight Drop Model, mimics diffuse TBI. Until recently, in comparison to other animal models used to study TBI,

the Impact–Acceleration Model, initially described by Marmarou et al., lacked precision or ease of reproducibility in results – typically desired in a well-studied animal model. However, this was disproven following Hsieh et al. (2017), who went on to demonstrate that by controlling both the impact height and pressure, it is possible to reliably induce injury of graded neurologic severity that strongly correlate with graded mechanical impact levels.

Protocol: Animals were anesthetized as per institutional protocol; then, their heads were shaved and inserted into a stereotaxic frame. Strict sterile technique is maintained throughout the course of the surgical procedure. A 3-mm craniotomy was performed and localized either in the midcoronal plane between the bregma and lambda on the sagittal suture (i.e., midline injury) or 1–2 mm lateral of midline in the midcoronal plane (i.e., lateral injury). A weight-drop device was placed on the stereotactic arm over the dura and centered over the desired area of impact. A brass weight was dropped from various heights above the exposed, intact dura to achieve the desired severity of neurologic injury. The scalp was sutured closed and animals were returned to housing for recovery (Bodnar et al., 2019; Golarai et al., 2001; Marmarou et al., 1994). Studies have indicated that graduations of mechanical impact level reproduces progressing degrees of injury severity, and thus, varying degrees of severity of TBI models simply by altering the heights by which the weights are dropped (Hsieh et al., 2017). Slight variations to the protocol for the Impact–Acceleration Model have been used as described by Bodnar et al. (2019), to include use of a metal disc helmet over the exposed dura at the location of impact to diffuse the blow and reduce both skull fractures and focal lesions; fixation of the animal's head during delivery of the impact; weight of projectile; and projectile drop height.

21.4.6 Penetrating Head Trauma

Penetrating head trauma has occurred with increasing prevalence over the last decade, with an estimated 35,000 civilian deaths annually and a high-associated morbidity and mortality. Post-traumatic complications associated with penetrating head trauma differ compared to blunt TBI, including: CSF leak, traumatic intracranial aneurysms, intraventricular hemorrhage, dural venous sinus thrombosis, bullet fragment migration, intracranial infections, and increased risk of post-traumatic epilepsy (Kendirli et al., 2014; Vakil and Singh, 2017).

Protocol: Animals are anesthetized as per institutional protocol; then, their heads are shaved and inserted into a stereotaxic frame. Strict sterile technique is maintained throughout the course of the surgical procedure. The skull was exposed, and a high-speed drill was mounted vertically on the stereotactic arm. A hardened steel burr (1.5 mm diameter) was introduced through the skull, dura, and brain at 1000 RPM using the stereotactic arm (anteroposterior: −4.9 mm, mediolateral: 4.5 mm to the bregma) to a depth of 8 mm below the brain surface. Copper wire (0.02 mm diameter, 5 mm length) or stainless-steel wire (0.03 mm diameter, 5 mm length) was introduced into the lesion immediately after it had been created and the scalp was closed (Bolkvadze and Pitkänen, 2012).

21.4.7 Pediatric Traumatic Brain Injury

Pediatric TBI studies are limited and, until recently, clinically relevant models in the pediatric population were lacking; however, previous studies have worked to develop preclinical models of pediatric TBI and post-traumatic epilepsy with some success, as described below (Kochanek et al., 2017). Furthermore, the development of pediatric models of TBI remain important as many age-dependent changes have been shown to differ in the development of secondary damage following TBI in the pediatric population, including: myelination, neurotransmitter development, apoptosis, synaptogenesis, synaptic reorganization, BBB dysfunction, CSF dynamics, and cerebral metabolism (Kochanek et al., 2017). For example, studies have demonstrated that the developing brain exhibits remarkably lower levels of antioxidant activities, particularly in clearing hydrogen peroxide, leading to accumulation of harmful free radicals (Bayır et al., 2006), increased vulnerability to apoptotic neurodegeneration via both intrinsic and extrinsic pathways secondary to age-dependent expression of caspase 3 (Yakovlev et al., 2001), and markedly increased neuroinflammatory response in infants and children as compared to the adult population (Hagberg et al., 2002). In general, rodents post-natal days (PND) 7–11 are used to model term infants and rodents PND 17–21 to model toddlers (Kochanek et al., 2017).

Protocol: Litters of Sprague–Dawley Rats were housed with lactating females until weaning on PND 21, at which time they were segregated and housed in a temperature- and light-controlled environment. Animals are anesthetized as per institutional protocol; then, their heads are shaved and inserted into a stereotaxic frame. A 6 mm ×

6 mm craniotomy was performed over the left parietal cortex centered around 4 mm anterior, 4 mm lateral to the bregma. Rats underwent CCI as per protocol centered over the left parietal cortex 4 mm rostral to lambda and 4 mm left of midline with a 5 mm round-tip at 4 m/s velocity with 2 mm deformation and 100 ms duration on PND 16–18 (Statler et al., 2009).

21.5 Conclusions

Undoubtedly, the variation in underlying mechanisms of injury, clinical presentation, degree of latency, and severity of TBI poses difficulties in diagnosis and management of TBI. Translation of successful in-vitro research studies into clinical therapeutics is a major challenge, with the potential for costly and prolonged clinical trials. Despite the important advances we have accomplished in understanding TBI, clinical evidence for management, particularly with the significant variations in TBI, remains elusive. Although the current animal models of TBI provide key evidence in understanding the underlying pathophysiology, no current model to date fully recapitulates TBI. Therefore, understanding the strengths and weaknesses of each animal model may be key in the determination of which animal model provides the necessary requirements for the evaluation of specific research questions.

Figure acknowledgements

The following images are credited to the authors of this chapter: Figures 21.1-21.2

References

Alder J, Fujioka W, Lifshitz J, Crockett DP, Thakker-Varia S. Lateral fluid percussion: model of traumatic brain injury in mice. *J Vis Exp* 2011;54:3063. https://doi.org/10.3791/3063.

Ansari MA, Roberts KN, Scheff SW. Oxidative stress and modification of synaptic proteins in hippocampus after traumatic brain injury. *Free Radic Biol Med* 2008;45(4):443–52. https://doi.org/10.1016/j.freeradbiomed.2008.04.038

Bales JW, Ma X, Yan HQ, Jenkins LW, Dixon CE. Expression of protein phosphatase 2B (calcineurin) subunit A isoforms in rat hippocampus after traumatic brain injury. *J Neurotrauma* 2010;27(1):109–20. https://doi.org/10.1089/neu.2009.1072.

Bayır H, Kochanek PM, Kagan VE. Oxidative stress in immature brain after traumatic brain injury. *Dev Neurosci* 2006;28(4–5):420–31. https://doi.org/10.1159/000094168.

Bodnar CN, Roberts KN, Higgins EK, Bachstetter AD. A systematic review of closed head injury models of mild traumatic brain injury in mice and rats. *J Neurotrauma* 2019;**36**(11):1683–706. https://doi.org/10.1089/neu.2018.6127.

Bolkvadze T, Pitkänen A. Development of post-traumatic epilepsy after controlled cortical impact and lateral fluid-percussion-induced brain injury in the mouse. *J Neurotrauma* 2012;**29**(5):789–812. https://doi.org/10.1089/neu.2011.1954.

Capizzi A, Woo J, Verduzco-Gutierrez M. Traumatic brain injury. *Med Clin N Am* 2020;**104**(2):213–38. https://doi.org/10.1016/j.mcna.2019.11.001.

Centers for Disease Control and Prevention, U.S. Department of Health and Human Services. Surveillance Report of Traumatic Brain Injury-related Emergency Department Visits, Hospitalizations, and Deaths – United States, 2014. [Internet]. www.cdc.gov/traumaticbraininjury/get_the_facts.html.

Cernak I. The importance of systemic response in the pathobiology of blast-induced neurotrauma. *Front Neur* [Internet] 2010;**1**:151. http://journal.frontiersin.org/article/10.3389/fneur.2010.00151/abstract

Cernak I. Understanding blast-induced neurotrauma: how far have we come? *Concussion* 2017;**2**(3):CNC42. https://doi.org/10.2217/cnc-2017-0006.

Dewan MC, Rattani A, Gupta S, et al. Estimating the global incidence of traumatic brain injury. *J Neurosurg* 2019;**130**(4):1080–97. https://doi.org/10.3171/2017.10.JNS17352.

Dixon CE, Clifton GL, Lighthall JW, Yaghmai AA, Hayes RL. A controlled cortical impact model of traumatic brain injury in the rat. J Neurosci Methods 1991;**39**(3):253–62. https://doi.org/10.1016/0165-0270(91)90104-8.

Faden A, Demediuk P, Panter S, Vink R. The role of excitatory amino acids and NMDA receptors in traumatic brain injury. *Science* 1989;**244**(4906):798–800. https://doi.org/10.1126/science.2567056

Folkerts MM, Parks EA, Dedman JR, Kaetzel MA, Lyeth BG, Berman RF. Phosphorylation of calcium calmodulin-dependent protein kinase II following lateral fluid percussion brain injury in rats. *J Neurotrauma* 2007;**24**(4):638–50. https://doi.org/10.1089/neu.2006.0188.

Frati A, Cerretani D, Fiaschi A, et al. Diffuse axonal injury and oxidative stress: a comprehensive review. *Int J Mol Sci* 2017;**18**(12):2600. https://doi.org/10.3390/ijms18122600.

Golarai G, Greenwood AC, Feeney DM, Connor JA. Physiological and structural evidence for hippocampal involvement in persistent seizure susceptibility after traumatic brain injury. *J Neurosci* 2001;**21**(21):8523–37. https://doi.org/10.1523/JNEUROSCI.21-21-08523.2001.

Hagberg H, Peebles D, Mallard C. Models of white matter injury: comparison of infectious, hypoxic–ischemic, and excitotoxic insults. *Ment Retard Dev Disabil Res Rev* 2002;**8**(1):30–8. https://doi.org/10.1002/mrdd.10007.

Hall ED, Detloff MR, Johnson K, Kupina NC. Peroxynitrite-mediated protein nitration and lipid peroxidation in a mouse model of traumatic brain injury. *J Neurotrauma* 2004;**21**(1):9–20. https://doi.org/10.1089/089771504772695904.

Hergenroeder GW, Moore AN, McCoy JP, et al. Serum IL-6: a candidate biomarker for intracranial pressure elevation following isolated traumatic brain injury. *J Neuroinflamm* 2010;**7**(1):19. https://doi.org/10.1186/1742-2094-7-19.

Hill RL, Singh IN, Wang JA, Hall ED. Time courses of post-injury mitochondrial oxidative damage and respiratory dysfunction and neuronal cytoskeletal degradation in a rat model of focal traumatic brain injury. *Neurochem Int* 2017;**111**:45–56. https://doi.org/10.1016/j.neuint.2017.03.015.

Hsieh T-H, Kang J-W, Lai J-H, et al. Relationship of mechanical impact magnitude to neurologic dysfunction severity in a rat traumatic brain injury model. *PLoS One* 2017;**12**(5):e0178186. https://doi.org/10.1371/journal.pone.0178186.

Hunt RF, Haselhorst LA, Schoch KM, et al. Posttraumatic mossy fiber sprouting is related to the degree of cortical damage in three mouse strains. *Epilepsy Res* 2012;**99**(1–2):167–70. https://doi.org/10.1016/j.eplepsyres.2011.10.011.

Kaur P, Sharma S. Recent advances in pathophysiology of traumatic brain injury. *Curr Neuropharmacol* 2018;**16**(9):1224–38. https://doi.org/10.2174/1570159X15666170613083606.

Kendirli MT, Rose DT, Bertram EH. A model of posttraumatic epilepsy after penetrating brain injuries: effect of lesion size and metal fragments. *Epilepsia* 2014;**55**(12):1969–77. https://doi.org/10.1111/epi.12854.

Kochanek PM, Wallisch JS, Bayır H, Clark RSB. Pre-clinical models in pediatric traumatic brain injury – challenges and lessons learned. *Childs Nerv Syst* 2017;**33**(10):1693–701. https://doi.org/10.1007/s00381-017-3474-2.

Landeghem FKHV, Weiss T, Oehmichen M, Deimling AV. Decreased expression of glutamate transporters in astrocytes after human traumatic brain injury. *J Neurotrauma* 2006;**23**(10):1518–28. https://doi.org/10.1089/neu.2006.23.1518.

Lu K-T, Cheng N-C, Wu C-Y, Yang Y-L. NKCC1-mediated traumatic brain injury-induced brain edema and neuron death via Raf/MEK/MAPK cascade. *Crit Care Med* 2008;**36**(3):917–22. https://doi.org/10.1097/CCM.0B013E31816590C4.

Marmarou A, Foda MAA-E, van den Brink W, Campbell J, Kita H, Demetriadou K. A new model of diffuse brain injury in rats: Part I: pathophysiology and biomechanics. *J Neurosurg* 1994;**80**(2):291–300. https://doi.org/10.3171/jns.1994.80.2.0291.

Meldrum BS. Glutamate as a neurotransmitter in the brain: review of physiology and pathology. *J Nutr* 2000;**130**(4):1007S–1015S. https://doi.org/10.1093/jn/130.4.1007S.

Mendez MF, Owens EM, Reza Berenji G, Peppers DC, Liang L-J, Licht EA. Mild traumatic brain injury from primary blast vs. blunt forces: post-concussion consequences and functional neuroimaging. *NeuroRehabilitation* 2013;**32**(2):397–407. https://doi.org/10.3233/NRE-130861.

Namjoshi DR, Cheng W, McInnes KA, et al. Merging pathology with biomechanics using CHIMERA (Closed-Head Impact Model of Engineered Rotational Acceleration): a novel, surgery-free model of traumatic brain injury. *Mol Neurodegen* 2014;9(1):55. https://doi.org/10.1186/1750-1326-9-55.

Ng SY, Lee AYW. Traumatic brain injuries: pathophysiology and potential therapeutic targets. *Front Cell Neurosci* 2019;13:528. https://doi.org/10.3389/fncel.2019.00528.

Osier ND, Dixon CE. The controlled cortical impact model: applications, considerations for researchers, and future directions. *Front Neurol* [Internet] 2016;7:134. http://journal.frontiersin.org/Article/10.3389/fneur.2016.00134/abstract

Raghavendra Rao VL, Başkaya MK, Doğan A, Rothstein JD, Dempsey RJ. Traumatic brain injury down-regulates glial glutamate transporter (GLT-1 and GLAST) proteins in rat brain. *J Neurochem* 2002;70(5):2020–7. https://doi.org/10.1046/j.1471-4159.1998.70052020.x.

Ray SK, Dixon CE, Banik NL. Molecular mechanisms in the pathogenesis of traumatic brain injury. *Histol Histopathol* 2002;17:1137–52. https://doi.org/10.14670/HH-17.1137.

Sapan HB, Paturusi I, Jusuf I, et al. Pattern of cytokine (IL-6 and IL-10) level as inflammation and anti-inflammation mediator of multiple organ dysfunction syndrome (MODS) in polytrauma. *Int J Burns Trauma* 2016;6(2):37–43.

Sauerbeck AD, Fanizzi C, Kim JH, et al. modCHIMERA: a novel murine closed-head model of moderate traumatic brain injury. *Sci Rep* 2018;8(1):7677. https://doi.org/10.1038/s41598-018-25737-6.

Shively SB, Horkayne-Szakaly I, Jones RV, Kelly JP, Armstrong RC, Perl DP. Characterisation of interface astroglial scarring in the human brain after blast exposure: a post-mortem case series. *Lancet Neurol* 2016;15(9):944–53. https://doi.org/10.1016/S1474-4422(16)30057-6.

Shively SB, Perl DP. Viewing the invisible wound: novel lesions identified in postmortem brains of U.S. service members with military blast exposure. *Military Med* 2017;182(1):1461–3. https://doi.org/10.7205/MILMED-D-16-00239.

Skandsen T, Kvistad KA, Solheim O, Strand IH, Folvik M, Vik A. Prevalence and impact of diffuse axonal injury in patients with moderate and severe head injury: a cohort study of early magnetic resonance imaging findings and 1-year outcome. *J Neurosurg* 2010;113(3):556–63. https://doi.org/10.3171/2009.9.JNS09626.

Statler KD, Scheerlinck P, Pouliot W, Hamilton M, White HS, Dudek FE. A potential model of pediatric posttraumatic epilepsy. *Epilepsy Res* 2009;86(2–3):221–3. https://doi.org/10.1016/j.eplepsyres.2009.05.006

Sullivan PG, Thompson MB, Scheff SW. Cyclosporin A attenuates acute mitochondrial dysfunction following traumatic brain injury. *Exp Neurol* 1999;160(1):226–34. https://doi.org/10.1006/exnr.1999.7197.

Thompson HJ, Lifshitz J, Marklund N, et al. Lateral fluid percussion brain injury: a 15-year review and evaluation. *J Neurotrauma* 2005;22(1):42–75. https://doi.org/10.1089/neu.2005.22.42.

Vakil MT, Singh AK. A review of penetrating brain trauma: epidemiology, pathophysiology, imaging assessment, complications, and treatment. *Emerg Radiol* 2017;24(3):301–09. https://doi.org/10.1007/s10140-016-1477-z.

Valiyaveettil M, Alamneh Y, Wang Y, et al. Contribution of systemic factors in the pathophysiology of repeated blast-induced neurotrauma. *Neurosci Lett* 2013;539:1–6. https://doi.org/10.1016/j.neulet.2013.01.028.

Weber JT. Altered calcium signaling following traumatic brain injury. Front Pharmacol [Internet] 2012;3:60. http://journal.frontiersin.org/article/10.3389/fphar.2012.00060/abstract

Woodcock T, Morganti-Kossmann MC. The role of markers of inflammation in traumatic brain injury. *Front Neurol* [Internet] 2013;4:18. http://journal.frontiersin.org/article/10.3389/fneur.2013.00018/abstract

Woodroofe MN, Sarna GS, Wadhwa M, et al. Detection of interleukin-1 and interleukin-6 in adult rat brain, following mechanical injury, by in vivo microdialysis: evidence of a role for microglia in cytokine production. *J Neuroimmunol* 1991;33(3):227–36. https://doi.org/10.1016/0165-5728(91)90110-s.

Xiong Y, Mahmood A, Chopp M. Animal models of traumatic brain injury. *Nat Rev Neurosci* 2013;14(2):128–42. https://doi.org/10.1038/nrn3407.

Yakovlev AG, Ota K, Wang G, et al. Differential expression of apoptotic protease-activating factor-1 and caspase-3 genes and susceptibility to apoptosis during brain development and after traumatic brain injury. *J Neurosci* 2001;21(19):7439–46. https://doi.org/10.1523/JNEUROSCI.21-19-07439.2001.

Yang L, Afroz S, Michelson HB, Goodman JH, Valsamis HA, Ling DSF. Spontaneous epileptiform activity in rat neocortex after controlled cortical impact injury. *J Neurotrauma* 2010;27(8):1541–8. https://doi.org/10.1089/neu.2009.1244.

Chapter 22

Vascular Neurosurgery

Karol P. Budohoski and Adib A. Abla

22.1 Introduction

Vascular neurosurgery is a diverse field focused on surgical and interventional treatment of cerebrovascular disease, both the manifestations as well as the underlying causes. Specifically, the common diseases that fall in the domain of vascular neurosurgery include cerebral ischemia and ischemic stroke including occlusive vascular disease, non-lesional hemorrhagic vascular disease – which includes spontaneous, hypertensive and angiopathic intracerebral hemorrhage (ICH) – and lesional hemorrhagic vascular disease – which includes cerebral aneurysms, arteriovenous malformations, and cavernomas.

Given this diverse disease pool, vascular neurosurgery spans multiple fields, including neurology, cardiology, intensive care, interventional radiology, and clinical genetics, and can affect involve both adult and pediatric patients. Furthermore, both cerebral ischemia and stroke, as well as intracranial hemorrhage, can be a manifestation of systemic disease, such as atherosclerosis or hypertension and amyloid angiopathy, respectively.

While research has led to significant improvements in understanding, preventions, and treatment of cerebrovascular disease, very few specific interventions were successfully translated from basic sciences and animal research into clinical practice. Tissue plasminogen activator (tPA) is widely known as the only medical intervention, out of more than 1000 studied in various animal models (Jickling and Sharp, 2015), that was successfully translated from animal research to an FDA-approved treatment (The National Institute of Neurological Disorders and Stroke rt-PA Stroke Study Group, 1995; Zivin et al., 1985). Similarly, the Gugliemi Detachable Coil (GDC) for the treatment of cerebral aneurysm is the only surgical intervention that has been shown to be efficacious in animal models as well as human trials (Guglielmi, 2009; Molyneaux et al., 2002). However, both these treatments have led a major shift in the management of patient with cerebrovascular disease and improved outcomes, demonstrating the value of basic research and animal models in treating patients with cerebrovascular pathology. Furthermore, basic research has contributed to significant improvements in understanding of the pathophysiology of cerebrovascular diseases and important changes in management, which were never evaluated in animal models, such as intensive care management of subarachnoid hemorrhage (SAH) and invasive brain monitoring. Therefore, clinicians should be familiar with opportunities as well as the challenges related to it.

The basic science of cerebrovascular disease is a very extensive topic and exceeds the scope of this chapter. Below we will focus on specific aspects of vascular neurosurgery where animal models of both the disease pathobiology as well as treatment have come to play a significant part. These include SAH and the associated early and delayed brain injury, as well as the biology of cerebral aneurysm formation and growth.

22.2 Pathobiology

22.2.1 Subarachnoid Hemorrhage

The incidence of spontaneous SAH is around 6–11 per 100,000 persons per year (Linn et al., 1996), out of which 85% of cases are due to a ruptured intracranial aneurysm. Approximately one in every 20 strokes is caused by aneurysmal SAH. Nevertheless, due to the relatively young age of the affected population and the high rates of disability, the burden to society is high, with a reported loss of productive years similar to that of ischemic and hemorrhagic strokes (Johnston et al., 1998; van Gijn et al., 2007).

The mortality rate after SAH is approximately 2.8 per 100,000 persons per year (Johnston et al., 1998); however, the case fatality is between 32% and 67%, with about 10–15% of patients dying before ever reaching the hospital (ACROSS, 2000; Hop et al., 1997; Kassell et al., 1990; van Gijn et al., 2007). Over the past two decades the advancement of understanding of the pathophysiology of SAH and its sequalae has led to a considerable reduction in the mortality of patients who survive the initial ictus (Lovelock et al., 2010). The latest figures from the International Subarachnoid Aneurysm Trial (ISAT) found that one-year mortality was 8.1% and 10.1% for endovascular and surgical treatments, respectively (Molyneaux et al., 2002). Despite the advancements, about 30% of patients following SAH will not regain full independence, while 69% will report a reduced quality of life (Hop et al., 1998).[13]

Early brain injury (EBI) and delayed cerebral ischemia (DCI) are recognized as the leading causes of death and disability following SAH. This suggests that improvements in treating EBI, as well as identifying patients at risk of DCI and the clinical management of DCI, could translate into considerable benefits for patients (Hop et al., 1997; Kassell et al., 1990; Rabinstein et al., 2004; Rosengart et al., 2007; Vergouwen et al., 2011b).

22.2.1.1 The Pathophysiology of Early Brain Injury and Delayed Cerebral Ischemia Following Subarachnoid Hemorrhage

Delayed cerebral ischemia is one of the most severe complications of aneurysmal SAH. It accounts for a large proportion of morbidity and mortality (Hop et al., 1997; Johnston et al., 1998; Vergouwen et al., 2011b). DCI has been shown to occur in approximately 30% of patients, typically between days 4 and 10 after bleeding (Hijdra et al., 1986; Vergouwen et al., 2011a). The pathophysiology of DCI is complex and not fully understood. While traditionally cerebral vasospasm (CVS) was treated as the primary cause, a clear paradigm shift to a multifactorial etiology can be observed with EBI playing a significant role contributing to vulnerability to subsequent ischemic insults (Macdonald et al., 2007; Pluta et al., 2009; Rabinstein, 2011).

Ecker and Riemenschneider (1951) first documented the presence of CVS in relation to a ruptured aneurysm. Subsequently, Allcock and Drake (1963) demonstrated a clear relationship between arterial narrowing a clinical symptoms. While CVS and DCI have been recognized entities for over 70 years, the precise mechanism for vessel narrowing has not been established. Numerous compounds have been proposed.

- Blood degradation products, with oxyhemoglobin being the most widely recognized, have been proposed as the trigger of a molecular cascade that leads to CVS (Macdonald et al., 1991a; Toda, 1990; Toda et al., 1980).
- Diminished levels of nitric oxide (NO) and nitrous oxide synthase (NOS), both potent vasodilators, have been demonstrated after SAH (Hino et al., 1996; Pluta et al., 2005).
- Endothelin-1 (ET-1), a potent vasoconstrictor, has been shown to increase after SAH (Juvela, 2000; Seifert et al., 1995), and its administration has been shown to reduce vasospasm (Macdonald et al., 2012; Vatter et al., 2005). However, in a multicenter trial ET-1 antagonists have failed to demonstrate outcome benefits (Macdonald et al., 2011).
- Blood–brain barrier (BBB) breakdown and an inflammatory response has been shown to occur following SAH (Doczi et al., 1986; Fassbender et al., 2001).

Recent reports suggest that the events occurring before the onset of DCI, during the first 72 hours after the ictus, may significantly contribute to outcome following SAH (Cahill et al., 2006; Claassen et al., 2002; Hop et al., 1999; Schubert et al., 2009). The effect of EBI may or may not be independent of DCI. It is recognized that aneurysm rupture is accompanied by a severe rise of intracranial pressure (ICP) and decreases in cerebral perfusion pressure (CPP), often to the point of cerebral circulatory arrest (Nornes, 1973; Trojanowski, 1984a, 1984b; Voldby and Enevoldsen, 1982). These mechanisms may be responsible for cessation of bleeding; therefore, having a beneficial effect (Nornes, 1973). The ensuing global cerebral ischemia, however, causes activation of several key pathophysiological pathways that may, in consequence, lead to direct nervous tissue injury as well as increased tissue vulnerability to secondary insults. These include initiation of cell death mechanisms, BBB disruption, inflammation, development of cerebral edema, loss of autoregulation, and cortical spreading depolarization (Figure 22.1; Budohoski et al., 2012; De Oliveira Manoel and Macdonald, 2018; Dreier et al., 2009; Geraghty et al., 2019; Gules et al., 2003; Hanafy et al., 2010; Schöller et al., 2007).

22.2.1.2 Animal Models of Subarachnoid Hemorrhage and Delayed Cerebral Ischemia

While significant information about disease process can be obtain from clinical and post-mortem material, it remains challenging to conduct research directly on nervous tissue and cerebral vasculature in live humans (Conway and McDonald, 1972; Crompton, 1964; Eldevik et al., 1981; Hughes and Schianchi, 1978). In-vitro and in-vivo animal models have been developed for this purpose. In-vitro models involve removing an artery from an experimental animal and subjecting it to various substances while

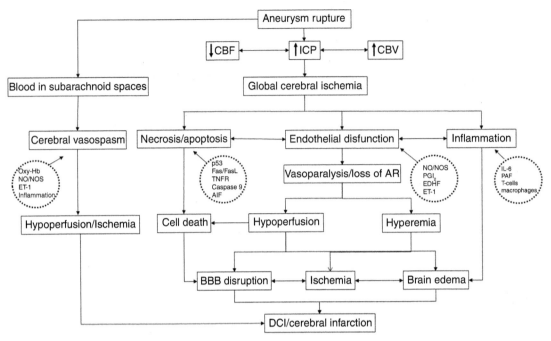

Figure 22.1 Mechanisms of EBI and DCI. *Abbreviations*: AIF, apoptosis inducing factor; BBB, blood–brain barrier; CBF, cerebral blood flow; CBV, cerebral blood volume; DCI, delayed cerebral ischemia; EDHF, endothelial derived growth factor; ET-1, endothelin-1; IL-6, interleukin-6; NO/NOS, nitric oxide/nitric oxide synthase; Oxy-Hb, oxyhemoglobin; PAF, platelet activating factor; PGI$_2$, prostaglandin I$_2$; TNFR, tumor necrosis factor receptor.

observing its physiological responses (Allen et al., 1974; Fukuroda et al., 1992). Although described in the context of SAH, this method has significant limitations due to the inability to accurately reproduce the environment following a SAH in vitro.

In order to study cerebral vasculature in its true environment and allow for observation of longitudinal changes, in-vivo models have been developed. The specifics of an animal model of SAH depend of the nature of the experiment. However, an adequate model of SAH should have extravasated blood in the subarachnoid space surrounding an intracranial vessel and should reliably elicit delayed vasospasm (Megyesi et al., 2000). Furthermore, the model should allow for adequate survival of animals to allow conduct of observations and for a control group where sham procedures are performed. Numerous models have been developed in the mouse, rat, rabbit, dog, cat, pig, goat, and primate (Figure 22.2). Extensive reviews of all models used can be found in Megyesi et al. (2000) and Marbacher et al. (2010, 2019). Fundamentally, the models that are most reliable and consistently used rely on:

- Injection of autologous blood into the subarachnoid space, typically cisterna magna
- In-situ arterial puncture using open or endovascular techniques
- Surgical application of autologous blood around an exposed intracranial vessel

Table 22.1 summarizes the most commonly used models of SAH along with the most commonly used animal species.

22.2.1.2.1 Subarachnoid Injection Model

The cisterna magna blood injection model, which was introduced by Solomon et al. (1985) in rats, is the most common animal model of SAH used in experimental studies (Marbacher et al., 2010). Subsequently, injection of blood was tried in the prechiasmatic cistern (Echlin, 1971), as well as directly next to an intracranial artery (Tsuji et al., 1996) The drawback of the initial technique in the rat is the unreliability of the time course of vasospasm, which does not correlate with that seen in humans after SAH (Solomon et al., 1985; Verlooy et al., 1992). This led to expansion of the model into different species, as well as development of the second

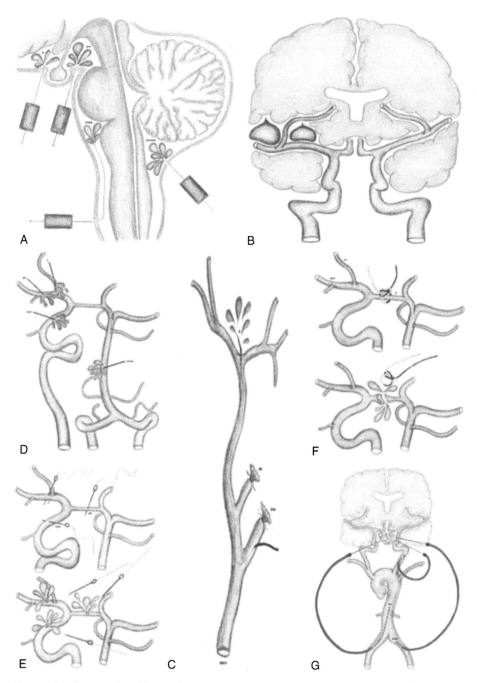

Figure 22.2 Diagram of models used for experimental SAH.

injection technique, whereby a second application of blood into the same subarachnoid cistern is performed 24–48 h after the first. The second injection resulted in a more reliable vasospasm period, peaking at day 5 in the rat (Vatter et al., 2006). Similar results were observed

with different animals, confirming the reliability of the model. Clinical assessment of vasospasm in the rat remains challenging. Quantitative assessment of angiography is difficult due to the caliber of vessels; therefore, often casting methods are used, requiring sacrifice of

Table 22.1 Animal models of SAH (Marbacher et al., 2010)

Animal	SAH technique	Blood amount	CVS peak	Degree of narrowing	CVS assessment
Mouse	Endovascular puncture	Various	Day 3	20–62%	Casting method
Rat	Single cisterna magna blood injection	0.3 ml	Day 2	19–29%	Casting method
	Double cisterna magna blood injection	2 × 0.3 ml	Day 7	28–57%	Casting method
Rabbit	Single cisterna magna blood injection	3 ml	Day 3	19–55%	Angiography
	Double cisterna magna blood injection	Various	Day 5	–	–
Canine	Double cisterna magna blood injection	2 × 4–5 ml	Day 7	45–66%	Angiography
Primate	Craniotomy and blood clot placement	5 ml	Day 7	32–52%	Angiography

CVS, cerebral vasospasm

animals and precluding longer-term observation (Turowski et al., 2007).

The subarachnoid injection model was applied to the rabbit and canine with good results (Edvinsson et al., 1982; Kuwayama et al., 1972; Varsos et al., 1983; Zhou et al., 2007). Interestingly, the second injection technique was proven to be beneficial in the dog (Varsos et al., 1983) but not in the rabbit (Zhang et al., 2007). Subarachnoid blood injection remains the most common method used in canines. The temporal profile of vasospasm is very well documented in this species, with onset at day 4 and resolution at day 10 (Yoshimoto et al., 1993). Furthermore, the significant similarities of SAH induced in the canine model with that of humans, including the lack of angiographic response to treatment with calcium channel blockers, makes it attractive for research (Varsos et al., 1983). Angiographic assessment of vessel diameter is easily obtained in the dog. Similarly, neurological assessment has been proven to be reliable and standardized, making the canine injection model one of the most commonly used in SAH research (White et al., 1979; Yatsushige et al., 2005).

A common drawback for all traditional subarachnoid injection models is its inability to reproduce the acute injury accompanying SAH, i.e., early brain injury consisting of mechanical trauma, transient, global reduction of blood flow, and the subsequent pathological events. Sehba et al. (2013) have described a method to overcome this shortfall. They propose a controlled injection of blood in the cisterna magna with concomitant monitoring of ICP to allow targeting of a specific CPP reduction, resulting in transient global ischemia, thus mimicking human SAH (Nornes, 1973; Trojanowksi, 1984b). While few studies have used this method, it provides an attempt at standardizing the end point of the induced SAH. Currently, there is no consensus as to the desired duration of infusion and volume of blood to be deposited in the subarachnoid space, leading to difficulty in comparing results.

Subarachnoid hemorrhage does not start in the cisterna magna in humans and, therefore, uncertainty exists whether some observed physiologic changes in the injection models described may be a result of direct irritation to the brain stem, e.g., blood pressure elevation (Schwartz et al., 2000). Secondly, measurement of ICP from the cisterna magna during infusion of blood may not give reliable information. Finally, the degree of ICP elevation is slower and artificially controlled with the rate of blood infusion, and does not mimic the acute nature of SAH.

22.2.1.2.2 Direct and Endovascular Arterial Puncture

The main limitation of the subarachnoid injection method related to the lack of a distinct ictal event and associated physiologic alterations has been addressed with the development of the direct arterial puncture method. First described by Barry et al. (1979) using an open transclival approach to access the basilar artery, more recently, endovascular techniques using a microfilament have been used to puncture either the basilar artery, the internal carotid artery, or the middle cerebral artery (Bederson et al., 1995; Parra et al., 2002; Schwartz et al., 2000; Veelken et al., 1995).

The direct puncture model, whether using an open approach or endovascular techniques, results in significant rates of vasospasm (Parra et al., 2002; Saito et al., 2001). The degree of vessel constriction has been demonstrated to be between 20% and 62% (Kamii et al., 1999; McGirt et al., 2002). The time course of vessel constriction after SAH using the endovascular puncture method in mice demonstrated an initial phase on day 1 and a second phase on day 3 after puncture (Kamii et al., 1999; Lin et al., 2003). The endovascular puncture has also been performed using rat (Bederson et al., 1995; Veelken et al., 1995), rabbit (Logothetis et al., 1983), and primate (Landau and Ransohoff, 1968; Simeone et al., 1972) models with similar high rates and predictable time course of vasospasm.

Mouse models, due to size constraints, do not allow assessment of vasculature by means of angiography. The corrosion casting method, in which a polymer is used to replace blood in the cerebral vasculature, has been introduced to study the degree of vasospasm in mice. The corrosion casting method requires sacrificing the animals, precluding longitudinal follow-up and exact, real-time assessment of the degree of spasm, clinical symptoms, and response to proposed treatment (Hossler and Douglas, 2001). In the arterial puncture technique, the severity of the hemorrhage cannot be reliably controlled. Whether performed endovascularly or through a surgical exposure the model results in 26–50% mortality (Barry et al., 1979; Bederson et al., 1995; Logothetis et al., 1983; Parra et al., 2002). Furthermore, due to the varied severity of hemorrhage, results are often difficult to interpret. Schwartz et al. (2000) aimed to address this by introducing a "modified filament model," where the severity of hemorrhage could be controlled by altering the diameter of the filament used to make the arterial puncture. They report being able to obtain two distinct severities of hemorrhage. Furthermore, the group where a smaller puncture was used on post-mortem examination had smaller SAH volumes than the cisterna magna injection group. However, there are no data on mortality of either group. Finally, the arterial puncture method suffers from the intrinsic limitation of not being compatible with a sham control.

On the other hand, there is now a standardized post-mortem SAH grading scale to determine the degree of hemorrhage caused during an arterial puncture (Parra et al., 2002). Furthermore, reliable neurobehavioral

assessment batteries have been used and show a good correlation with the degree if spasm in the mouse, allowing for study of therapeutic interventions (Parra et al., 2002). Finally, the benefits of using mice models, where the arterial puncture technique predominates, are related to the very well characterized murine genome. Readily available tools allow accurately mapping of the molecular alterations following SAH, as well as introduction of "knockout" or "transgenic" mice to determine the functions of specific genes and proteins.

22.2.1.2.3 Surgical Application of Blood Around an Exposed Vessel

Echlin (1965) first used the primate model for the study of SAH and vasospasm. Using a transoral approach, the basilar artery was exposed and autologous blood was directly placed in the prepontine cistern around the vessel. The author reliably demonstrated vasoconstriction of the basilar artery using this model. Subsequently, numerous other techniques have been tried in the primate, including the previously described subarachnoid blood injection and direct arterial puncture (Delgado-Zygmunt et al., 1992; Landau and Ransohoff, 1968; Sahlin et al., 1987; Simeone et al., 1972). In 1984, Espinosa and colleagues developed a model of direct placement of autologous blood over the internal carotid artery and its branches using a frontal craniotomy, mimicking closely the distribution of blood seen in humans with SAH (Espinosa et al., 1984). The authors demonstrated significant angiographic spasm, with a mean 47% reduction in vessel caliber, with a reproducible time course, peaking at day 7 and no mortalities. This model has been consistently used in the primate.

Similarly to the subarachnoid injection models, the shortfall of directly placing autologous blood over exposed vessels is related to the lack of an ictal event and the associated pathological mechanisms. On the other hand, direct placement of blood over exposed vessels allows tight control of degree of hemorrhage and for sham operations, providing the foundations for rigorous standardization and control of experimental findings. Furthermore, the reliability of inducing arterial spasm has allowed numerous investigations into the mechanisms of cerebral vasospasm. The ultrastructural changes within the tunica media during vasospasm were first described using this model (Findlay et al., 1989), as was the role of oxyhemoglobin as the primary factor driving vasospasm (Macdonald et al., 1991b).

Despite more than half a century of research into the nature of DCI after SAH, no useful treatment has been developed. While the role of extravasated blood and specifically oxyhemoglobin as the inciting factor has been widely accepted, treatments aimed to address the presence of a subarachnoid clot have not yielded clinical benefit and have not been widely adopted (Al-Tamimi et al., 2012; Findlay et al., 1995; Kramer and Fletcher, 2011). Systemic medical treatment targeting DCI has not shown clinical benefit. Nimodpine remains the only FDA-approved preventive treatment for DCI. Interestingly, while its benefit on outcome has been demonstrated in large randomized controlled trials (Pickard et al., 1989), there was no documented effect on cerebral vasospasm in animal models (Espinosa et al., 1984; Nosko et al., 1985).

More recently, emphasis has changed from large-vessel spasm to early brain injury and the multifactorial effects of SAH, including microvascular changes, inflammatory cascade, and loss of autoregulation. To this effect, new models of SAH that allow study of the acute ictal event need to be developed and standardized. An example of this is the recent modification of the subarachnoid injection model to target a drop of CPP to zero and a transient cerebral circulatory arrest (Sehba and Pluta, 2013). Similarly, there is a steady increase in laboratories studying the acute phase after SAH using the murine endovascular filament model.

22.2.2 Unruptured Cerebral Aneurysm

Equally important to the treatment of patients with SAH is the understanding of the biology of cerebral aneurysm formation. Their global prevalence is estimated at 2–6% in the general population, making them relatively common (Weir, 2002). The most frequently reported risk factors for harboring aneurysms and their risk of causing a hemorrhage have been identified as increased age, female sex, smoking, alcohol intake, hypertension, Japanese and Finnish ancestry, and most importantly, size of aneurysm (Weir, 2002). However, debate remains as to which aneurysms pose a risk of bleeding and, therefore, which aneurysms require treatment (International Study of Unruptured Intracranial Aneurysms Investigators, 1998; Wiebers et al., 2003).

The biology of aneurysm formation has not been fully understood. It is thought that hemodynamic stress leading to endothelial dysfunction, macrophage infiltration, and vessel wall inflammation and subsequent loss of smooth muscle cells and remodeling lead to the formation and growth of aneurysms (Chalouhi et al., 2013). Numerous clinical studies have established genetic association with genetic syndromes, e.g., autosomal polycystic

kidney disease, Ehlers–Danlos syndrome, Marfan syndrome, etc. (Samuel and Radovanovic, 2019). However, most aneurysms occur sporadically, and are not hereditary. However, significantly less is known about genetic predisposition and somatic mutations that drive aneurysm formation. Large-scale genome-wide association studies on humans have identified numerous polymorphisms in genes related to endothelial function, extracellular matrix, and inflammation (Alg et al., 2013; Samuel and Radovanovic, 2019). Animal models utilizing "knockout" and "overexpression" animals will form a large part of the inquiry to the molecular mechanisms of aneurysm formation, growth, and subsequent rupture. Furthermore, these models will likely play a role in developing target treatments. Table 22.2 summarizes the current understanding of cerebral aneurysm formation borne out of animal models.

Numerous aneurysm formation models have been developed in various animal species, including mice,

Table 22.2 Mechanisms of aneurysm formation (Chalouhi et al., 2013)

Mechanism	Mediators
Endothelial dysfunction	IL-1β NF-κB MCP-1 Reactive oxygen species Nitric oxide Nitric oxide synthase Angiotensin II Phosphodiesterase-4 Prostaglandin E2 Vascular cell adhesion protein 1 Intercellular adhesion molecule 1
Macrophage infiltration and vessel wall inflammation	MCP-1 NF-κB Ets-1 MMPs IL-1β TNF-α IL-8 IL-17
Loss of smooth muscle cells/vessel remodeling	TNF-α IL-1β MCP-1 MMPs Adhesion molecules Complement FGF, TGF, VEGF

FGF, fibroblast growth factor; IL-1β, interleukin 1β; IL-6, interleukin 6; IL-8, interleukin 8; TGF, transforming growth factor; MCP-1, monocyte chemoattractant protein-1; MMP, matrix metalloproteinase; NF-κB, nuclear factor-κ B; TNFα, tumor necrosis factor-α; VEGF, vascular endothelial growth factor.

rats, rabbits, canine, swine, and primates. The models can be broadly divided into:

- Models developed to understand the biology of aneurysm formation, growth, and factors leading to rupture
- Models developed to test specific treatment modalities, typically endovascular. In these models an aneurysm is surgically formed using autologous tissue, allografts, xenografts, or artificial materials. Pathophysiologically, these lesions have no resemblance to real intracranial aneurysms and are used to serve as a target for aneurysm treatment. These models will not be discussed here.

Small animal models, typically, have been developed to understand the biology of cerebral aneurysms, while large animal models more often focus on developing new endovascular treatment approaches.

22.2.2.1 Small Animal Models

Small animal models primarily utilize induced hypertension, increased blood flow, and weakening of vessel wall to promote aneurysm formation (Figure 22.3). The first model was created by Hashimoto et al. (1978) in the rodent. This model requires numerous surgical procedures to achieve the goals stated above. Increased hemodynamic stress is achieved by unilateral ligation of the common carotid artery. Hypertension is induced by unilateral nephrectomy followed by treatment with deoxycorticosterone acetate and a high salt diet. Finally, the vessel wall is weakened by oral administration of a lysyl oxidase inhibitor, which prevents collagen and elastase cross-linking. Histologically, aneurysms formed this way resemble human aneurysms with degenerative changes in the media; namely, fragmentation of internal elastic lamina and thinning of the smooth muscle layer (Hashimoto et al., 1978, Morimoto et al., 2002). However, the majority of these lesions are small and detectable on light or electron microscopy only.

Histologically, degeneration and disruption of the elastic lamina are key characteristics of human intracranial aneurysms (Cajander and Hassler, 1976; Schievink, 1997). To limit surgical intervention, the elastase and angiotensin II model was developed (Nuki et al., 2009). In this model the authors utilized stereotactic injection of elastase into the basal cisterns and induced hypertension with administration of angiotensin II. This technique led to 77% of animals developing aneurysms at the circle of Willis. Again, histological analysis confirmed severely disorganized elastic lamina and reduction in the smooth muscle layer, in keeping with human pathological specimens.

The limitations of these models relate to a relative lack of atherosclerotic degeneration seen commonly in human cerebral aneurysms (Frösen et al., 2013; Ollikainen et al., 2016). Furthermore, the introduction of elastase into the system may not represent naturally occurring mechanisms, and hence may limit the applicability of the models in developing medical treatment strategies.

More recently, due to wide availability of genetically modified mice, efforts have intensified to investigate the molecular basis for aneurysm formation. Combining "knockout" animals for specific genes with the above-described techniques of inducing aneurysm formation has the potential to identify specific treatment targets that can translate into clinically useful therapies. NF-κB p50 subunit-deficient mice have shown less aneurysm formation and less macrophage wall infiltration, suggesting the NF-κB p50 subunit could become a target for treatment (Aoki et al., 2007). Similarly, using "knockout" mice monocyte chemoattractant protein-1 (MCP-1) has been shown to be a key factor in the progression of vessel wall inflammation leading to aneurysm formation (Aoki et al., 2009). Multiple other genes and proteins have been studied to date, leading to an improved understanding of the pathophysiology of cerebral aneurysm formation (for review, see Chalouhi et al., 2013).

22.3 Challenges

Despite the accumulation of vast amounts of knowledge about the pathophysiology of aneurysmal SAH and the development of cerebral aneurysms, there has been very little translation into routine clinical practice. Similar to other diseases where emphasis needs to be placed on

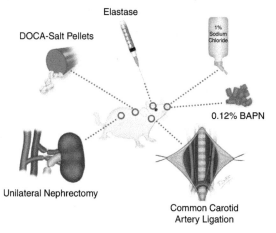

Figure 22.3 Diagram of models of cerebral aneurysm formation in rodents.

prevention of secondary injury, such as traumatic brain injury and stroke, neuroprotection in SAH has not, thus far, proven successful. The only medical treatment available for SAH remains nimodipine, with multiple failed clinical trials demonstrating a poor success rate in translation from animal models to humans.

It remains unclear whether the lack of benefit in human clinical trials, where initial efficacy has been shown in animal studies, is related to the intrinsic differences between humans and experimental animals used in the preclinical studies or to the inadequacy of the models.

It remains a challenge to produce a reliable, standardized SAH model that would account for the initial ictus and resultant early brain injury as well as lead to development of DCI. Furthermore, it is difficult to replicate the intensive care management that patients receive after sustaining SAH, which undoubtedly has contributed to improved outcomes and limitation of the DCI and its negative effects (Connolly Jr et al., 2012; Lovelock et al., 2010). Many recent advances in the pathophysiology of SAH have come from clinical studies where invasive monitoring has been used (Budohoski et al., 2012; Chen et al., 2011; Dreier et al., 2009; Jaeger et al., 2005), or from implementation of specific goal-directed therapies (Anetsberger et al., 2020; Connolly Jr et al., 2012; Diringer et al., 2011). Nevertheless, these have not yielded new treatments, rather modifications or a stricter implementation of standard practices.

There remains a need for basic research into the pathophysiology of SAH if major breakthroughs are to be had. With molecular biology playing an increasing role in elucidating the pathobiology of disease states, there needs to be a renewed focus on identifying the mechanisms of early and delayed brain injury following SAH. New animal models may be required to account for the early injury seen in clinical SAH. With improved imaging techniques and endovascular methods, producing reliable SAH and longitudinal imaging using angiography should become possible.

Currently available models of cerebral aneurysm formation are complicated and require physical or chemical destruction of vessel walls. It remains uncertain whether this has the potential to confound results. It is expected that molecular biology will become the standard method of investigating the pathophysiology of cerebral aneurysm formation. Molecular biology techniques and single-cell sequencing of surgical specimens should provide insight into the genetic composition of cells within aneurysmal walls, leading to the development of refined models of aneurysm formation. Genetically engineered animals with either an overexpression or "knockout" of desired genes can lead to the discovery of specific driving forces for formation and/or growth of aneurysms.

Figure acknowledgements

The following image is credited to the authors of this chapter: Figure 22.1
The following image has been reprinted from Marbacher et al., 2010, with permission: Figure 22.2
The following image has been reprinted from Thompson et al., 2019, with permission: Figure 22.3

References

ACROSS. Epidemiology of aneurysmal subarachnoid hemorrhage in Australia and New Zealand: incidence and case fatality from the Australasian Cooperative Research on Subarachnoid Hemorrhage Study (ACROSS). *Stroke* 2000;**31**(8):1843–50. www.ncbi.nlm.nih.gov/entrez/query.fcgi?cmd=Retrieve&db=PubMed&dopt=Citation&list_uids=10926945

Alg VS, Sofat R, Houlden H, Werring DJ. Genetic risk factors for intracranial aneurysms: a meta-analysis in more than 116,000 individuals. *Neurology* 2013;**80**(23):2154. www.ncbi.nlm.nih.gov/pmc/articles/PMC3716358/

Allcock JM, Drake CG. Postoperative angiography in cases of ruptured intracranial aneurysm. *J Neurosurg* 1963;**20**:752–9. www.ncbi.nlm.nih.gov/entrez/query.fcgi?cmd=Retrieve&db=PubMed&dopt=Citation&list_uids=14184993

Allen G, Henderson L, Chou S, French L. Cerebral arterial spasm. 1. In vitro contractile activity of vasoactive agents on canine basilar and middle cerebral arteries. *J Neurosurg* 1974;**40**(4):433–41. https://pubmed.ncbi.nlm.nih.gov/4360691/

Al-Tamimi YZ, Bhargava D, Feltbower RG, et al. Lumbar drainage of cerebrospinal fluid after aneurysmal subarachnoid hemorrhage: a prospective, randomized, controlled trial (LUMAS). *Stroke* 2012;**43**(3):677–82. www.ncbi.nlm.nih.gov/entrez/query.fcgi?cmd=Retrieve&db=PubMed&dopt=Citation&list_uids=22282887

Anetsberger A, Gempt J, Blobner M, et al. Impact of goal-directed therapy on delayed ischemia after aneurysmal subarachnoid hemorrhage. *Stroke* 2020;**51**(8):2287–96. www.ahajournals.org/doi/10.1161/STROKEAHA.120.029279

Aoki T, Kataoka H, Ishibashi R, Nozaki K, Egashira K, Hashimoto N. Impact of monocyte chemoattractant protein-1 deficiency on cerebral aneurysm formation. *Stroke* 2009;**40**(3):942–51. www.ahajournals.org/doi/10.1161/STROKEAHA.108.532556

Aoki T, Kataoka H, Shimamura M, et al. NF-κB is a key mediator of cerebral aneurysm formation. *Circulation* 2007;**116**(24):2830–40. www.ahajournals.org/doi/10.1161/CIRCULATIONAHA.107.728303

Barry K, Gogjian M, Stein B. Small animal model for investigation of subarachnoid hemorrhage and cerebral vasospasm. *Stroke* 1979;**10**(5). https://pubmed.ncbi.nlm.nih.gov/505495/

Bederson J, Germano I, Guarino L. Cortical blood flow and cerebral perfusion pressure in a new noncraniotomy model of subarachnoid hemorrhage in the rat. *Stroke* 1995;**26**(6):1086–91. https://pubmed.ncbi.nlm.nih.gov/7762027/

Budohoski KP, Czosnyka M, Smielewski P, et al. Impairment of cerebral autoregulation predicts delayed cerebral ischemia after subarachnoid hemorrhage: a prospective observational study. *Stroke* 2012;**43**(12):3230–7. www.ncbi.nlm.nih.gov/entrez/query.fcgi?cmd=Retrieve&db=PubMed&dopt=Citation&list_uids=23150652

Cahill J, Calvert JW, Zhang JH. Mechanisms of early brain injury after subarachnoid hemorrhage. *J Cereb Blood Flow Metab* 2006;**26**(11):1341–53. www.ncbi.nlm.nih.gov/entrez/query.fcgi?cmd=Retrieve&db=PubMed&dopt=Citation&list_uids=16482081

Cajander S, Hassler O. Enzymatic destruction of the elastic lamella at the mouth of cerebral berry aneurysm? *Acta Neurol Scand* 1976;**53**(3):171–81. http://doi.wiley.com/10.1111/j.1600-0404.1976.tb04335.x

Chalouhi N, Hoh B, Hasan D. Review of cerebral aneurysm formation, growth, and rupture. *Stroke* 2013;**44**(12):3613–22. https://pubmed.ncbi.nlm.nih.gov/24130141/

Chen HI, Stiefel MF, Oddo M, et al. Detection of cerebral compromise with multimodality monitoring in patients with subarachnoid hemorrhage. *Neurosurgery* 2011;**69**(1):53–63; discussion 63. www.ncbi.nlm.nih.gov/pubmed/21796073

Claassen J, Carhuapoma JR, Kreiter KT, Du EY, Connolly ES, Mayer SA. Global cerebral edema after subarachnoid hemorrhage: frequency, predictors, and impact on outcome. *Stroke* 2002;**33**(5):1225–32. www.ncbi.nlm.nih.gov/entrez/query.fcgi?cmd=Retrieve&db=PubMed&dopt=Citation&list_uids=11988595

Connolly Jr ES, Rabinstein AA, Carhuapoma JR, et al. Guidelines for the management of aneurysmal subarachnoid hemorrhage: a guideline for healthcare professionals from the American Heart Association/American Stroke Association. *Stroke* 2012;**43**(6):1711–37. www.ncbi.nlm.nih.gov/entrez/query.fcgi?cmd=Retrieve&db=PubMed&dopt=Citation&list_uids=22556195

Conway L, McDonald L. Structural changes of the intradural arteries following subarachnoid hemorrhage. *J Neurosurg* 1972;**37**(6):715–23. https://pubmed.ncbi.nlm.nih.gov/4654701/

Crompton M. The pathogenesis of cerebral infarction following the rupture of cerebral berry aneurysms. *Brain* 1964;**87**:491–510. https://pubmed.ncbi.nlm.nih.gov/14215175/

Delgado-Zygmunt T, Arbab M, Shiokawa Y, Svendgaard N. A primate model for acute and late cerebral vasospasm: angiographic findings. *Acta Neurochir (Wien)* 1992;**118**(3–4):130–6. https://pubmed.ncbi.nlm.nih.gov/1456096/

De Oliveira Manoel AL, Macdonald RL. Neuroinflammation as a target for intervention in subarachnoid hemorrhage. *Front Neurol* 2018;**9**:292. www.ncbi.nlm.nih.gov/pmc/articles/PMC5941982/

Diringer MN, Bleck TP, Hemphill 3rd JC, et al. Critical care management of patients following aneurysmal subarachnoid hemorrhage: recommendations from the Neurocritical Care Society's Multidisciplinary Consensus Conference. *Neurocrit Care* 2011;**15**(2):211–40. www.ncbi.nlm.nih.gov/entrez/query.fcgi?cmd=Retrieve&db=PubMed&dopt=Citation&list_uids=21773873

Doczi T, Joo F, Adam G, Bozoky B, Szerdahelyi P. Blood–brain barrier damage during the acute stage of subarachnoid hemorrhage, as exemplified by a new animal model. *Neurosurgery* 1986;**18**(6):733–9. www.ncbi.nlm.nih.gov/entrez/query.fcgi?cmd=Retrieve&db=PubMed%26dopt=Citation%26list_uids=3736802

Dreier JP, Major S, Manning A, et al. Cortical spreading ischaemia is a novel process involved in ischaemic damage in patients with aneurysmal subarachnoid haemorrhage. *Brain* 2009;**132**(Pt7):1866–81. www.ncbi.nlm.nih.gov/entrez/query.fcgi?cmd=Retrieve&db=PubMed&dopt=Citation&list_uids=19420089

Echlin F. Spasm of basilar and vertebral arteries caused by experimental subarachnoid hemorrhage. *J Neurosurg* 1965;**23**(1):1–11. https://pubmed.ncbi.nlm.nih.gov/4953757/

Echlin F. Experimental vasospasm, acute and chronic, due to blood in the subarachnoid space. *J Neurosurg* 1971;**35**(6):646–56. https://pubmed.ncbi.nlm.nih.gov/5000661/

Ecker A, Riemenschneider PA. Arteriographic demonstration of spasm of the intracranial arteries, with special reference to saccular arterial aneurysms. *J Neurosurg* 1951;**8**(6):660–7. www.ncbi.nlm.nih.gov/entrez/query.fcgi?cmd=Retrieve&db=PubMed&dopt=Citation&list_uids=14889314

Edvinsson L, Egund N, Owman O, Sahlin C, Svendgaard N. Reduced noradrenaline uptake and retention in cerebrovascular nerves associated with angiographically visible vasoconstriction following experimental subarachnoid hemorrhage in rabbits. *Brain Res Bull* 1982;**9**(1–6):799–805. https://pubmed.ncbi.nlm.nih.gov/7172049/

Eldevik O, Kristiansen K, Torvik A. Subarachnoid hemorrhage and cerebrovascular spasm. Morphological study of intracranial arteries based on animal experiments and human autopsies. *J Neurosurg* 1981;**55**(6):869–76. https://pubmed.ncbi.nlm.nih.gov/7299462/

Espinosa F, Weir B, Overton T, Castor W, Grace M, Boisvert D. A randomized placebo-controlled double-blind trial of nimodipine after SAH in monkeys. Part 1: Clinical and radiological findings. *J Neurosurg* 1984;**60**(6):1167–75. https://pubmed.ncbi.nlm.nih.gov/6726360/

Fassbender K, Hodapp B, Rossol S, et al. Inflammatory cytokines in subarachnoid haemorrhage: association with abnormal blood flow velocities in basal cerebral arteries. *J Neurol Neurosurg Psychiatry* 2001;**70**(4):534–7. www.ncbi.nlm.nih.gov/entrez/query.fcgi?cmd=Retrieve&db=PubMed&dopt=Citation&list_uids=11254783

Findlay J, Weir B, Kanamaru K, Espinosa F. Arterial wall changes in cerebral vasospasm. *Neurosurgery* 1989;**25**(5):736–45. https://pubmed.ncbi.nlm.nih.gov/2586727/

Findlay JM, Kassell NF, Weir BK, et al. A randomized trial of intraoperative, intracisternal tissue plasminogen activator for the prevention of vasospasm. *Neurosurgery* 1995;**37**(1):168. www.ncbi.nlm.nih.gov/entrez/query.fcgi?cmd=Retrieve&db=PubMed&dopt=Citation&list_uids=8587685

Frösen J, Tulamo R, Heikura T, et al. Lipid accumulation, lipid oxidation, and low plasma levels of acquired antibodies against oxidized lipids associate with degeneration and rupture of the intracranial aneurysm wall. *Acta Neuropathol Commun* 2013;**1**(1):71. https://actaneurocomms.biomedcentral.com/articles/10.1186/2051-5960-1-71

Fukuroda T, Nishikibe M, Ohta Y, et al. Analysis of responses to endothelins in isolated porcine blood vessels by using a novel endothelin antagonist, BQ-153. *Life Sci* 1992;**50**(15):PL107–12. https://pubmed.ncbi.nlm.nih.gov/1313516/

Geraghty JR, Davis JL, Testai FD. Neuroinflammation and microvascular dysfunction after experimental subarachnoid hemorrhage: emerging components of early brain injury related to outcome. *Neurocrit Care* 2019;**31**(2):373. www.ncbi.nlm.nih.gov/pmc/articles/PMC6759381/

Guglielmi G. History of the genesis of detachable coils. A review. *J Neurosurg* 2009;**111**(1):1–8. https://pubmed.ncbi.nlm.nih.gov/19284239/

Gules I, Satoh M, Nanda A, Zhang JH. Apoptosis, blood–brain barrier, and subarachnoid hemorrhage. *Acta Neurochir Suppl* 2003;**86**:483–7. www.ncbi.nlm.nih.gov/entrez/query.fcgi?cmd=Retrieve&db=PubMed&dopt=Citation&list_uids=14753491

Hanafy KA, Morgan Stuart R, Fernandez L, et al. Cerebral inflammatory response and predictors of admission clinical grade after aneurysmal subarachnoid hemorrhage. *J Clin Neurosci* 2010;**17**(1):22–5. www.pubmedcentral.nih.gov/articlerender.fcgi?artid=2830726&tool=pmcentrez&rendertype=abstract

Hashimoto N, Handa H, Hazama F. Experimentally induced cerebral aneurysms in rats. *Surg Neurol* 1978;**10**(1):3–8. https://europepmc.org/article/med/684603

Hijdra A, Van Gijn J, Stefanko S, Van Dongen KJ, Vermeulen M, Van Crevel H. Delayed cerebral ischemia after aneurysmal subarachnoid hemorrhage: clinicoanatomic correlations. *Neurology* 1986;**36**(3):329–33. www.ncbi.nlm.nih.gov/entrez/query.fcgi?cmd=Retrieve&db=PubMed&dopt=Citation&list_uids=3951698

Hino A, Tokuyama Y, Weir B, et al. Changes in endothelial nitric oxide synthase mRNA during vasospasm after subarachnoid hemorrhage in monkeys. *Neurosurgery* 1996;**39**(3):562–8. www.ncbi.nlm.nih.gov/entrez/query.fcgi?cmd=Retrieve&db=PubMed&dopt=Citation&list_uids=8875487

Hop JW, Rinkel GJ, Algra A, van Gijn J. Case-fatality rates and functional outcome after subarachnoid hemorrhage: a systematic review. *Stroke* 1997;**28**(3):660–4. www.ncbi.nlm.nih.gov/entrez/query.fcgi?cmd=Retrieve&db=PubMed&dopt=Citation&list_uids=9056628

Hop JW, Rinkel GJ, Algra A, van Gijn J. Initial loss of consciousness and risk of delayed cerebral ischemia after aneurysmal subarachnoid hemorrhage. *Stroke* 1999;**30**(11):2268–71. www.ncbi.nlm.nih.gov/entrez/query.fcgi?cmd=Retrieve&db=PubMed&dopt=Citation&list_uids=10548655

Hop JW, Rinkel GJ, Algra A, van Gijn J. Quality of life in patients and partners after aneurysmal subarachnoid hemorrhage. *Stroke* 1998;**29**(4):798–804. www.ncbi.nlm.nih.gov/entrez/query.fcgi?cmd=Retrieve&db=PubMed&dopt=Citation&list_uids=9550514

Hossler FE, Douglas JE. Vascular corrosion casting: review of advantages and limitations in the application of some simple quantitative methods. *Microsc Microanal* 2001;**7**(3):253–64. www.cambridge.org/core/product/identifier/S1431927601010261/type/journal_article

Hughes J, Schianchi P. Cerebral artery spasm. A histological study at necropsy of the blood vessels in cases of subarachnoid hemorrhage. *J Neurosurg* 1978;**48**(4):515–25. https://pubmed.ncbi.nlm.nih.gov/632876/

International Study of Unruptured Intracranial Aneurysms Investigators. Unruptured intracranial aneurysms – risk of rupture and risks of surgical intervention. *N Engl J Med* 1998;**339**(24):1725–33. https://pubmed.ncbi.nlm.nih.gov/9867550/

Jaeger M, Soehle M, Schuhmann MU, Winkler D, Meixensberger J. Correlation of continuously monitored regional cerebral blood flow and brain tissue oxygen. *Acta Neurochir* 2005;**147**(1):51–6; discussion 56. www.ncbi.nlm.nih.gov/entrez/query.fcgi?cmd=Retrieve&db=PubMed&dopt=Citation&list_uids=15565486

Jickling GC, Sharp FR. Improving the translation of animal ischemic stroke studies to humans. *Metab Brain Dis* 2015;**30**(2):461. www.ncbi.nlm.nih.gov/pmc/articles/PMC4186910/

Johnston SC, Selvin S, Gress DR. The burden, trends, and demographics of mortality from subarachnoid hemorrhage. *Neurology* 1998;**50**(5):1413–8. www.ncbi.nlm.nih.gov/entrez/query.fcgi?cmd=Retrieve&db=PubMed&dopt=Citation&list_uids=9595997

Juvela S. Plasma endothelin concentrations after aneurysmal subarachnoid hemorrhage. *J Neurosurg* 2000;**92**(3):390–400. www.ncbi.nlm.nih.gov/entrez/query.fcgi?cmd=Retrieve&db=PubMed&dopt=Citation&list_uids=10701524

Kamii H, Kato I, Kinouchi H, et al. Amelioration of vasospasm after subarachnoid hemorrhage in transgenic mice overexpressing CuZn-superoxide dismutase. *Stroke* 1999;**30** (4):867–71. https://pubmed.ncbi.nlm.nih.gov/10187893/

Kassell NF, Torner JC, Jane JA, Haley Jr. EC, Adams HP. The International Cooperative Study on the Timing of Aneurysm Surgery. Part 2: Surgical results. *J Neurosurg* 1990;**73**(1):37–47. www.ncbi.nlm.nih.gov/entrez/query.fcgi?cmd=Retrieve&db=PubMed&dopt=Citation&list_uids=2191091

Kramer AH, Fletcher JJ. Locally-administered intrathecal thrombolytics following aneurysmal subarachnoid hemorrhage: a systematic review and meta-analysis. *Neurocrit Care* 2011;**14**(3):489–99. www.ncbi.nlm.nih.gov/entrez/query.fcgi?cmd=Retrieve&db=PubMed&dopt=Citation&list_uids=20740327

Kuwayama K, Zervas N, Belson R, Shintani A, Pickren K. A model for experimental cerebral arterial spasm. *Stroke* 1972;**3** (1):49–56. https://pubmed.ncbi.nlm.nih.gov/5008305/

Landau B, Ransohoff J. Prolonged cerebral vasospasm in experimental subarachnoid hemorrhage. *Neurology* 1968;**18** (11):1056–65. https://pubmed.ncbi.nlm.nih.gov/4975163/

Lin C, Calisaneller T, Ukita N, Dumont A, Kassell N, Lee K. A murine model of subarachnoid hemorrhage-induced cerebral vasospasm. *J Neurosci Methods* 2003;**123**(1):89 97. https://pubmed.ncbi.nlm.nih.gov/12581852/

Linn FH, Rinkel GJ, Algra A, van Gijn J. Incidence of subarachnoid hemorrhage: role of region, year, and rate of computed tomography: a meta-analysis. *Stroke* 1996;**27**(4):625–9. www.ncbi.nlm.nih.gov/entrez/query.fcgi?cmd=Retrieve&db=PubMed&dopt=Citation&list_uids=8614919

Logothetis J, Karacostas D, Karoutas G, Artemis N, Mansouri A, Milonas I. A new model of subarachnoid hemorrhage in experimental animals with the purpose to examine cerebral vasospasm. *Exp Neurol* 1983;**81**(2):257–78. https://pubmed.ncbi.nlm.nih.gov/6873215/

Lovelock CE, Rinkel GJ, Rothwell PM. Time trends in outcome of subarachnoid hemorrhage: population-based study and systematic review. *Neurology* 2010;**74**(19):1494–501. www.ncbi.nlm.nih.gov/entrez/query.fcgi?cmd=Retrieve&db=PubMed&dopt=Citation&list_uids=20375310

Macdonald RL, Higashida RT, Keller E, et al. Clazosentan, an endothelin receptor antagonist, in patients with aneurysmal subarachnoid haemorrhage undergoing surgical clipping: a randomised, double-blind, placebo-controlled phase 3 trial (CONSCIOUS-2). *Lancet Neurol* 2011;**10**(7):618–25. www.ncbi.nlm.nih.gov/entrez/query.fcgi?cmd=Retrieve&db=PubMed&dopt=Citation&list_uids=21640651

Macdonald RL, Higashida RT, Keller E, et al. Randomized trial of clazosentan in patients with aneurysmal subarachnoid hemorrhage undergoing endovascular coiling. *Stroke* 2012;**43** (6):1463–9. www.ncbi.nlm.nih.gov/entrez/query.fcgi?cmd=Retrieve&db=PubMed&dopt=Citation&list_uids=22403047

Macdonald RL, Pluta RM, Zhang JH. Cerebral vasospasm after subarachnoid hemorrhage: the emerging revolution. *Nat Clin Pr Neurol* 2007;**3**(5):256–63. www.ncbi.nlm.nih.gov/entrez/query.fcgi?cmd=Retrieve&db=PubMed&dopt=Citation&list_uids=17479073

Macdonald RL, Weir BK, Grace MG, Martin TP, Doi M, Cook DA. Morphometric analysis of monkey cerebral arteries exposed in vivo to whole blood, oxyhemoglobin, methemoglobin, and bilirubin. *Blood Vessels* 1991a;**28** (6):498–510. www.ncbi.nlm.nih.gov/entrez/query.fcgi?cmd=Retrieve&db=PubMed&dopt=Citation&list_uids=1782405

Macdonald RL, Weir BK, Runzer TD, et al. Etiology of cerebral vasospasm in primates. *J Neurosurg* 1991b;**75**(3):415–24. www.ncbi.nlm.nih.gov/entrez/query.fcgi?cmd=Retrieve&db=PubMed&dopt=Citation&list_uids=1869943

Marbacher S, Fandino J, Kitchen ND. Standard intracranial in vivo animal models of delayed cerebral vasospasm. *Br J Neurosurg* 2010;**24**(4):415–34.

Marbacher S, Grüter B, Schöpf S, et al. Systematic review of in vivo animal models of subarachnoid hemorrhage: species, standard parameters, and outcomes. *Transl Stroke Res* 2019;**10** (3):250–8.

McGirt M, Parra A, Sheng H, et al. Attenuation of cerebral vasospasm after subarachnoid hemorrhage in mice overexpressing extracellular superoxide dismutase. *Stroke* 2002;**33**(9):2317–23. https://pubmed.ncbi.nlm.nih.gov/12215605/

Megyesi JF, Vollrath B, Cook DA, Findlay JM. In vivo animal models of cerebral vasospasm: a review. *Neurosurgery* 2000;**46** (2):448–61. https://academic.oup.com/neurosurgery/article/46/2/448/2931531

Molyneux A, Kerr R, Stratton I, et al. International Subarachnoid Aneurysm Trial (ISAT) of neurosurgical clipping versus endovascular coiling in 2143 patients with ruptured intracranial aneurysms: a randomised trial. *Lancet* 2002;**360** (9342):1267–74. www.ncbi.nlm.nih.gov/entrez/query.fcgi?cmd=Retrieve&db=PubMed&dopt=Citation&list_uids=12414200

Morimoto M, Miyamoto S, Mizoguchi A, Kume N, Kita T, Hashimoto N. Mouse model of cerebral aneurysm: experimental induction by renal hypertension and local hemodynamic changes. *Stroke* 2002;**33**(7):1911–5. https://pubmed.ncbi.nlm.nih.gov/12105374/

Nornes H. The role of intracranial pressure in the arrest of hemorrhage in patients with ruptured intracranial aneurysm. *J Neurosurg* 1973;**39**(2):226–34. www.ncbi.nlm.nih.gov/entrez/query.fcgi?cmd=Retrieve&db=PubMed&dopt=Citation&list_uids=4719700

Nosko M, Weir B, Krueger C, et al. Nimodipine and chronic vasospasm in monkeys: Part 1. Clinical and radiological findings. *Neurosurgery* 1985;**16**(2):129–36. https://pubmed.ncbi.nlm.nih.gov/3974822/

Nuki Y, Tsou T-L, Kurihara C, Kanematsu M, Kanematsu Y, Hashimoto T. Elastase-induced intracranial aneurysms in hypertensive mice. *Hypertension* 2009;**54**(6):1337–44. www.aha journals.org/doi/10.1161/HYPERTENSIONAHA.109.138297

Ollikainen E, Tulamo R, Lehti S, et al. Smooth muscle cell foam cell formation, apolipoproteins, and ABCA1 in intracranial aneurysms: implications for lipid accumulation as a promoter of aneurysm wall rupture. *J Neuropathol Exp Neurol* 2016;**75** (7):689–99. https://academic.oup.com/jnen/article-lookup/doi/10.1093/jnen/nlw041

Parra A, McGirt M, Sheng H, Laskowitz D, Pearlstein R, Warner D. Mouse model of subarachnoid hemorrhage associated cerebral vasospasm: methodological analysis. *Neurol Res* 2002;**24**(5):510–6. https://pubmed.ncbi.nlm.nih.gov/12117325/

Pickard JD, Murray GD, Illingworth R, et al. Effect of oral nimodipine on cerebral infarction and outcome after subarachnoid haemorrhage: British aneurysm nimodipine trial. *BMJ* 1989;**298** (6674):636–42. www.ncbi.nlm.nih.gov/entrez/query.fcgi?cmd=Retrieve&db=PubMed&dopt=Citation&list_uids=2496789

Pluta RM, Dejam A, Grimes G, Gladwin MT, Oldfield EH. Nitrite infusions to prevent delayed cerebral vasospasm in a primate model of subarachnoid hemorrhage. *JAMA* 2005;**293** (12):1477–84. www.ncbi.nlm.nih.gov/entrez/query.fcgi?cmd=Retrieve&db=PubMed&dopt=Citation&list_uids=15784871

Pluta RM, Hansen-Schwartz J, Dreier J, et al. Cerebral vasospasm following subarachnoid hemorrhage: time for a new world of thought. *Neurol Res* 2009;**31**(2):151–8. www.ncbi.nlm.nih.gov/entrez/query.fcgi?cmd=Retrieve&db=PubMed&dopt=Citation&list_uids=19298755

Rabinstein AA. Secondary brain injury after aneurysmal subarachnoid haemorrhage: more than vasospasm. *Lancet Neurol* 2011;**10**(7):593–5. www.ncbi.nlm.nih.gov/entrez/query.fcgi?cmd=Retrieve&db=PubMed&dopt=Citation&list_uids=21640652

Rabinstein AA, Friedman JA, Weigand SD, et al. Predictors of cerebral infarction in aneurysmal subarachnoid hemorrhage. *Stroke* 2004;**35**(8):1862–6. www.ncbi.nlm.nih.gov/entrez/query.fcgi?cmd=Retrieve&db=PubMed&dopt=Citation&list_uids=15218156

Rosengart AJ, Schultheiss KE, Tolentino J, Macdonald RL. Prognostic factors for outcome in patients with aneurysmal subarachnoid hemorrhage. *Stroke* 2007;**38**(8):2315–21. www.ncbi.nlm.nih.gov/entrez/query.fcgi?cmd=Retrieve&db=PubMed&dopt=Citation&list_uids=17569871

Sahlin C, Brismar J, Delgado T, Owman C, Salford L, Svendgaard N. Cerebrovascular and metabolic changes during the delayed vasospasm following experimental subarachnoid hemorrhage in baboons, and treatment with a calcium antagonist. *Brain Res* 1987;**403**(2):313–32. https://pubmed.ncbi.nlm.nih.gov/3828823/

Saito A, Kamii H, Kato I, et al. Transgenic CuZn-superoxide dismutase inhibits NO synthase induction in experimental subarachnoid hemorrhage. *Stroke* 2001;**32**(7):1652–7. https://pubmed.ncbi.nlm.nih.gov/11441215/

Samuel N, Radovanovic I. Genetic basis of intracranial aneurysm formation and rupture: clinical implications in the postgenomic era. *Neurosurg Focus* 2019;**47**(1):E10. https://pubmed.ncbi.nlm.nih.gov/31261114/

Schievink WI. Intracranial aneurysms. *N Engl J Med* 1997;**336** (1):28–40. www.ncbi.nlm.nih.gov/entrez/query.fcgi?cmd=Retrieve&db=PubMed&dopt=Citation&list_uids=8970938

Schöller K, Trinkl A, Klopotowski M, et al. Characterization of microvascular basal lamina damage and blood–brain barrier dysfunction following subarachnoid hemorrhage in rats. *Brain Res* 2007;**1142**:237–46. www.ncbi.nlm.nih.gov/pubmed/17303089

Schubert GA, Seiz M, Hegewald AA, Manville J, Thome C. Acute hypoperfusion immediately after subarachnoid hemorrhage: a xenon contrast-enhanced CT study. *J Neurotrauma* 2009;**26**(12):2225–31. www.ncbi.nlm.nih.gov/entrez/query.fcgi?cmd=Retrieve&db=PubMed&dopt=Citation&list_uids=19929373

Schwartz AY, Masago A, Sehba FA, Bederson JB. Experimental models of subarachnoid hemorrhage in the rat: a refinement of the endovascular filament model. *J Neurosci Methods* 2000;**96** (2):161–7.

Sehba FA, Pluta RM. Aneurysmal subarachnoid hemorrhage models: do they need a fix? *Stroke Res Treat* 2013;**2013**:615154. https://doi.org/10.1155/2013/615154

Seifert V, Loffler BM, Zimmermann M, Roux S, Stolke D. Endothelin concentrations in patients with aneurysmal subarachnoid hemorrhage. Correlation with cerebral vasospasm, delayed ischemic neurological deficits, and volume of hematoma. *J Neurosurg* 1995;**82**(1):55–62. www.ncbi.nlm.nih.gov/entrez/query.fcgi?cmd=Retrieve&db=PubMed&dopt=Citation&list_uids=7815135

Simeone FA, Trepper PJ, Brown DJ. Cerebral blood flow evaluation of prolonged experimental vasospasm. *J Neurosurg* 1972;**37**(3):302–11. www.ncbi.nlm.nih.gov/entrez/query.fcgi?cmd=Retrieve&db=PubMed&dopt=Citation&list_uids=4627019

Solomon R, Antunes J, Chen R, Bland L, Chien S. Decrease in cerebral blood flow in rats after experimental subarachnoid hemorrhage: a new animal model. *Stroke* 1985;**16**(1):58–64. https://pubmed.ncbi.nlm.nih.gov/3966267/

The National Institute of Neurological Disorders and Stroke rt-PA Stroke Study Group. Tissue plasminogen activator for acute ischemic stroke. *N Engl J Med* 1995;**333**(24):1581–7. https://pubmed.ncbi.nlm.nih.gov/7477192/

Thompson JW, Elwardany O, McCarthy DJ, Shelnberg DL, Alvarez CM, Nada A, Snelling BM, Chen SH, Sur S, Starke RM. In vIvo cerebral aneurysm models. Neurosurg Focus. 2019; 1; **47** (1): E20. doi: 10.3171/2019.4.FOCUS19219.

Toda N. Mechanisms of contracting action of oxyhemoglobin in isolated monkey and dog cerebral arteries. *Am J Physiol* 1990;**258**(1

Pt 2):H57–63. www.ncbi.nlm.nih.gov/entrez/query.fcgi?cmd=Retrieve&db=PubMed&dopt=Citation&list_uids=2105667

Toda N, Shimizu K, Ohta T. Mechanism of cerebral arterial contraction induced by blood constituents. *J Neurosurg* 1980;**53**(3):312–22. www.ncbi.nlm.nih.gov/entrez/query.fcgi?cmd=Retrieve&db=PubMed&dopt=Citation&list_uids=7420146

Trojanowski T. Early effects of experimental arterial subarachnoid haemorrhage on the cerebral circulation. Part I: Experimental subarachnoid haemorrhage in cat and its pathophysiological effects. Methods of regional cerebral blood flow measurement and evaluation of microcirulation. *Acta Neurochir (Wien)* 1984a;**72**(1–2):79–94. https://pubmed.ncbi.nlm.nih.gov/6741649/

Trojanowski T. Early effects of experimental arterial subarachnoid haemorrhage on the cerebral circulation. Part II: Regional cerebral blood flow and cerebral microcirculation after experimental subarachnoid haemorrhage. *Acta Neurochir (Wien)* 1984b;**72**(3–4):241–55. https://pubmed.ncbi.nlm.nih.gov/6475579/

Tsuji T, Cook D, Weir B, Handa Y. Effect of clot removal on cerebrovascular contraction after subarachnoid hemorrhage in the monkey: pharmacological study. *Heart Vessels* 1996;**11**(2):69–79. https://pubmed.ncbi.nlm.nih.gov/8836754/

Turowski B, Hänggi D, Beck A, Aurich V, Steiger H, Moedder U. New angiographic measurement tool for analysis of small cerebral vessels: application to a subarachnoid haemorrhage model in the rat. *Neuroradiology* 2007;**49**(2):129–37. https://pubmed.ncbi.nlm.nih.gov/17111162/

van Gijn J, Kerr RS, Rinkel GJ. Subarachnoid haemorrhage. *Lancet* 2007;**369**(9558):306–18. www.ncbi.nlm.nih.gov/entrez/query.fcgi?cmd=Retrieve&db=PubMed&dopt=Citation&list_uids=17258671

Varsos V, Liszczak T, Han D, et al. Delayed cerebral vasospasm is not reversible by aminophylline, nifedipine, or papaverine in a "two-hemorrhage" canine model. *J Neurosurg* 1983;**58**(1):11–7. https://pubmed.ncbi.nlm.nih.gov/6847896/

Vatter H, Weidauer S, Konczalla J, et al. Time course in the development of cerebral vasospasm after experimental subarachnoid hemorrhage: clinical and neuroradiological assessment of the rat double hemorrhage model. *Neurosurgery* 2006;**58**(6):1190–7. https://pubmed.ncbi.nlm.nih.gov/16723899/

Vatter H, Zimmermann M, Tesanovic V, Raabe A, Schilling L, Seifert V. Cerebrovascular characterization of clazosentan, the first nonpeptide endothelin receptor antagonist clinically effective for the treatment of cerebral vasospasm. Part I: inhibitory effect on endothelin(A) receptor-mediated contraction. *J Neurosurg* 2005;**102**(6):1101–7. www.ncbi.nlm.nih.gov/entrez/query.fcgi?cmd=Retrieve&db=PubMed&dopt=Citation&list_uids=16028770

Veelken J, Laing R, Jakubowski J. The Sheffield model of subarachnoid hemorrhage in rats. *Stroke* 1995;**26**(7):1279–83. https://pubmed.ncbi.nlm.nih.gov/7604426/

Vergouwen MD, Etminan N, Ilodigwe D, Macdonald RL. Lower incidence of cerebral infarction correlates with improved functional outcome after aneurysmal subarachnoid hemorrhage. *J Cereb Blood Flow Metab* 2011a;**31**(7):1545–53. www.ncbi.nlm.nih.gov/entrez/query.fcgi?cmd=Retrieve&db=PubMed&dopt=Citation&list_uids=21505477

Vergouwen MD, Ilodigwe D, Macdonald RL. Cerebral infarction after subarachnoid hemorrhage contributes to poor outcome by vasospasm-dependent and -independent effects. *Stroke* 2011b;**42**(4):924–9. www.ncbi.nlm.nih.gov/entrez/query.fcgi?cmd=Retrieve&db=PubMed&dopt=Citation&list_uids=21311062

Verlooy J, Van Reempts J, Haseldonckx M, Borgers M, Selosse P. The course of vasospasm following subarachnoid haemorrhage in rats. A vertebrobasilar angiographic study. *Acta Neurochir (Wien)* 1992;**117**(1–2):48–52. https://pubmed.ncbi.nlm.nih.gov/1514428/

Voldby B, Enevoldsen EM. Intracranial pressure changes following aneurysm rupture. Part 1: clinical and angiographic correlations. *J Neurosurg* 1982;**56**(2):186–96. www.ncbi.nlm.nih.gov/entrez/query.fcgi?cmd=Retrieve&db=PubMed&dopt=Citation&list_uids=7054427

Weir B. Unruptured intracranial aneurysms: a review. *J Neurosurg* 2002;**96**(1):3–42. https://pubmed.ncbi.nlm.nih.gov/11794601/

White R, Hagen A, Robertson J. Effect of nonsteroid anti-inflammatory drugs on subarachnoid hemorrhage in dogs. *J Neurosurg* 1979;**51**(2):164–71. https://pubmed.ncbi.nlm.nih.gov/582181/

Wiebers D, Whisnant J, Huston J, et al. Unruptured intracranial aneurysms: natural history, clinical outcome, and risks of surgical and endovascular treatment. *Lancet* 2003;**362**(9378):103–10. https://pubmed.ncbi.nlm.nih.gov/12867109/

Yatsushige H, Yamaguchi M, Zhou C, Calvert J, Zhang J. Role of c-Jun N-terminal kinase in cerebral vasospasm after experimental subarachnoid hemorrhage. *Stroke* 2005;**36**(7):1538–43. https://pubmed.ncbi.nlm.nih.gov/15947258/

Yoshimoto Y, Kim P, Sasaki T, Takakura K. Temporal profile and significance of metabolic failure and trophic changes in the canine cerebral arteries during chronic vasospasm after subarachnoid hemorrhage. *J Neurosurg* 1993;**78**(5):807–12. https://pubmed.ncbi.nlm.nih.gov/8468611/

Zhang X, Fei Z, Zhang W, et al. Emergency transsphenoidal surgery for hemorrhagic pituitary adenomas. *Surg Oncol* 2007;**16**(2):115–20. www.ncbi.nlm.nih.gov/pubmed/17643985

Zhou M, Shi J, Zhu J, et al. Comparison between one- and two-hemorrhage models of cerebral vasospasm in rabbits. *J Neurosci Methods* 2007;**159**(2):318–24. https://pubmed.ncbi.nlm.nih.gov/16942802/

Zivin J, Fisher M, DeGirolami U, Hemenway C, Stashak J. Tissue plasminogen activator reduces neurological damage after cerebral embolism. *Science* 1985;**230**(4731):1289–92. https://pubmed.ncbi.nlm.nih.gov/3934754/

Chapter 23

Pediatric Vascular Malformations

Alaa Montaser and Edward R. Smith

23.1 Introduction

Pediatric vascular malformations are a heterogeneous group of disorders that can generally be categorized into structural lesions and arteriopathies. Aneurysms are one of the most common vascular disorders of the central nervous system (CNS); however, they are predominantly a disease of the adult population and therefore are outside the scope of this chapter. The most common structural lesions encountered in pediatric neurosurgery include high-flow malformations involving abnormal connections between arteries and veins (c) and low-flow malformations of aberrant capillary development (cavernous malformations, CM). The term "moyamoya" is used to encompass a diverse group of arteriopathies characterized by the shared finding of progressive stenosis of the intracranial internal carotid arteries resulting in stroke. Here we will define these lesions, discuss epidemiology to put the scope of the disease in context, and then review the pathobiology in detail, with current genetic screening recommendations.

23.2 High-Flow Malformations

23.2.1 Definition and Clinical Overview

Arteriovenous fistulae, vein of Galen malformations, and arteriovenous malformations can be grouped together logically when viewed as an anatomic spectrum of abnormal arterial to venous connections – a concept that is supported by emerging scientific data. An AVF is the simplest, single-point fistula, followed by VOGM, which essentially is a cluster of multiple abnormal connections between arteries and the vein of Galen and, lastly, AVMs, which are discrete lesions entirely composed of numerous arterio-venous fistulae (Figure 23.1).

Arteriovenous fistulae are the simplest lesions anatomically, consisting of a direct connection between a cortical artery and a cortical vein, leading to venous engorgement and potential hemorrhage (Walcott et al.,

2013a, 2013b). In rare cases, high-flow shunts can lead to problems similar to VOGMs, with "melting brain" and mass effect on the surrounding parenchyma. Treatment can include embolization or surgical obliteration.

In contrast to AVFs, which are single-point fistulae, VOGMs are high-flow lesions that involve multiple direct communications between arteries of the limbic system (predominately choroidal branches of the posterior and anterior circulation) into a dilated vein of Galen (Raybaud et al., 1989). The engorged vein of Galen is sometimes termed an "aneurysm" or varix. There are two embryological variants of VOGM – choroidal, which has multiple connections to a primitive vein of the prosencephalon and often presents with high-output cardiac failure in neonates, and mural, with smaller numbers of fistulae directly to the vein of Galen, often with an outflow obstruction leading to a markedly dilated varix and a slower clinical decline marked by hydrocephalus, venous stasis and subsequent cerebral ischemia with "melting brain" over months to years. Treatment of VOGMs is now nearly exclusively embolization of the lesion to obliterate the fistulae.

An AVM is a tangle of dysplastic vessels (nidus) consisting of direct arterial-to-venous connections without intervening capillaries, forming a high-flow low-resistance shunt between the arterial and venous systems (Lawton et al., 2015). Central nervous system AVMs lack functional neural tissue within the lesions. Arteriovenous malformations are an important cause of intracerebral hemorrhage in children and adolescents; with an overall bleeding rate of 1–3% per year for unruptured malformations, which increases to fivefold once ruptured; and a 25% fatality risk with each bleed (Mohr et al., 2014; Riordan et al., 2018; Rutledge et al., 2014). The likelihood and severity of hemorrhage are multifactorial depending on the AVM size, anatomical location, hemodynamics, and angio-architectural characteristics. Although AVMs have been historically thought to be congenital, recent data from novel genetic studies and animal models

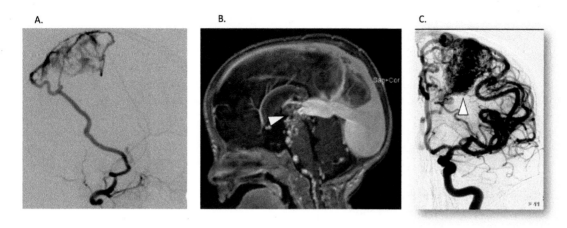

Figure 23.1 Three radiographic images demonstrating high-flow vascular malformations of the brain. (A) Lateral arteriogram with injection of the external carotid artery revealing an arteriovenous fistula between the middle meningeal artery and cortical vessels. (B) Sagittal T₁ MRI with contrast showing a vein of Galen malformation with multiple small arterial fistulous connections marked by the arrowhead. (C) A-P projection of an angiogram with injection of the internal carotid artery demonstrating a large AVM with multiple feeders from both the anterior and middle cerebral territories, with the nidus denoted by the arrowhead.

suggest that they arise from aberrant angiogenesis coupled with genetic mutations.

Intracerebral AVM is usually an isolated lesion, but it can be associated with other types of vascular malformations. In a study of 280 intracranial vascular malformations, 14 cases of combined malformations were noted, with CM found most often (Awad et al., 1993). Multiple AVMs are most commonly found in two conditions (Willinsky et al., 1990). First is hereditary hemorrhagic telangiectasia (HHT), an autosomal dominant disorder with telangiectasias of the skin in association with AVMs of deep structures including the lungs and CNS. Second is Wyburn–Mason syndrome, characterized by ipsilateral retinal and optic pathway cerebral AVMs with cutaneous capillary malformations (Willinsky et al., 1990). Treatment of AVMs may involve surgical resection, radiation, and/or embolization.

23.2.2 Epidemiology

Intracranial hemorrhage (ICH) comprises about half of pediatric stroke, with an incidence of ~1/100,000/year, caused by either structural lesions or hematological disorders (Fullerton et al., 2003). Non-traumatic, spontaneous ICH are caused by structural lesions in up to ~75% of cases, with AVM found most commonly and ~10% of hemorrhage remaining idiopathic (Adil et al., 2015; Al-Jarallah et al., 2000; Beslow et al., 2010; Broderick et al., 1993; Jordan et al., 2009; Liu et al., 2015). Vein of Galen malformations are far more rare, comprising <1% of all pediatric vascular cases in the US, with 1–2 cases on average per high-volume center annually (Recinos et al., 2012). The prevalence of AVFs ranges between 0.1/100,000 and 1/100,000 with no clear sex predilection (Hetts et al., 2012; Tomlinson et al., 1993; Weon et al., 2005; Yoshida et al., 2004). Arteriovenous fistulae comprise about 4% of pediatric cerebral vascular malformations (Cooke et al., 2012; Tomlinson et al., 1993).

23.2.3 Pathogenesis and Laboratory Models

The pathogenesis of high-flow vascular lesions of the CNS appears to be heterogeneous and multifactorial, with etiologies ranging from genetic drivers to trauma. However, a number of recent investigations from different centers have started to identify a series of common pathways that influence the formation of these lesions. In particular, molecules associated with angiogenesis, including the Notch family, *RASA-1*, vascular endothelial growth factor (VEGF), and axonal guidance factors (including ephrins and neuropilins) are increasingly observed to be interconnected and associated with high-flow vascular malformations.

Starting with AVFs, it appears that a significant number of patients with HHT may also have AVFs, ranging between 0.5% and 25% (Garcia-Monaco et al., 1995; Weon et al., 2005; Woodall et al., 2014). Mutations in the *RASA-1* gene have been linked to pial AVFs, with one series demonstrating that about 1/3 of pediatric patients with AVF also have concomitant *RASA-1* mutations (Walcott et al., 2013b). The capillary malformation–AVM (CM-AVM) syndrome is one of the most notable of these *RASA-1* mutation subgroups with CNS AVFs (Chee et al., 2010; Eerola et al., 2003; Thieux et al., 2010). The recently characterized CLOVES syndrome (congenital lipomatous overgrowth, vascular malformations, epidermal nevi, and skeletal/scoliosis/spinal anomalies) is known to be associated with a wide range of CNS vascular lesions, including AVFs and AVMs. CLOVES is caused by a mutation in *PIK3CA* and, unlike *RASA-1* or HHT, manifests as a sporadic, post-zygotic activating mutation that is not inherited (Kurek et al., 2012).

Vein of Galen malformations and AVMs share clinical and anatomic findings and these similarities extend to some shared genetic mutations in ephrins. Venous endothelial cells respond to VEGF with a pathway that suppresses Notch signaling and promotes expression of the venous marker Ephrin B4 (EphB4). Recent data have implicated mutations in *RASA-1* and ephrin genes, including Ephrin B2 and its receptor, Eph B4 (Duran et al., 2018; Goss et al., 2019; Vivanti et al., 2018; Zeng et al., 2019). These findings are important as they serve to bridge the gap between clinical observations on the spectrum of disease and linking anatomic findings to specific molecular pathways.

This same network is implicated in the development of AVMs, with data indicating that genetic imbalances in ephrin B2/EphB4 signaling may contribute to AVM pathogenesis (Fehnel et al., 2020; Goss et al., 2019; Pricola Fehnel et al., 2016). When combined with previous reports associating *KRAS*, *RASA-1*, *ALK*-1 and endoglin mutations with AVMs, a more coherent picture of structural, high-flow vascular lesion development emerges, predicated on embryologic errors in the construction of normal arterial to venous transitions (Boon et al., 2005; Fehnel et al., 2020; Fish et al., 2020; Goss et al., 2019; Seki et al., 2003; Thieux et al., 2010). The normal pathways that designate the developing vasculature as arterial, capillary or venous are disrupted by mutation, leading to imbalances in patterning the circulation and result in pathologic connections between arteries and veins. For example, increasing the ratio of EphrinB2 to EphB4 (either by supplementing EphrinB2 or blockade of EphB4; Protack et al., 2017) leads to loss of normal endothelial function, characterized by increased, but markedly disorganized, tube formation and increased invasion, mimicking the behavior of AVM cells (Fehnel et al., 2020). These data are tantalizing in suggesting possible biomarkers for detecting disease, measuring therapeutic effect, and ultimately novel therapeutic targets.

Animal models are increasingly available that leverage these novel findings (Duran et al., 2018; Fish et al., 2020; Garrido-Martin et al., 2014; Gauden et al., 2020; Kim et al., 2018; Protack et al., 2017; Raj and Stoodley, 2015). Zebrafish allow in-vitro cell imaging while murine and other animal models enable studies in mammalian systems. These molecular-based models differ from earlier techniques that relied on surgical creation of direct arteriovenous fistulae, but these surgical models offer utility in study of specific flow-related phenomena (Jia et al., 2015; Somarathna et al., 2020).

23.2.4 Screening

The current expansion of research linking specific genetic mutations with high-flow CNS vascular lesions has accelerated the indications for patient and family screening. In patients with documented AVF, recent data suggest that about 9% will harbor known mutations (Saliou et al., 2017; Walcott et al., 2013a, 2013b). *RASA-1* and HHT-related mutations (*ENG* and *ACVRL1*) were most common, with clinical findings including multiple cranial lesions, spinal AVF/AVM, hypercoagulable states, and capillary hemangioma (in *RASA-1*) (Saliou et al., 2017; Thieux et al., 2010; Walcott et al., 2013a, 2013b). However, in VOGM, there are very limited indications for familial screening (Duran et al., 2018).

While most AVMs are thought to be isolated developmental lesions, there are known genetic conditions predisposing individuals to multiple AVMs. Mutations in *RASA-1* are associated with problems in vessel development, including familial high-flow arteriovenous lesions (Thieux et al., 2010). Hereditary hemorrhagic telangectasia is a genetic condition that predisposes affected individuals to AVMs throughout the body (Lasjaunias, 1997). Hereditary hemorrhagic telangectasia guidelines recommend AVM screening with MRI of the brain in the first 6 months of life or at the time of diagnosis (Faughnan et al., 2011). A general review of screening recommendations for pediatric cerebrovascular disease is summarized in the current American Stroke Association guidelines (Ferriero et al., 2019).

23.3 Low-Flow Malformations

23.3.1 Definition and Clinical Overview

Cavernous malformations consist of compact clusters of sponge-like vascular spaces without intervening neural parenchyma (Gault et al., 2004; Vanaman et al., 2010; Figure 23.2). The nomenclature for these malformations

A.

B.

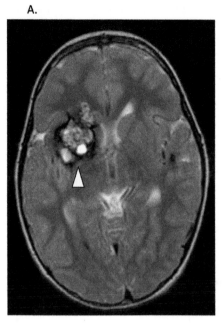
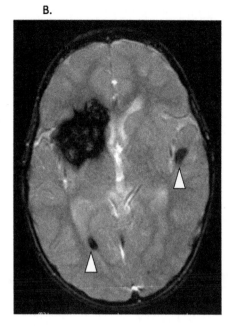

Figure 23.2 (A) T$_2$ axial MRI of the brain showing a large cavernous malformation of the frontal lobe with characteristic multiple lobules of lesion (arrowhead) and dark ring of hemosiderin staining around periphery. (B) Axial susceptibility-weighted image of the same patient demonstrating other, smaller cavernous malformations (arrowhead) in familial case.

can be confusing as they have been called cavernomas, cavernous angiomas, and cavernous hemangiomas. Cavernous malformations can cause symptoms from hemorrhage or progressive enlargement with mass effect (Gross et al., 2016). Seizure as the presenting symptom is found in 25–30% of cases (Gross et al., 2013b, 2016). However, many CMs are asymptomatic and are frequently found incidentally. These lesions can be familial with a number of associated germline mutations, but the majority are spontaneous lesions. Developmental venous anomalies (DVA) are commonly seen in association with CMs (Mottolese et al., 2001; Rigamonti et al., 1988).

Treatment of CMs is either surgical resection or observation, with data supporting excision of symptomatic lesions, lesions with recurrent hemorrhage or lesions with high risk of neurological deficit (such as large lesions or those located in the posterior fossa; Gross et al., 2013a, 2013b, 2016). For patients with multiple CMs, resection should be limited to symptomatic lesions or lesions with documented expansion over time (Frim and Scott, 1999; Zabramski et al., 1994). Radiation therapy is controversial and generally reserved for surgically inaccessible lesions with a demonstrated malignant natural history (Di Rocco et al., 1997; Scott, 1990; Scott et al., 1992).

Research into novel pharmacologic agents is ongoing, with some early clinical trials, but to date there is no medical therapy approved for obliteration of CMs. It is common to observe lesions that are small, asymptomatic, or located in areas of high potential surgical morbidity (Ferriero et al., 2019; Gross et al., 2016).

23.3.2 Epidemiology

Most cases are sporadic (50–80%), although familial variants exist, with most familial cases demonstrating multiple lesions on imaging (Zabramski et al., 1994). If multiple CMs are seen on imaging, a familial or postradiation etiology should be considered (Baumgartner et al., 2003). Very few (~10%) sporadic cases will have multiple lesions (Gault et al., 2004; Gross et al., 2016). Multiple CMs can also be found in association with cranial irradiation (Gross et al., 2016; Larson et al., 1998; Singla et al., 2013; Vanaman et al., 2010). Cavernous malformations are found with a prevalence of about 0.5% in autopsy studies (Barnes et al., 2002; Gault et al., 2004; Hang et al., 1996; Zabramski et al., 1994). An incidence of 0.43 diagnoses per 100,000 people per year has been reported (Al-Shahi et al., 2003). There is no difference in sex incidence.

23.3.3 Pathogenesis and Laboratory Models

Cavernous malformations are lesions that have long been known to have familial associations, and this clinical knowledge has spurred laboratory investigation. Advances have been made in understanding how specific mutations influence the development of these lesions. Three genes have been most strongly associated with the formation of CMs. *CCM1* (also known as *KRIT1* [*Krev-1 interaction trapped 1*], located on chromosome 7q), *CCM2* (also known as *malcaverin*, found on 7p), and *CCM3* (also known as *Programmed Cell Death 10*, on chromosome 3p) are well-described (Chen et al., 2009; Craig et al., 1998; Dubovsky et al., 1995; Dupre et al., 2003; Gil-Nagel et al., 1996; Gunel et al., 1995, 1996; Labauge et al., 1999; Laberge et al., 1999; Laberge-le Coutelx et al., 1999; Laurans et al., 2003; Marchuk et al., 1995; Shenkar et al., 2003; Tanriover et al., 2008; Zhang et al., 2007). Investigations into *CCM1* function have revealed that the gene product is essential for normal embryonic vascular development, with loss-of-function mutations found in hereditary cases of CM (Whitehead et al., 2004). In patients with these *CCM1* mutations, nearly all will have radiographic evidence of multiple CMs, but only about 60% of patients will develop symptoms, making this a relatively mild variant of familial CM (Hayman et al., 1982).

De-novo CMs can develop over the life of a given patient. The *CCM1* genotype is associated with a higher number of lesions with increased age than the *CCM2* or *CCM3* genotypes (Denier et al., 2006). In contrast, while *CCM3* mutation carriers generally have fewer lesions, the CMs they harbor appear to have a higher risk of hemorrhage during childhood. This results in ~50% of *CCM3* patients exhibiting symptoms before age 15, and about half of *CCM3* mutation patients who were symptomatic presented with hemorrhage (Denier et al., 2006). Other systems may be affected including skin, eyes, and visceral organs, most commonly found with *CCM1* mutations (Sirvente et al., 2009; Toll et al., 2009).

Overall, recent research advances have started to present a unified thematic picture of the CCM mutations in that they all seem to overlap in loss of function affecting cell adhesion, leading to impaired cell–cell connections and smooth muscle activity in the vessels with concomitant "bubbles" of vasculature prone to growth and bleeding, involving a limited number of overlapping pathways shared with high-flow lesions, such as *NOTCH* mutations (Awad and Polster, 2019;

Bacigaluppi et al., 2013; Cavalcanti et al., 2012; Fish et al., 2020; Kim, 2016; Spiegler et al., 2018; Wang et al., 2019). *CCM1* (*KRIT1*) suppresses RhoA-GTPase in normal state, but mutation of *CCM1* leads to over-activation of the RhoA-GTPase, which increases actin fiber activity and loss of cell–cell junctions. *CCM2* (*malcaverin*) also creates a complex that regulates RhoA-GTPase, but when this gene is mutated, the end result is a similar increased RhoA/actin activity akin to *CCM1* mutations. In addition, it appears that *CCM2* also affects angiogenesis and this may affect bleeding and vessel growth within the lesion. *CCM3* (*PDCD10*) has a more poorly defined role in cell adhesion and also appears to be involved with apoptosis regulation.

A remarkable recent series of reports have linked the gut microbiome with bleeding risk of CMs (Awad and Polster, 2019; Starke et al., 2017; Tang et al., 2017). The hypothesis centers on the premise that Gram-negative bacteria in the gut flora produce lipopolysaccharide which stimulates TLR4, an endothelial cell surface receptor that interacts with the CCM protein complex that regulates cell adhesion. Alterations in gut microbiome flora lead to subsequent changes in CM endothelial cell permeability and can influence the rate of bleeding of these lesions. These data suggest that dietary and antibiotic changes can potentially impact the risk of intracranial hemorrhage.

Advances in the study of CMs have been aided by development of animal models. The ability to create specific genetic mutations in rodents has expanded in recent years, along with other vertebrates (Chan et al., 2010; Starke et al., 2017; Tang et al., 2017; Wetzel-Strong et al., 2017). These models have advanced the understanding of multiorgan involvement in bleeding risk and lesion evolution (Tang et al., 2017).

23.3.4 Screening

Screening of first-degree relatives with genetic counseling should be considered for patients who have multiple CMs on imaging or if there is a known family history of CMs, as a germline mutation is likely, with *CCM1*, *CCM2*, or *CCM3* found in >90% of familial cases (Merello et al., 2016). If multiple intracranial lesions are seen on imaging, the likelihood of a familial form of the disease approaches 85%, while single lesions only have a ~16% likelihood of harboring a germline mutation (Merello et al., 2016). Current screening recommendations are summarized in the recent American Stroke Association guidelines (Ferriero et al., 2019).

23.4 Arteriopathy – Moyamoya

23.4.1 Definition and Clinical Overview

Moyamoya disease is a cerebrovascular condition characterized by idiopathic chronic progressive steno-occlusive changes of the terminal portions of internal carotid arteries (ICAs) and their proximal branches. These changes results in reduction of the blood flow through the anterior circulation of the brain which can induce the formation of a network of collateral vasculature to compensate for the progressive cerebral ischemia. This collateral network is the "puff of smoke" that the term moyamoya means in Japanese (Scott and Smith, 2009; Figure 23.3). Recently, it has become increasingly apparent that the term "moyamoya" actually encompasses many different arteriopathies with distinct genetic and environmental drivers that share a common end-stage radiographic appearance.

The natural history of moyamoya is variable; however, moyamoya inevitably progresses in the majority of cases. In general, it has been estimated that up to two thirds of patients with moyamoya disease demonstrate symptomatic progression, and that progression cannot be halted by medical treatment alone, with 66–90% experiencing symptomatic stroke within 5 years if untreated (Ferriero et al., 2019; Scott and Smith, 2009). Therapy is predicated on surgical revascularization and this approach is supported by the recent American Stroke Association guidelines (Ferriero et al., 2019).

23.4.2 Epidemiology

First described in Japan, moyamoya has now been identified in patients worldwide, ranging from 3/100,000 to 1/1,000,000 (Scott and Smith, 2009). Asian ancestry is an increased risk factor for moyamoya, with up to 56% of Asian-American moyamoya patients found to harbor a specific mutation of *RNF213* (Cecchi et al., 2014). In contrast, non-Asian moyamoya patients only had *RNF213* mutations in 3.6–29% of individuals (Cecchi et al., 2014). Associations exist between moyamoya and radiotherapy of the head or neck (especially for optic gliomas, craniopharyngiomas, and pituitary tumors), Down syndrome (26-fold increased likelihood of moyamoya), neurofibromatosis type 1 (with or without hypothalamic–optic pathway tumors; ~2.5% prevalence of moyamoya), and sickle cell anemia (Adil et al., 2015; Al-Jarallah et al., 2000; Broderick et al., 1993; Jordan et al., 2009; Liu et al., 2015). Caucasian moyamoya patients in the US have a higher rate of autoimmune disorders, including type I diabetes (8.5% versus 0.4% in the general population) and thyroid disease (17% versus 8%) (Bower et al., 2013).

23.4.3 Pathogenesis and Laboratory Models

The angiographic findings of moyamoya result from a wide range of genetic and acquired conditions. Pathologic analysis has demonstrated that affected vessels generally do not exhibit arteriosclerotic or inflammatory changes (Scott and Smith, 2009). Rather, vessel occlusion results from a combination of both hyperplasia of smooth muscle cells and luminal thrombosis. The moyamoya collaterals are dilated perforating arteries believed to be a combination of pre-existing and newly developed vessels. A number of growth factors, enzymes, and other peptides have been reported in association with moyamoya, including basic fibroblast growth factor, transforming growth factor-β1, hepatocyte growth factor, vascular endothelial growth factor, matrix metalloproteinases, intracellular adhesion molecules, and hypoxia-inducing factor-1α, among others (Fujimura et al., 2009; Kang et al., 2010; Smith, 2015; Soriano et al., 2002). At present, it is difficult to discern which of these peptides are pathologic primary causal agents of disease and which are present merely as part of a normal response to ischemia.

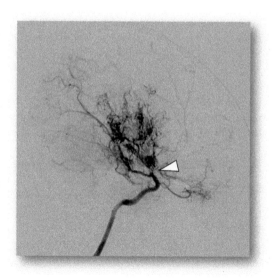

Figure 23.3 Lateral arteriogram with injection of the internal carotid artery (ICA) demonstrating typical findings of moyamoya, with marked narrowing of the apex of the ICA (arrowhead) and marked collateral development distal to the narrowing ("puff of smoke").

Data support the premise that some type of environmental factor may precipitate the syndrome's clinical emergence in susceptible patients and suggest that the angiographic changes of moyamoya are the result of a complex interplay between genetic predisposition and external stimuli (Ganesan and Smith, 2015). There has been considerable progress made in genetic association studies in moyamoya disease.

Associations between moyamoya and loci on chromosomes 3, 6, 8, and 17 (*MYMY1*, *MYMY2*, *MYMY3*), as well as specific HLA haplotypes, have been described (Duran et al., 2018; Fehnel et al., 2020; Goss et al., 2019; Pricola-Fehnel et al., 2016; Vivanti et al., 2018; Zeng et al., 2019). A major finding has been the correlation between mutations in *RNF213* in patients of Asian ancestry (and other ethnicities) with moyamoya disease (Gauden et al., 2020; Kim et al., 2018; Raj and Stoodley, 2015; Somarathna et al., 2020). In North America, only a small minority of pediatric moyamoya cases (<5%) appear to have clear mutational associations, unless the children have Asian heritage (who have *RNF213* mutations in 30–50%) (Cecchi et al., 2014; Gaillard et al., 2017; Guey et al., 2015; Lee et al., 2015). The presence of an *RNF213* mutation with moyamoya has marked significance for familial screening, as data suggest that familial penetrance is ~23% and, if an individual carries the mutation, there is a near 50% likelihood of manifesting arteriopathy (Lee et al., 2015; Matsuda et al., 2017). Other mutations are rarer, but may be detected by specific clinical or radiographic phenotypes (*ACTA2* carriers with distinctive stellate arteries branching from a dilated proximal internal carotid, *GUCY* mutations with achalasia, etc.) (Cecchi et al., 2014; Ganesan and Smith, 2015; Guey et al., 2015; Lee et al., 2015; Matsuda et al., 2017; Miskinyte et al., 2011; Munot et al., 2012; Wallace et al., 2016; Warejko et al., 2018). In addition, *TIMP-2* (a MMP inhibitor), *ACTA2* (a smooth muscle peptide) and mutations on chromosome 17 (near the *NF1* gene) have all been identified in select moyamoya patients (Jia et al., 2015; Raj and Stoodley, 2015; Somarathna et al., 2020). Other work has revealed genes associated with chromatin remodeling (*CHD4*, *CNOT3*, *SETD5*) (Pinard et al., 2020).

The mutations associated with moyamoya are heterogeneous, but they can be generally categorized into groups that suggest that some may be primary drivers of the pathology (such as those influence smooth muscle cell function like *ACTA2*, *GUCY*, and *RNF213*) and those that may be secondary and perhaps more responsible for aberrant responses to epigenetic factors (such as *TIMP-2*, *CNOT3*, *SEDT5*, and *CHD4*). These sorts of distinctions are important not only for identifying distinct subgroups of moyamoya patients (presumably with differing clinical profiles) but also for the development of tailored therapies. These efforts are aided by spontaneous and surgically induced animal models of moyamoya, including both rodents and zebrafish (Hyacinth et al., 2019; Mansour et al., 2018; Roberts et al., 2018; Wen et al., 2016).

23.4 Screening

Initial screening is commonly defined as MRI and MRA, looking for the defining radiographic characteristics of moyamoya (Fukui, 1997; Gaillard et al., 2017; Research Committee on the Pathology, Treatment and Spontaneous Occlusion of the Circle of Willis and Health Labour Sciences Research Grant for Research on Measures for Infractable Diseases, 2012; Smith and Scott, 2012). Indications for radiographic screening are in evolution, but are summarized in the recent stroke guidelines (Ferriero et al., 2019).

Genetic testing and counseling is relevant to children and families diagnosed with moyamoya, particularly in that there is generally high penetrance of the phenotype with most mutations and there is a potential surgical treatment if identified. In North America, only a small minority of pediatric moyamoya cases (<5%) appear to have clear mutational associations (Cecchi et al., 2014; Gaillard et al., 2017; Guey et al., 2015; Lee et al., 2015).

23.5 Conclusions

There has been significant evolution in the understanding of the pathogenesis of pediatric cerebrovascular disease; from genes, to proteins, to the interplay between complex molecular pathways. This research has directly translated into improved diagnostic, prognostic and therapeutic advances in the clinical setting. Continued progress in this field will increasingly rely on multi-disciplinary and multi-center collaboration to advance the knowledge of these rare disorders.

Figure acknowledgements

The following images obtained with consent are credited to the authors of this chapter: Figures 23.1-23.3

References

Adil MM, Qureshi AI, Beslow LA, Malik AA, Jordan LC. Factors associated with increased in-hospital mortality among children with intracerebral hemorrhage. *J Child Neurol* 2015;**30**(8):1024–8. https//doi.org/10.1177/0883073814552191.

Al-Jarallah A, Al-Rifai MT, Riela AR, Roach ES. Nontraumatic brain hemorrhage in children: etiology and presentation. *J Child Neurol* 2000;**15**:284–9. https://doi.org/10.1177/088307380001500503.

Al-Shahi R, Bhattacharya JJ, Currie DG, et al. Prospective, population-based detection of intracranial vascular malformations in adults: the Scottish Intracranial Vascular Malformation Study (SIVMS). *Stroke* 2003;**34**:1163–9. https//doi.org/10.1161/01.STR.0000069018.90456.C9.

Awad IA, Polster SP. Cavernous angiomas: deconstructing a neurosurgical disease. *J Neurosurg* 2019;**131**:1–13. https//doi.org/10.3171/2019.3.JNS181724.

Awad IA, Robinson JR, Jr., Mohanty S, Estes ML. Mixed vascular malformations of the brain: clinical and pathogenetic considerations. *Neurosurgery* 1993;**33**:179–88; discussion 88. https://doi.org/10.1227/00006123-199308000-00001.

Bacigaluppi S, Retta SF, Pileggi S, et al. Genetic and cellular basis of cerebral cavernous malformations: implications for clinical management. *Clin Genet* 2013;**83**:7–14. https//doi.org/10.1111/j.1399-0004.2012.01892.x.

Barnes B, Cawley CM, Barrow DL. Intracerebral hemorrhage secondary to vascular lesions. *Neurosurg Clin N Am* 2002;**13**:289–97, v. https//doi.org/10.1016/s1042-3680(02)00015-3.

Baumgartner JE, Ater JL, Ha CS, et al. Pathologically proven cavernous angiomas of the brain following radiation therapy for pediatric brain tumors. *Pediatr Neurosurg* 2003;**39**:201–07. https//doi.org/10.1159/000072472.

Beslow LA, Licht DJ, Smith SE, et al. Predictors of outcome in childhood intracerebral hemorrhage: a prospective consecutive cohort study. *Stroke* 2010;**41**:313–8. https//doi.org/10.1161/STROKEAHA.109.568071.

Boon LM, Mulliken JB, Vikkula M. *RASA1*: variable phenotype with capillary and arteriovenous malformations. *Curr Opin Genet Dev* 2005;**15**:265–9. https://doi.org/10.1016/j.gde.2005.03.004.

Bower RS, Mallory GW, Nwojo M, Kudva YC, Flemming KD, Meyer FB. Moyamoya disease in a primarily white, Midwestern US population: increased prevalence of autoimmune disease. *Stroke* 2013;**44**:1997–9. https//doi.org/10.1161/STROKEAHA.111.000307.

Broderick J, Talbot GT, Prenger E, Leach A, Brott T. Stroke in children within a major metropolitan area: the surprising importance of intracerebral hemorrhage. *J Child Neurol* 1993;**8**:250–5. https//doi.org/10.1177/088307389300800308.

Cavalcanti DD, Kalani MY, Martirosyan NL, Eales J, Spetzler RF, Preul MC. Cerebral cavernous malformations: from genes to proteins to disease. *J Neurosurg* 2012;**116**:122–32. https//doi.org/10.3171/2011.8.JNS101241.

Cecchi AC, Guo D, Ren Z, et al. *RNF213* rare variants in an ethnically diverse population with Moyamoya disease. *Stroke* 2014;**45**:3200–07. https//doi.org/10.1161/STROKEAHA.114.006244.

Chan AC, Li DY, Berg MJ, Whitehead KJ. Recent insights into cerebral cavernous malformations: animal models of CCM and the human phenotype. *FEBS J* 2010;**277**:1076–83. https//doi.org/10.1111/j.1742-4658.2009.07536.x.

Chee D, Phillips R, Maixner W, Southwell BR, Hutson JM. The potential of capillary birthmarks as a significant marker for capillary malformation–arteriovenous malformation syndrome in children who had nontraumatic cerebral hemorrhage. *J Pediatr Surg* 2010;**45**:2419–22. https//doi.org/10.1016/j.jpedsurg.2010.08.043.

Chen L, Tanriover G, Yano H, Friedlander R, Louvi A, Gunel M. Apoptotic functions of *PDCD10/CCM3*, the gene mutated in cerebral cavernous malformation 3. *Stroke* 2009;**40**:1474–81. https//doi.org/10.1161/STROKEAHA.108.527135.

Cooke D, Tatum J, Farid H, Dowd C, Higashida R, Halbach V. Transvenous embolization of a pediatric pial arteriovenous fistula. *J Neurointerv Surg* 2012;**4**:e14. https//doi.org/10.1136/neurintsurg-2011-010028.

Craig HD, Gunel M, Cepeda O, et al. Multilocus linkage identifies two new loci for a mendelian form of stroke, cerebral cavernous malformation, at 7p15-13 and 3q25.2-27. *Hum Mol Genet* 1998;**7**:1851–8. https//doi.org/10.1093/hmg/7.12.1851.

Denier C, Labauge P, Bergametti F, et al. Genotype–phenotype correlations in cerebral cavernous malformations patients. *Ann Neurol* 2006;**60**:550–6. https//doi.org/10.1002/ana.20947.

Di Rocco C, Iannelli A, Tamburrini G. Cavernous angiomas of the brain stem in children. *Pediatr Neurosurg* 1997;**27**:92–9. https//doi.org/10.1159/000121233.

Dubovsky J, Zabramski JM, Kurth J, et al. A gene responsible for cavernous malformations of the brain maps to chromosome 7q. *Hum Mol Genet* 1995;**4**:453–8. https//doi.org/10.1093/hmg/4.3.453.

Dupre N, Verlaan DJ, Hand CK, et al. Linkage to the *CCM2* locus and genetic heterogeneity in familial cerebral cavernous malformation. *Can J Neurol Sci* 2003;**30**:122–8. https//doi.org/10.1017/s0317167100053385.

Duran D, Karschnia P, Gaillard JR, et al. Human genetics and molecular mechanisms of vein of Galen malformation. *J Neurosurg Pediatr* 2018;**21**:367–74. https//doi.org/10.3171/2017.9.PEDS17365.

Eerola I, Boon LM, Mulliken JB, et al. Capillary malformation–arteriovenous malformation, a new clinical and genetic disorder caused by *RASA1* mutations. *Am J Hum Genet* 2003;**73**:1240–9. https//doi.org/10.1086/379793.

Faughnan ME, Palda VA, Garcia-Tsao G, et al. International guidelines for the diagnosis and management of hereditary haemorrhagic telangiectasia. *J Med Genet* 2011;**48**:73–87. https//doi.org/10.1136/jmg.2009.069013.

Fehnel KP, Penn DL, Duggins-Warf M, et al. Dysregulation of the EphrinB2–EphB4 ratio in pediatric cerebral arteriovenous malformations is associated with endothelial cell dysfunction in vitro and functions as a novel noninvasive biomarker in patients. *Exp Mol Med* 2020;**52**:658–71. https//doi.org/10.1038/s12276-020-0414-0.

Ferriero DM, Fullerton HJ, Bernard TJ, et al. Management of stroke in neonates and children: a scientific statement from the American Heart Association/American Stroke Association. *Stroke* 2019;**50**:e51–e96. https//doi.org/10.1161/STR.0000000000000183.

Fish JE, Flores-Suarez CP, Boudreau E, et al. Somatic gain of *KRAS* function in the endothelium is sufficient to cause vascular malformations that require *MEK* but not *PI3K* signaling. *Circ Res* 2020;**127**(6):727–43. https://doi.org/10.1161/CIRCRESAHA.

Frim DM, Scott RM. Management of cavernous malformations in the pediatric population. *Neurosurg Clin N Am* 1999;**10**:513–8. https//doi.org/10.1016/S1042-3680(18)30182-7.

Fujimura M, Watanabe M, Narisawa A, Shimizu H, Tominaga T. Increased expression of serum matrix metalloproteinase-9 in patients with moyamoya disease. *Surg Neurol* 2009;**72**:476–80; discussion 80. https//doi.org/10.1016/j.surneu.2008.10.009.

Fukui M. Guidelines for the diagnosis and treatment of spontaneous occlusion of the circle of Willis ('moyamoya' disease). Research Committee on Spontaneous Occlusion of the Circle of Willis (Moyamoya Disease) of the Ministry of Health and Welfare, Japan. *Clin Neurol Neurosurg* 1997;**99**(Suppl 2):S238–40.

Fullerton HJ, Wu YW, Zhao S, Johnston SC. Risk of stroke in children: ethnic and gender disparities. *Neurology* 2003;**61**:189–94. https//doi.org/10.1212/01.wnl.0000078894.79866.95.

Gaillard J, Klein J, Duran D, et al. Incidence, clinical features, and treatment of familial moyamoya in pediatric patients: a single-institution series. *J Neurosurg Pediatr* 2017;**19**:553–9. https//doi.org/10.3171/2016.12.PEDS16468.

Ganesan V, Smith ER. Moyamoya: defining current knowledge gaps. *Dev Med Child Neurol* 2015;**57**:786–7. https//doi.org/10.1111/dmcn.12708.

Garcia-Monaco R, Taylor W, Rodesch G, et al. Pial arteriovenous fistula in children as presenting manifestation of Rendu–Osler–Weber disease. *Neuroradiology* 1995;**37**:60–4. https//doi.org/10.1007/BF00588522.

Garrido-Martin EM, Nguyen HL, Cunningham TA, et al. Common and distinctive pathogenetic features of arteriovenous malformations in hereditary hemorrhagic telangiectasia 1 and hereditary hemorrhagic telangiectasia 2 animal models – brief report. *Arterioscler Thromb Vasc Biol* 2014;**34**:2232–6. https//doi.org/10.1161/ATVBAHA.114.303984.

Gauden AJ, McRobb LS, Lee VS, et al. Occlusion of animal model arteriovenous malformations using vascular targeting. *Transl Stroke Res* 2020;**11**:689–99. https//doi.org/10.1007/s12975-019-00759-y.

Gault J, Sarin H, Awadallah NA, Shenkar R, Awad IA. Pathobiology of human cerebrovascular malformations: basic mechanisms and clinical relevance. *Neurosurgery* 2004;**55**:1–16; discussion 16–7. https//doi.org/10.1227/01.neu.0000440729.59133.c9.

Gil-Nagel A, Dubovsky J, Wilcox KJ, et al. Familial cerebral cavernous angioma: a gene localized to a 15-cM interval on chromosome 7q. *Ann Neurol* 1996;**39**:807–10. https//doi.org/10.1002/ana.410390619.

Goss JA, Huang AY, Smith E, et al. Somatic mutations in intracranial arteriovenous malformations. *PLoS One* 2019;**14**:e0226852. https://doi.org/10.1371/journal.pone.0226852.

Gross BA, Du R, Orbach DB, Scott RM, Smith ER. The natural history of cerebral cavernous malformations in children. *J Neurosurg Pediatr* 2016;**17**(2):123–8. https://doi.org/10.3171/2015.2.PEDS14541.

Gross BA, Smith ER, Goumnerova L, Proctor MR, Madsen JR, Scott RM. Resection of supratentorial lobar cavernous malformations in children: clinical article. *J Neurosurg Pediatr* 2013a;**12**:367–73. https//doi.org/10.3171/2013.7.PEDS13126.

Gross BA, Smith ER, Scott RM. Cavernous malformations of the basal ganglia in children. *J Neurosurg Pediatr* 2013b;**12**:171–4. https://doi.org/10.3171/2013.5.PEDS1335.

Guey S, Tournier-Lasserve E, Herve D, Kossorotoff M. Moyamoya disease and syndromes: from genetics to clinical management. *Appl Clin Genet* 2015;**8**:49–68. https//doi.org/10.2147/TACG.S42772.

Gunel M, Awad IA, Anson J, Lifton RP. Mapping a gene causing cerebral cavernous malformation to 7q11.2-q21. *Proc Natl Acad Sci U S A* 1995;**92**:6620–4. https://doi.org/10.1073/pnas.92.14.6620.

Gunel M, Awad IA, Finberg K, et al. A founder mutation as a cause of cerebral cavernous malformation in Hispanic Americans. *N Engl J Med* 1996;**334**:946–51. https//doi.org/10.1056/NEJM199604113341503.

Hang Z, Shi Y, Wei Y. [A pathological analysis of 180 cases of vascular malformation of brain]. *Zhonghua Bing Li Xue Za Zhi* 1996;**25**:135–8.

Hayman LA, Evans RA, Ferrell RE, Fahr LM, Ostrow P, Riccardi VM. Familial cavernous angiomas: natural history and genetic study over a 5-year period. *Am J Med Genet* 1982;**11**:147–60. https//doi.org/10.1002/ajmg.1320110205.

Hetts SW, Keenan K, Fullerton HJ, et al. Pediatric intracranial nongalenic pial arteriovenous fistulas: clinical features, angioarchitecture, and outcomes. *Am J Neuroradiol* 2012;**33**:1710–9. https//doi.org/10.3174/ajnr.A3194.

Hyacinth HI, Sugihara CL, Spencer TL, Archer DR, Shih AY. Higher prevalence of spontaneous cerebral vasculopathy and cerebral infarcts in a mouse model of sickle cell disease. *J Cereb Blood Flow Metab* 2019;**39**:342–51. https//doi.org/10.1177/0271678X17732275.

Jia L, Wang L, Wei F, et al. Effects of wall shear stress in venous neointimal hyperplasia of arteriovenous fistulae. *Nephrology (Carlton)* 2015;**20**:335–42. https//doi.org/10.1111/nep.12394.

Jordan LC, Kleinman JT, Hillis AE. Intracerebral hemorrhage volume predicts poor neurologic outcome in children. *Stroke*

2009;**40**:1666–71. https//doi.org/10.1161/STROKEAHA.108.541383.

Kang HS, Kim JH, Phi JH, et al. Plasma matrix metalloproteinases, cytokines and angiogenic factors in moyamoya disease. *J Neurol Neurosurg Psychiatry* 2010;**81**:673–8. https//doi.org/10.1136/jnnp.2009.191817.

Kim J. Introduction to cerebral cavernous malformation: a brief review. *BMB Rep* 2016;**49**:255–62. https//doi.org/10.5483/bmbrep.2016.49.5.036.

Kim YH, Choe SW, Chae MY, Hong S, Oh SP. *SMAD4* deficiency leads to development of arteriovenous malformations in neonatal and adult mice. *J Am Heart Assoc* 2018;**7**:e009514. https//doi.org/10.1161/JAHA.118.009514.

Kurek KC, Luks VL, Ayturk UM, et al. Somatic mosaic activating mutations in *PIK3CA* cause CLOVES syndrome. *Am J Hum Genet* 2012;**90**:1108–15. https//doi.org/10.1016/j.ajhg.2012.05.006.

Labauge P, Enjolras O, Bonerandi JJ, et al. An association between autosomal dominant cerebral cavernomas and a distinctive hyperkeratotic cutaneous vascular malformation in 4 families. *Ann Neurol* 1999;**45**:250–4. https//doi.org/10.1002/1531-8249(199902)45:2<250::aid-ana17>3.0.co;2-v.

Laberge S, Labauge P, Marechal E, Maciazek J, Tournier-Lasserve E. Genetic heterogeneity and absence of founder effect in a series of 36 French cerebral cavernous angiomas families. *Eur J Hum Genet* 1999;**7**:499–504. https//doi.org/10.1038/sj.ejhg.5200324.

Laberge-le Couteulx S, Jung HH, Labauge P, et al. Truncating mutations in *CCM1*, encoding *KRIT1*, cause hereditary cavernous angiomas. *Nat Genet* 1999;**23**:189–93. https//doi.org/10.1038/13815.

Larson JJ, Ball WS, Bove KE, Crone KR, Tew JM, Jr. Formation of intracerebral cavernous malformations after radiation treatment for central nervous system neoplasia in children. *J Neurosurg* 1998;**88**:51–6. https//doi.org/10.3171/jns.1998.88.1.0051.

Lasjaunias P. *Vascular Diseases in Neonates, Infants and Children*. Springer Verlag; 1997.

Laurans MS, DiLuna ML, Shin D, et al. Mutational analysis of 206 families with cavernous malformations. *J Neurosurg* 2003;**99**:38–43. https//doi.org/10.3171/jns.2003.99.1.0038.

Lawton MT, Rutledge WC, Kim H, et al. Brain arteriovenous malformations. *Nat Rev Dis Primers* 2015;**1**:15008. https//doi.org/10.1038/nrdp.2015.8.

Lee MJ, Chen YF, Fan PC, et al. Mutation genotypes of *RNF213* gene from moyamoya patients in Taiwan. *J Neurol Sci* 2015;**353**:161–5. https//doi.org/10.1016/j.jns.2015.04.019.

Liu J, Wang D, Lei C, et al. Etiology, clinical characteristics and prognosis of spontaneous intracerebral hemorrhage in children: a prospective cohort study in China. *J Neurol Sci* 2015;**358**:367–70. https//doi.org/10.1016/j.jns.2015.09.366.

Mansour A, Niizuma K, Rashad S, et al. A refined model of chronic cerebral hypoperfusion resulting in cognitive impairment and a low mortality rate in rats. *J Neurosurg* 2018;**131**:892–902. https//doi.org/10.3171/2018.3.JNS172274.

Marchuk DA, Gallione CJ, Morrison LA, et al. A locus for cerebral cavernous malformations maps to chromosome 7q in two families. *Genomics* 1995;**28**:311–4. https//doi.org/10.1006/geno.1995.1147.

Matsuda Y, Mineharu Y, Kimura M, et al. *RNF213* p.R4810K variant and intracranial arterial stenosis or occlusion in relatives of patients with moyamoya disease. *J Stroke Cerebrovasc Dis* 2017;**26**:1841–7. https//doi.org/10.1016/j.jstrokecerebrovasdis.2017.04.019.

Merello E, Pavanello M, Consales A, et al. Genetic screening of pediatric cavernous malformations. *J Mol Neurosci* 2016;**60**:232–8. https//doi.org/10.1007/s12031-016-0806-8.

Miskinyte S, Butler MG, Herve D, et al. Loss of BRCC3 deubiquitinating enzyme leads to abnormal angiogenesis and is associated with syndromic moyamoya. *Am J Hum Genet* 2011;**88**:718–28. https//doi.org/10.1016/j.ajhg.2011.04.017.

Mohr JP, Parides MK, Stapf C, et al. Medical management with or without interventional therapy for unruptured brain arteriovenous malformations (ARUBA): a multicentre, non-blinded, randomised trial. *Lancet* 2014;**383**:614–21. https//doi.org/10.1016/S0140-6736(13)62302-8.

Mottolese C, Hermier M, Stan H, et al. Central nervous system cavernomas in the pediatric age group. *Neurosurg Rev* 2001;**24**:55–71; discussion 2–3. https//doi.org/10.1007/pl00014581.

Munot P, Saunders DE, Milewicz DM, et al. A novel distinctive cerebrovascular phenotype is associated with heterozygous Arg179 *ACTA2* mutations. *Brain* 2012;**135**:2506–14. https//doi.org/10.1093/brain/aws172.

Pinard A, Guey S, Guo D, et al. The pleiotropy associated with de novo variants in *CHD4*, *CNOT3*, and *SETD5* extends to moyamoya angiopathy. *Genet Med* 2020;**22**:427–31. https//doi.org/10.1038/s41436-019-0639-2.

Pricola Fehnel K, Duggins-Warf M, Zurakowski D, et al. Using urinary bFGF and TIMP3 levels to predict the presence of juvenile pilocytic astrocytoma and establish a distinct biomarker signature. *J Neurosurg Pediatr* 2016;**18**:396–407. https//doi.org/10.3171/2015.12.PEDS15448.

Protack CD, Foster TR, Hashimoto T, et al. Eph-B4 regulates adaptive venous remodeling to improve arteriovenous fistula patency. *Sci Rep* 2017;**7**:15386. https//doi.org/10.1038/s41598-017-13071-2.

Raj JA, Stoodley M. Experimental animal models of arteriovenous malformation: a review. *Vet Sci* 2015;**2**:97–110. https//doi.org/10.3390/vetsci2020097.

Raybaud CA, Strother CM, Hald JK. Aneurysms of the vein of Galen: embryonic considerations and anatomical features relating to the pathogenesis of the malformation.

Neuroradiology 1989;**31**:109–28. https//doi.org/10.1007/BF00698838.

Recinos PF, Rahmathulla G, Pearl M, et al. Vein of Galen malformations: epidemiology, clinical presentations, management. *Neurosurg Clin N Am* 2012;**23**:165–77. https//doi.org/10.1016/j.nec.2011.09.006.

Research Committee on the Pathology and Treatment of Spontaneous Occlusion of the Circle of Willis, and Health Labour Sciences Research Grant for Research on Measures for Infractable Diseases. Guidelines for diagnosis and treatment of moyamoya disease (spontaneous occlusion of the circle of Willis). *Neurol Med Chir (Tokyo)* 2012;**52**:245–66. https://doi.org/10.2176/nmc.52.245.

Rigamonti D, Hadley MN, Drayer BP, et al. Cerebral cavernous malformations. Incidence and familial occurrence. *N Engl J Med* 1988;**319**:343–7. https//doi.org/10.1056/NEJM198808113190605.

Riordan CP, Orbach DB, Smith ER, Scott RM. Acute fatal hemorrhage from previously undiagnosed cerebral arteriovenous malformations in children: a single-center experience. *J Neurosurg Pediatr* 2018;**22**:244–50. https//doi.org/10.3171/2018.3.PEDS1825.

Roberts JM, Maniskas ME, Fraser JF, Bix GJ. Internal carotid artery stenosis: a novel surgical model for moyamoya syndrome. *PLoS One* 2018;**13**:e0191312. https//doi.org/10.1371/journal.pone.0191312

Rutledge WC, Abla AA, Nelson J, Halbach VV, Kim H, Lawton MT. Treatment and outcomes of ARUBA-eligible patients with unruptured brain arteriovenous malformations at a single institution. *Neurosurg Focus* 2014;**37**:E8. https//doi.org/10.3171/2014.7.FOCUS14242.

Saliou G, Eyries M, Iacobucci M, et al. Clinical and genetic findings in children with CNS arteriovenous fistulas. *Ann Neurol* 2017;**82**(6):972–80. https://doi.org/10.1002/ana.25106.

Scott RM. Brain stem cavernous angiomas in children. *Pediatr Neurosurg* 1990;**16**:281–6. https//doi.org/10.1159/000120543.

Scott RM, Barnes P, Kupsky W, Adelman LS. Cavernous angiomas of the central nervous system in children. *J Neurosurg* 1992;**76**:38–46. https//doi.org/10.3171/jns.1992.76.1.0038.

Scott RM, Smith ER. Moyamoya disease and moyamoya syndrome. *N Engl J Med* 2009;**360**:1226–37. https//doi.org/10.1056/NEJMra0804622.

Seki T, Yun J, Oh SP. Arterial endothelium-specific activin receptor-like kinase 1 expression suggests its role in arterialization and vascular remodeling. *Circ Res* 2003;**93**:682–9. https://doi.org/10.1161/01.RES.0000095246.40391.3B.

Shenkar R, Elliott JP, Diener K, et al. Differential gene expression in human cerebrovascular malformations. *Neurosurgery* 2003;**52**:465–77; discussion 77–8. https//doi.org/10.1227/01.neu.0000044131.03495.22.

Singla A, Brace O'Neill JE, Smith E, Scott RM. Cavernous malformations of the brain after treatment for acute lymphocytic leukemia: presentation and long-term follow-up. *J Neurosurg Pediatr* 2013;**11**:127–32. https://doi.org/10.3171/2012.11.PEDS12235.

Sirvente J, Enjolras O, Wassef M, Tournier-Lasserve E, Labauge P. Frequency and phenotypes of cutaneous vascular malformations in a consecutive series of 417 patients with familial cerebral cavernous malformations. *J Eur Acad Dermatol Venereol* 2009;**23**(9):1066–72. https://www/doi/10.1111/j.1468-3083.2009.03263.x.

Smith ER. Moyamoya biomarkers. *J Korean Neurosurg Soc* 2015;**57**:415–21. https//doi.org/10.3340/jkns.2015.57.6.415.

Smith ER, Scott RM. Spontaneous occlusion of the circle of Willis in children: pediatric moyamoya summary with proposed evidence-based practice guidelines. A review. *J Neurosurg Pediatr* 2012;**9**:353–60. https//doi.org/10.3171/2011.12.PEDS1172.

Somarathna M, Isayeva-Waldrop T, Al-Balas A, Guo L, Lee T. A Novel Model of balloon angioplasty injury in rat arteriovenous fistula. *J Vasc Res* 2020;**57**(4):223–35. https://doi.org/10.1159/000507080.

Soriano SG, Cowan DB, Proctor MR, Scott RM. Levels of soluble adhesion molecules are elevated in the cerebrospinal fluid of children with moyamoya syndrome. *Neurosurgery* 2002;**50**:544–9. https://doi.org/10.1097/00006123-200203000-00022.

Spiegler S, Rath M, Paperlein C, Felbor U. Cerebral cavernous malformations: an update on prevalence, molecular genetic analyses, and genetic counselling. *Mol Syndromol* 2018;**9**:60–9. https://doi.org/10.1159/000486292.

Starke RM, McCarthy DJ, Komotar RJ, Connolly ES. Gut microbiome and endothelial *TLR4* activation provoke cerebral cavernous malformations. *Neurosurgery* 2017;**81**:N44–N6. https://doi.org/10.1093/neuros/nyx450.

Tang AT, Choi JP, Kotzin JJ, et al. Endothelial *TLR4* and the microbiome drive cerebral cavernous malformations. *Nature* 2017;**545**:305–10. https://doi.org/10.1038/nature22075.

Tanriover G, Boylan AJ, Diluna ML, Pricola KL, Louvi A, Gunel M. *PDCD10*, the gene mutated in cerebral cavernous malformation 3, is expressed in the neurovascular unit. *Neurosurgery* 2008;**62**:930–8; discussion 8. https//doi.org/10.1227/01.neu.0000318179.02912.ca.

Thiex R, Mulliken JB, Revencu N, et al. A novel association between *RASA1* mutations and spinal arteriovenous anomalies. *Am J Neuroradiol* 2010;**31**:775–9. https://doi.org/10.3174/ajnr.A1907.

Toll A, Parera E, Gimenez-Arnau AM, et al. Cutaneous venous malformations in familial cerebral cavernomatosis caused by *KRIT1* gene mutations. *Dermatology* 2009;**218**:307–13. https//doi.org/10.1159/000199461.

Tomlinson FH, Rufenacht DA, Sundt TM, Jr., Nichols DA, Fode NC. Arteriovenous fistulas of the brain and the spinal cord. *J Neurosurg* 1993;**79**:16–27. https://doi.org/10.3171/jns.1993.79.1.0016

Vanaman MJ, Hervey-Jumper SL, Maher CO. Pediatric and inherited neurovascular diseases. *Neurosurg Clin N Am* 2010;**21**:427–41. https//doi.org/10.1016/j.nec.2010.03.001.

Vivanti A, Ozanne A, Grondin C, et al. Loss of function mutations in *EPHB4* are responsible for vein of Galen aneurysmal malformation. *Brain* 2018;**141**:979–88. https//doi.org/10.1093/brain/awy020.

Walcott BP, Smith ER, Scott RM, Orbach DB. Dural arteriovenous fistulae in pediatric patients: associated conditions and treatment outcomes. *J Neurointerv Surg* 2013a;**5**(1):6–9. https://doi.org/10.1136/neurintsurg-2011-010169.

Walcott BP, Smith ER, Scott RM, Orbach DB. Pial arteriovenous fistulae in pediatric patients: associated syndromes and treatment outcome. *J Neurointerv Surg* 2013b;**5**(1):10–4. https://doi.org/10.1136/neurintsurg-2011-010168.

Wallace S, Guo DC, Regalado E, et al. Disrupted nitric oxide signaling due to *GUCY1A3* mutations increases risk for moyamoya disease, achalasia and hypertension. *Clin Genet* 2016;**90**:351–60. https//doi.org/10.1111/cge.12739.

Wang K, Zhou HJ, Wang M. *CCM3* and cerebral cavernous malformation disease. *Stroke Vasc Neurol* 2019;**4**:67–70. https//doi.org/10.1136/svn-2018-000195.

Warejko JK, Schueler M, Vivante A, et al. Whole exome sequencing reveals a monogenic cause of disease in approximately 43% of 35 families with midaortic syndrome. *Hypertension* 2018;**71**:691–9. https//doi.org/10.1161/HYPERTENSIONAHA.117.10296.

Wen J, Sun X, Chen H, et al. Mutation of *rnf213a* by TALEN causes abnormal angiogenesis and circulation defects in zebrafish. *Brain Res* 2016;**1644**:70–8. https//doi.org/10.1016/j.brainres.2016.04.051.

Weon YC, Yoshida Y, Sachet M, et al. Supratentorial cerebral arteriovenous fistulas (AVFs) in children: review of 41 cases with 63 non choroidal single-hole AVFs. *Acta Neurochir (Wien)* 2005;**147**:17–31. https//doi.org/10.1007/s00701-004-0341-1.

Wetzel-Strong SE, Detter MR, Marchuk DA. The pathobiology of vascular malformations: insights from human and model organism genetics. *J Pathol* 2017;**241**:281–93. https//doi.org/10.1002/path.4844.

Whitehead KJ, Plummer NW, Adams JA, Marchuk DA, Li DY. *Ccm1* is required for arterial morphogenesis: implications for the etiology of human cavernous malformations. *Development* 2004;**131**:1437–48. https//doi.org/10.1242/dev.01036.

Willinsky RA, Lasjaunias P, Terbrugge K, Burrows P. Multiple cerebral arteriovenous malformations (AVMs). Review of our experience from 203 patients with cerebral vascular lesions. *Neuroradiology* 1990;**32**:207–10. https://doi.org/10.1007/BF00589113.

Woodall MN, McGettigan M, Figueroa R, Gossage JR, Alleyne CH, Jr. Cerebral vascular malformations in hereditary hemorrhagic telangiectasia. *J Neurosurg* 2014;**120**:87–92. https//doi.org/10.3171/2013.10.JNS122402.

Yoshida Y, Weon YC, Sachet M, et al. Posterior cranial fossa single-hole arteriovenous fistulae in children: 14 consecutive cases. *Neuroradiology* 2004;**46**:474–81. https://doi.org/10.1007/s00234-004-1176-4.

Zabramski JM, Wascher TM, Spetzler RF, et al. The natural history of familial cavernous malformations: results of an ongoing study. *J Neurosurg* 1994;**80**:422–32. https://doi.org/10.3171/jns.1994.80.3.0422.

Zeng X, Hunt A, Jin SC, Duran D, Gaillard J, Kahle KT. EphrinB2–EphB4–RASA1 signaling in human cerebrovascular development and disease. *Trends Mol Med* 2019;**25**:265–86. https//doi.org/10.1016/j.molmed.2019.01.009.

Zhang J, Rigamonti D, Dietz HC, Clatterbuck RE. Interaction between *krit1* and *malcavernin*: implications for the pathogenesis of cerebral cavernous malformations. *Neurosurgery* 2007;**60**:353–9; discussion 9. https//doi.org/10.1227/01.NEU.0000249268.11074.83.

24 Craniofacial Neurosurgery

John T. Smetona and John A. Persing

24.1 Definition

Craniosynostosis is a condition associated with the pathologic premature fusion of one or more cranial sutures. The incidence is 1 in 2000–2500 live births (Boulet et al., 2008; Di Rocco et al., 2009; Selber et al., 2008). The metopic suture closes early in infancy (physiologic closure can occur as early as 3 months of age). In craniosynostosis, characteristic calvarial deformity first appears on ultrasound in the second trimester and precedes identifiable suture fusion by 4–16 weeks (Delahaye et al., 2003; Tonni et al., 2011). When this premature closure occurs, it is associated with restriction of calvarial growth perpendicular to the fused suture, with compensatory increase in growth at the remaining sutures (Delashaw et al., 1989). Previously there was debate as to whether the suture fusion itself drives this restriction of growth, or whether a cranial base deformity drives the abnormal development through tension bands in the dura. Currently there is a preponderance of evidence from human and rabbit studies supporting the idea that suture fusion is at least a significant contributor to the overall skull shape abnormality (Christensen and Clark, 1970; Delashaw et al., 1989; Fellows-Mayle et al., 2006; Mooney et al., 1998; Moss and Salentijn, 1969; Persing and Jane, 1989; Persing et al., 1986; Persson et al., 1979). The natural history of the disease is such that the deformity observed in infancy increases in severity if not surgically corrected (Heller et al., 2008).

24.2 Categories of Disease; Associated Manifestations

Craniosynostosis is commonly classified into two categories: syndromic and non-syndromic. Syndromic cases comprise approximately 15% of craniosynostosis. Over 180 defined syndromes exist, with Apert, Crouzon, Pfeiffer, Saethre–Chotzen, and Muenke syndromes being the most common. Syndromic cases are typically inherited in Mendelian fashion, are associated with decreased intelligence or other cognitive abnormalities, and include characteristic extracranial manifestations (Agochukwu et al., 2012; Ciurea and Toader, 2009; Da Costa et al., 2006; de Jong et al., 2012; Passos-Bueno et al., 2008). Well-defined genetic mutations drive the disease in most instances, often from those in the Fibroblast Growth Factor Receptor family. There has also been recent evidence demonstrating that mutations in the Transcription Factor AP-2 Beta (*TFAP2B*), K acetyltransferase 6A (*KAT6A*), GLI Family Zinc Finger 2 (*GLI2*), SRY-Box Transcription Factor 11 (*SOX11*), Catenin Alpha 1 (*CTNNA1*), Glypican 4 (*GPC4*) gene families are causative agents in cases of syndromic synostosis without mutation in the most common genetically recognized loci. This implies genetic underpinnings of syndromic cases even when the common causative genes are the wild type (Timberlake et al., 2019). Even in the well-recognized syndromes, presentation can vary significantly. For example, in addition to the obvious clinical differences that may be seen between individuals, Crouzon syndrome can display four major patterns of suture fusion, with corresponding differences in the cranial base length and facial skeleton (Lu et al., 2020). Thus, the spectrum of presentation may be additionally influenced by environmental factors, epigenetics, and normal alleles that confer susceptibility or mutations in genes that will not cause craniosynostosis in isolation (Azoury et al., 2017).

Non-syndromic craniosynostosis (NSC), comprising approximately 85% of the disease, is less well understood. Increasing recent evidence points toward a polygenic inheritance, with a confluence of rare mutations and common genetic variants that confer susceptibility coinciding in a single individual to drive the disease process (Timberlake et al., 2016, 2018). Timberlake et al. have demonstrated that many different mutations, particularly those in BMP, Wnt, and Ras/ERL pathways, are associate with NSC (Timberlake et al., 2018). While patients with NSC are typically of normal IQ, they have been demonstrated to have a range of more subtle abnormalities in cognition, leading to learning difficulties and varying irregularities in executive function and emotional regulation (Chuang et al., 2018; Da Costa et al., 2006; Klajić et al., 2019; Lajeunie et al., 1998; Magge et al., 2002; Thwin et al., 2015).

24.3 Etiology of Neural Dysfunction

In addition to characteristic structural and esthetic deformities, craniosynostosis is associated with cognitive dysfunction. The etiology and, correspondingly, the treatment of these abnormalities has been an area of extensive debate and ongoing investigation.

The first potential explanation for this abnormal function was the observation of increased intracranial pressure (ICP), which is found in up to 50% of syndromic cases (Renier et al., 1982, 2000). It was hypothesized that this increased pressure might decrease cerebral perfusion and therefore disrupt normal cognitive development. However, further studies demonstrated that only at most 12–14% of NSC (Cohen and Persing, 1998; Renier et al., 2000) patients exhibited elevated ICP, while 50% display learning disabilities or other cognitive dysfunction (Becker et al., 2005; Bolthauser et al., 2003; Bottero et al., 1998; Collett et al., 2017; Cradock et al., 2015; Kapp-Simon et al., 2007; Magge et al., 2002). Additional studies have suggested that there is no association between elevated ICP and cognitive outcome (Thiele-Nygaard et al., 2020); however, the manner and duration of ICP recording has yet to be defined optimally.

24.4 Theory 1: Regional Constraint

There are now two leading theories to explain the cognitive abnormalities observed in craniosynostosis. The first holds that the restriction of growth imposed on the brain by the fused suture interrupts normal development. This is supported by the fact that abnormal calvarial shape enforces an abnormal brain shape, altering the relative distribution of gray matter and the length of white matter tracts, thus altering the functional networks that comprise cognition. In addition, it may cause localized areas of increased pressure, producing changes in cortical metabolism and blood flow.

24.5 Theory 2: Modular Developmental Abnormality

The second theory suggests that there is a primary development abnormality of the cranium, including both the brain and the bony encasement, and fused calvarial sutures are just one manifestation of this process rather than a driver of it. This is supported by the observation that the brain and calvarium share some common embryological tissues of origin, and particularly in syndromic cases genes that play a role in suture fusion are also important in neural development (particularly the FGF family of cytokines).

24.6 Developmental Evidence for Modular Abnormality

Brain parenchyma, meninges, and calvarium have overlapping embryological origins. Neural crest tissue gives rise to the frontal bones, metopic, and sagittal sutures (Lenton et al., 2005), and also contributes to the meninges (Adeeb et al., 2012) and parenchyma (Creuzet et al., 2006) of forebrain and midbrain. Thus, a developmental abnormality in neural crest tissue might simultaneously affect bony, sutural, and brain parenchymal development.

24.7 Genetic Evidence for Modular Abnormality

There is evidence to suggest a component of genetically driven primary developmental abnormality of the brain in syndromic craniosynostosis. *FGFR1* is essential for formation and migration of nerve cells in the brain (Hebert, 2003). Mutations in this gene are also associated with nerve dysfunction in conditions such as Kallman's syndrome (Cariboni and Maggi, 2006). *FGFR3*, the causative mutation in Muenke syndrome, has been shown to be critical to regulating brain size in mice, which it does by controlling apoptosis and proliferation. *FGFR3* mutant mice developed markedly increased cortical thickness, while *FGFR2* knockouts demonstrate cortical thinning (Inglis- Broadgate et al., 2005). Of note, *FGFR 2* mutations drive the most common craniosynostotic syndromes, including Crouzon's, Apert's, and Pfieffer's syndrome. These effects may be due to the importance of *FGFR* family genes for the action of L1 cell adhesion molecule (L1CAM). Mutations in *L1CAM* cause Bickers–Adams syndrome, and *L1CAM* requires FGFR family interaction to function (Doherty and Walsh, 1996; Kamiguchi and Lemmon, 1997). The full array of presenting symptoms may rely on environmental or epigenetic factors, or on the interaction with other normal variants that increase risk.

Non-syndromic craniosynostosis, however, has no clear genetic causation of primary brain malformation. The genetic underpinning of NSC is less well understood, but recent data indicating that is polygenic have not identified genes with equally critical roles in neural development (Boyadjiev, 2007; Lajeunie et al., 1996, 2005; Timberlake et al., 2016). As the type role of individual genetic mutations and their interactions are not yet defined, a definitive assessment of the role of primary brain malformation in NSC will require much more detailed understanding of the genetic etiology of the disease.

24.8 Intrinsic Brain Malformation in Syndromic Craniosynostosis

In syndromic craniosynostosis, key brain structures including the corpus callosum, hippocampus, septum pellucidum, cortex, cerebellum, and ventricular system are distinctly abnormal (Collmann et al., 2005; Proudman et al., 1995; Quintero-Rivera et al., 2006; Raybaud and Di Rocco, 2007; Tokumaru et al., 1996; Yacubian-Fernandes et al., 2004). In addition, regional distribution of brain matter will also be forced to conform to the bony construct within which it resides (Aldridge et al., 2005; Richtsmeier et al., 2006). In Crouzon syndrome, for example, the anterior cranial fossa is increased in volume, the middle cranial fossa is normal, and the posterior cranial fossa is reduced, while the overall volume is normal (Lu et al., 2019). The anteroposterior length is reduced, primarily due to the reduction in posterior cranial fossa length (Lu et al., 2019).

24.9 Calvarial Deformity Enforces Brain Distortion in Non-Syndromic Craniosynostosis

In NSC, these distinctive brain irregularities are not yet visible; however, the brain architecture changes in conformity with the vault structure (Aldridge et al., 2005; Engel et al., 2012; Hukki et al., 2012; Richtsmeier et al., 2006). The specific pattern of deformity will then depend on the pattern of suture fusion, and it has been demonstrated that these patterns of deformity may correct with the surgical normalization of the skull. For example, in sagittal NSC, the brain is elongated in the sagittal plain and constricted in the coronal plane, following the pattern of skull deformity. After surgical treatment, however, most of these changes normalize, and this normalization persists into adolescence (Brooks et al., 2016). This suggests that fusion of the suture has a definite impact on brain growth, and that deformity of brain is not purely intrinsic to its own genetic programming.

24.10 Brain Distortion May Disrupt Functional Circuit Connectivity

The abnormal configuration of brain matter may impact the development of functional circuits. Skull restriction becomes evident on ultrasound in the second trimester (Delahaye et al., 2003; Tonni et al., 2011), when early synaptogenesis is occurring simultaneously with neuronal proliferation, differentiation, and migration (Kostović et al., 1995). Neural circuits are established in conjunction with and following the development of structural substrate (Jessell and Sanes, 2000; Kostović et al., 1995; Levitt, 2003). This is corroborated by electrophysiologic data showing that electrical activity patterns change as structural development continues between gestational weeks 20 and 40 (Graziani et al., 1968; Kostović et al., 1995; Kurtzberg et al., 2008; Novak et al., 1989). This may therefore constitute a critical period for circuit development, and restriction of growth by physical limitation, in addition to possibly localized intracranial hypertension and decreased perfusion, may constitute an irreversible insult to the developing brain circuits. Abnormal circuitry is associated with cognitive abnormalities at maturity (Churchill et al., 2002; Morton and Munakata, 2005; Munakata et al., 2008).

24.11 Cortical Metabolism and Blood Flow Are Altered Beneath Fused Sutures

With the advent of PET-CT and functional magnetic resonance imaging (FMRI), it has become possible to non-invasively measure intracranial metabolism. This has made it possible to assess localized areas of brain beneath fused sutures. Multiple studies with PET-CT have demonstrated that patients with both syndromic and NSC have reduced blood flow in the area compressed by suture fusion, which is largely normalized after surgical release (David et al., 1996; Satoh et al., 1990; Sen et al., 1995). Non-invasive near-infrared spectroscopy (NIRS) study has provided additional evidence that cerebral oxygenation is regionally compromised in craniosynostosis, and that this compromise is generally relieved by surgical decompression (Martini et al., 2014). A rabbit model of early onset craniosynostosis demonstrated abnormally increased blood flow in the superficial cortex at 25 days of age, which was normalized by suturectomy (Grandhi et al., 2018). By 42 days of age, blood flow in all areas had normalized regardless of treatment. While generalized mild ICP elevation may not cause intellectual dysfunction, focal compression may cause local perfusion abnormalities which may impair synaptic development. A study looking a cerebral blood flow (CBF) in humans with syndromic craniosynostosis demonstrated that untreated patients less than one year of age had reduced CBF compared to controls, which increased significantly after surgery and normalized with increasing age (Doerga et al., 2020). The peak in CBF seen at age 4 in normal individuals occurred at age 5–6 in affected patients (Doerga et al., 2020). This provides additional evidence that an abnormal perfusion pattern may occur transiently but still have long-term effects by restricting growth and development in critical periods.

24.12 White Matter Microstructure Is Atypical in Syndromic Craniosynostosis

Studies using diffusion tensor imaging (DTI) have identified radiologic differences in the white matter in patients with craniosynostosis, involving both diffusivity and anisotropy, suggesting different microstructural properties (Florisson et al., 2011; Rijken et al., 2015). These changes may occur in syndromic patients due to the importance of FGFR genes in myelination. A rabbit model showed that characteristic white matter changes occurred in rabbits with familial coronal craniosynostosis. These changes increased with age and were sufficiently distinctive that by age 42 days, rabbits could be identified as wild-type or fused with 100% accuracy (Bonfield et al., 2015). Rabbits treated with early suturectomy displayed no differences from wild-type (Bonfield et al., 2015). However, human SC patients do not display this normalization with age (Florisson et al., 2011). Similar findings of white matter disruption have not been widely reported in NSC. Given that both NSC and syndromic cases demonstrate abnormal blood flow, the presence of marked white matter abnormalities only in syndromic cases suggests an intrinsic developmental abnormality in syndromic craniosynostosis that may not be present in NSC.

24.13 Electrophysiologic Data Provide an Early Indication of Cognitive Dysfunction

Unlike traditional assessments of infant development, event-related potential (ERP) data have been demonstrated to correlate with cognitive function at maturity (Guttorm et al., 2010; Hack et al., 2005; Molfese, 2000). Electrophysiologic study has shown abnormal responses to a range of stimuli in SC as well as improvement or normalization after surgical treatment. There is evidence

of rare improvement in response to decompression in auditory responses and up to 100% improvement in visually evoked potentials (VEP) (Church et al., 2007; Donati et al., 1997; Liasis, 2006; Mursch et al., 1998; Thompson et al., 2006). In spite of the previously discussed evidence of intrinsic abnormality, this suggests an additive developmental insult from local cranial distortion.

While the correlation of severity of metopic craniosynostosis (mCSO) and functional outcomes has been debated, ERP data have shown that severe mCSO patients have reduced ERP response to language in the left frontal scalp, while mild cases demonstrated no difference compared to normal controls (Yang et al., 2017). Another study demonstrated that infants with single-suture synostosis demonstrate an atypical neural response to language, which normalizes after whole vault cranioplasty (Chuang et al., 2018). These observations support the idea that bony constriction plays a role in cognitive dysfunction, and that relieving this constriction may improve cognitive development.

24.14 Altered Functional Circuits in Craniosynostosis

Functional magnetic resonance imaging studies have demonstrated abnormal connectivity in brains with craniosynostosis. A 2014 study demonstrated that surgically treated sagittal non-syndromic craniosynostosis (sNSC) displayed a broadly altered pattern of functional connectivity in many cortical areas, including increases in negative connectivity between Brodmann's Area (BA) 8 and the prefrontal cortex and the anterior cingulate cortex (Beckett et al., 2014). Later FMRI data illustrated that metopic with sagittal synostosis demonstrated a connectivity pattern similar to that seen in attention deficit hyperactivity disorder (ADHD), while those with only sagittal synostosis (SSO) showed increased connectivity in areas of attention and auditory processing compared to patients with ADHD (Cabrejo et al., 2019a, 2019b). A further study showed that SSO have decreased connectivity in areas of visuomotor integration and attention; coronal synostosis (CSO) patients demonstrated decreased connectivity in areas responsible for cognition and executive function (Sun et al., 2019). Brain regions responsible for emotional regulation have also been shown to be abnormal, with unilateral coronal synostosis linked to abnormal response to frustration, and mCSO-related brains, showing a muted response to emotional stimuli (Wu et al., 2019). These studies demonstrate a consistent pattern of functional network abnormality in craniosynostosis, which may explain cognitive deficiencies and also suggest neurocognitive profiles specific to suture fusion patterns. However these findings must be considered as preliminary, as the studies done to date are with either a relatively limited number of patients, or utilized anesthetic agents during the analysis, which may influence the validity of the data.

24.15 Functional Assessment Reveals Cognitive Deficiency at Maturity

While ERP and FMRI provide early assessments of abnormal cortical function, neurocognitive assessment at maturity provides the most definitive assessment of cognitive ability. Tests including the Beery–Buktenica Developmental Test of Visual–Motor Integration, the Wechsler Abbreviated Scale of Intelligence, and the Wechsler Fundamentals demonstrate neurocognitive deficiencies in children with NSC in spite of treatment in infancy (Gabrick et al., 2020; Hashim et al., 2014; Patel

et al., 2014; Wu et al., 2020). In addition, a small but growing body of evidence supports the idea that the timing and type of vault remodeling may influence the ultimate extent of cognitive dysfunction (Hashim et al., 2014; Patel et al., 2014).

A morphological assessment of the link between severity of cranial dysmorphology and neurocognitive outcomes demonstrated that infants with severe frontal restriction as measured by the endocranial bifrontal angle narrowing, ultimately performed worse than those with mild deformity (Gabrick et al., 2020). A study in 2014 showed that patients with isolated sagittal synostosis who were treated with whole vault cranioplasty showed better cognitive outcomes than those treated with strip craniectomy across scales including full scale IQ, verbal IQ, reading comprehension, and visuomotor integration (Hashim et al., 2014). Patients who were treated prior to 6 months of age also demonstrated superior outcomes to those treated later, with a higher percentage of the latter cohort demonstrating one or more reading-related disabilities (Patel et al., 2014). On the other hand, another neurocognitive assessment found that, in patients with midline synostosis, those with *SMAD-6* mutations (Figure 24.1)

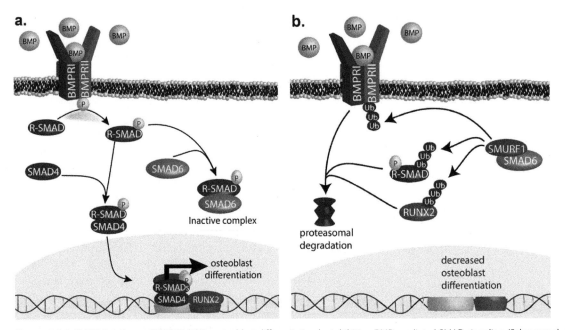

Figure 24.1 *SMAD-6* pathway. *SMAD6* inhibits osteoblast differentiation by inhibiting BMP-mediated SMAD signaling (Salazar et al., 2016). (a) BMP ligands activate BMP receptors, leading to phosphorylation of receptor-regulated SMADs (R-SMADs), which complex with SMAD4 and enter the nucleus, cooperating with RUNX2 to induce osteoblast differentiation. SMAD6 inhibits this signal by competing with SMAD4 for binding to R-SMADs, preventing nuclear translocation. (b) SMAD6 also cooperates with SMURF1, an E3 ubiquitin ligase, to induce ubiquitin-mediated proteasomal degradation of R-SMADs, BMP receptor complexes, and RUNX2.

had higher incidence of intellectual disability than those without, suggesting that a genetically driven intrinsic brain development anomaly is also contributing to intellectual disability in NSC craniosynostosis (Wu et al., 2020).

24.16 Summary

In syndromic craniosynostosis, well-defined genetic drivers cause severe deformity as well as intrinsic brain malformation. In NSC, emerging data suggest a polygenic etiology. Surgical release does not just address esthetic concerns and the occasional symptomatic intracranial hypertension, but also provides a potential for cognitive benefit. Surgery should be performed as early as safely possible, in order to provide the greatest possible relief of cortical compression and distortion. Further study is needed to elucidate the full genetic role in the non-syndromic craniosynostosis, and to begin to develop treatments that can address the developmental anomalies, potentially in brain matter.

Figure acknowledgement

The following image has been reproduced from Timberlake et al., 2016, with permission: Figure 24.1

References

Adeeb N, Mortazavi MM, Tubbs RS, Cohen-Gadol AA. The cranial dura mater: a review of its history, embryology, and anatomy. *Childs Nerv Syst* 2012;**28**(6):827–37. https://doi.org/10.1007/s00381-012-1744-6.

Agochukwu NB, Solomon BD, Muenke M. Impact of genetics on the diagnosis and clinical management of syndromic craniosynostoses. *Childs Nerv Syst* 2012;**28**(9):1447–63. https://doi.org/10.1007/s00381-012-1756-2.

Aldridge K, Kane AA, Marsh JL, Yan P, Govier D, Richtsmeier JT. Relationship of brain and skull in pre- and postoperative sagittal synostosis. *J Anat* 2005;**206**(4):373–85. https://doi.org/10.1111/j.1469-7580.2005.00397.x.

Azoury SC, Reddy S, Shukla V, Deng C-X. Fibroblast Growth Factor Receptor 2 (*FGFR2*) mutation related syndromic craniosynostosis. *Int J Biol Sci* 2017;**13**(12):1479–88. https://doi.org/10.7150/ijbs.22373.

Becker DB, Petersen JD, Kane AA, Cradock MM, Pilgram TK, Marsh JL. Speech, cognitive, and behavioral outcomes in nonsyndromic craniosynostosis. *Plast Reconstr Surg* 2005;**116**(2):400–7. https://doi.org/10.1097/01.prs.0000172763.71043.b8.

Beckett JS, Brooks ED, Lacadie C, et al. Altered brain connectivity in sagittal craniosynostosis. *J Neurosurg Pediatr* 2014;**13**(6):690–8. https://doi.org/10.3171/2014.3.PEDS13516.

Bolthauser E, Ludwig S, Dietrich F, Landolt MA. Sagittal craniosynostosis: cognitive development, behaviour, and quality of life in unoperated children. *Neuropediatrics* 2003;**34**(6):293–300. https://doi.org/10.1055/s-2003-44667.

Bonfield CM, Foley LM, Kundu S, et al. The influence of surgical correction on white matter microstructural integrity in rabbits with familial coronal suture craniosynostosis. *Neurosurg Focus* 2015;**38**(5):E3. https://doi.org/10.3171/2015.2.FOCUS14849.

Bottero L, Lajeunie E, Arnaud E, Marchac D, Renier D. Functional outcome after surgery for trigonocephaly. *Plast Reconstr Surg* 1998;**102**(4):952–8; discussion 959–60.

Boulet SL, Rasmussen SA, Honein MA. A population-based study of craniosynostosis in metropolitan Atlanta, 1989–2003. *Am J Med Genet A* 2008;**146A**(8):984–91. https://doi.org/10.1002/ajmg.a.32208.

Boyadjiev S, for the International Craniosynostosis Consortium. Genetic analysis of non-syndromic craniosynostosis. *Orthod Craniofac Res* 2007;**10**(3):129–37. https://doi.org/10.1111/j.1601-6343.2007.00393.x.

Brooks ED, Yang J, Beckett JS, et al. Normalization of brain morphology after surgery in sagittal craniosynostosis. *J Neurosurg Pediatr* 2016;**17**(4):460–8. https://doi.org/10.3171/2015.7.PEDS15221.

Cabrejo R, Lacadie C, Brooks E, et al. Understanding the learning disabilities linked to sagittal craniosynostosis. *J Craniofac Surg* 2019a;**30**(2):497–502. https://doi.org/10.1097/SCS.0000000000005194.

Cabrejo R, Lacadie C, Chuang C, et al. What is the functional difference between sagittal with metopic and isolated sagittal craniosynotosis? *J Craniofac Surg* 2019b;**30**(4):968–73. https://doi.org/10.1097/SCS.0000000000005288.

Cariboni A, Maggi R. Kallmann's syndrome, a neuronal migration defect. *Cell Mol Life Sci* 2006;**63**(21):2512–26. https://doi.org/10.1007/s00018-005-5604-3.

Christensen FK, Clark DB. The effect of restricted suture growth on brain growth in dogs. *Surg Forum* 1970;**21**:439–40. https://doi.org/10.3389/fcell.2021.653579.

Chuang C, Rolison M, Yang JF, et al. Normalization of speech processing after whole-vault cranioplasty in sagittal synostosis: *J Craniofac Surg* 2018;**29**(5):1132–6. https://doi.org/10.1097/SCS.0000000000004474.

Church MW, Parent-Jenkins L, Rozzelle AA, Eldis FE, Kazzi SNJ. Auditory brainstem response abnormalities and hearing loss in children with craniosynostosis. *Pediatrics* 2007;**119**(6):e1351–60. https://doi.org/10.1542/peds.2006-3009.

Churchill JD, Grossman AW, Irwin SA, et al. A converging-methods approach to fragile X syndrome. *Dev Psychobiol* 2002;**40**(3):323–338. https://doi.org/10.1002/dev.10036.

Ciurea AV, Toader C. Genetics of craniosynostosis: review of the literature. *J Med Life* 2009;**2**(1):5–17.

Cohen SR, Persing JA. Intracranial pressure in single-suture craniosynostosis. *Cleft Palate–Craniofacial J* 1998;**35**(3):194–6. https://doi.org/10.1597/1545-1569_1998_035_0194_ipissc_2 .3.co_2.

Collett BR, Kapp-Simon KA, Wallace E, Cradock MM, Buono L, Speltz ML. Attention and executive function in children with and without single-suture craniosynostosis. *Child Neuropsychol* 2017;**23**(1):83–98. https://doi.org/10.1080/09297049 .2015.1085005.

Collmann H, Sörensen N, Krauß J. Hydrocephalus in craniosynostosis: a review. *Childs Nerv Syst* 2005;**21**(10):902–12. https://doi.org/10.1007/s00381-004-1116-y.

Cradock MM, Gray KE, Kapp-Simon KA, Collett BR, Buono LA, Speltz ML. Sex differences in the neurodevelopment of school-age children with and without single-suture craniosynostosis. *Childs Nerv Syst* 2015;**31**(7):1103–11. https:// doi.org/10.1007/s00381-015-2671-0.

Creuzet SE, Martinez S, Le Douarin NM. The cephalic neural crest exerts a critical effect on forebrain and midbrain development. *Proc Natl Acad Sci* 2006;**103**(38):14033–8. https:// doi.org/10.1073/pnas.0605899103.

Da Costa AC, Walters I, Savarirayan R, Anderson VA, Wrennall JA, Meara JG. Intellectual outcomes in children and adolescents with syndromic and nonsyndromic craniosynostosis. *Plast Reconstr Surg* 2006;**118**(1):175–81. https://doi.org/10.1097/01.prs.0000221009.93022.50.

David LR, Wilson JA, Watson NE, Argenta LC. Cerebral perfusion defects secondary to simple craniosynostosis. *J Craniofac Surg* 1996;**7**(3):177–85. https://doi.org/10.1097/000 01665-199605000-00003.

de Jong T, Maliepaard M, Bannink N, Raat H, Mathijssen IMJ. Health-related problems and quality of life in patients with syndromic and complex craniosynostosis. *Childs Nerv Syst* 2012;**28**(6):879–82. https://doi.org/10.1007/s00381-012-1681-4.

Delahaye S, Bernard JP, Rénier D, Ville Y. Prenatal ultrasound diagnosis of fetal craniosynostosis: fetal craniosynostosis. *Ultrasound Obstet Gynecol* 2003;**21**(4):347–53. https://doi.org/ 10.1002/uog.91.

Delashaw JB, Persing JA, Broaddus WC, Jane JA. Cranial vault growth in craniosynostosis. *J Neurosurg* 1989;**70**(2):159–65. https://doi.org/10.3171/jns.1989.70.2.0159.

Di Rocco F, Arnaud E, Renier D. Evolution in the frequency of nonsyndromic craniosynostosis: clinical article. *J Neurosurg Pediatr* 2009;**4**(1):21–5. https://doi.org/10.3171/2009.3 .PEDS08355.

Doerga PN, Lequin MH, Dremmen MHG, et al. Cerebral blood flow in children with syndromic craniosynostosis: cohort arterial spin labeling studies. *J Neurosurg Pediatr* 2020;**25** (4):340–50. https://doi.org/10.3171/2019.10.PEDS19150.

Doherty P, Walsh FS. CAM–FGF receptor interactions: a model for axonal growth. *Mol Cell Neurosci* 1996;**8**(2–3):99–111. https://doi.org/10.1006/mcne.1996.0049.

Donati R, Landi A, Rovati LC, et al. Neurophysiological evaluation with multimodality evoked potentials in craniostenosis and craniofacial stenosis. *J Craniofac Surg* 1997;**8** (4):286–9. https://doi.org/10.1097/00001665-199707000-00011.

Engel M, Hoffmann J, Mühling J, Castrillón-Oberndorfer G, Seeberger R, Freudlsperger C. Magnetic resonance imaging in isolated sagittal synostosis. *J Craniofac Surg* 2012;**23**(4):e366–9. https://doi.org/10.1097/SCS.0b013e3182543258.

Fellows-Mayle W, Hitchens TK, Simplaceanu E, et al. Testing causal mechanisms of nonsyndromic craniosynostosis using path analysis of cranial contents in rabbits with uncorrected craniosynostosis. *Cleft Palate Craniofac J* 2006;**43**(5):524–31. https://doi.org/10.1597/05-107.

Florisson JMG, Dudink J, Koning IV, et al. Assessment of white matter microstructural integrity in children with syndromic craniosynostosis: a diffusion-tensor imaging study. *Radiology* 2011;**261**(2):534–41. https://doi.org/10.1148/radiol.11101024.

Gabrick KS, Wu RT, Singh A, Persing JA, Alperovich M. Radiographic severity of metopic craniosynostosis correlates with long-term neurocognitive outcomes. *Plast Reconstr Surg* 2020;**145**(5):1241–8. https://doi.org/10.1097/PRS .0000000000006746.

Grandhi R, Peitz GW, Foley LM, et al. The influence of suturectomy on age-related changes in cerebral blood flow in rabbits with familial bicoronal suture craniosynostosis: a quantitative analysis. *PLoS One* 2018;**13**(6):e0197296. https:// doi.org/10.1371/journal.pone.0197296.

Graziani LJ, Weitzman ED, Velasco MS. Neurologic maturation and auditory evoked responses in low birth weight infants. *Pediatrics* 1968;**41**(2):483–94.

Guttorm TK, Leppänen PHT, Hämäläinen JA, Eklund KM, Lyytinen HJ. Newborn event-related potentials predict poorer pre-reading skills in children at risk for dyslexia. *J Learn Disabil* 2010;**43**(5):391–401. https://doi.org/:10.1177/002221 9409345005.

Hack M, Taylor HG, Drotar D, et al. Poor predictive validity of the Bayley Scales of Infant Development for cognitive function of extremely low birth weight children at school age. *Pediatrics* 2005;**116**(2):333–41. https://doi.org/10 .1542/peds.2005-0173.

Hashim PW, Patel A, Yang JF, et al. The effects of whole-vault cranioplasty versus strip craniectomy on long-term neuropsychological outcomes in sagittal craniosynostosis. *Plast Reconstr Surg* 2014;**134**(3):491–501. https://doi.org/10.1097/PR S.0000000000000420.

Hebert JM. FGF signaling through *FGFR1* is required for olfactory bulb morphogenesis. *Development* 2003;**130**(6):1101– 11. https://doi.org/10.1242/dev.00334.

Heller JB, Heller MM, Knoll B, Gabbay JS, Duncan C, Persing JA. Intracranial volume and cephalic index outcomes for total calvarial reconstruction among nonsyndromic sagittal synostosis patients. *Plast Reconstr Surg* 2008;**121**(1):187–95. https://doi.org/10.1097/01.prs.0000293762.71115.c5.

Hukki A, Koljonen V, Karppinen A, Valanne L, Leikola J. Brain anomalies in 121 children with non-syndromic single suture craniosynostosis by MR imaging. *Eur J Paediatr Neurol* 2012;**16** (6):671–5. https://doi.org/10.1016/j.ejpn.2012.04.003.

Inglis-Broadgate SL, Thomson RE, Pellicano F, et al. *FGFR3* regulates brain size by controlling progenitor cell proliferation and apoptosis during embryonic development. *Dev Biol* 2005;**279** (1):73–85. https://doi.org/10.1016/j.ydbio.2004.11.035.

Jessell TM, Sanes JR. Development. *Curr Opin Neurobiol* 2000;**10** (5):599–611. https://doi.org/10.1016/S0959-4388(00)00136-7.

Kamiguchi H, Lemmon V. Neural cell adhesion molecule L1: signaling pathways and growth cone motility. *J Neurosci Res* 1997;**49**(1):1–8. https://doi.org/10.1002/(sici)1097-4547(19970701)49:1<1::aid-jnr1>3.0.co;2-h.

Kapp-Simon KA, Speltz ML, Cunningham ML, Patel PK, Tomita T. Neurodevelopment of children with single suture craniosynostosis: a review. *Childs Nerv Syst* 2007;**23**(3):269–81. https://doi.org/10.1007/s00381-006-0251-z.

Kljajić M, Maltese G, Tarnow P, Sand P, Kölby L. The cognitive profile of children with nonsyndromic craniosynostosis. *Plast Reconstr Surg* 2019;**143**(5):1037e–52e. https://doi.org/10.1097/PRS.0000000000005515.

Kostović I, Judaš M, Petanjek Z, Šimić G. Ontogenesis of goal-directed behavior: anatomo-functional considerations. *Int J Psychophysiol* 1995;**19**(2):85–102. https://doi.org/10.1016/0167-8760(94)00081-O.

Kurtzberg D, Hitpert PL, Kreuzer JA, Vaughan HG. Differential maturation of cortical auditory evoked potentials to speech sounds in normal fullterm and very low-birthweight infants. *Dev Med Child Neurol* 2008;**26**(4):466–75. https://doi.org/10.1111/j.1469-8749.1984.tb04473.x.

Lajeunie E, Crimmins DW, Arnaud E, Renier D. Genetic considerations in nonsyndromic midline craniosynostoses: a study of twins and their families. *J Neurosurg Pediatr* 2005;**103** (4):353–6. https://doi.org/10.3171/ped.2005.103.4.0353.

Lajeunie E, Le Merrer M, Bonaïti-Pellie C, Marchac D, Renier D. Genetic study of scaphocephaly. *Am J Med Genet* 1996;**62**(3):282–5. https://doi.org/10.1002/(SICI)1096-8628(19960329)62:3<282::AID-AJMG15>3.0.CO;2-G.

Lajeunie E, Le Merrer M, Marchac D, Renier D. Syndromal and nonsyndromal primary trigonocephaly: analysis of a series of 237 patients. *Am J Med Genet* 1998;**75**(2):211–5. https://doi.org/10.1002/(sici)1096-8628(19980113)75:2<211::aid-ajmg19>3.0.co;2-s.

Lenton KA, Nacamuli RP, Wan DC, Helms JA, Longaker MT. Cranial suture biology. *Curr Topics Devel Biol* 2005;**66**:287–328. https://doi.org/10.1016/S0070-2153(05)66009-7.

Levitt P. Structural and functional maturation of the developing primate brain. *J Pediatr* 2003;**143**(4):35–45. https://doi.org/10.1067/S0022-3476(03)00400-1.

Liasis A. Monitoring visual function in children with syndromic craniosynostosis: a comparison of 3 methods. *Arch Ophthalmol* 2006;**124**(8):1119. https://doi.org/10.1001/archopht.124.8.1119.

Lu X, Forte AJ, Steinbacher DM, Alperovich M, Alonso N, Persing JA. Enlarged anterior cranial fossa and restricted posterior cranial fossa, the disproportionate growth of basicranium in Crouzon syndrome. *J Cranio-Maxillofac Surg* 2019;**47**(9):1426–35. https://doi.org/10.1016/j.jcms.2019.06.003.

Lu X, Sawh-Martinez R, Forte AJ, et al. Classification of subtypes of Crouzon syndrome based on the type of vault suture synostosis. *J Craniofac Surg* 2020;**31**(3):678–84. https://doi.org/10.1097/SCS.0000000000006173.

Magge SN, Westerveld M, Pruzinsky T, Persing JA. Long-term neuropsychological effects of sagittal craniosynostosis on child development. *J Craniofac Surg* 2002;**13**(1):99–104. https://doi.org/10.1097/00001665-200201000-00023.

Martini M, Röhrig A, Wenghoefer M, Schindler E, Messing-Jünger AM. Cerebral oxygenation and hemodynamic measurements during craniosynostosis surgery with near-infrared spectroscopy. *Childs Nerv Syst* 2014;**30**(8):1367–74. https://doi.org/10.1007/s00381-014-2418-3.

Molfese DL. Predicting dyslexia at 8 years of age using neonatal brain responses. *Brain Lang* 2000;**72**(3):238–45. https://doi.org/10.1006/brln.2000.2287.

Mooney MP, Siegel MI, Burrows AM, et al. A rabbit model of human familial, nonsyndromic unicoronal suture synostosis I. Synostotic onset, pathology, and sutural growth patterns. *Childs Nerv Syst* 1998;**14**(6):236–46. https://doi.org/10.1007/s003810050219.

Morton JB, Munakata Y. What's the difference? Contrasting modular and neural network approaches to understanding developmental variability. *J Dev Behav Pediatr* 2005;**26**(2):128–39. https://doi.org/10.1097/00004703-200504000-00010.

Moss ML, Salentijn L. The primary role of functional matrices in facial growth. *Am J Orthod* 1969;**55**(6):566–77. https://doi.org/10.1016/0002-9416(69)90034-7.

Munakata Y, Casey BJ, Diamond A. Developmental cognitive neuroscience: progress and potential. *Trends Cogn Sci* 2004;**8** (3):122–8. https://doi.org/10.1016/j.tics.2004.01.005.

Mursch K, Brockmann K, Lang JK, Markakis E, Behnke-Mursch J. Visually evoked potentials in 52 children requiring operative repair of craniosynostosis. *Pediatr Neurosurg* 1998;**29** (6):320–3. https://doi.org/10.1159/000028746.

Novak GP, Kurtzberg D, Kreuzer JA, Vaughan HG. Cortical responses to speech sounds and their formants in normal infants: maturational sequence and spatiotemporal analysis. *Electroencephalogr Clin Neurophysiol* 1989;**73**(4):295–305. https://doi.org/10.1016/0013-4694(89)90108-9.

Passos-Bueno MR, Sertié AL, Jehee FS, Fanganiello R, Yeh E. Genetics of craniosynostosis: genes, syndromes, mutations and genotype–phenotype correlations. In Rice DP (Ed.), *Frontiers of Oral Biology*, Vol **12**. S. KARGER AG; 2008; pp. 107–43. https://doi.org/10.1159/000115035.

Patel A, Yang JF, Hashim PW, et al. The impact of age at surgery on long-term neuropsychological outcomes in sagittal craniosynostosis. *Plast Reconstr Surg* 2014;**134**(4):608e–17e. https://doi.org/10.1097/PRS.0000000000000511.

Persing JA, Babler WJ, Jane JA, Duckworth PF. Experimental unilateral coronal synostosis in rabbits. *Plast Reconstr Surg* 1986;**77**(3):369–76. https://doi.org/10.1097/00006534-198603000-00003.

Persing JA, Jane JA. Craniosynostosis. *Semin Neurol* 1989;**9**(3):200–09. https://doi.org/10.1055/s-2008-1041326.

Persson KM, Roy WA, Persing JA, Rodeheaver GT, Winn HR. Craniofacial growth following experimental craniosynostosis and craniectomy in rabbits. *J Neurosurg* 1979;**50**(2):187–97. https://doi.org/10.3171/jns.1979.50.2.0187.

Proudman TW, Clark BE, Moore MH, Abbott AH, David DJ. Central nervous system imaging in Crouzon's syndrome: *J Craniofac Surg* 1995;**6**(5):401–05. https://doi.org/10.1097/00001665-199509000-00016.

Quintero-Rivera F, Robson CD, Reiss RE, et al. Intracranial anomalies detected by imaging studies in 30 patients with Apert syndrome. *Am J Med Genet A* 2006;**140A**(12):1337–8. https://doi.org/10.1002/ajmg.a.31277.

Raybaud C, Di Rocco C. Brain malformation in syndromic craniosynostoses, a primary disorder of white matter: a review. *Childs Nerv Syst* 2007;**23**(12):1379–88. https://doi.org/10.1007/s00381-007-0474-7.

Renier D, Lajeunie E, Arnaud E, Marchac D. Management of craniosynostoses. *Childs Nerv Syst* 2000;**16**(10–11):645–58. https://doi.org/10.1007/s003810000320.

Renier D, Sainte-Rose C, Marchac D, Hirsch J-F. Intracranial pressure in craniostenosis. *J Neurosurg* 1982;**57**(3):370–7. https://doi.org/10.3171/jns.1982.57.3.0370.

Richtsmeier JT, Aldridge K, DeLeon VB, et al. Phenotypic integration of neurocranium and brain. *J Exp Zoolog B Mol Dev Evol* 2006;**306B**(4):360–78. https://doi.org/10.1002/jez.b.21092.

Rijken BFM, Leemans A, Lucas Y, van Montfort K, Mathijssen IMJ, Lequin MH. Diffusion tensor imaging and fiber tractography in children with craniosynostosis syndromes. *Am J Neuroradiol* 2015;**36**(8):1558–64. https://doi.org/10.3174/ajnr.A4301.

Salazar V, Gamer L, Rosen V. BMP signalling in skeletal development, disease and repair. *Nat Rev Endocrinol* 2016;**12**:203–21. https://doi.org/10.1038/nrendo.2016.1.

Satoh M, Ishikawa N, Enomoto T, Takeda T, Yoshizawa T, Nose T. [Study by I-123-IMP-SPECT before and after surgery for craniosynostosis]. *Kaku Igaku* 1990;**27**(12):1411–8.

Selber J, Reid RR, Chike-Obi CJ, et al. The changing epidemiologic spectrum of single-suture synostoses. *Plast Reconstr Surg* 2008;**122**(2):527–33. https://doi.org/10.1097/PRS.0b013e31817d548c.

Sen A, Dougal P, Padhy AK, et al. Technetium-99m-HMPAO SPECT cerebral blood flow study in children with craniosynostosis. *J Nucl Med* 1995;**36**(3):394–8.

Sun AH, Eilbott J, Chuang C, et al. An investigation of brain functional connectivity by form of craniosynostosis. *J Craniofac*

Surg 2019;**30**(6):1719–23. https://doi.org/10.1097/SCS.0000000000005537.

Thiele-Nygaard AE, Foss-Skiftesvik J, Juhler M. Intracranial pressure, brain morphology and cognitive outcome in children with sagittal craniosynostosis. *Childs Nerv Syst* 2020;**36**(4):689–95. https://doi.org/10.1007/s00381-020-04502-z.

Thompson DA, Liasis A, Hardy S, et al. Prevalence of abnormal pattern reversal visual evoked potentials in craniosynostosis. *Plast Reconstr Surg* 2006;**118**(1):184–92. https://doi.org/10.1097/01.prs.0000220873.72953.3e.

Thwin M, Schultz TJ, Anderson PJ. Morphological, functional and neurological outcomes of craniectomy versus cranial vault remodeling for isolated nonsyndromic synostosis of the sagittal suture: a systematic review. *JBI Database Syst Rev Implement Rep* 2015;**13**(9):309–68. https://doi.org/10.11124/jbisrir-2015-2470.

Timberlake AT, Choi J, Zaidi S, et al. Two locus inheritance of non-syndromic midline craniosynostosis via rare *SMAD6* and common *BMP2* alleles. *eLife* 2016;**5**. https://doi.org/10.7554/eLife.20125.

Timberlake AT, Jin SC, Nelson-Williams C, et al. Mutations in *TFAP2B* and previously unimplicated genes of the BMP, Wnt, and Hedgehog pathways in syndromic craniosynostosis. *Proc Natl Acad Sci U S A* 2019;**116**(30):15116–21. https://doi.org/10.1073/pnas.1902041116.

Timberlake AT, Persing JA. Genetics of nonsyndromic craniosynostosis. *Plast Reconstr Surg* 2018;**141**(6):1508–16. https://doi.org/10.1097/PRS.0000000000004374.

Tokumaru AM, Barkovich AJ, Ciricillo SF, Edwards MS. Skull base and calvarial deformities: association with intracranial changes in craniofacial syndromes. *Am J Neuroradiol* 1996;**17**(4):619–30.

Tonni G, Panteghini M, Rossi A, et al. Craniosynostosis: prenatal diagnosis by means of ultrasound and SSSE-MRI. Family series with report of neurodevelopmental outcome and review of the literature. *Arch Gynecol Obstet* 2011;**283**(4):909–16. https://doi.org/10.1007/s00404-010-1643-6.

Wu RT, Timberlake AT, Abraham PF, et al. *SMAD6* genotype predicts neurodevelopment in nonsyndromic craniosynostosis. *Plast Reconstr Surg* 2020;**145**(1):117e–25e. https://doi.org/10.1097/PRS.0000000000006319.

Wu RT, Yang JF, Zucconi W, et al. Frustration and emotional regulation in nonsyndromic craniosynostosis: a functional magnetic resonance imaging study. *Plast Reconstr Surg* 2019;**144**(6):1371–83. https://doi.org/10.1097/PRS.0000000000005850.

Yacubian-Fernandes A, Palhares A, Giglio A, et al. Apert syndrome: analysis of associated brain malformations and conformational changes determined by surgical treatment. *J Neuroradiol* 2004;**31**(2):116–22. https://doi.org/10.1016/S0150-9861(04)96978-7.

Yang JF, Brooks ED, Hashim PW, et al. The severity of deformity in metopic craniosynostosis is correlated with the degree of neurologic dysfunction. *Plast Reconstr Surg* 2017;**139**(2):442–7. https://doi.org/10.1097/PRS.0000000000002952.

Chapter 25

Hydrocephalus

Benjamin C. Reeves, Jason K. Karimy, Phan Q. Duy, and Kristopher T. Kahle

25.1 Introduction

Hydrocephalus was historically defined according to Dandy's bulk flow model as the progressive distension of the brain's ventricular system that results from inadequate passage of cerebrospinal fluid (CSF) from its main site of production at the choroid plexus epithelium (CPe) to its site(s) of reabsorption into the systemic circulation (Rekate, 2009). Alternative hydrodynamic models that account for additional factors such as cardiac pulsatility (Benveniste et al., 2017; Brinker et al., 2014) and emerging data regarding proposed alternative sources of both CSF production and reabsorption (e.g., glymphatic pathways) are modifying this model and revealing the complexity of CSF homeostasis. In addition, genetic analyses are uncovering novel mechanisms of primary (congenital) hydrocephalus in humans, indicating that many inherited and spontaneous forms of hydrocephalus may reflect altered regulation of neural stem cell fate (Furey et al., 2018). Regardless of etiology, hydrocephalus is often characterized by increased intracranial pressure, ventricular enlargement from CSF build-up, and structural brain damage that, left untreated, can lead to progressive neurological decline, coma, and death (Kahle et al., 2016).

Hydrocephalus is a frequent complication of multiple CNS insults associated with neuroinflammation, including hemorrhage, infection, and trauma (Dewan et al., 2018; Kahle et al., 2016; Karimy et al., 2016, 2017). Post-hemorrhagic hydrocephalus (PHH) and post-infectious hydrocephalus (PIH) constitute two of the most common forms of hydrocephalus worldwide (Dewan et al., 2018; Kahle et al., 2016). Although many patients with these disorders have no discernible physical impediment to CSF flow in the ventricular and subarachnoid spaces, the traditional paradigm of these disorders has predominately centered on obstructive mechanisms that prevent CSF reabsorption (Cherian et al., 2004; Strahle et al., 2012). In line with such understanding, surgical CSF diversion – achieved primarily by permanent, implantable ventricular shunts – remains a mainstay of care for many patients requiring neurosurgical management. While these procedures are life-saving, they carry significant morbidity due to their high failure and complication rates (Reddy et al., 2014). Additionally, these treatments are often not available in many lower-income countries due to lack of resources and specialized personnel, including neuro-intensivists and neurosurgeons (Kahle et al., 2016).

One fundamental obstacle to developing more effective treatments for hydrocephalus, including non-surgical medical therapies, is our limited knowledge of the molecular physiology of the CPe. The CPe is a remarkable but historically neglected brain structure that serves, at least in animals, both as the principal blood–CSF immune barrier and the main source of CSF (Damkier et al., 2013). Choroid plexus epithelium "immuno-secretory" plasticity, manifest as an inflammatory CSF hypersecretory response dependent on toll-like receptor-4 (TLR4) signaling and SPAK-NKCC1-mediated CSF secretion, appears important to development of acute ventriculomegaly in experimental PHH (Karimy et al., 2017). Common features of PIH and PHH include CPe inflammation (Barichello et al., 2013; Gram et al., 2013, 2014; Karimy et al., 2017; Simard et al., 2011), increased CSF levels of TLR4-NF-κB-regulated cytokines, and increased immune cells (Barichello et al., 2013; Fassbender et al., 1997; Gram et al., 2013, 2014; Habiyaremye et al., 2017; Karimy et al., 2017; Krebs et al., 2005; Lahrtz et al., 1998; Simard et al., 2011), suggesting the question: might acute PIH and PHH be driven by similar mechanisms?

In this chapter, we briefly review the current epidemiology, etiology, and clinical treatment paradigms of PHH and PIH. Within this context, we highlight several recent findings that demonstrate the important role of CPe inflammation in pathogenesis of acute PHH and suggest this may also play an important role in PIH. We suggest that the concept of "inflammatory hydrocephalus" may better account for shared mechanisms and therapeutic vulnerabilities of PHH/PIH. We propose that two critical functions of the CPe – immune function and CSF secretion – become maladaptively entangled in an epithelial "response-to-injury" that manifests as the acute inflammation-dependent hypersecretion of CSF. We also speculate that sustained, chronic inflammation propagated by ongoing injury to CPe, ependymal cells, and brain tissue, with resulting release of host-derived damage-associated molecular patterns (DAMPs), likely impacts other resorptive aspects of CSF homeostasis. The mechanism of impaired CSF homeostasis at this stage may be due to intraventricular obstruction from secondary ependymal scar formation or extraventricular obstruction via arachnoidal scar impairment of glymphatic pathways. This model may describe the *dynamic* pathologic changes in PHH/PIH across time (acute versus chronic) and space (CPe versus ependyma versus aqueduct versus glymphatics, etc.) better than previous models. Nonetheless, we emphasize that *inflammation*, a common pathologic driver throughout this complex process, is mediated by specific molecules that may serve as therapeutic targets. As such, an improved understanding of the shared pathophysiology of these forms of secondary hydrocephalus may catalyze discovery of agents relevant for both PHH/PIH.

25.2 Post-Hemorrhagic and Post–Infectious Hydrocephalus: Diseases of Prosperity and Poverty

Despite an apparent myriad of etiologies, hydrocephalus has historically been classified into categories of primary (i.e., congenital) or secondary (e.g., due to hemorrhage, infection, trauma, or tumor) hydrocephalus. Hydrocephalus affects individuals of all age groups and imposes a heavy physical, emotional, and socioeconomic burden worldwide (Isaacs et al., 2018). Until recently, worldwide statistics have been difficult to estimate due to lack of consistent reporting (Dewan et al., 2018). A recent global meta-analysis from Dewan et al. (2018) has revealed interesting differences between higher- and lower-income countries in burden of hydrocephalus. The epidemiology of PHH and PIH (secondary forms of hydrocephalus) appears driven by socioeconomic status, with PIH predominating among children of poorer countries in which neonatal and infant infections are more common (Dewan et al., 2018). Together, PHH/PIH likely account for the majority of hydrocephalus cases worldwide.

Post-hemorrhagic hydrocephalus is the most common cause of acquired pediatric hydrocephalus in higher-income countries (Warf et al., 2011), occurring in ~38 neonates per 100,000 live births (Dewan et al., 2018; Warf et al., 2011). It occurs primarily in very low birth weight (VLBW) preterm neonates (<1500 g) due to germinal matrix hemorrhage (Chen et al., 2017; Tsitouras and Sgouros, 2011), and is often fatal in the absence of adequate prenatal, neonatal intensive, and neurosurgical care (Murphy et al., 2002). Accordingly, infant PHH is underrepresented in countries that lack these resources (Dewan et al., 2018; Warf et al., 2011). For example, in East Africa, with sparse neonatal resources and 1 neurosurgeon per ~10,000,000 people (Warf, 2010), most VLBW neonates do not survive (Warf et al., 2011). Post-hemorrhagic hydrocephalus is also a common cause of adult hydrocephalus (Bir et al., 2016; Chahlavi et al., 2001; Chen et al., 2017), often associated with intraventricular hemorrhage (IVH) due to hypertensive hemorrhage, aneurysm rupture, and traumatic brain injury (Cioca et al., 2014). As lifespan increases worldwide, and poor countries increasingly adopt Westernized diets with associated increases in hypertension and diabetes (Sacks et al., 2001; Shang et al., 2012), the prevalence of adult PHH will likely also grow.

Post-infectious hydrocephalus is the most common cause of pediatric hydrocephalus worldwide (Kahle et al., 2016), with highest prevalence in Africa, Latin America, and Southeast Asia (Dewan et al., 2018). The combination of increased peripartum infections, hygienically challenging neonatal environments, and lack of advanced obstetric care likely explain why PIH is more common than PHH in lower income countries (Muir et al., 2016; Warf, 2010). The complex bacterial diversity of CSF samples from PHH patients in developing countries, with their limited access to more advanced clinical microbiological diagnostics, has contributed to difficulties in identifying individual causative organisms (Li et al., 2011). This is likely reflects regional differences in bacteria flora associated with living conditions (e.g., proximity to farm animals; Li et al., 2011), access to prenatal care (Dewan et al., 2018; Li et al., 2011), and seasonal changes in rainfall (Schiff et al., 2012). Seasonal meningitis within the African meningitis belt is also associated with PIH (Aziz, 1976). Interestingly, congenital Zika virus has been shown to cause severe hydrocephalus in Brazil (van der Linden et al., 2019). In endemic areas such as South Africa (Kamat et al., 2018), India (Aranha et al., 2018; Rajshekar, 2009), China (Li et al., 2017), and Philippines (Lee, 2000), post-tuberculosis hydrocephalus constitutes a considerable disease burden. In higher-income countries, PIH due to prenatal infections is often caused by *Toxoplasma gondii* and cytomegalovirus (CMV), whereas typical neonatal etiologies include bacterial sepsis from *Escherichia coli*, *Streptococcus agalactiae*, and *Listeria monocytogenes* (Kahle et al., 2016; Li et al., 2011; Kulkarni et al., 2017). Among adults, the most common causes of bacterial PIH include *Neisseria meningitidis* and *Streptococcus pneumoniae* (Thigpen et al., 2011), although viral, fungal, and protozoan infections have been implicated in immunocompromised patients (Liu et al., 2018; Pyrgos et al., 2013).

25.3 Current Hydrocephalus Treatments: Neurosurgery, When Available

The current treatment paradigm for hydrocephalus involves CSF ventriculo-peritoneal shunting or endoscopic third ventriculostomy, with or without choroid plexus cauterization (ETV/CPC; i.e., endoscopic fenestration of the third ventricular floor to provide an alternate pathway for CSF reabsorption, coupled with electrothermal destruction of the CPe; see below). Shunting is perhaps the most common treatment for PHH and PIH among all age groups (Kahle et al., 2016; Kulkarni, 2016; Kulkarni et al., 2017; Stagno et al., 2013; Warf, 2005a, 2005b). This generally involves subcutaneously tunneling silastic tubing from the cerebral ventricles to the peritoneal cavity, with an interposed valve to prevent CSF over drainage (Kahle et al., 2016). The benefits of shunting include lower rate of failure in the early months following surgery (Kulkarni, 2016; Kulkarni et al., 2010), immediate decrease in ventricular size on imaging (Kahle et al., 2016; Kulkarni, 2016), and the requirement for only moderate technical expertise (Baird, 2016). However, shunts are often plagued with mechanical obstructions/malfunction, tubing complications, and infections. The high likelihood of shunt failure creates for shunt-dependent patients a lifelong need for access to immediate neurosurgical care (Kulkarni et al., 2010). Indeed, shunt failure is the most common medical device failure in the US, with 2- and 10-year failure rates of >50% and 70%, respectively, significantly decreasing quality of life (Kahle et al., 2016; Kulkarni et al., 2013).

The alternative to shunting is ETV/CPC, which has been increasingly utilized used for the treatment of infants with both PHH and PIH worldwide (Drake et al., 2009; Kulkarni et al., 2009). Benefits of ETV/CPC include lower chance of failure long term (Kulkarni et al., 2010), elimination of hardware complications (Pindrik et al., 2013), and, in infants below 6 months of age, cognitive development outcomes and brain growth comparable to shunting, although with lesser reduction in imaged ventricular size (Kulkarni et al., 2017; Limbrick et al., 2014). Drawbacks to ETV/CPC include the requirement for more advanced technical expertise (Kulkarni et al., 2014), a higher rate of short-term failure, and an unclear impact on other critical functions of the CPe, including immune function, nutrient reabsorption, and neurodevelopment (Marques et al., 2017). However, recent data indicate that ETV/CPC is the preferred option in poorer countries with limited access to urgent neurosurgical care, as well as in some other countries (Kulkarni et al., 2017).

25.4 Pathobiology of Post-Hemorrhagic and Post-Infectious Hydrocephalus: Beyond the "Plugged Drain"

It is widely accepted that PHH and PIH result from intraventricular CSF accumulation due to failed homeostasis mechanisms. Classical models of CSF dynamics hold that PHH/PIH result from a primary decrease in CSF reabsorption due to obstruction of intraventricular CSF flow and/or dysfunction of extraventricular arachnoid granulations (Murphy et al., 2002; Strahle et al., 2012). Some older case series reported occlusion of the fourth ventricular outflow tracts by fibrous thickening of the leptomeninges, creating "tetra-ventricular" hydrocephalus following hemorrhage (Larroche, 1972; Omar et al., 2018). Others suggested that blood and its breakdown products acutely obstruct narrow CSF passages such as the cerebral aqueduct (Lategan et al., 2010; Whitelaw, 2001). Some authors have implicated the arachnoid granulations in an attempt to explain cases of communicating hydrocephalus following IVH. Microthrombi and debris from IVH may plug arachnoid villi and impair CSF reabsorption; obliterative arachnoiditis at the posterior fossa may hinder CSF flow (Hill et al., 1984). Indeed, in some cases of PIH and PHH, frank obstruction from intraventricular blood clot, or a scarred-over aqueduct are apparent and causative, and combinations of the above mechanisms likely contribute to development of hydrocephalus, especially in the chronic setting (see below).

Despite these reports, however, the above paradigm: (i) is supported by sparse experimental evidence (Chen et al., 2017; Karimy et al., 2017); (ii) neglects potential roles of increased CSF secretion (Karimy et al., 2016, 2017); (iii) overlooks CPe inflammation in human tissue and/or animal models of PHH/PIH (Barichello et al., 2013; Gram et al., 2013, 2014; Karimy et al., 2017; Krebs et al., 2005; Simard et al., 2011); (iv) fails to acknowledge the gradual development of arachnoid granulations (believed to reabsorb much of adult CSF) in human infants and most hydrocephalus animal models (Bateman and Brown, 2012; Oi and Di Rocco, 2006); and (v) does not account for other sites of CSF reabsorption such as the ventricular ependyma, perineural space, leptomeninges, glymphatics, and nasal mucosa (Bateman and Brown, 2012; Hill et al., 1984; Lohrberg and Eilting, 2016; Miyajima and Arai, 2015; Oreskovic et al., 2017), or the role of ependymal ciliary beating on CSF bulk flow (Olstad et al., 2019). Moreover, CSF hypersecretion caused by CPe villous hyperplasia or CP tumors suffices to cause non-obstructive hydrocephalus, although these tumors may impact CSF protein composition (Karimy et al., 2016). In addition, intracerebroventricular (ICV) injection of blood metabolites suffices to cause CPe inflammation (Gram et al., 2013, 2014; Karimy et al., 2017; Krebs et al., 2005; Simard et al., 2011) and hydrocephalus (Gao et al., 2014) in animal models. These observations collectively suggest that decreased CSF reabsorption alone is probably insufficient to adequately explain PHH/PIH, and demonstrate the need for alternate, or complimentary mechanism(s) of pathogenesis.

25.5 Choroid Plexus Epithelium Immunosecretory Plasticity

The CPe consists of a single cell layer of polarized cuboidal epithelial cells surrounding fenestrated capillaries located within the cerebral ventricles. These epithelial cells are responsible for the majority of CSF production in animals (~80%; Brinker et al., 2014), and probably in humans, actively secreting sodium (Na^+), potassium (K^+), chloride (Cl^-), bicarbonate (HCO_3^-), and other ions, along with osmotically driven transport of water between blood and the ventricular space. The remainder of CSF is likely contributed by brain interstitial fluid (Brinker et al., 2014). The CPe is the most actively secreting epithelium in the human body, producing CSF at a rate of ~400–500 mL per day (~25 mL/h; Damkier et al., 2013). As such, the CPe receives more blood flow per gram of tissue than any other tissue in the body (Damkier et al., 2013; Keep and Jones, 1990), and metabolizes more ATP than any other epithelium. Accordingly, CSF secretion is subject to strict regulation and can be dynamically modified by multiple neurohumoral mechanisms (Damkier et al., 2013).

Epithelial barrier cells are constantly exposed to microbial and other environmental insults that may compromise tissue function, either by excessive activation of inflammation or by direct cell damage. The immune system's major challenge is to neutralize foreign invaders and resolve injury without inflicting collateral damage that perpetuates a chronic inflammatory cycle. Immune homeostasis is particularly challenging at barrier sites where constant exposure to immunogenic agents may induce destructive inflammation. While the role of the innate immune system has been well studied in barrier epithelia in the intestine, skin, and respiratory tract, immune functions of blood–CSF barrier (CPe) and brain–CSF barrier (ependyma) have lagged far behind.

The CPe exhibits a unique immunological plasticity that allows it to function as a tightly regulated gate separating blood and CSF compartments, and through which circulating systemic immune cells enter the brain for defense and repair in response to bleeding, infection, and injury (Praetorius and Damkier, 2017). The CPe, like other epithelia, expresses Toll-like receptors (TLRs) on both apical and basolateral membranes, along with other pattern recognition receptors, e.g., nucleotide-binding oligomerization domain-like receptors (NOD-like receptors) that bind pathogen-associated molecular patterns (PAMPs) to activate non-specific innate immune responses (Coorens et al., 2017; Medzhitov, 2007). For example, TLR4 (Karimy et al., 2017) and other TLRs (Gram et al., 2014; Skipor et al., 2015) are highly expressed in the CPe and exhibit ligand-specific regulation in response to proinflammatory stimuli (Gram et al., 2013, 2014; Karimy et al., 2017); TLRs also recognize damage-associated molecular patterns (DAMPs), or "alarmins" – molecules released from host tissue in response to injury and interpreted by adjacent cells as foreign danger signals (Miyake, 2007). TLR4 DAMPs include heat shock proteins, matrix degradation products, S100A8/S100A9 (Ehrchen et al., 2009), lysophosphatidic acid (LPA; Yang et al., 2016), and other IVH-derived blood-breakdown products (e.g., methemoglobin [metHgb] and iron) present in PHH (Fang et al., 2011; Gao et al., 2014; Kwon et al., 2015; Tsan and Gao, 2004). The Gram-negative bacterial cell wall component lipopolysaccharide (LPS), prominent in PIH cases in Western countries, is a classic PAMP and canonical TLR4 ligand that activates NF-κB-dependent cytokine production and immune cell recruitment (Praetorius and Damkier, 2017; Rivest, 2003).

25.6 TLR4-Dependent Choroid Plexus Epithelium Hypersecretion in Post-Hemorrhagic Hydrocephalus

The CPe is one of the first brain structures to encounter extravasated blood after IVH (Demeestere et al., 2015; Gram et al., 2014; Kleine and Benes, 2006). Recent animal models have shown that ICV injection of autologous blood into the lateral ventricles is sufficient to cause ventriculomegaly and intense NF-κB activation and cytokine production in CPe cells (Karimy et al., 2017; Simard et al., 2011). In rabbit pups and human infants with IVH, CSF cell-free metHgb, a blood breakdown product, strongly correlates with the TLR4-dependent cytokine TNFα, and in-vivo ICV delivery of metHgb is sufficient to cause ventriculomegaly, with associated increases in the CPe of TLR4-NF-κB, TNF-α, and IL-1β (Gram et al., 2013, 2014). At physiological concentrations, metHgb activates TLR4 homodimers or TLR4/2 heterodimers (Cox et al., 2012; Wang et al., 2014). MetHgb injected in vivo into CSF acts as a TLR4 DAMP, promoting TNF-α secretion and TLR4-dependent neuroinflammation (Cox et al., 2012; Kwon et al., 2015; Wang et al., 2014).

Interestingly, many systemic secretory epithelia respond to pro-inflammatory stimuli by increasing fluid secretion (Berkes et al., 2003). This helps maintain homeostasis by clearing pathogens or debris from the epithelial surface (Doyle et al., 1994; Wilson et al., 1987). However, the attendant inflammation, inappropriately initiated or sustained, can lead to disease vulnerabilities (Kotas and Medzhitov, 2015; Nowarski et al., 2017). For example, dysregulated epithelial inflammation and associated fluid hypersecretion can accompany chemical, autoimmune, or infectious pleuritis, colitis, pancreatitis, and other conditions (Barichello et al., 2013; Gram et al., 2014). In addition, chronic inflammation can cause tissue damage, propagating and amplifying the initial inflammatory response via the release of host-derived DAMPs from damaged barrier epithelia and other tissues. Unfortunately, the impact of inflammation on the secretory capacity of the CPe has until recently been difficult to study, reflecting a relative paucity of adequate techniques to measure and manipulate rates of CSF secretion in vivo.

However, the recent development of a novel microneurosurgical technique that directly measures real-time CSF secretion rates in live rats (Karimy et al., 2015) has allowed several novel observations of CSF dynamics in the context of experimental PHH (Karimy et al., 2017). Strikingly, autologous experimental IVH was shown to cause a TLR4-NF-κB-dependent CPe inflammatory response associated with a >3-fold increase in bumetanide-sensitive CSF secretion measured at 24 h after IVH, and lasting until at least 7 days after IVH, a period sufficient to cause ventriculomegaly (Karimy et al., 2017). Choroid plexus epithelium inflammation was characterized by greatly up-regulated phosphorylation of NF-κB, production of TNF-α and IL-1β, as well as infiltration of activated ED-1[+] microglia and macrophages (Karimy et al., 2017).

IVH-induced CSF hypersecretion resulted from TLR4-dependent activation of the NF-κB-regulated STE20/SPS1-related, proline-alanine-rich kinase (SPAK), which binds, phosphorylates, and stimulates the bumetanide-target cotransporter NKCC1 at the CPe apical membrane (Alessi et al., 2014; Karimy et al., 2017; Thastrup et al., 2012). SPAK integrates and transduces environmental stress signals, including NF-κB-dependent inflammatory signals (Piechotta et al., 2003; Shekarabi et al., 2017; Yan and Merlin, 2008; Yan et al., 2008). Interestingly, TNF-α (Yan et al., 2008) and IFN-γ (Yan et al., 2007) have been shown to stimulate SPAK in an NF-κB-dependent manner to increase epithelial transport in models of colitis (Thiagarajah et al., 2015), IgA nephropathy (Lin et al., 2016), and hypoxic lung injury (Lan et al., 2017). SPAK directly interacts with TNFα receptor RELT to activate both p38 and JNK1/2 signaling pathways (Polek et al., 2006). NF-κB is itself a transcriptional regulator of SPAK (Yan et al., 2008).

SPAK is more abundant in CPe than in other epithelia, localizing predominantly to the CPe apical membrane (Piechotta et al., 2002). In addition to its *upstream* regulation by TLR4-NF-κB signaling, SPAK kinase binds and regulates multiple *downstream* ion transporters, in addition to NKCC1 (de Los et al., 2014). Therefore, SPAK appears to be a critical link between TLR4-dependent CPe inflammation and CSF hypersecretion. In the CPe, NKCC1 is probably SPAK's most important ion transport target, as this transporter has been shown to account for >50% of total CSF production (Karimy et al., 2017; Steffenson et al., 2018). Genetic inhibition of TLR4 or SPAK normalized hyperactive CSF secretion and prevented PHH by decreasing IVH-induced phosphorylation of NKCC1, as did treatment before IVH onset with inhibitors of TLR4-NF-κB or SPAK-NKCC1 (Karimy et al., 2017). These data suggest that CPe immunosecretory plasticity is central to pathogenesis of acute PHH, and that pharmacologically targeting TLR4 or SPAK may be a promising non-invasive treatment approach.

25.7 Reparative Versus Pathological Inflammation: More to the Story Than Cerebrospinal Fluid Hypersecretion?

While these recent studies have begun to elucidate inflammatory mediators in PHH (Gram et al., 2013, 2014; Karimy et al., 2017; Kwon et al., 2015; Simard et al., 2011; Sveinsdottir et al., 2014), numerous remaining gaps in our understanding include: (i) the identities of IVH-induced metabolite(s) signaling through TLR4 (although metHgb has been shown to be a TLR4 ligand; Kwon et al., 2015); (ii) the identities of acute and chronic IVH-induced signaling components of the TLR4 signaling cascade; (iii) the dynamic spectra and profiles of TLR4-dependent cytokines and immune cells; (iv) whether inflammation-induced CPe hypersecretion is a sustained phenomenon, and whether other inflammation-dependent mechanisms (e.g., due to accompanying tissue injury) contribute to pathogenesis; and (v) whether TLR4 inhibition at clinically relevant times post-IVH can prevent PHH.

It seems most likely that a CSF hypersecretory response from an inflamed CPe contributes to development of *acute* hydrocephalus. This accords with the acute timing of hydrocephalus development following PHH (and PIH) that is often seen in human patients, often too soon for chronic inflammation-induced scarring to take place. However, it is possible other TLR-dependent or innate immune mechanisms (e.g., NOD-like receptors [NLRs] found on microglia; Gharagozloo et al., 2017; White et al., 2017) triggered by inflammation-induced tissue damage of CNS barrier epithelia (the CPe and ependyma) and associated DAMP release, could propagate and sustain the neuroinflammatory reaction and potentially impact other CSF homeostatic pathways, such as the recently characterized glymphatic system. The glymphatic system has been shown to be another portal of entry for immune cells (Schiefenhövel et al., 2017) and is involved in CSF drainage, immune cell trafficking, and neuroinflammation (Louveau et al., 2015, 2017).

Following injury, microglial- and epithelial-derived cytokines promote reparative inflammation by induction of cytokines and growth factors in underlying connective tissue fibroblasts, promoting epithelial proliferation and repair (Eming et al., 2009). As in the intestine and respiratory tract, it is tempting to speculate that chronic tissue damage or inflammation in the CPe and ependyma, such as that associated with extensive IVH (e.g., grade IV germinal matrix hemorrhage) and with partially treated ventriculitis, may drive the conversion of activated connective tissue fibroblasts to extracellular matrix (ECM)-producing myofibroblasts. This could lead to fibrosis, recruitment of inflammatory cells, and excessive production of inflammatory mediators, thus driving pathological inflammation that exacerbates tissue damage. This concept would be consistent with neurosurgical observations from neuroendoscopic procedures of damaged, "burnt out" CPe, intraventricular fibrosis and septations, and friable ependyma in chronic cases of PIH/PHH. Additional support includes the recent experimental demonstration of ependymal denudation and ventricular zone disruption in both human and experimental chronic PHH (McAllister et al., 2017).

At present, our ability to investigate these questions in human pathological cases is limited by the paucity of non-invasive molecular imaging tools. Phase contrast magnetic resonance imaging (PC-MRI) has been used to assess CSF flow in the Sylvian aqueduct between the third and fourth ventricles. In some cases of communicating hydrocephalus, PC-MRI measurements have shown up to sixfold increased orthograde fluid flow through the aqueduct during the cardiac cycle. However, other reports suggest a reversal of flow direction (reviewed in Hladky and Barrand, 2014), underscoring gaps in methodology and/or understanding. Innovative imaging reagents such as "bis-5-hydroxytryptamide-diethylenetriaminepentaacetate gadolinium with cross-linked iron oxide nanoparticles" (Hoffmann et al., 2019) or "europium-doped very small superparamagnetic iron oxide particles" (Millward et al., 2019) appear to be particularly sensitive detectors of choroid plexus neuroinflammation. However, these techniques have not yet been applied to inflammatory hydrocephalus.

25.8 Shared Mechanisms and Therapeutic Targets in Post-Hemorrhagic and Post-Infectious Hydrocephalus: Advances and Future

Bacterial CNS infection is probably the most common cause of PIH (Dewan et al., 2018; Kahle et al., 2016). Bacteria may cross the blood–brain barrier (BBB) and blood–CSF barrier (CPe) to gain entry into the CNS (Kim, 2008), replicate within subarachnoid and ventricular CSF spaces, and cause intense CPe, ependymal, and CSF inflammation by releasing highly immunogenic cell wall fragments (Koedel et al., 2010). The robust acute inflammatory response associated with PIH has been assumed to cause non-communicating (i.e., obstructive) hydrocephalus due to blockage of the aqueduct, of the fourth ventricle outlets, or of the basal subarachnoid spaces around the fourth ventricle. However, the *acute* onset of PIH (often within 12 hours) precedes the time normally required for post-inflammatory scarring and aqueductal obstruction.

Pathogen-associated molecular patterns contained in PIH-causing organisms promote local inflammation through recognition by antigen-presenting cells (e.g., microglia and CPe) expressing cell surface pattern-recognition receptors (e.g., TLRs; Sellner et al., 2010). TLR4 and other CPe TLRs (Gram et al., 2014; Skipor et al., 2015) exhibit ligand-specific regulation in response to pro-inflammatory stimuli from PIH-associated microorganisms, including LPS found on Gram-negative bacterial cell walls (; Gram et al., 2013, 2014; Karimy et al., 2017; Li et al., 2011). TLR4 also recognizes *S. pneumoniae*-derived pneumolysin (Malley et al., 2003). TLR4 activation results in production of inflammatory cytokines such as TNF-α, IL-1β, and IL-6 (Krebs et al., 2005; Lahrtz et al., 1998; van Furth et al., 1996) and recruitment of additional immune cells into the CNS from across the BBB and CPe (Grandgirard and Leib, 2010). TLR2 recognizes lipoteichoic acids from *S. pneumoniae* (Dessing et al., 2008), *L. monocytogenes* (Flo et al., 2000; Janot et al., 2008; Seki et al., 2002) and *S. agalactiae* (Mook-Kanamori et al., 2011), whereas TLR5 recognizes flagellin of flagellated bacteria (Hayashi et al., 2001). Thus, PIH and PHH may share common pathogenic mechanisms driven by PAMP- and DAMP-triggered innate immune responses, raising the compelling possibility that anti-inflammatory therapeutics could modulate development of hydrocephalus in both conditions.

How would such a therapeutic approach work? Many patients with PIH and PHH require urgent placement of temporary CSF diversion devices such as external ventricular drains, implanted access reservoirs, or lumbar drains prior to permanent CSF shunting. In these settings, intraventricular administration of medications targeting TLR4-dependent inflammation seems particularly attractive. Such agents could include Tak242 (already effective in acute experimental PHH (Karimy et al., 2017) and subjected to clinical trial in human sepsis patients (Rice et al., 2010)) or other anti-inflammatory agents targeting the TLR4-NF-κB pathway, such as pyrrolidine dithiocarbamate (Liu et al., 1999) or melatonin (Hu et al., 2017; Robinson et al., 2018). Data in experimental PHH suggest that systemic administration of Tak242 and similar agents might also be effective

(Karimy et al., 2017). Additional agents such as neutralizing antibodies or decoy receptor "sponges" to sequester other DAMPs/PAMPs or cytokines might also be efficacious, and perhaps better tolerated. Obviously, these concepts are speculative and require experimental validation in models of PIH.

The NKCC1 inhibitor, bumetanide has been used successfully in trials of children with autism (Lemonnier and Ben-Ari, 2010; Lemonnier et al., 2012, 2017), but the low CNS penetration of bumetanide and its derivatives argues against their systemic administration to reduce increased CSF secretion in the acute setting of inflammation (Erker et al., 2016; Karimy et al., 2017). In contrast, ICV delivery of bumetanide via the systems discussed above might prove effective in the acute timeframe. However, bumetanide administration to neonatal brain is probably unwise, given its association with hearing loss when added to phenobarbital for treatment of seizures (Pressler et al., 2015). The above considerations suggest that SPAK may be preferable to NKCC1 as a therapeutic target, as SPAK is more highly expressed in CPe than in any other human epithelial tissue, serving as amplifier of TLR4-dependent inflammatory reaction and cytokine production (Karimy et al., 2017) and as master regulator of multiple ion transporters (Alessi et al., 2014). We nonetheless propose that targeting inflammation (relative to CPe ion transport) might be a more promising therapy, because this process drives not only the initial hypersecretory response, but is also responsible for the ensuing tissue damage and release of DAMPs that ultimately lead to a sustained hydrocephalic phenotype.

25.9 Conclusions

Emerging data on the pathophysiology of hydrocephalus suggest that prevention of PIH/PHH is a feasible goal. We propose that the concept of "inflammatory hydrocephalus" more accurately conveys the shared pathogenic mechanisms and therapeutic vulnerabilities pf PHH and PIH than does the term "secondary hydrocephalus." We believe this nomenclature change could catalyze a shift in our view of these types of hydrocephalus from that of lifelong neurosurgical brain plumbing disorders to one of treatable neuroinflammatory conditions. Nonetheless, much future work remains before any treatment strategies can be considered, including: (i) continued identification of specific inflammatory mechanisms and targets that contribute to the pathogenesis of PHH and PIH; (ii) development of pharmacologic agents that modulate these targets; and (iii) preclinical trial of these drugs in relevant experimental models. An approach addressing neuroinflammation may not only prevent shunt dependence, but also ameliorate associated neurodevelopmental sequelae including cerebral palsy and secondary inflammation-induced tissue damage that are not addressed by surgical CSF diversion. Such an approach would reduce the lifelong morbidity and economic burden associated with hydrocephalus surgery, and could be life-saving in regions with limited neurosurgical access.

References

Alessi DR, Zhang J, Khanna A, Hochdorfer T, Shang Y, Kahle KT. The WNK–SPAK/OSR1 pathway: master regulator of cation–chloride cotransporters. *Sci Signal* 2014;**7**(334): re3. https://doi.org/10.1126/scisignal.2005365.

Aranha A, Choudhary A, Bhaskar S, Gupta LN. A randomized study comparing endoscopic third ventriculostomy versus ventriculoperitoneal shunt in the management of hydrocephalus due to tuberculous meningitis. *Asian J Neurosurg* 2018;**13**(4):1140–7. https://doi.org/10.4103/ajns.AJNS_107_18.

Aziz IA. Hydrocephalus in the Sudan. *J R Coll Surg Edinb* 1976;**21**(4):222–4.

Baird LC. First treatment in infants with hydrocephalus: the case for endoscopic third ventriculostomy/choroid plexus cauterization. *Neurosurgery* 2016;**63**(Suppl 1):78–82. https://doi.org/10.1227/NEU.0000000000001299.

Barichello T, Fagundes GD, Generoso JS, Elias SG, Simoes LR, Teixeira AL. Pathophysiology of neonatal acute bacterial meningitis. *J Med Microbiol* 2013;**62**(Pt 12):1781–9. https://doi.org/10.1099/jmm.0.059840-0.

Bateman GA, Brown KM. The measurement of CSF flow through the aqueduct in normal and hydrocephalic children: from where does it come, to where does it go? *Childs Nerv Syst* 2012;**28**(1):55–63. http://doi.org/10.1007/s00381-011-1617-4.

Benveniste H, Lee H, Volkow ND. The glymphatic pathway: waste removal from the CNS via cerebrospinal fluid transport. *Neuroscientist* 2017;**23**(5):454–65. https://doi.org/10.1177/1073858417691030.

Berkes J, Viswanathan VK, Savkovic SD, Hecht G. Intestinal epithelial responses to enteric pathogens: effects on the tight junction barrier, ion transport, and inflammation. *Gut* 2003;**52**(3):439–51. https://doi.org/10.1136/gut.52.3.439.

Bir SC, Patra DP, Maiti TK, et al. Epidemiology of adult-onset hydrocephalus: institutional experience with 2001 patients. *Neurosurg Focus* 2016;**41**(3):E5. https://doi.org/10.3171/2016.7.FOCUS16188.

Brinker T, Stopa E, Morrison J, Klinge P. A new look at cerebrospinal fluid circulation. *Fluids Barriers CNS* 2014;**11**:10. https://doi.org/10.1186/2045-8118-11-10.

Chahlavi A, El-Babaa SK, Luciano MG. Adult-onset hydrocephalus. *Neurosurg Clin N Am* 2001;**12**(4):753–60, ix.

Chen Q, Feng Z, Tan Q, et al. Post-hemorrhagic hydrocephalus: recent advances and new therapeutic insights. *J Neurol Sci* 2017;**375**:220–30. https://doi.org/10.1016/j.jns.2017.01.072.

Cherian S, Whitelaw A, Thoresen M, Love S. The pathogenesis of neonatal post-hemorrhagic hydrocephalus. *Brain Pathol* 2004;**14**(3):305–11. https://doi.org/10.1111/j.1750-3639.2004.tb00069.x.

Cioca A, Gheban D, Perju-Dumbrava D, Chiroban O, Mera M. Sudden death from ruptured choroid plexus arteriovenous malformation. *Am J Forens Med Pathol* 2014;**35**(2):100–02. https://doi.org/10.1097/PAF.0000000000000091.

Coorens M, Schneider VAF, de Groot AM, et al. Cathelicidins inhibit *Escherichia coli*-induced TLR2 and TLR4 activation in a viability-dependent manner. *J Immunol* 2017;**199**(4):1418–28. https://doi.org/10.4049/jimmunol.1602164.

Cox KH, Cox ME, Woo-Rasberry V, Hasty DL. Pathways involved in the synergistic activation of macrophages by lipoteichoic acid and hemoglobin. *PLoS One* 2012;**7**(10):e47333. https://doi.org/10.1371/journal.pone.0047333.

Damkier HH, Brown PD, Praetorius J. Cerebrospinal fluid secretion by the choroid plexus. *Physiol Rev* 2013;**93**(4):1847–92. https://doi.org/10.1152/physrev.00004.2013.

de Los HP, Alessi DR, Gourlay R, et al. The WNK-regulated SPAK/OSR1 kinases directly phosphorylate and inhibit the K^+–Cl^- co-transporters. *Biochem J* 2014;**458**(3):559–73. https://doi.org/10.1042/BJ20131478.

Demeestere D, Libert C, Vandenbroucke RE. Clinical implications of leukocyte infiltration at the choroid plexus in (neuro)inflammatory disorders. *Drug Discov Today* 2015;**20** (8):928–41. https://doi.org/10.1016/j.drudis.2015.05.003.

Dessing MC, Schouten M, Draing C, Levi M, von Aulock S, van der Poll T. Role played by Toll-like receptors 2 and 4 in lipoteichoic acid-induced lung inflammation and coagulation. *J Infect Dis* 2008;**197**(2):245–52. https://doi.org/10.1086/524873.

Dewan MC, Rattani A, Mekary R, et al. Global hydrocephalus epidemiology and incidence: systematic review and meta-analysis. *J Neurosurg* 2018: online ahead of publication. https://doi.org/10.3171/2017.10.JNS17439.

Doyle WJ, Skoner DP, Hayden F, Buchman CA, Seroky JT, Fireman P. Nasal and otologic effects of experimental influenza A virus infection. *Ann Otol Rhinol Laryngol* 1994;**103**(1):59–69. https://doi.org/10.1177/000348949410300111.

Drake JM, Kulkarni AV, Kestle J. Endoscopic third ventriculostomy versus ventriculoperitoneal shunt in pediatric patients: a decision analysis. *Childs Nerv Syst* 2009;**25**(4):467–72. https://doi.org/10.1007/s00381-008-0761-y.

Ehrchen JM, Sunderkotter C, Foell D, Vogl T, Roth J. The endogenous Toll-like receptor 4 agonist S100A8/S100A9 (calprotectin) as innate amplifier of infection, autoimmunity, and cancer. *J Leukocyte Biol* 2009;**86**(3):557–66. https://doi.org /10.1189/jlb.1008647.

Eming SA, Hammerschmidt M, Krieg T, Roers A. Interrelation of immunity and tissue repair or regeneration. *Semin Cell Dev Biol* 2009;**20**(5):517–27. https://doi.org/10.1016/j .semcdb.2009.04.009.

Erker T, Brandt C, Tollner K, et al. The bumetanide prodrug BUM5, but not bumetanide, potentiates the antiseizure effect of phenobarbital in adult epileptic mice. *Epilepsia* 2016;**57** (5):698–705. https://doi.org/10.1111/epi.13346.

Fang H, Wu Y, Huang X, et al. Toll-like receptor 4 (TLR4) is essential for Hsp70-like protein 1 (HSP70L1) to activate dendritic cells and induce Th1 response. *J Biol Chem* 2011;**286** (35):30393–400. https://doi.org/10.1074/jbc.M111.266528.

Fassbender K, Schminke U, Ries S, et al. Endothelial-derived adhesion molecules in bacterial meningitis: association to cytokine release and intrathecal leukocyte-recruitment. *J Neuroimmunol* 1997;**74**(1–2):130–4. https://doi.org/10.1016/ s0165-5728(96)00214-7.

Flo TH, Halaas O, Lien E, et al. Human toll-like receptor 2 mediates monocyte activation by *Listeria monocytogenes*, but not by group B streptococci or lipopolysaccharide. *J Immunol* 2000;**164**(4):2064–9. https://doi.org/10.4049/jimmunol.164.4 .2064.

Furey CG, Choi J, Jin SC, et al. De novo mutation in genes regulating neural stem cell fate in human congenital hydrocephalus. *Neuron* 2018;**99**(2):302–14. https://doi.org/10 .1016/j.neuron.2018.06.019.

Gao C, Du H, Hua Y, Keep RF, Strahle J, Xi G. Role of red blood cell lysis and iron in hydrocephalus after intraventricular hemorrhage. *J Cerebr Blood Flow Metab* 2014;**34**(6):1070–5. https://doi.org/10.1038/jcbfm.2014.56.

Gharagozloo M, Gris KV, Mahvelati T, Amrani A, Lukens JR, Gris D. NLR-dependent regulation of inflammation in multiple sclerosis. *Front Immunol* 2017;**8**:2012. https://doi.org/10.3389/f immu.2017.02012.

Gram M, Sveinsdottir S, Cinthio M, et al. Extracellular hemoglobin – mediator of inflammation and cell death in the choroid plexus following preterm intraventricular hemorrhage. *J Neuroinflam* 2014;**11**:200. https://doi.org/10.1186/s12974-014- 0200-9.

Gram M, Sveinsdottir S, Ruscher K, et al. Hemoglobin induces inflammation after preterm intraventricular hemorrhage by methemoglobin formation. *J Neuroinflam* 2013;**10**:100. https:// doi.org/10.1186/1742-2094-10-100.

Grandgirard D, Leib SL. Meningitis in neonates: bench to bedside. *Clin Perinatol* 2010;**37**(3):655–76. https://doi.org/10 .1016/j.clp.2010.05.004.

Habiyaremye G, Morales DM, Morgan CD, et al. Chemokine and cytokine levels in the lumbar cerebrospinal fluid of preterm infants with post-hemorrhagic hydrocephalus. *Fluids Barriers CNS* 2017;**14**(1):35. https://doi.org/10.1186/s12987-017-0083-0.

Hayashi F, Smith KD, Ozinsky A, et al. The innate immune response to bacterial flagellin is mediated by Toll-like receptor 5. *Nature* 2001;**410**(6832):1099–103. https://doi.org/10.1038 /35074106.

Hill A, Shackelford GD, Volpe JJ. A potential mechanism of pathogenesis for early posthemorrhagic hydrocephalus in the premature newborn. *Pediatrics* 1984;**73**(1):19–21.

Hladky SB, Barrand MA. Mechanisms of fluid movement into, through and out of the brain: evaluation of the evidence. *Fluids Barriers CNS* 2014;**11**(1):26. https://doi.org/10.1186/2045-8118- 11-26.

Hoffmann A, Pfeil J, Mueller AK, et al. MRI of iron oxide nanoparticles and myeloperoxidase activity links inflammation to brain edema in experimental cerebral malaria. *Radiology* 2019;**290**(2):359–67. https://doi.org/10.1148/radiol .2018181051.

Hu Y, Wang Z, Pan S, et al. Melatonin protects against blood–brain barrier damage by inhibiting the TLR4/ NF-κB signaling pathway after LPS treatment in neonatal rats. *Oncotarget* 2017;**8** (19):31638–54. https://doi.org/10.18632/oncotarget.15780.

Isaacs AM, Riva-Cambrin J, Yavin D, et al. Age-specific global epidemiology of hydrocephalus: systematic review, metanalysis and global birth surveillance. *PLoS One* 2018;**13**(10):e0204926. https://doi.org/10.1371/journal.pone.0204926.

Janot L, Secher T, Torres D, et al. CD14 works with toll-like receptor 2 to contribute to recognition and control of *Listeria monocytogenes* infection. *J Infect Dis* 2008;**198**(1):115–24. https:// doi.org/10.1086/588815.

Kahle KT, Kulkarni AV, Limbrick DD, Jr., Warf BC. Hydrocephalus in children. *Lancet* 2016;**387**(10020):788–99. https://doi.org/10.1016/S0140-6736(15)60694-8.

Kamat AS, Gretschel A, Vlok AJ, Solomons R. CSF protein concentration associated with ventriculoperitoneal shunt obstruction in tuberculous meningitis. *Int J Tuberc Lung Dis* 2018;**22**(7):788–92. https://doi.org/10.5588/ijtld.17.0008.

Karimy JK, Duran D, Hu JK, et al. Cerebrospinal fluid hypersecretion in pediatric hydrocephalus. *Neurosurg Focus* 2016;**41**(5):E10. https://doi.org/10.3171/2016.8.FOCUS16278.

Karimy JK, Kahle KT, Kurland DB, Yu E, Gerzanich V, Simard JM. A novel method to study cerebrospinal fluid dynamics in rats. *J Neurosci Methods* 2015;**241**:78–84. https:// doi.org/10.1016/j.jneumeth.2014.12.015.

Karimy JK, Zhang J, Kurland DB, et al. Inflammation-dependent cerebrospinal fluid hypersecretion by the choroid plexus epithelium in posthemorrhagic hydrocephalus. *Nature Med* 2017;**23**(8):997–1003. https://doi.org/10.1038/ nm.4361.

Keep RF, Jones HC. A morphometric study on the development of the lateral ventricle choroid plexus, choroid plexus capillaries and ventricular ependyma in the rat. *Brain Res Dev Brain Res* 1990;**56**(1):47–53. https://doi.org/10.1016/0165-3806(90) 90163-s.

Kim KS. Mechanisms of microbial traversal of the blood–brain barrier. *Nature Rev Microbiol* 2008;**6**(8):625–34. https://doi.org/10.1038/nrmicro1952.

Kleine TO, Benes L. Immune surveillance of the human central nervous system (CNS): different migration pathways of immune cells through the blood–brain barrier and blood–cerebrospinal fluid barrier in healthy persons. *Cytometry Part A* 2006;**69**(3):147–51. https://doi.org/10.1002/cyto.a.20225.

Koedel U, Klein M, Pfister H-W. New understandings on the pathophysiology of bacterial meningitis. *Curr Opin Infect Dis* 2010;**23**(3):217–23. https://doi.org/10.1097/QCO.0b013e328337f49e.

Kotas ME, Medzhitov R. Homeostasis, inflammation, and disease susceptibility. *Cell* 2015;**160**(5):816–27. https://doi.org/10.1016/j.cell.2015.02.010.

Krebs VL, Okay TS, Okay Y, Vaz FA. Tumor necrosis factor-alpha, interleukin-1beta and interleukin-6 in the cerebrospinal fluid of newborn with meningitis. *Arq Neuropsiquiatr* 2005;**63**(1):7–13. https://doi.org/10.1590/s0004-282x2005000100002.

Kulkarni AV. First treatment in infants with hydrocephalus: the case for shunt. *Neurosurgery* 2016;**63**(Suppl 1):73–7. https://doi.org/10.1227/NEU.0000000000001287.

Kulkarni AV, Drake JM, Kestle JR, Mallucci CL, Sgouros S, Constantini S. Endoscopic third ventriculostomy vs cerebrospinal fluid shunt in the treatment of hydrocephalus in children: a propensity score-adjusted analysis. *Neurosurgery* 2010;**67**(3):588–93. https://doi.org/10.1227/01.NEU.0000373199.79462.21.

Kulkarni AV, Drake JM, Mallucci CL, Sgouros S, Roth J, Constantini S. Endoscopic third ventriculostomy in the treatment of childhood hydrocephalus. *J Pediatrics* 2009;**155**(2):254–9. https://doi.org/10.1016/j.jpeds.2009.02.048.

Kulkarni AV, Riva-Cambrin J, Browd SR, et al. Endoscopic third ventriculostomy and choroid plexus cauterization in infants with hydrocephalus: a retrospective Hydrocephalus Clinical Research Network study. *J Neurosurg Pediatr* 2014;**14**(3):224–9. https://doi.org/10.3171/2014.6.PEDS13492.

Kulkarni AV, Riva-Cambrin J, Butler J, et al. Outcomes of CSF shunting in children: comparison of Hydrocephalus Clinical Research Network cohort with historical controls. *J Neurosurg Pediatr* 2013;**12**(4):334–8. https://doi.org/10.3171/2013.7.PEDS12637.

Kulkarni AV, Schiff SJ, Mbabazi-Kabachelor E, et al. Endoscopic treatment versus shunting for infant hydrocephalus in Uganda. *New Engl J Med* 2017;**377**(25):2456–64. https://doi.org/10.1056/NEJMoa1707568.

Kwon MS, Woo SK, Kurland DB, et al. Methemoglobin is an endogenous toll-like receptor 4 ligand-relevance to subarachnoid hemorrhage. *Int J Molec Sci* 2015;**16**(3):5028–46. https://doi.org/10.3390/ijms16035028.

Lahrtz F, Piali L, Spanaus KS, Seebach J, Fontana A. Chemokines and chemotaxis of leukocytes in infectious meningitis. *J Neuroimmunol* 1998;**85**(1):33–43. https://doi.org/10.1016/s0165-5728(97)00267-1.

Lan CC, Peng CK, Tang SE, et al. Inhibition of Na–K–Cl cotransporter isoform 1 reduces lung injury induced by ischemia–reperfusion. *J Thorac Cardiovasc Surg* 2017;**153**(1):206–15. https://doi.org/10.1016/j.jtcvs.2016.09.068.

Larroche JC. Post-haemorrhagic hydrocephalus in infancy. Anatomical study. *Biol Neonate* 1972;**20**(3):287–99. https://doi.org/10.1159/000240472.

Lategan B, Chodirker BN, Del Bigio MR. Fetal hydrocephalus caused by cryptic intraventricular hemorrhage. *Brain Pathol* 2010;**20**(2):391–8. https://doi.org/10.1111/j.1750-3639.2009.00293.x.

Lee LV. Neurotuberculosis among Filipino children: an 11-year experience at the Philippine Children's Medical Center. *Brain Dev* 2000;**22**(8):469–74. https://doi.org/10.1016/s0387-7604(00)00190-x.

Lemonnier E, Ben-Ari Y. The diuretic bumetanide decreases autistic behaviour in five infants treated during 3 months with no side effects. *Acta Paediatr* 2010;**99**(12):1885–8. https://doi.org/10.1111/j.1651-2227.2010.01933.x.

Lemonnier E, Degrez C, Phelep M, et al. A randomised controlled trial of bumetanide in the treatment of autism in children. *Transl Psychiatry* 2012;**2**:e202. https://doi.org/10.1038/tp.2012.124.

Lemonnier E, Villeneuve N, Sonie S, et al. Effects of bumetanide on neurobehavioral function in children and adolescents with autism spectrum disorders. *Transl Psychiatry* 2017;**7**(3):e1056. https://doi.org/10.1038/tp.2017.10.

Li K, Tang H, Yang Y, et al. Clinical features, long-term clinical outcomes, and prognostic factors of tuberculous meningitis in West China: a multivariate analysis of 154 adults. *Expert Rev Anti Infect Ther* 2017;**15**(6):629–35. https://doi.org/10.1080/14787210.2017.1309974.

Li L, Padhi A, Ranjeva SL, et al. Association of bacteria with hydrocephalus in Ugandan infants. *J Neurosurg Pediatr* 2011;**7**(1):73–87. https://doi.org/10.3171/2010.9.PEDS10162.

Limbrick DD, Jr., Baird LC, Klimo P, Jr., Riva-Cambrin J, Flannery AM. Pediatric hydrocephalus: systematic literature review and evidence-based guidelines. Part 4: Cerebrospinal fluid shunt or endoscopic third ventriculostomy for the treatment of hydrocephalus in children. *J Neurosurg Pediatr* 2014;**14**(Suppl 1):30–4. https://doi.org/10.3171/2014.7.PEDS14324.

Lin TJ, Yang SS, Hua KF, Tsai YL, Lin SH, Ka SM. SPAK plays a pathogenic role in IgA nephropathy through the activation of NF-kappaB/MAPKs signaling pathway. *Free Rad Biol Med* 2016;**99**:214–24. https://doi.org/10.1016/j.freeradbiomed.2016.08.008.

Liu J, Chen ZL, Li M, et al. Ventriculoperitoneal shunts in non-HIV cryptococcal meningitis. *BMC Neurol* 2018;**18**(1):58. https://doi.org/10.1186/s12883-018-1053-0.

Liu SF, Ye X, Malik AB. Inhibition of NF-B activation by pyrrolidine dithiocarbamate prevents in vivo expression of proinflammatory genes. *Circulation* 1999;**100**(12):1330–7. https://doi.org/10.1161/01.cir.100.12.1330.

Lohrberg M, Wilting J. The lymphatic vascular system of the mouse head. *Cell Tissue Res* 2016;**366**(3):667–77. https://doi.org/10.1007/s00441-016-2493-8.

Louveau A, Plog BA, Antila S, Alitalo K, Nedergaard M, Kipnis J. Understanding the functions and relationships of the glymphatic system and meningeal lymphatics. *J Clin Invest* 2017;**127**(9):3210–9. https://doi.org/10.1172/JCI90603.

Louveau A, Smirnov I, Keyes TJ, et al. Structural and functional features of central nervous system lymphatic vessels. *Nature* 2015;**523**(7560):337–41. https://doi.org/10.1038/nature14432.

Malley R, Henneke P, Morse SC, et al. Recognition of pneumolysin by Toll-like receptor 4 confers resistance to pneumococcal infection. *Proc Natl Acad Sci U S A* 2003;**100**(4):1966–71. https://doi.org/10.1073/pnas.0435928100.

Marques F, Sousa JC, Brito MA, et al. The choroid plexus in health and in disease: dialogues into and out of the brain. *Neurobiol Dis* 2017;**107**:32–40. https://doi.org/10.1016/j.nbd.2016.08.011.

McAllister JP, Guerra MM, Ruiz LC, et al. Ventricular zone disruption in human neonates with intraventricular hemorrhage. *J Neuropathol Exp Neurol* 2017;**76**(5):358–75. https://doi.org/10.1093/jnen/nlx017.

Medzhitov R. TLR-mediated innate immune recognition. *Semin Immunol* 2007;**19**(1):1–2. https://doi.org/10.1016/j.smim.2007.02.001.

Millward JM, Ariza de Schellenberger A, Berndt D, et al. Application of europium-doped very small iron oxide nanoparticles to visualize neuroinflammation with MRI and fluorescence microscopy. *Neuroscience* 2019;**403**:136–144. https://doi.org/10.1016/j.neuroscience.2017.12.014

Miyajima M, Arai H. Evaluation of the production and absorption of cerebrospinal fluid. *Neurol Med Chir (Tokyo)* 2015;**55**(8):647–56. https://doi.org/10.2176/nmc.ra.2015-0003.

Miyake K. Innate immune sensing of pathogens and danger signals by cell surface Toll-like receptors. *Semin Immunol* 2007;**19**(1):3–10. https://doi.org/10.1016/j.smim.2006.12.002.

Mook-Kanamori BB, Geldhoff M, van der Poll T, van de Beek D. Pathogenesis and pathophysiology of pneumococcal meningitis. *Clin Microbiol Rev* 2011;**24**(3):557–91. https://doi.org/10.1128/CMR.00008-11.

Muir RT, Wang S, Warf BC. Global surgery for pediatric hydrocephalus in the developing world: a review of the history, challenges, and future directions. *Neurosurg Focus* 2016;**41**(5):E11. https://doi.org/10.3171/2016.7.FOCUS16273.

Murphy BP, Inder TE, Rooks V, et al. Posthaemorrhagic ventricular dilatation in the premature infant: natural history and predictors of outcome. *Arch Dis Child Fetal Neonatal Ed* 2002;**87**(1):F37–41. https://doi.org/10.1136/fn.87.1.f37.

Nowarski R, Jackson R, Flavell RA. The stromal intervention: regulation of immunity and inflammation at the epithelial-mesenchymal barrier. *Cell* 2017;**168**(3):362–75. https://doi.org/10.1016/j.cell.2016.11.040.

Oi S, Di Rocco C. Proposal of "evolution theory in cerebrospinal fluid dynamics" and minor pathway hydrocephalus in developing immature brain. *Childs Nerv Syst* 2006;**22**(7):662–9. https://doi.org/10.1007/s00381-005-0020-4.

Olstad EW, Ringers C, Hansen JN, et al. Ciliary beating compartmentalizes cerebrospinal fluid flow in the brain and regulates ventricular development. *Curr Biol* 2019;**29**(2):229–41. https://doi.org/10.1016/j.cub.2018.11.059.

Omar AT, 2nd, Bagnas MAC, Del Rosario-Blasco KAR, Diestro JDB, Khu KJO. Shunt surgery for neurocutaneous melanosis with hydrocephalus: case report and review of the literature. *World Neurosurg* 2018;**120**:583–9. https://doi.org/10.1016/j.wneu.2018.09.002.

Oreskovic D, Rados M, Klarica M. Role of choroid plexus in cerebrospinal fluid hydrodynamics. *Neuroscience* 2017;**354**:69–87. https://doi.org/10.1016/j.neuroscience.2017.04.025.

Piechotta K, Garbarini N, England R, Delpire E. Characterization of the interaction of the stress kinase SPAK with the $Na^+-K^+-2Cl^-$ cotransporter in the nervous system: evidence for a scaffolding role of the kinase. *J Biol Chem* 2003;**278**(52):52848–56. https://doi.org/10.1074/jbc.M309436200.

Piechotta K, Lu J, Delpire E. Cation chloride cotransporters interact with the stress-related kinases Ste20-related proline-alanine-rich kinase (SPAK) and oxidative stress response 1 (OSR1). *J Biol Chem* 2002;**277**(52):50812–9. https://doi.org/10.1074/jbc.M208108200.

Pindrik J, Jallo GI, Ahn ES. Complications and subsequent removal of retained shunt hardware after endoscopic third ventriculostomy: case series. *J Neurosurg Pediatr* 2013;**11**(6):722–6. https://doi.org/10.3171/2013.3.PEDS12489.

Polek TC, Talpaz M, Spivak-Kroizman T. The TNF receptor, RELT, binds SPAK and uses it to mediate p38 and JNK activation. *Biochem Biophys Res Commun* 2006;**343**(1):125–34. https://doi.org/10.1016/j.bbrc.2006.02.125.

Praetorius J, Damkier HH. Transport across the choroid plexus epithelium. *Am J Physiol Cell Physiol* 2017;**312**(6):C673–86. https://doi.org/10.1152/ajpcell.00041.2017.

Pressler RM, Boylan GB, Marlow N, et al. Bumetanide for the treatment of seizures in newborn babies with hypoxic ischaemic encephalopathy (NEMO): an open-label, dose finding, and feasibility phase 1/2 trial. *Lancet Neurol* 2015;**14**(5):469–77. https://doi.org/10.1016/S1474-4422(14)70303-5.

Pyrgos V, Seitz AE, Steiner CA, Prevots DR, Williamson PR. Epidemiology of cryptococcal meningitis in the US: 1997–2009. *PLoS One* 2013;8(2):e56269. https://doi.org/10.1371/journal.pone.0056269.

Rajshekhar V. Management of hydrocephalus in patients with tuberculous meningitis. *Neurol India* 2009;57(4):368–74. https://doi.org/10.4103/0028-3886.55572.

Reddy GK, Bollam P, Caldito G. Long-term outcomes of ventriculoperitoneal shunt surgery in patients with hydrocephalus. *World Neurosurg* 2014;81(2):404–10. https://doi.org/10.1016/j.wneu.2013.01.096.

Rekate HL. A contemporary definition and classification of hydrocephalus. *Semin Pediatr Neurol* 2009;16(1):9–15. https://doi.org/10.1016/j.spen.2009.01.002.

Rice TW, Wheeler AP, Bernard GR, et al. A randomized, double-blind, placebo-controlled trial of TAK-242 for the treatment of severe sepsis. *Crit Care Med* 2010;38(8):1685–94. https://doi.org/10.1097/CCM.0b013e3181e7c5c9.

Rivest S. Molecular insights on the cerebral innate immune system. *Brain Behav Immun* 2003;17(1):13–9. https://doi.org/10.1016/s0889-1591(02)00055-7.

Robinson S, Conteh FS, Oppong AY, et al. Extended combined neonatal treatment with erythropoietin plus melatonin prevents posthemorrhagic hydrocephalus of prematurity in rats. *Front Cell Neurosci* 2018;12:322. https://doi.org/10.3389/fncel.2018.00322.

Sacks FM, Svetkey LP, Vollmer WM, et al. Effects on blood pressure of reduced dietary sodium and the Dietary Approaches to Stop Hypertension (DASH) diet. DASH-Sodium Collaborative Research Group. *N Engl J Med* 2001;344(1):3–10. https://doi.org/10.1056/NEJM200101043440101.

Schiefenhövel F, Immig K, Prodinger C, Bechmann I. Indications for cellular migration from the central nervous system to its draining lymph nodes in CD11c-GFP+ bone-marrow chimeras following EAE. *Exp Brain Res* 2017;235(7):2151–66. https://doi.org/10.1007/s00221-017-4956-x.

Schiff SJ, Ranjeva SL, Sauer TD, Warf BC. Rainfall drives hydrocephalus in East Africa. *J Neurosurg Pediatr* 2012;10(3):161–7. https://doi.org/10.3171/2012.5.PEDS11557.

Seki E, Tsutsui H, Tsuji NM, et al. Critical roles of myeloid differentiation factor 88-dependent proinflammatory cytokine release in early phase clearance of *Listeria monocytogenes* in mice. *J Immunol* 2002;169(7):3863–8. https://doi.org/10.4049/jimmunol.169.7.3863.

Sellner J, Tauber MG, Leib SL. Pathogenesis and pathophysiology of bacterial CNS infections. *Handb Clin Neurol* 2010;96:1–16. https://doi.org/10.1016/S0072-9752(09)96001-8.

Shang X, Li Y, Liu A, et al. Dietary pattern and its association with the prevalence of obesity and related cardiometabolic risk factors among Chinese children. *PLoS One* 2012;7(8):e43183. https://doi.org/10.1371/journal.pone.0043183.

Shekarabi M, Zhang J, Khanna AR, Ellison DH, Delpire E, Kahle KT. WNK kinase signaling in ion homeostasis and human disease. *Cell Metab* 2017;25(2):285–99. https://doi.org/10.1016/j.cmet.2017.01.007.

Simard PF, Tosun C, Melnichenko L, Ivanova S, Gerzanich V, Simard JM. Inflammation of the choroid plexus and ependymal layer of the ventricle following intraventricular hemorrhage. *Transl Stroke Res* 2011;2(2):227–31. https://doi.org/10.1007/s12975-011-0070-8.

Skipor J, Szczepkowska A, Kowalewska M, Herman AP, Lisiewski P. Profile of toll-like receptor mRNA expression in the choroid plexus in adult ewes. *Acta Vet Hung* 2015;63(1):69–78. https://doi.org/10.1556/AVet.2014.027.

Stagno V, Navarrete EA, Mirone G, Esposito F. Management of hydrocephalus around the world. *World Neurosurg* 2013;79(2 Suppl):S23.e17–20. https://doi.org/10.1016/j.wneu.2012.02.004.

Steffensen AB, Oernbo EK, Stoica A, et al. Cotransporter-mediated water transport underlying cerebrospinal fluid formation. *Nature Commun* 2018;9(1):2167. https://doi.org/10.1038/s41467-018-04677-9.

Strahle J, Garton HJ, Maher CO, Muraszko KM, Keep RF, Xi G. Mechanisms of hydrocephalus after neonatal and adult intraventricular hemorrhage. *Transl Stroke Res* 2012;3(Suppl 1):25–38. https://doi.org/10.1007/s12975-012-0182-9.

Sveinsdottir S, Gram M, Cinthio M, Sveinsdottir K, Morgelin M, Ley D. Altered expression of aquaporin 1 and 5 in the choroid plexus following preterm intraventricular hemorrhage. *Dev Neurosci* 2014;36(6):542–51. https://doi.org/10.1159/000366058.

Thastrup JO, Rafiqi FH, Vitari AC, et al. SPAK/OSR1 regulate NKCC1 and WNK activity: analysis of WNK isoform interactions and activation by T-loop trans-autophosphorylation. *Biochem J* 2012;441(1):325–37. https://doi.org/10.1042/BJ20111879.

Thiagarajah JR, Donowitz M, Verkman AS. Secretory diarrhoea: mechanisms and emerging therapies. *Nat Rev Gastroenterol Hepatol* 2015;12(8):446–57. https://doi.org/10.1038/nrgastro.2015.111.

Thigpen MC, Whitney CG, Messonnier NE, et al. Bacterial meningitis in the United States, 1998–2007. *New Engl J Med* 2011;364(21):2016–25. https://doi.org/10.1056/NEJMoa1005384.

Tsan MF, Gao B. Endogenous ligands of Toll-like receptors. *J Leukocyte Biol* 2004;76(3):514–9. https://doi.org/10.1189/jlb.0304127.

Tsitouras V, Sgouros S. Infantile posthemorrhagic hydrocephalus. *Child Nervous Syst* 2011;27(10):1595–608. https://doi.org/10.1007/s00381-011-1521-y.

van der Linden V, de Lima Petribu NC, Pessoa A, et al. Association of severe hydrocephalus with congenital Zika syndrome. *JAMA Neurol* 2019;76(2):203–10. http://doi.org/10.1001/jamaneurol.2018.3553.

van Furth AM, Roord JJ, van Furth R. Roles of proinflammatory and anti-inflammatory cytokines in pathophysiology of bacterial meningitis and effect of adjunctive therapy. *Infect Immun* 1996;**64**(12):4883–90. https://doi.org/10.1128/iai .64.12.4883 4890.1996.

Wang YC, Zhou Y, Fang H, et al. Toll-like receptor 2/4 heterodimer mediates inflammatory injury in intracerebral hemorrhage. *Ann Neurol* 2014;**75**(6):876–89. https://doi.org/10 .1002/ana.24159.

Warf BC. Hydrocephalus in Uganda: the predominance of infectious origin and primary management with endoscopic third ventriculostomy. *J Neurosurg* 2005a;**102**(1 Suppl):1–15. https://doi.org/10.3171/ped.2005.102.1.0001.

Warf BC. Comparison of endoscopic third ventriculostomy alone and combined with choroid plexus cauterization in infants younger than 1 year of age: a prospective study in 550 African children. *J Neurosurg* 2005b;**103**(6 Suppl):475–81. https://doi.org /10.3171/ped.2005.103.6.0475.

Warf BC, East African Neurosurgical Research Collaboration. Pediatric hydrocephalus in East Africa: prevalence, causes, treatments, and strategies for the future. *World Neurosurg* 2010;**73**(4):296–300. https://doi.org/10.1016/j .wneu.2010.02.009.

Warf BC, Campbell JW, Riddle E. Initial experience with combined endoscopic third ventriculostomy and choroid plexus cauterization for post-hemorrhagic hydrocephalus of prematurity: the importance of prepontine cistern status and the predictive value of FIESTA MRI imaging. *Childs Nerv Syst* 2011;**27**(7):1063–71. https://doi.org/10.1007/s00381-011- 1475-0.

White CS, Lawrence CB, Brough D, Rivers-Auty J. Inflammasomes as therapeutic targets for Alzheimer's disease. *Brain Pathol* 2017;**27**(2):223–34. https://doi.org/10.1111/bpa .12478

Whitelaw A. Intraventricular haemorrhage and posthaemorrhagic hydrocephalus: pathogenesis, prevention and future interventions. *Semin Neonatol* 2001;**6**(2):135–46. https://doi.org/10.1053/siny.2001.0047.

Wilson R, Alton E, Rutman A, et al. Upper respiratory tract viral infection and mucociliary clearance. *Eur J Respir Dis* 1987;**70** (5):272–9.

Yan Y, Dalmasso G, Nguyen HT, et al. Nuclear factor-kappaB is a critical mediator of Ste20-like proline-/alanine-rich kinase regulation in intestinal inflammation. *Am J Pathol* 2008;**173** (4):1013–28. https://doi.org/10.2353/ajpath.2008.080339.

Yan Y, Merlin D. Ste20-related proline/alanine-rich kinase: a novel regulator of intestinal inflammation. *World J Gastroenterol* 2008;**14**(40):6115–21. https://doi.org/10.3748/ wjg.14.6115.

Yan Y, Nguyen H, Dalmasso G, Sitaraman SV, Merlin D. Cloning and characterization of a new intestinal inflammation-associated colonic epithelial Ste20-related protein kinase isoform. *Biochim Biophys Acta* 2007;**1769** (2):106–16. https://doi.org/10.1016/j.bbaexp.2007.01.003.

Yang B, Zhou Z, Li X, Niu J. The effect of lysophosphatidic acid on Toll-like receptor 4 expression and the nuclear factor- κB signaling pathway in THP-1 cells. *Mol Cell Biochem* 2016;**422**(1–2):41–9. https://doi.org/10.1007/s11010-016- 2804-0.

Peripheral Nerve Injury Response Mechanisms

Andrew S. Jack and Line Jacques

26.1 Introduction

The peripheral nervous system (PNS) is made up of spinal and cranial nerves which include motor, sensory, and autonomic nerves, as well as their roots, trunks, plexuses, ganglia, and accompanying supportive connective tissue distal to the brain and spinal cord (Caillaud et al., 2019; Vallat et al., 2009). As its name implies it is located peripheral to the central nervous system (CNS), and unlike some other organ systems has very little in the way of protection from injury (as the skull and spinal column may help protect the CNS from external trauma, for example). Also in contrast to the CNS, the PNS has a much higher innate capacity for repair and recovery after injury. Despite its physiological diversity, the PNS has a highly organized and choreographed injury response mechanism partially explaining its improved outcomes post-injury. In this chapter, we discuss the pathophysiology of peripheral nerve injury (PNI) and its ensuing reparative response. This shall serve as a preface for understanding some of the foundational basic science underpinning clinical PNIs in the subsequent chapter. However, before delving into these PNIs and their classifications, it is first important to review the basic anatomic organization of the PNS, its key cellular components, and supporting connective tissue.

26.2 Peripheral Nerve Injury Anatomy, Classification, and Response to Injury

26.2.1 Peripheral Nerve Anatomy

Because of the shear diversity of the PNS, an in-depth description and discussion of all of the various PNS cellular components, their functions, and molecular signaling mechanisms is beyond the scope of this chapter. Here, we aim to provide a brief overview as a reminder of PNS anatomy and its organization. The PNS is broadly made up of somatic, autonomic, and enteric subdivisions. In each of these, there are three primary cell types:

neurons, glial cells, and stromal cells. Neurons are the principle functioning cell in the PNS; they are responsible for relaying afferent sensory information regarding the external and internal environment to the CNS, as well as efferent information conveying a response from the CNS to an end-target effector. Neurons can be further subcategorized into several basic functional components, including:

- Dendrites: area in which incoming electrical signals are received
- Cell body/soma: compartment where cellular machinery is housed governing various functions such as gene expression from nucleic acids into a protein product
- Axon hillock: unmyelinated proximal area of an axon between it and the cell body believed to be the site of summation of incoming action potentials (APs) and initial site of further AP propagation
- Axon: site of AP propagation conveying the electrical impulse toward or away from the CNS, typically consisting of a long cellular process that may be myelinated or unmyelinated and have several different configurations
- Axon terminal: terminus of the neuronal axon where it communicates with another cell or target effector typically through a chemical or electrical synapse

PNS neurons are also typically categorized based on their axonal configuration (unipolar, pseudounipolar, bipolar, and multipolar). Glial cells and stromal cells play a key role in supporting neurons and ensuring their efficacious functioning (Kurosinski and Gotz, 2002). Schwann cells are an example of glial cells that ensheathe some axons in myelin, supporting them through the production and secretion of trophic factors, in addition to insulating them in order to increase their speed of AP propagation. The latter is called saltatory conduction (AP "jumping" from one small, unmyelinated, section of the axon (node of Ranvier) to the next toward the axon terminal). As will be discussed later in this chapter, Schwann cells also play a key role in the neuronal response to injury and its subsequent regeneration.

Schwann cells insulate individual axons. Around each of these axons is a series of connective tissue layers that also support and protect individual axons (endoneurium), axons bundled together in nerve fascicles (perineurium), and nerve fascicles bundled together as whole nerves (epineurium). The endoneurium is the innermost connective tissue layer encircling a nerve axon within a fascicle. Within the endoneurium, microvasculature and capillaries supply and remove necessary axonal metabolites for functioning. Furthermore, these endothelial cells are linked via tight junctions creating an isolated environment around the axons and making up one part of the blood–nerve barrier. The perineurium makes up the second component of the blood–nerve barrier, again through tight endothelial junctions of vessels found within it (Mizisin and Weerasuriya, 2011; Weerasuriya and Mizisin, 2011). The perineurium is the connective tissue layer that surrounds bundles of axons, grouping them into nerve fascicles. Fascicles change position as they travel within nerves toward their end target, even moving from one nerve to another, and also become more specialized the more distal they are (often existing as a pure motor or pure sensory nerve fascicle the more distal to the spinal cord they are). The outermost connective tissue layer is the epineurium, which is predominantly made up collagen and elastic fibers (Tassler et al., 1994; Topp and Boyd, 2006). The epineurium binds nerve fascicles together into nerves by both encircling them, as well as holding them together in a scaffold-like nature as the interfascicular epineurium. This layer has a relatively high tensile strength and helps protect nerves from mechanical stretching.

26.2.2 Classification

Two main PNI classification systems exist, and are based on the severity of injury occurring to not only the neuronal axon, but the connective tissue layers surrounding them as well. The first classification system was proposed by Seddon (1943) and consists of three grades: neuropraxia, axonotmesis, and neurotmesis. Neuropraxia is the mildest from of PNI and is strictly an injury to the myelin sheath with preservation of the underlying axon. The effect of this can vary depending on severity from impaired conduction to complete conduction block. This type of injury pattern is typically seen in cases of mild compression or trauma to the nerve and is completely reversible upon Schwann cells proliferating and remyelinating the axon (thus taking less time than cases in which there is axonal damage and Wallerian degeneration ensues). Axonotmesis is the next most severe grade of injury and results in demyelination, as well as injury to the axon. In the original description by Seddon, this type of injury was described as sparing the internal nerve architecture (or with very little injury to the surrounding connective tissue layers), and was seen to subsequently have excellent recovery after axonal regeneration to their end-target (Seddon, 1943). In contrast, neurotmesis is the most severe type of nerve injury in this schema, and is the result of injury to both the axon and its surrounding connective tissue. Although complete nerve disruption may occur as in a transection, rupture, or avulsion type of injury, it is not always required. The epineurium may be intact, holding the nerve in physical continuity; however, subsequent fibroblastic scar tissue within the nerve results in impaired function and prevents axonal regeneration such that the nerve is effectively transected (Table 26.1).

Subsequent to Seddon reporting this PNI classification system, in 1951 Sunderland elaborated on it by expanding and describing the various degrees of injury that can occur to the nerve connective tissue (essentially expanding Seddon's axonometsis category). As shown in Figure 26.1, the result was a five-grade PNI classification (later becoming six grades by the introduction of a "mixed levels of injury" category) (Mackinnon and Dellon, 1988; Sunderland, 1951). Grade 1 injuries correspond to Seddon's neuropraxia injuries, grade 5 to neurotmesis injuries, and grades 2–4 varying degrees of connective tissue injury (2: axonal injury; 3: accompanying endoneurial injury; 4: accompanying perineurial injury). As will be discussed in Chapter 27, this classification system provided further insight into the outcome and appropriate timing of intervention after PNI. Grades 1 and 2 injuries were described as having excellent recovery and no intervention often being required, grades 4 and 5 resulting in poor recovery without intervention, and grade 3 injuries potentially resulting in good recovery, although requiring close observation for potential interventional repair being required.

26.2.3 Pathophysiology: Response to Injury

26.2.3.1 Zone of Injury and Distal Segment

The peripheral nerve response to injury (illustrated in Figure 26.2), including its sequence of events and the timing of these changes, depend on the severity of

Table 26.1 Peripheral Nerve Injury Classification (Seddon, 1943)

Seddon	Sunderland	Mackinnon	Description	Schematic
1: Neuropraxia	1: Neuropraxia	1: Neuropraxia	Focal conduction block ± demyelination	
	2: Axonotmesis	2: Axonotmesis	Demyelination with axonal injury	
2: Axonotmesis	3: Axonotmesis + endoneurium	3: Axonotmesis + endoneurium	Demyelination, axonal and endoneurial injury	
	4: Axonotmesis + perineurium	4: Axonotmesis + perineurium	Demyelination, axonal, endoneurial, and perineurial injury	
3: Neurotmesis	5: Axonotmesis + epineurium	5: Axonotmesis + epineurium	Demyelination, axonal, endoneurial, perineurial, and epineurial injury	
		6: Combination of above within the same nerve	Combinations of demyelination, axonal, endo-/peri-/epineurial injury	

injury and can be thought of in terms of neuronal cell components (axon – both proximal and distal to the injury – and the neuronal soma). Before (and if) regeneration occurs, first degeneration must occur. For neuropraxic injuries, no axonal degeneration occurs because no axonal injury has occurred. These injuries recover quickly because all that is required is remyelination. In grade 2 axonotmesis injuries, there is damage to the axon resulting in degeneration of its distal process through Wallerian degeneration (anterograde degeneration of the axon distal to the site of injury). Within hours of the injury, axonal and myelin fragmentation occurs with breakdown of its cytoskeletal components and subsequent loss of conductivity by 2–4 days post-injury, and the terminal, injured, axonal end sealing itself off (Burnett and Zager, 2004). Due to this process taking several days, it is possible that immediately after the injury APs can continue to be transmitted in the injured axon resulting in no detectable electrophysiological abnormality.

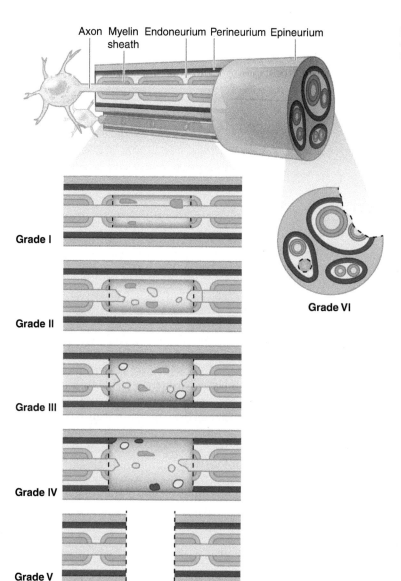

Axon Myelin Endoneurium Perineurium Epineurium
sheath

Grade I

Grade II

Grade III

Grade IV

Grade V

Grade VI

Figure 26.1 Diagrammatic representation of the different Sunderland (grades 1–5) and Mackinnon (grade 6) grades of nerve injury.

As axoplasmic transport slows and ceases, organelles and proteins/metabolites-in-transport accumulate in the proximal stump, resulting in its swelling. Schwann cells respond to the injury immediately by proliferating and upregulating gene expression essential to their function in Wallerian degeneration. Macrophages (having migrated into the zone of injury from nearby blood vessels) phagocytose the axonal and myelin debris preparing it for axonal regeneration. Local inflammatory cells such as endoneurial mast cells help by releasing histamine and serotonin inducing further capillary permeability (in addition to that caused by the injury itself; Burnett and Zager, 2004). This allows other inflammatory cells such as the previously mentioned macrophages to gain entry into the site and begin phagocytosing the debris, which can take several weeks to several months post-injury. As endoneurial connective tissue tubes are not irreversibly damaged, they return to their normal conformation by 2 weeks with Wallerian degeneration of the distal process continuing over the subsequent weeks to months.

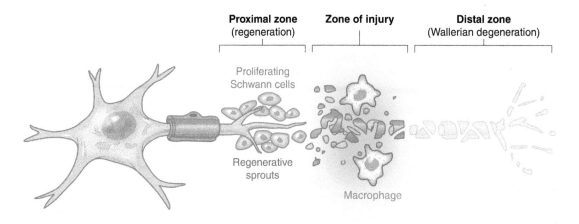

Proximal zone (regeneration) **Zone of injury** **Distal zone** (Wallerian degeneration)

Proliferating Schwann cells

Regenerative sprouts

Macrophage

Figure 26.2 Diagrammatic representation showing the nerve zone proximal to the injury (where nerve outgrowth occurs – whether regeneration or collateralization), the nerve injury zone, and nerve distal to the injury (where Wallerian degeneration occurs).

When injuries are more severe and there is disruption of the nerve's supporting connective tissue (Sunderland grade injuries >2), the inflammatory response is typically much more vigorous with subsequent necrosis, cellular infiltration, and proliferation that correlates with the severity of the initial injury. Endoneurial vascular disruption also occurs resulting in hemorrhage, edema, and influx of neutrophils and fibroblasts. The latter ultimately results in intraneural scarring with collagen deposition. In the distal segment, Schwann cells aggregate to form distinct columns within the basal lamina of the distal endoneurial tube (Bands of Bunger) after the axonal remnants have degenerated and been cleared. These Schwann cell columns act as a guidance tube for regenerating axons providing neurotrophic support for the incoming regenerating axons. Wallerian degeneration in the distal segment occurs (as in grade 2 injuries); however, the scarring within the zone of injury slows and impedes axonal regeneration resulting in the distal endoneurial tubes being denervated for longer periods of time. By 3–4 months post-injury, the distal segment endoneurial tubes have begun shrinking and if no regenerating axon re-innervates them, they eventually obliterate with their supportive Schwann cell columns due to progressive collagen deposition (Burnett and Zager, 2004). In the case of severe injuries (grades 4 and 5), the extent of intraneural and intrafascicular scarring from fibroblastic infiltration and proliferation is pronounced. In these circumstances, without intervention regenerating axons are often not able to penetrate the dense collagenous scar, ending blindly with subsequent obliteration of the distal nerve segment due to lack of re-innervation.

26.2.3.2 Proximal Segment and Neuronal Cell Body

Depending on the severity of the inciting injury, a variable amount of nerve degeneration more proximally occurs (up to the next node of Ranvier in the mildest of cases and potentially all the way back to the cell body in the most severe). This proximal segment involved undergoes Wallerian degeneration (with the entire axon degenerating if the cell body is involved). Immediately after injury, the neuronal soma swells, undergoes chromatolysis, and is isolated by processes from surrounding glial cells undergoing proliferation (Burnett and Zager, 2004). The proximal axonal segment shrinks as well, dependent both on the amount of injury to the neuronal cell body and the severity of the injurious stimulus. Neuronal cell body changes in response to PNI is an area of active research. The influence of the peripheral nerve microenvironment, including the role of Schwann cells and neurotrophins like nerve growth factor (NGF) and brain-derived neurotrophic factor (BDNF) on the neuronal cell body survival (which in turn dictates the regenerative capacity of its axon) and how this can be manipulated holds much promise in improving outcomes after PNI.

26.2.4 Regeneration

Much like the degenerative phase of PNI, the regenerative phase can also be thought of in terms of neuronal segment and PNI severity (which dictates to a degree the quality of regeneration and timing thereof). Typically, the regenerative process begins after Wallerian degeneration has been completed. However, in milder forms of injury (Sunderland grades 1 and 2 in which endoneurial tubes remain intact) regeneration may begin almost immediately after injury without the clearance of myelin and axonal debris. In more severe injuries, Wallerian degeneration occurs followed by regeneration across the zone of injury and into the distal endoneurial tube toward the end target. However, this may be delayed on account of several prerequisite factors and steps, including: reversal of nuclear chromatolysis (which has reprogrammed its cellular machinery from synaptic transmission to repair and regrowth functions); re-establishment of cytoskeletal axoplasmic transport (both fast and slow components); which is rate limiting and is thought to dictate the heuristic of 1–2 mm of regrowth/day (Jack et al., 2018); the length of proximal segment regeneration required to reach the zone of injury (which is again dependent on the severity of injury); regenerative fibers having to cross the scarred zone of injury, which may even prevent the axonal growth cone from reaching the distal segment before endoneurial tube obliteration; misdirection of axonal growth through the zone of injury or into inappropriate endoneurial tubes; the length of the distal segment needed to regenerate through in order to re-establish synaptic connections (i.e., with the neuromuscular end-plate) upon reaching the end target; and remyelination and axonal maturation, which then allows for functional recovery. A myriad of other factors may also influence the ability of a peripheral nerve axon to regenerate. These may include, for example, the age of the patient (which may be related to the intrinsic capacity of a PNS axon to produce neurotrophins or second messengers such as cyclic adenosine monophosphate, cAMP) or their comorbidities (such as smoking or diabetes, which may affect the neovascularization process also required for regeneration), to name a few.

At the tip of the regenerating axon, numerous axonal outgrowth sprouts extend distally with growth cone tips at each one. Through neurotropic chemotaxis, one or more of these growth cones can grow into the distal endoneurial tubes (either the same or different tubes) and continue down toward the end target via contact-mediated cues between filopodia found at their distal tip and Schwann cell basal lamina(Burnett and Zager, 2004; Dodd and Jessell, 1988; Gundersen and Barrett, 1980). Several factors also influence the re-establishment of a meaningful end-target connection. If a regenerating sprout grows into a functionally unrelated endoneurial tube, no connection is made. Furthermore, if too much time has passed between injury and end-target re-innervation, a functional connection is also not made. Depending on a plethora of factors similar to those discussed above (for

example, the presence or ability of collateral sprouts from adjacent uninjured axons at the end target to grow and maintain a functional connection while the regenerating axon grows toward it – termed collateralization), after a certain time window without innervation the end-organ target is no longer receptive to re-innervation (even if a newly regenerated axon reaches it). This time window is generally believed to be 1–2 years. Muscle fiber atrophy begins soon after denervation with cells losing 70% of their cross-sectional area by 2 months (Burnett and Zager, 2004). Moreover, synaptic folds at the neuromuscular junction end-plate are lost, and fibroblastic infiltration and proliferation results in collagen deposition between atrophied muscle fibers, which become separated by thickened connective tissue bands. Eventually these muscle fibers may be lost as a result (Burden et al., 1979; Burnett and Zager, 2004; Pestronk and Drachman, 1978). This is in part why physical therapy (PT) plays such an important role after PNI to try to prevent and delay irreversible muscle and joint atrophy, as well as contractures which hamper recovery if re-innervation does occur. Sensory re-innervation and cross-innervation is another impediment to a meaningful functional outcome in which fast-twitch muscle fibers may become re-innervated by a slow-twitch motor unit (the nerve fiber and all of the muscle cells it innervates) or vice versa, leading to inefficient muscle contraction. Sensory re-innervation and re-establishment of proprioception also have an important role to play in determining a meaningful functional outcome. Like motor re-innervation, sensory re-innervation is modality-specific; however, less so than motor re-innervation. This results in increased cross-innervation, and may also partly explain the occurrence of post-injury neuropathic pain (to be discussed later in the chapter).

Approximately 2 weeks after the start of regeneration, remyelination commences and continues at a rate much slower than regeneration. Schwann cells encircle the newly regenerated axon, wrapping around it to form a multi-laminated sheath which increases in diameter once it establishes a connection with its end target. However, differences between it and the original axon do exist, such as decreased internodal distances, a newly regenerated axon being typically smaller and more tortuous, as well as it having a higher g-ratio (axon diameter: axon + myelin diameter) indicating a thinner myelin sheath (Pham and Gupta, 2009). Despite the successful completion of all of these steps of axonal regeneration and remyelination in response to PNIs, it should be evident that a successful functional outcome is not guaranteed.

26.3 Conclusion

As discussed, a multitude of factors can influence the functional outcome of a patient after PNI. These factors may be intrinsic to the patient and non-modifiable (e.g., patient age), whereas others may be modifiable (e.g., timing of surgical intervention). Although the PNS has a remarkable capacity for regeneration and recovery post-injury with a relatively stereotyped choreography of promoting this, complete functional recovery is never guaranteed. Even with positive prognostic factors for recovery, it can be difficult to predict who will recover and over what time frame with a lot hinging on the mechanism of injury. In Chapter 27 we discuss different experimental PNI models, including: acute traumatic PNIs (such as nerve crush, stretch, and transection), entrapment nerve injury, tumor-related PNI, and models of neuropathic pain. Furthermore, repair strategies are also discussed.

Figure acknowledgements

The following images are credited to the authors of this chapter: Figures 26.1-26.2

References

Burden SJ, Sargent PB, McMahan UJ. Acetylcholine receptors in regenerating muscle accumulate at original synaptic sites in the absence of the nerve. *J Cell Biol* 1979;**82**(2):412–25. https://doi.org/10.1083/jcb.82.2.412

Burnett MG, Zager EL. Pathophysiology of peripheral nerve injury: a brief review. *Neurosurg Focus* 2004;**16**(5):E1. https://doi.org/10.3171/foc.2004.16.5.2

Caillaud M, Richard L, Vallat JM, Desmouliere A, Billet F. Peripheral nerve regeneration and intraneural revascularization. *Neural Regen Res* 2019;**14**(1):24–33. https://doi.org/10.4103/1673-5374.243699

Dodd J, Jessell TM. Axon guidance and the patterning of neuronal projections in vertebrates. *Science* 1988;**242**(4879):692–9. https://doi.org/10.1126/science.3055291

Gundersen RW, Barrett JN. Characterization of the turning response of dorsal root neurites toward nerve growth factor. *J Cell Biol* 1980;**87**(3 Pt 1):546–54. https://doi.org/10.1083/jcb.87.3.546

Jack AS, Hurd C, Forero J, et al. Cortical electrical stimulation in female rats with a cervical spinal cord injury to promote axonal outgrowth. *J Neurosci Res* 2018;**96**(5):852–62. https://doi.org/10.1002/jnr.24209

Kurosinski P, Gotz J. Glial cells under physiologic and pathologic conditions. *Arch Neurol* 2002;**59**(10):1524–8. https://doi.org/10.1001/archneur.59.10.1524

Mackinnon S, Dellon A. *Surgery of the Peripheral Nerve.* New York: Thieme, 1988.

Mizisin AP, Weerasuriya A. Homeostatic regulation of the endoneurial microenvironment during development, aging and in response to trauma, disease and toxic insult. *Acta Neuropathol* 2011;**121**(3):291–312. https://doi.org/10.1007/s00401-010-0783-x

Pestronk A, Drachman DB. Motor nerve sprouting and acetylcholine receptors. *Science* 1978;**199**(4334):1223–5. https://doi.org/10.1126/science.204007

Pham K, Gupta R. Understanding the mechanisms of entrapment neuropathies. *Neurosurg Focus* 2009;**26**(2):E7. https://doi.org/10.3171/FOC.2009.26.2.E7

Seddon H. Three types of nerve injury. *Brain* 1943;**66**:237.

Sunderland S. A classification of peripheral nerve injuries producing loss of function. *Brain* 1951;**74**(4):491–516. https://doi.org/10.1093/brain/74.4.491

Tassler PL, Dellon AL, Canoun C. Identification of elastic fibres in the peripheral nerve. *J Hand Surg Br* 1994;**19**(1):48–54. https://doi.org/10.1016/0266-7681(94)90049-3

Topp KS, Boyd BS. Structure and biomechanics of peripheral nerves: nerve responses to physical stresses and implications for physical therapist practice. *Phys Ther* 2006;**86**(1):92–109. https://doi.org/10.1093/ptj/86.1.92

Vallat JM, Tazir M, Calvo J, Funalot B. [Hereditary peripheral neuropathies]. *Presse Med* 2009;**38**(9):1325–34. https://doi.org/10.1016/j.lpm.2009.01.014

Weerasuriya A, Mizisin AP. The blood–nerve barrier: structure and functional significance. *Methods Mol Biol* 2011;**686**:149–73. https://doi.org/10.1007/978-1-60761-938-3_6

Clinical Peripheral Nerve Injury Models

Andrew S. Jack, Charlotte J. Huie, and Line Jacques

27.1 Introduction

Peripheral nerve injuries (PNIs) come in many varieties and their mechanism of injury can have a tremendous impact on a patient's expected outcome. As discussed in the last chapter, depending on the mechanism, PNIs have a relatively well-choreographed response to injury. However, much of this sequence will be influenced by both modifiable and non-modifiable prognostic factors. Furthermore, this mechanism of injury and its severity will also help dictate the appropriate treatment of the injury. In this chapter, basic science principles and models addressing PNIs are more specifically examined as they occur in the context of trauma, entrapment, tumors, and the changes occurring in acute and chronic pain states. Moreover, clinical case examples of such injuries will be discussed to conclude each section, including their respective management.

27.2 Peripheral Nerve Injury Models: Trauma, Entrapment, Tumors, and Pain

27.2.1 Acute Traumatic Injury

Acute traumatic nerve injuries may result in any category of Seddon or Sunderland injury, although typical experimental injury models studied include grades 2 to 5. Both in-vitro and in-vivo models have been used to study this type of PNI, and they can be categorized based on the mechanism of injury (crush, lacerating, stretch, to name a few), nerve studied, and/or animal species. Typical in-vitro models include cell cultures, 3D organotypic cultures, and glial cell cultures, whereas in-vivo models typically include sciatic and femoral nerve injuries from several different animal species, including: rats, mice, dogs, rabbits, among others (Menorca et al., 2013). Nerve crush models act to impart axonal damage and thus induce Wallerian degeneration while maintaining connective tissue continuity (resulting in typically better

outcomes; Caillaud et al., 2019; Geuna et al., 2009). Even within the nerve crush models previously used there exists substantial heterogeneity depending on how granular of detail is considered. For example, nerve crush models using a variety of surgical instruments for imparting the crush injury have been devised to study this type of PNI, which creates substantial heterogeneity and thus outcomes reported in the available literature (Caillaud et al., 2019; Chen et al., 1993; Kingery et al., 1994; Savastano et al., 2014). However, the advent and use of non-serrated surgical clamps applying a standardized force and pressure to the sciatic nerve have helped to normalize this heterogeneity (Beer et al., 2001; Varejao et al., 2004). Low interanimal variability with respect to regeneration and recovery has resulted in this type of sciatic-crush injury being ideal for studying nerve regeneration (Caillaud et al., 2019). However, its applicability to humans is questionable due to the sciatic nerve being a rare site of nerve crush injury (due to its relatively protected anatomical site; Menorca et al., 2013), most surgically relevant human sciatic nerve injuries involving partial transection or laceration and not necessarily a crush injury (Geuna, 2015), and the presence of extensive intraneural fibrosis that occurs after crush injury mandating early surgical intervention and often the use of nerve grafts and conduits for repair (Caillaud et al., 2019; Geuna, 2015; Tos et al., 2012).

Traumatic human PNI may include stretch injuries that result in irreversible damage upon the nerve's elastic properties being exceeded (which may also result in rupture or avulsion if the tensile force is high enough). Examples of this include brachial plexus birthing injuries (Teixera et al., 2015), spinal cord-root avulsion (Jack et al., 2020a, 2020b), and postoperative C5 palsy (Jack et al., 2019, 2020c), among others. Stretch injuries typically result in impaired axoplasmic flow and electrophysiological AP conduction abnormalities, as well as impaired intraneural perfusion leading to ischemia and potential infarct (Driscoll et al., 2002; Jack et al., 2019;

Keir and Rempel, 2005; Kwan et al., 1992; Lundborg and Rydevik,1973; Wall et al., 1992; Watanabe et al., 2001). Historically, most PNI animal models have focused on crush and transection injuries. However, more recently, several groups have devised stretch injury models, again involving the rat sciatic nerve (Alant et al., 2012, 2013; Kwan et al., 1992; Mahan, 2019; Ray et al., 2017; Wall et al., 1992). Although a comprehensive review of this model and its history is beyond the scope of this chapter, these models consist of both rapid and slow nerve stretch injury. Considering stretch injuries are the commonest form of traumatic nerve injury, these newer animal models will hopefully provide crucial information pertaining to nerve regenerative potential (Mahan, 2019; Ray et al., 2017).

One of the most commonly studied PNIs is a laceration or transection injury. In humans, this may occur cleanly as in the case of an iatrogenic injury at the time of surgery or more bluntly as in the case of traumatic transection after animal bite (Caillaud et al., 2019; Martyn and Hughes, 1997). This often results in a Seddon neurotmetic (or Sunderland grade 5) lesion. In these cases, functional recovery will almost certainly never be complete. It is because of the poor functional outcome without surgical intervention that these injuries are typically repaired either acutely or subacutely. In the case of a clean, sharp nerve laceration/transection with relatively little damage to the surrounding tissues, repair is typically undertaken within the first 3 days. However, in the setting of a dirty, blunt laceration/transection with the possibility of more damage to the surrounding tissues, repair is typically undertaken after a delay of 2–3 weeks. The latter type of injury often incites more inflammation and more widespread injury to the nerve. Both of these then require more time for the full extent of nerve injury to be delineated in order for the surgeon to determine how much of the affected nerve then requires repair.

In contrast, the previously discussed crush injuries are typically repaired in a more delayed fashion (typically ≥3-months post-injury). The reason for the delay in repair (if it is required) is because of the difficult in clinically and/or electrophysiologically determining the severity of the closed nerve injury that has occurred (which then dictates if and when PNI recovery will occur and thus whether surgical intervention will be required). If the injury is a Sunderland grade 1–3, then some electrophysiological and/or clinical recovery should be seen by that time and the patient can continue to be followed. However, if the injury is a Sunderland grade 4 or 5 injury, no recovery is likely to be seen and surgical intervention may be warranted. Unfortunately, nerve injuries in reality may not be this simplistic and a mixed type of injury severities can exist which can complicate this algorithmic approach (Mackinnon and Dellon, 1988). Furthermore, even at 3 months' time, despite there being no electrophysiological evidence of recovery, upon surgical intervention nerve action potentials (NAPs) through the damaged segment may be evident. In general, simple external neurolysis should be completed in this case without a need for internal neurolysis or direct nerve repair. That being said, however, akin to the 3-day, 3-week, 3-month heuristic described for the timing of injury repair, the former is merely a guide with many factors determining the best surgical treatment and repair adjuncts (such as the use of nerve transfers) to be used for different types of injuries. For example, traumatic laceration/transection injuries may also result in a gap between the proximal and distal ends requiring the use of a nerve graft (such as a sural nerve graft) or conduit (biological or synthetic) to bridge the two ends (Berger and Millesi, 1978; Caillaud et al., 2019; Hastert-Talini et al., 2013; Johansson and Dahlin, 2014; Reid et al., 2013; Stossel et al., 2018; Tos et al., 2012). The rat sciatic nerve is the most frequently used to study this type of transection injury. This is in part because of the model's versatility in being able to accommodate the study of various aspects of nerve regeneration and repair techniques such as both early and late effects of muscular denervation, strategies in preventing muscle atrophy, direct neurorrhaphy, scar tissue formation, the use and efficacy of nerve grafts, conduits, decellularized allografts, as well as various tissue glues, among others (Battiston et al., 2009; Blom et al., 2014; Brooks et al., 2012; Felix et al., 2013; Caillaud et al., 2019; Geuna, 2015; Geuna et al., 2009; Gordon and Borschel, 2017; Karsidag et al., 2012; Moimas et al., 2013; Que et al., 2013; Siemionow and Brzezicki, 2009; Whitlock et al., 2009). Other animal nerve models such as the femoral nerve (often used to study the effects of pure motor or sensory injury and recovery; Al-Majed et al., 2000a, 2000b; Brushart et al., 2002; Gordon et al., 2008; Madison et al., 1996; Menorca et al., 2013) and the median nerve (for studying grasping) have also been used to study laceration/transection injuries (Menorca et al., 2013; Papalia et al., 2003; Tos et al., 2008). However, these have been much less commonplace than the sciatic due to their innate technical difficulty (Menorca et al., 2013).

27.2.1.1 Case Example

A 36-year-old man presented 6 months after being involved in a motorcycle collision in which he was dragged under another vehicle. As a result, he suffered a right elbow dislocation. At the time of injury, he experienced immediate onset, electric-like pain radiating down his entire right arm, was unable to feel his dorsal forearm and entire hand, and was unable to move his hand. He subsequently regained some function with physiotherapy to the point where at presentation as an outpatient his neurological deficits were confined to a radial nerve distribution and included: weakness to forearm supination, paralysis of his wrist and fingers, as well as decreased dorsal hand sensation. Nerve conduction and electromyography (EMG) studies were in keeping with a neurotmetic lesion localized just proximal to the patient's elbow and a magnetic resonance imaging neurogram (MRN) showed an avulsion of the patient's radial nerve just above his elbow (Figure 27.1). The patient underwent exploration and operative repair of his radial nerve with an interpositional graft being used to bridge a 6.5-cm gap between the proximal nerve stump just above the elbow to his posterior interosseus nerve.

27.2.2 Compression

Unlike acute traumatic PNIs due to stretch, crush, or laceration/transection, chronic compression injuries do not typically involve axonal injury until late in the disease course. Furthermore, although chronic nerve compression (CNC) injuries are the most prevalent type of injury clinically (as seen in cases of carpal tunnel syndrome (CTS) or cubital tunnel syndrome (CuTS)), research into

CNC pathophysiological mechanisms has been much more recently established. Several animal models (including different species and nerves studied) for this type of PNI have been created including circumferential nerve compression with silastic tubes and inflatable cuffs (Gelberman et al., 1983a, 1983b; Gupta and Steward, 2003; Lundborg et al., 1982; O'Brien et al., 1987; Ochoa et al., 1972; Pham and Gupta, 2009; Rydevik and Lundborg, 1977; Rydevik et al., 1981; Szabo and Sharkey, 1993), nerve flattening and compression with cyanoacrylate (Dong et al., 2019), vibration-induced nerve injury (Chang et al., 1994; Dahlin et al., 1987, 1993; Dahlin and Kanje, 1992; Dahlin and Thambert, 1993; Lundborg et al., 1990), repetitive animal grasping (Clark et al., 2003, 2004), chemical-induced inflammation (Rosen et al., 1992), nerve excursion and strain-based models (Sommerich et al., 2007; Tricaud et al., 2005; Yamaguchi et al., 2008), among others. Although the latter is more in keeping with a stretch-based PNI, evidence suggests that both it and CNC models may involve (at least in part) an ischemia-based mechanism.

Upon compression of a nerve, mechanical shear forces at the nerve surface are more responsible for the peripheral/external nerve damage and may lead to ischemia-based injury to the inner part of the nerve, which seems to be more related to the duration of compression rather than the magnitude (Ochoa et al., 1972; Rydevik and Lundborg, 1977; Rydevik et al., 1981). This creates a vicious cycle in which intraneural edema also develops and is sustained long after the compression is released (also helping to explain the prolonged deficits seen after brief episodes of compression; Dyck et al., 1990; Lundborg et al.,

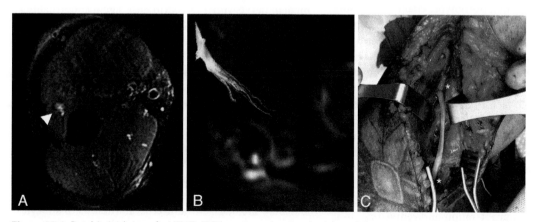

Figure 27.1 Panel A: Axial view of a MRN T_2 FLEX sequence showing the right radial nerve ending in a T_2 hyperintense neuromatous stump (white arrowhead) just proximal to the elbow. Panel B: MRN diffusion tensor imaging sequence showing the avulsed right radial nerve. Panel C: Intraoperative image (top: proximal and bottom: distal) of the radial nerve repair after coaptation (white asterisks) of the proximal radial nerve to the distal posterior interosseus nerve with an interpositional nerve graft.

1983; Rydevik and Lundborg, 1977; Rydevik et al., 1981). This increased intraneural pressure is then thought to translate into myelin-based axonal changes and cytoskeletal-based changes, both of which result in abnormal electrophysiological AP conduction (Dahlin et al., 1993; Dahlin and Kanje, 1992; Dahlin and Thambert, 1993; Gupta et al, 2004; Ludwin and Maitland, 1984; Mackinnon et al., 1986; O'Brien et al., 1987). With ongoing and repetitive compression, more extensive axonal injury will ensue, resulting in degeneration and regeneration, remyelination, fibrosis, as well as vascular and connective tissue hypertrophy.

In addition to the cytoskeletal changes observed, Schwann cell-driven demyelination and remyelination is thought to be one of the primary pathophysiological processes in CNC PNI. Like acute traumatic injuries, CNC results in characteristic changes such as an increased g-ratio and decreased internodal distance; however, in CNC conditions, increased Schmidt–Lanterman incisures are also seen (Gupta et al, 2004; Ludwin and Maitland, 1984; Mackinnon et al., 1986; O'Brien et al., 1987; Tricaud et al., 2005). The increased Schmidt–Lanterman incisures are thought to be indicative of an increased axonal metabolic demand with both Schwann cell proliferation and apoptosis being observed soon after CNC injury (Gupta and Steward, 2003). Furthermore, this proliferative–apoptotic response occurs without any evidence of axonal injury or Wallerian degeneration (Pham and Gupta, 2009). Other changes observed include myelin-associated glycoprotein (MAG) downregulation (presumably to allow for axonal sprouting, even in the absence of axonal injury), growth-associated protein (GAP-43) upregulation (involved in actin molecule regulation at the growth cone), phenotypic change in sensory neurons from neurofilament-200 neurons to isolectin B4-binding and calcitonin gene-related peptide neurons (suggesting a change from proprioceptive to nociceptive neurons and discussed in the pain section of this chapter), which is likely Schwann cell-mediated through glial cell-derived neurotrophic factor (GDNF) (Chao et al., 2008; Jacobson et al., 1986; Molliver et al., 1997).

Unlike traumatic injuries, macrophage infiltration in CNC injuries occurs much more gradually over a period of several weeks, and does not seem to be responsible for Schwann cell proliferation (Bruck, 1997; Gray et al., 2007; Gupta and Channual, 2006; Taskinen and Roytta, 1997). Instead, Schwann cell proliferation and remyelination is thought to be mediated through direct, mechanical, contact-based cues (Gupta et al., 2005; Nodari et al., 2008; Previtali et al., 2001; Salzer and Bunge, 1980; Schwartz

and DeSimone, 2008). The exact mechanism for this, however, is still under investigation. Although acute traumatic PNIs and CNC PNIs share some common characteristics, it is evident that the two have very distinct pathophysiological processes. Whereas in acute traumatic injuries in which the neuron dictates the glial cell response leading to Wallerian degeneration, evidence suggests that CNC results in primarily a Schwann cell-directed response that then dictates neuronal changes. It is also likely that CNC represents a spectrum of dysfunction in which the response and result depend on the compression duration and magnitude, among other factors, which then dictate the degree of ischemia and Schwann cell dysfunction (and/or axonal cytoskeletal degeneration) that occurs. Regardless of mechanism, both represent unfortunately common modalities of PNI resulting not only in significant neurological deficit, but significant neuropathic pain.

27.2.2.1 Case Example

A 56-year-old man presented as an outpatient with ongoing numbness, tingling, and pain in his left hand after undergoing a left carpal tunnel release (CTR) 2 months prior. He stated that he had awoken after his previous CTR with severe pain in his hand that had subsequently progressed over the last 2 months to include numbness and tingling to the point where he would burn his index and middle finger without noticing. Upon examination, the patient was found to have severe palmar-sparing numbness (almost insensate) in a median nerve distribution with thenar muscle weakness and wasting. Nerve conduction and EMG studies revealed severe median neuropathy at the wrist with MRN revealing an enlarged median nerve with T_2 hyperintense signal abnormality at the wrist (Figure 27.2). Intraoperatively, repeat CTR was performed with incomplete release of the flexor retinaculum being seen and the median nerve appearing hyperemic, indurated, and focally enlarged, in keeping with a neuroma-in-continuity (NIC).

27.2.3 Tumor

The first description of what we now know as a peripheral nerve sheath tumor (PNST) was in 1741 (Kim et al., 2011). Peripheral nerve sheath tumors are tumors that arise from cells surrounding an axon or nerve fascicle, and may include Schwann cells, fibroblasts, histiocytes, and macrophage-like cells, among others. These tumors can be classified based on their cell of origin (e.g., perineurioma, schwannoma, neurofibroma), in addition to

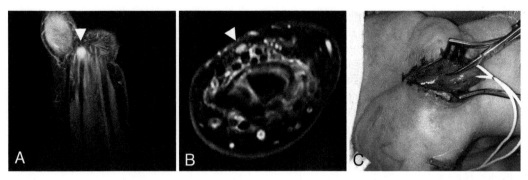

Figure 27.2 Panel A: Coronal view of a MRN T$_2$ FLEX sequence showing a focally enlarged median nerve (white arrowhead) at the wrist with T$_2$ hyperintense signal abnormality. Panel B: Axial view of the same MRN showing the abnormal median nerve in-keeping with a neuroma-in-continuity (white arrowhead). Panel C: Intraoperative image of the focally enlarged and hyperemic median nerve after repeat carpal tunnel release.

being benign or malignant. Here, we discuss the most common types of PNSTs (neurofibromas and schwannomas) and some of the pathobiology and animal models underlying much of the research that has been done regarding their formation.

Neurofibromas are benign PNSTs and in adults comprise the second most common type of PNST after schwannomas (this ratio being reversed in the pediatric population). Furthermore, they can be subclassified as either solitary or plexiform and sporadic or syndromic in the context of neurofibromatosis type 1 or type 2 (NF-1, NF-2; Chick et al., 2000; Kim et al., 2011). Similarly, schwannomas can also occur sporadically or in association with a genetic syndrome (NF-1, NF-2, Schwannomatosis, Carney's complex). The natural history and malignant potential of both neurofibromas and schwannomas will depend on the presence or absence of a genetic predisposition (Longo et al., 2018).

In general, clinical indications for PNST surgical resection may include pain (usually failing conservative management), neurologic deficit (paresthesia/anesthesia or weakness), demonstrated growth (although tumor growth that remains asymptomatic can also be monitored with serial imaging and regular physical examination), diameter over 3 cm, and the possibility of malignancy (Desai, 2012; Spinner and Kline, 2000). Surgical resection is usually the treatment of choice for PNST, with gross total resection (GTR) often being curative (Stone and Spinner, 2020). However, this does not come without risks that must be weighed against the possibility of new or worsened motor deficit and painful paresthesia (Prudner et al., 2020; Stone and Spinner, 2020). The likelihood of GTR depends on several factors such as tumor size, location, and malignancy, among others,

and the difference between benign and malignant entities is not always clear cut. In order to better define benign and malignant tumors, a recently described malignant precursor has been introduced, termed atypical neurofibromatous neoplasm of uncertain biologic potential (ANNUBP; Miettinen et al., 2017). Epidemiologically, malignant transformation has been reported to occur in 10–15% of plexiform neurofibromas associated with NF-1, with 50% of all malignant PNSTs (MPNSTs) occurring in the context of NF-1 (Evans et al., 2002; Kolberg et al., 2013; Longo et al., 2018; McCaughan et al., 2007; Pasmant et al., 2010; Staedtke et al., 2017). Treatment of MPNSTs remains challenging, with many advocating multidisciplinary input and a combination of surgery, radiation therapy, and chemotherapeutic agents.

PNSTs occurring in the context of genetic syndromes such as neurofibromatosis are an area of active research. Genetically engineered mouse models (GEMMs) have been designed to address key questions about the cell lineage that is essential for tumorigenesis, the microenvironment that contributes to neoplasia, mutations implicated in the malignant transformation and progression of neurofibromas, the role of dysregulated growth factor signaling, as well as neurofibromin-regulated Ras proteins (Brossier and Carroll, 2012; Gottfried et al., 2010). Loss-of-function mutations in tumor suppressor and cell cycle genes such as *p53*, *CDNKN2A*, and *PTEN* have been long implicated in the formation and progression of MPNSTs (Laycock-van Spyk et al., 2011). However, further study is still needed to help elucidate several missing steps in these models, such as the role of paracrine signaling molecules. The role that cell cycle signaling molecules play in NF-1 MPNST progression such as Ras/ERK signaling has provided a strong rationale for creation and testing of novel biological therapeutics such as mitogen-activated protein kinase (MAPK) inhibitors in clinical trials. In GEMMS, oral dosing of selumetinib, an inhibitor of MEK1-2, has resulted in a reduction in number, size, and proliferation of neurofibromas. Moreover, Phase I and Phase II clinical trials (SPRINT) in children with inoperable plexiform neurofibromas in the context of NF-1 haVE resulted in a 72% response rate with respect to peripheral nerve-related pain and motor impairment (most responses being sustained ≥ 6 months). Selumetinib is now FDA-approved and indicated for the treatment of pediatric patients ≥2 years of age with NF-1 who have symptomatic, inoperable plexiform neurofibromas (Dombi et al., 2016; Gross et al., 2017, 2020a, 2020b).

The astonishing progress being made in basic science research techniques (specifically, molecular biology and genetic sequencing) has resulted in an equally impressive advancement of our understanding of the pathogenesis of the PNST pathobiology. This understanding has also led to a bench-to-bedside knowledge translation with the advent of novel tumor therapeutics. More accurate animal models and agents for targeted molecular therapy are currently being developed and show promising preliminary results for the treatment of traditionally difficult diseases such as MPNSTs.

27.2.3.1 Case Example

A 50-year-old man with known history of NF-1 was referred as an outpatient for left-sided electric-like, lancinating pain radiating down from his neck into his arm, dorsal forearm, and hand. He stated the pain had been relatively unchanged compared to a year prior, although seemed to be occurring more frequently now with movement of his arm and neck. He denied any history of constitutional symptoms or weakness; however, he did mention that he had started noticing some subtle numbness in the back of his hand. On examination, the patient had fullness to his left supraclavicular fossa with tenderness to palpation (eliciting the electric-like pain), and his neurological deficits included only subtle numbness to his dorsal hand in a radial nerve-like distribution. Nerve conduction and EMG studies were unremarkable and MRN revealed a large PNST emanating from the C7 nerve root (Figure 27.3). Intraoperatively, a left-supraclavicular brachial plexus approach was used with the help of neurophysiological monitoring for maximal safe tumor resection. Frozen-section pathology at the

time of surgery and permanent section both confirmed a neurofibroma.

27.2.4 Pain

The International Association for the Study of Pain (IASP) has described the taxonomy and defined pain as an "unpleasant sensory and emotional experience associated with, or resembling that associated with, actual or potential tissue damage" (Scholz et al., 2019). Its classification can be based on its timing (acute versus chronic), its pathophysiology (neuropathic versus nociceptive), and/or based on its anatomical localization (e.g., headache, back pain, etc.; Bouhassira, 2019; Scholz et al., 2019; Swieboda et al., 2013).

The mechanisms involved in the pathophysiology of neuropathic pain are numerous and can be thought of in terms of peripheral, spinal, and central localization. At a peripheral level, there is an increased production of sodium (Na) channels after injury. This accumulation of Na channels at the neuroma site and along the axon act as foci of hyperexcitability and ectopic discharges (responsible for a Tinel's sign, for instance, and the rationale behind the use of Na channel blockers as pain medication). Pain may also be sympathetically maintained post-injury. Axons express α-adrenergic receptors and become sensitive to the post-ganglionic sympathetic release of norepinephrine. After PNI, sympathetic axons sprout into the dorsal root ganglion (DRG) and can activate sensory neurons (explaining sympathectomy procedures for the treatment of pain). There is also a peripheral sensitization process that may occur involving inflammatory mediators such as bradykinin and/or prostaglandins. These mediators sensitize the peripheral nerve endings through phosphorylation of voltage-gated channels and produced greater excitation in the peripheral nerve by lowering the activation threshold of the neurons. For example, a damaged C-fiber may therefore begin to fire spontaneously (Alles and Smith, 2018; Hashmonai et al., 2016; Kramis et al., 1996; Tobbs et al., 2016). More proximally, at a spinal level, mechanisms involved in pain signal generation and propagation include decreased inhibition of dorsal horn sensory neurons, excitotoxic death of inhibitory interneurons in lamina II, gamma-aminobutyric-acid (GABA) reduction and GABA- and/or opioid-receptor downregulation, and cholycystokinin (opiate inhibitor) upregulation resulting in increased dorsal horn neuronal activity, to name a few (Sommer et al., 2018; Tsuda, 2016).

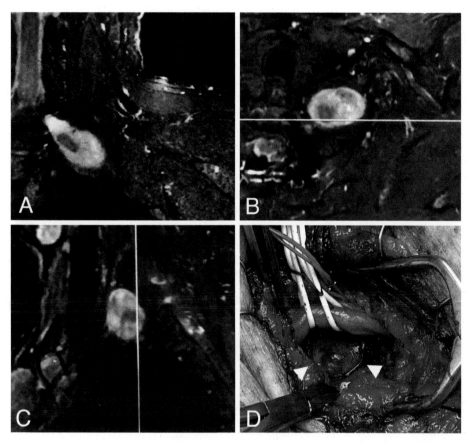

Figure 27.3 Panels A–C: Coronal (Panel A), axial (Panel B), and sagittal (Panel C) views of an MRN T$_2$ FLEX sequence showing a large, left, extraforaminal peripheral nerve sheath tumor emanating from the C7 nerve root extending down into the middle trunk. Panel D: Intraoperative image (left: distal and right: proximal) of the C7 neurofibroma (white arrowheads) after supraclavicular brachial plexus exposure (white vessel loops isolating the upper trunk and red vessel loop isolating the phrenic nerve).

Centrally, sensitization of nociceptive C-fiber input is a key factor in the mechanisms involved in pain generation. Prolonged depolarization and stimulation of C-fibers recruits N-methyl-D-aspartate (NMDA) receptors, which eventually cause greater excitation in the postsynaptic neurons of the dorsal horn (due to the NMDA receptors adding to the response). The central sensitization of dorsal horn neurons then results in an enlargement of the field to which they are responsive and results in them being hypersensitive. Sprouting of A-β-fibers into lamina II (which typically only receives A-δ and C-fibers) after injury, in conjunction with an A-β-fiber phenotypic switch from being responsive to met-enkephalin to substance P responsive (resulting in typically non-noxious stimuli from A-β-fibers being perceived as noxious), also results in central sensitization and pain signal amplification. Finally, cerebral plasticity alters the processing of pain and potentially amplifies it through the recruitment of new areas not normally involved in pain (Li et al., 2016; Penas and Navarro, 2018).

Spinal cord stimulation (SCS), peripheral nerve stimulation, and peripheral nerve field stimulation (PNFS) are all used to treat pain generated from PNIs, and are technologies that have been developed by understanding the mechanisms involved in pain such as the gate theory model by Melzach and Wall (1965) (Banks and Winfree, 2019; Deogaonkar and Slavin, 2014; Melzack, 1999; Mendell, 2014; Sdrulla et al., 2018). As mentioned, several electrical stimulation (ES)-based technologies have been devised to treat pain that are based on several different mechanisms. For example, SCS involves ES of the dorsal columns extradurally, which mediates the inhibition of spinal afferents depending on the stimulation frequency. Computational modeling has predicted that 30–80 Hz suppresses a wide dynamic range dorsal neuron activity. GABAergic mechanisms also modulate the activity of sensory neurons and SCS responses. Dorsal root ganglion stimulation is also an attractive target as the somata of primary sensory neurons in the DRG are important foci for changes that lead to neuropathic pain. The DRG

T-junction may normally impede the propagation of some action potentials arising in the periphery, thus acting as a filter which may be lost in states of chronic pain. Several in-vitro and in-vivo animal studies have reported an improvement in pain-related behavior following stimulation (Koopmeiners et al., 2013; Kovalsky et al., 2009; Vuka et al., 2018). Animal models such as these for DRG ES can be thought of based on the method of insult and their end-point measurements. For example, pain testing can be reflexive and includes pain-inducing insults such as thermal (Hargreaves, tail-flick, acetone), mechanical (Von Frey fibers, pressure), or electrical stimuli, whereas non-reflexive testing may include measuring behavioral changes to pain (e.g., spontaneous pain behavior or avoidance of evoked stimuli; Greogory et al., 2013). Conversely, these animal nerve injury pain models can be grouped according to their mechanism of injury: nerve transection, nerve root ligation, crush, or stretch. These injuries can often lead to painful

neuroma formation, which is also an active area of research. However, there is no consensus on the optimal way to treat the painful neuromas, and the role of surgery remains controversial.

Neuroma excision, excision and cap, excision and transposition into a vein/bone/muscle, and excision and nerve repair with or without interpositional auto- or allograft have all been described. A comparative meta-analysis concluded that 77% of painful neuroma cases had clinically meaningful improvement of pain regardless of the surgical technique. Future studies are necessary to facilitate the evidence-based treatment of patients with painful neuromas (Poppler et al., 2018). Targeted muscle re-innervation (TMR) is another more recent surgical technique developed for neuroma-induced pain treatment that consists of reassigning remaining arm or leg nerve stumps after amputation through coaptation to residual chest/arm or leg muscles that are no longer

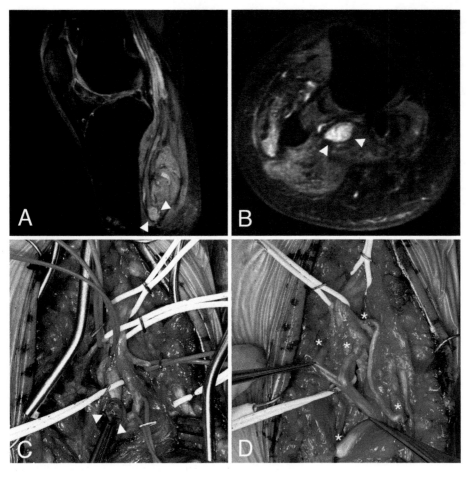

Figure 27.4 Sagittal (Panel A) and coronal (Panel B) view of a T_2-weighted, fat-suppressed and gadolinium-enhanced MRN revealing an ovoid and enhancing neuroma from the tibial nerve (white arrowheads). Intraoperative photographs (top: proximal and bottom: distal) showing the neuroma (white arrowheads) before resection (Panel C) and after resection with coaptation (white asterisks) to medial and lateral gastrocnemius muscle branches using an interpositional allograft (Panel D).

functional due to the loss of the limb. Targeted muscle re-innervation was initially developed to improve control of myoelectric upper limb prostheses; however, it was then found to improve pain control and as such has more recently been investigated as a method to prevent or treat painful amputation neuromas (Kuiken et al., 2017). A prospective randomized clinical trial was conducted on 28 amputees and showed that TMR improved the phantom limb pain and demonstrated a trend toward improving residual limb pain compared with conventional neurectomy (Dumanian et al., 2019). Further animal model research will hopefully improve our understanding and help clarify changes in pain pathways and neuronal regeneration induced by TMR.

Despite major advances being made in the investigational aspect of peripheral nerve injury and pain, there are a lot of questions that remain unanswered. Robust, well-validated, animal models research of neuropathic pain, in addition to well-constructed prospective randomized control clinical trials, will hopefully help shed light on some of these questions.

27.2.4.1 Case Example

A 59-year-old female had previously undergone a right below-knee amputation after a prolonged history of osteomyelitis. Approximately 1 year after the amputation she began experiencing a constant sharp pain from her stump with electric-like, lancinating pain whenever she put on her prosthetic for weight-bearing or palpated the area. The pain would radiate up her posterior thigh into her back. Examination revealed a well-healed below-knee amputation stump with a positive Tinel's sign close to the distal amputation site. Investigations including an MRN revealed a 1.0 cm × 0.7 cm ovoid neuroma in her right lower-extremity stump emanating from her tibial nerve (Figure 27.4A and 27.4B). Having failed more conservative pain management strategies, the patient was scheduled for a TMR procedure. Intraoperatively, the tibial nerve was identified, as well as the sural nerve, in the popliteal fossa and followed distally to the neuroma. The neuroma was then resected (Figure 27.4C) and branches from the medial and lateral gastrocnemius muscle identified and isolated with vessel loops. An interpositional allograft was coapted to the tibial nerve proximally and divided distally such that four branches were coapted to the gastrocnemius muscle branches (Figure 27.4D). Finally, the sural nerve was also divided and coapted with a lateral gastrocnemius muscle branch. At 9-month clinical follow-up, the patient had recovered without complication and was pain-free.

Figure acknowledgements

The following images obtained from patients with consent are credited to the authors of this chapter: Figures 27.1–27.4

References

Alant JD, Kemp SW, Khu KJ, Kumar R, Webb AA, Midha R. Traumatic neuroma in continuity injury model in rodents. *J Neurotrauma* 2012;**29**(8):1691–703. https://doi.org/10.1089/neu.2011.1857.

Alant JD, Senjaya F, Ivanovic A, Forden J, Shakhbazau A, Midha R. The impact of motor axon misdirection and attrition on behavioral deficit following experimental nerve injuries. *PLoS One* 2013;**8**(11):e82546. https://doi.org/10.1371/journal.pone.0082546.

Alles SRA, Smith PA. Etiology and pharmacology of neuropathic pain. *Pharmacol Rev* 2018;**70**(2):315–47. https://doi.org/10.1124/pr.117.014399.

Al-Majed AA, Brushart TM, Gordon T. Electrical stimulation accelerates and increases expression of BDNF and trkB mRNA in regenerating rat femoral motoneurons. *Eur J Neurosci* 2000a;**12**(12):4381–90.

Al-Majed AA, Neumann CM, Brushart TM, Gordon T. Brief electrical stimulation promotes the speed and accuracy of motor axonal regeneration. *J Neurosci* 2000b;**20**(7):2602–08.

Banks GP, Winfree CJ. Evolving techniques and indications in peripheral nerve stimulation for pain. *Neurosurg Clin N Am* 2019;**30**(2):265–73. https://doi.org/10.1016/j.nec.2018.12.011.

Battiston B, Raimondo S, Tos P, et al. Chapter 11: Tissue engineering of peripheral nerves. *Int Rev Neurobiol* 2009;**87**:227–49. https://doi.org/10.1016/S0074-7742(09)87011-6.

Beer GM, Steurer J, Meyer VE. Standardizing nerve crushes with a non-serrated clamp. *J Reconstr Microsurg* 2001;**17**(7):531–534. https://doi.org/10.1055/s-2001-17755.

Berger A, Millesi H. Nerve grafting. *Clin Orthop Relat Res* 1978;(133):49–55.

Blom CL, Martensson LB, Dahlin LB. Nerve injury-induced c-Jun activation in Schwann cells is JNK independent. *Biomed Res Int* 2014;**2014**:392971. https://doi.org/10.1155/2014/392971.

Bouhassira D. Neuropathic pain: definition, assessment and epidemiology. *Rev Neurol (Paris)* 2019;**175**(1–2):16–25. https://doi.org/10.1016/j.neurol.2018.09.016.

Brooks DN, Weber RV, Chao JD, et al. Processed nerve allografts for peripheral nerve reconstruction: a multicenter study of utilization and outcomes in sensory, mixed, and motor nerve reconstructions. *Microsurgery* 2012;**32**(1):1–14. https://doi.org/10.1002/micr.20975.

Brossier NM, Carroll SL. Genetically engineered mouse models shed new light on the pathogenesis of neurofibromatosis type

I-related neoplasms of the peripheral nervous system. *Brain Res Bull* 2012;**88**(1):58–71. https://doi.org/10.1016/j.brainresbull.2011.08.005.

Bruck W. The role of macrophages in Wallerian degeneration. *Brain Pathol* 1997;**7**(2):741–52. https://doi.org/10.1111/j.1750-3639.1997.tb01060.x.

Brushart TM, Hoffman PN, Royall RM, Murinson BB, Witzel C, Gordon T. Electrical stimulation promotes motoneuron regeneration without increasing its speed or conditioning the neuron. *J Neurosci* 2002;**22**(15):6631–8. https://doi.org/10.1523/JNEUROSCI.22-15-06631.2002.

Caillaud M, Richard L, Vallat JM, Desmouliere A, Billet F. Peripheral nerve regeneration and intraneural revascularization. *Neural Regen Res* 2019;**14**(1):24–33. https://doi.org/10.4103/1673-5374.243699.

Chang KY, Ho ST, Yu HS. Vibration induced neurophysiological and electron microscopical changes in rat peripheral nerves. *Occup Environ Med* 1994;**51**(2):130–5. https://doi.org/10.1136/oem.51.2.130.

Chao T, Pham K, Steward O, Gupta R. Chronic nerve compression injury induces a phenotypic switch of neurons within the dorsal root ganglia. *J Comp Neurol* 2008;**506**(2):180–93. https://doi.org/10.1002/cne.21537.

Chen LE, Seaber AV, Urbaniak JR. The influence of magnitude and duration of crush load on functional recovery of the peripheral nerve. *J Reconstr Microsurg* 1993;**9**(4):299–306; discussion 306–07. https://doi.org/10.1055/s-2007-1006671.

Chick G, Alnot JY, Silbermann-Hoffman O. [Benign solitary tumors of the peripheral nerves]. *Rev Chir Orthop Reparatrice Appar Mot* 2000;**86**(8):825–34.

Clark BD, Al-Shatti TA, Barr AE, Amin M, Barbe MF. Performance of a high-repetition, high-force task induces carpal tunnel syndrome in rats. *J Orthop Sports Phys Ther* 2004;**34**(5):244–53. https://doi.org/10.2519/jospt.2004.34.5.244.

Clark BD, Barr AE, Safadi FF, et al. Median nerve trauma in a rat model of work-related musculoskeletal disorder. *J Neurotrauma* 2003;**20**(7):681–95. https://doi.org/10.1089/089771503322144590.

Dahlin LB, Archer DR, McLean WG. Axonal transport and morphological changes following nerve compression. An experimental study in the rabbit vagus nerve. *J Hand Surg Br* 1993;**18**(1):106–10. https://doi.org/10.1016/0266-7681(93)90206-u.

Dahlin LB, Kanje M. Conditioning effect induced by chronic nerve compression. An experimental study of the sciatic and tibial nerves of rats. *Scand J Plast Reconstr Surg Hand Surg* 1992;**26**(1):37–41. https://doi.org/10.3109/02844319209035181.

Dahlin LB, Nordborg C, Lundborg G. Morphologic changes in nerve cell bodies induced by experimental graded nerve compression. *Exp Neurol* 1987;**95**(3):611–21. https://doi.org/10.1016/0014-4886(87)90303-7.

Dahlin LB, Thambert C. Acute nerve compression at low pressures has a conditioning lesion effect on rat sciatic nerves. *Acta Orthop Scand* 1993;**64**(4):479–81. https://doi.org/10.3109/17453679308993673.

Deogaonkar M, Slavin KV. Peripheral nerve/field stimulation for neuropathic pain. *Neurosurg Clin N Am* 2014;**25**(1):1–10. https://doi.org/10.1016/j.nec.2013.10.001.

Desai KI. Primary benign brachial plexus tumors: an experience of 115 operated cases. *Neurosurgery* 2012;**70**(1):220–33; discussion 233. https://doi.org/10.1227/NEU.0b013e31822d276a.

Dombi E, Baldwin A, Marcus LJ, et al. Activity of selumetinib in neurofibromatosis type 1-related plexiform neurofibromas. *N Engl J Med* 2016;**375**(26):2550–60. https://doi.org/10.1056/NEJMoa1605943.

Dong R, Liu Y, Yang Y, Wang H, Xu Y, Zhang Z. MSC-derived exosomes-based therapy for peripheral nerve injury: a novel therapeutic strategy. *Biomed Res Int* 2019;**2019**:6458237. https://doi.org/10.1155/2019/6458237.

Driscoll PJ, Glasby MA, Lawson GM. An in vivo study of peripheral nerves in continuity: biomechanical and physiological responses to elongation. *J Orthop Res* 2002;**20**(2):370–5. https://doi.org/10.1016/S0736-0266(01)00104-8.

Dumanian GA, Potter BK, Mioton LM, et al. Targeted muscle reinnervation treats neuroma and phantom pain in major limb amputees: a randomized clinical trial. *Ann Surg* 2019;**270**(2):238–46. https://doi.org/10.1097/SLA.0000000000003088.

Dyck PJ, Lais AC, Giannini C, Engelstad JK. Structural alterations of nerve during cuff compression. *Proc Natl Acad Sci U S A* 1990;**87**(24):9828–32. https://doi.org/10.1073/pnas.87.24.9828.

Evans DG, Baser ME, McGaughran J, Sharif S, Howard E, Moran A. Malignant peripheral nerve sheath tumours in neurofibromatosis 1. *J Med Genet* 2002;**39**(5):311–4. https://doi.org/10.1136/jmg.39.5.311.

Felix SP, Pereira Lopes FR, Marques SA, Martinez AM. Comparison between suture and fibrin glue on repair by direct coaptation or tubulization of injured mouse sciatic nerve. *Microsurgery* 2013;**33**(6):468–77. https://doi.org/10.1002/micr.22109.

Gelberman RH, Szabo RM, Williamson RV, Dimick MP. Sensibility testing in peripheral-nerve compression syndromes. An experimental study in humans. *J Bone Joint Surg Am* 1983a;**65**(5):632–8.

Gelberman RH, Szabo RM, Williamson RV, Hargens AR, Yaru NC, Minteer-Convery MA. Tissue pressure threshold for peripheral nerve viability. *Clin Orthop Relat Res* 1983b(178):285–91.

Geuna S. The sciatic nerve injury model in pre-clinical research. *J Neurosci Methods* 2015;**243**:39–46. https://doi.org/10.1016/j.jneumeth.2015.01.021.

Geuna S, Raimondo S, Ronchi G, et al. Chapter 3: Histology of the peripheral nerve and changes occurring during nerve regeneration. *Int Rev Neurobiol* 2009;**87**:27–46. https://doi.org/10.1016/S0074-7742(09)87003-7.

Gordon T, Borschel GH. The use of the rat as a model for studying peripheral nerve regeneration and sprouting after complete and partial nerve injuries. *Exp Neurol* 2017;**287**(Pt 3):331–47. https://doi.org/10.1016/j.expneurol.2016.01.014.

Gordon T, Brushart TM, Chan KM. Augmenting nerve regeneration with electrical stimulation. *Neurol Res* 2008;**30**(10):1012–22. https://doi.org/10.1179/174313208X362488.

Gottfried ON, Viskochil DH, Couldwell WT. Neurofibromatosis Type 1 and tumorigenesis: molecular mechanisms and therapeutic implications. *Neurosurg Focus* 2010;**28**(1):E8. https://doi.org/10.3171/2009.11.FOCUS09221.

Gray M, Palispis W, Popovich PG, van Rooijen N, Gupta R. Macrophage depletion alters the blood–nerve barrier without affecting Schwann cell function after neural injury. *J Neurosci Res* 2007;**85**(4):766–77. https://doi.org/10.1002/jnr.21166.

Gregory NS, Harris AL, Robinson CR, Dougherty PM, Fuchs PN, Sluka KA. An overview of animal models of pain: disease models and outcome measures. *J Pain* 2013;**14**(11):1255–69. https://doi.org/10.1016/j.jpain.2013.06.008.

Gross A, Bishop R, Widemann BC. Selumetinib in plexiform neurofibromas. *N Engl J Med* 2017;**376**(12):1195. https://doi.org/10.1056/NEJMc1701029.

Gross AM, Dombi E, Widemann BC. Current status of MEK inhibitors in the treatment of plexiform neurofibromas. *Childs Nerv Syst* 2020a;**36**(10):2443–52. https://doi.org/10.1007/s00381-020-04731-2.

Gross AM, Wolters PL, Dombi E, et al. Selumetinib in children with inoperable plexiform neurofibromas. *N Engl J Med* 2020b;**382**(15):1430–42. https://doi.org/10.1056/NEJMoa1912735.

Gupta R, Channual JC. Spatiotemporal pattern of macrophage recruitment after chronic nerve compression injury. *J Neurotrauma* 2006;**23**(2):216–26. https://doi.org/10.1089/neu.2006.23.216.

Gupta R, Rowshan K, Chao T, Mozaffar T, Steward O. Chronic nerve compression induces local demyelination and remyelination in a rat model of carpal tunnel syndrome. *Exp Neurol* 2004;**187**(2):500–08. https://doi.org/10.1016/j.expneurol.2004.02.009.

Gupta R, Steward O. Chronic nerve compression induces concurrent apoptosis and proliferation of Schwann cells. *J Comp Neurol* 2003;**461**(2):174–86. https://doi.org/10.1002/cne.10692.

Gupta R, Truong L, Bear D, Chafik D, Modafferi E, Hung CT. Shear stress alters the expression of myelin-associated glycoprotein (MAG) and myelin basic protein (MBP) in Schwann cells. *J Orthop Res* 2005;**23**(5):1232–9. https://doi.org/10.1016/j.orthres.2004.12.010.

Haastert-Talini K, Geuna S, Dahlin LB, et al. Chitosan tubes of varying degrees of acetylation for bridging peripheral nerve defects. *Biomaterials* 2013;**34**(38):9886–904. https://doi.org/10.1016/j.biomaterials.2013.08.074.

Hashmonai M, Cameron AE, Licht PB, Hensman C, Schick CH. Thoracic sympathectomy: a review of current indications. *Surg Endosc* 2016;**30**(4):1255–69. https://doi.org/10.1007/s00464-015-4353-0.

Jack A, Ramey WL, Dettori JR, et al. Factors associated with C5 palsy following cervical spine surgery: a systematic review. *Global Spine J* 2019;**9**(8):881–94. https://doi.org/10.1177/2192568219874771.

Jack AS, Chapman JR, Mummaneni PV, Gerard CS, Jacques L. Radiological data of brachial plexus avulsion injury associated spinal cord herniation (BPAI-SCH) and comparison to anterior thoracic spinal cord herniation (ATSCH). *Data Brief* 2020a;**29**:105333. https://doi.org/10.1016/j.dib.2020.105333.

Jack AS, Chapman JR, Mummaneni PV, Jacques LG, Gerard CS. Late cervical spinal cord herniation resulting from post-traumatic brachial plexus avulsion injury. *World Neurosurg* 2020b;**137**:1–7. https://doi.org/10.1016/j.wneu.2020.01.129.

Jack AS, Osburn BR, Tymchak ZA, et al. Foraminal ligaments tether upper cervical nerve roots: a potential cause of postoperative C5 palsy. *J Brachial Plex Peripher Nerve Inj* 2020c;**15**(1):e9–e15. https://doi.org/10.1055/s-0040-1712982.

Jacobson RD, Virag I, Skene JH. A protein associated with axon growth, GAP-43, is widely distributed and developmentally regulated in rat CNS. *J Neurosci* 1986;**6**(6):1843–55.

Johansson F, Dahlin LB. The multiple silicone tube device, "tubes within a tube," for multiplication in nerve reconstruction. *Biomed Res Int* 2014;**2014**:689127. https://doi.org/10.1155/2014/689127.

Karsidag S, Akcal A, Sahin S, Karsidag S, Kabukcuoglu F, Ugurlu K. Neurophysiological and morphological responses to treatment with acetyl-L-carnitine in a sciatic nerve injury model: preliminary data. *J Hand Surg Eur* 2012;**37**(6):529–36. https://doi.org/10.1177/1753193411426969.

Keir PJ, Rempel DM. Pathomechanics of peripheral nerve loading. Evidence in carpal tunnel syndrome. *J Hand Ther* 2005;**18**(2):259–69. https://doi.org/10.1197/j.jht.2005.02.001.

Kim DH, Friedman AH, Kitagawa RS, Kiline DG. Management of peripheral nerve tumors In Filler AG, Kline DG, Zager EL (Eds.), *Youmans Neurological Surgery*. 6th ed. Philadelphia, PA: Elsevier Saunders, 2011; p. 3264.

Kingery WS, Lu JD, Roffers JA, Kell DR. The resolution of neuropathic hyperalgesia following motor and sensory functional recovery in sciatic axonotmetic mononeuropathies. *Pain* 1994;**58**(2):157–68. https://doi.org/10.1016/0304-3959(94)90196-1.

Kolberg M, Holand M, Agesen TH, et al. Survival meta-analyses for >1800 malignant peripheral nerve sheath tumor patients with and without neurofibromatosis type 1. *Neuro Oncol* 2013;**15**(2):135–47. https://doi.org/10.1093/neuonc/nos287.

Koopmeiners AS, Mueller S, Kramer J, Hogan QH. Effect of electrical field stimulation on dorsal root ganglion neuronal function. *Neuromodulation* 2013;**16**(4):304–11; discussion 310–01. https://doi.org/10.1111/ner.12028.

Kovalsky Y, Amir R, Devor M. Simulation in sensory neurons reveals a key role for delayed Na⁺ current in subthreshold oscillations and ectopic discharge: implications for neuropathic pain. *J Neurophysiol* 2009;**102**(3):1430–42. https://doi.org/10.1152/jn.00005.2009.

Kramis RC, Roberts WJ, Gillette RG. Post-sympathectomy neuralgia: hypotheses on peripheral and central neuronal mechanisms. *Pain* 1996;**64**(1):1–9. https://doi.org/10.1016/0304-3959(95)00060-7.

Kuiken TA, Barlow AK, Hargrove L, Dumanian GA. Targeted muscle reinnervation for the upper and lower extremity. *Tech Orthop* 2017;**32**(2):109–16. https://doi.org/10.1097/BTO.0000000000000194.

Kwan MK, Wall EJ, Massie J, Garfin SR. Strain, stress and stretch of peripheral nerve. Rabbit experiments in vitro and in vivo. *Acta Orthop Scand* 1992;**63**(3):267–72. https://doi.org/10.3109/17453679209154780.

Laycock-van Spyk S, Thomas N, Cooper DN, Upadhyaya M. Neurofibromatosis type 1-associated tumours: their somatic mutational spectrum and pathogenesis. *Hum Genomics* 2011;**5**(6):623–90. https://doi.org/10.1186/1479-7364-5-6-623.

Li XY, Wan Y, Tang SJ, Guan Y, Wei F, Ma D. Maladaptive plasticity and neuropathic pain. *Neural Plast* 2016;**2016**:4842159. https://doi.org/10.1155/2016/4842159.

Longo JF, Weber SM, Turner-Ivey BP, Carroll SL. Recent advances in the diagnosis and pathogenesis of neurofibromatosis type 1 (NF1)-associated peripheral nervous system neoplasms. *Adv Anat Pathol* 2018;**25**(5):353–68. https://doi.org/10.1097/PAP.0000000000000197.

Ludwin SK, Maitland M. Long-term remyelination fails to reconstitute normal thickness of central myelin sheaths. *J Neurol Sci* 1984;**64**(2):193–8. https://doi.org/10.1016/0022-510x(84)90037-6.

Lundborg G, Dahlin LB, Hansson HA, Kanje M, Necking LE. Vibration exposure and peripheral nerve fiber damage. *J Hand Surg Am* 1990;**15**(2):346–51. https://doi.org/10.1016/0363-5023(90)90121-7.

Lundborg G, Gelberman RH, Minteer-Convery M, Lee YF, Hargens AR. Median nerve compression in the carpal tunnel–functional response to experimentally induced controlled pressure. *J Hand Surg Am* 1982;**7**(3):252–9. https://doi.org/10.1016/s0363-5023(82)80175-5.

Lundborg G, Myers R, Powell H. Nerve compression injury and increased endoneurial fluid pressure: a "miniature compartment syndrome". *J Neurol Neurosurg Psychiatry* 1983;**46**(12):1119–24. https://doi.org/10.1136/jnnp.46.12.1119.

Lundborg G, Rydevik B. Effects of stretching the tibial nerve of the rabbit. A preliminary study of the intraneural circulation and the barrier function of the perineurium. *J Bone Joint Surg Br* 1973;**55**(2):390–401.

Mackinnon S, Dellon A. *Surgery of the Peripheral Nerve*. New York: Thieme, 1988.

Mackinnon SE, Dellon AL, Hudson AR, Hunter DA. Chronic human nerve compression – a histological assessment. *Neuropathol Appl Neurobiol* 1986;**12**(6):547–65. https://doi.org/10.1111/j.1365-2990.1986.tb00159.x.

Madison RD, Archibald SJ, Brushart TM. Reinnervation accuracy of the rat femoral nerve by motor and sensory neurons. *J Neurosci* 1996;**16**(18):5698–703.

Mahan MA. Nerve stretching: a history of tension. *J Neurosurg* 2019;**132**(1):252–9. https://doi.org/10.3171/2018.8.JNS173181.

Martyn CN, Hughes RA. Epidemiology of peripheral neuropathy. *J Neurol Neurosurg Psychiatry* 1997;**62**(4):310–8. https://doi.org/10.1136/jnnp.62.4.310.

McCaughan JA, Holloway SM, Davidson R, Lam WW. Further evidence of the increased risk for malignant peripheral nerve sheath tumour from a Scottish cohort of patients with neurofibromatosis type 1. *J Med Genet* 2007;**44**(7):463–6. https://doi.org/10.1136/jmg.2006.048140.

Melzack R. From the gate to the neuromatrix. *Pain* 1999;(Suppl 6):S121–6. https://doi.org/10.1016/s0304-3959(99)00145-1.

Melzack R, Wall PD. Pain mechanisms: a new theory. *Science* 1965;**150**:971–9. https://doi.org/10.1126/science.150.3699.971.

Mendell LM. Constructing and deconstructing the gate theory of pain. *Pain* 2014;**155**(2):210–6. https://doi.org/10.1016/j.pain.2013.12.010.

Menorca RM, Fussell TS, Elfar JC. Nerve physiology: mechanisms of injury and recovery. *Hand Clin* 2013;**29**(3):317–30. https://doi.org/10.1016/j.hcl.2013.04.002.

Miettinen MM, Antonescu CR, Fletcher CDM, et al. Histopathologic evaluation of atypical neurofibromatous tumors and their transformation into malignant peripheral nerve sheath tumor in patients with neurofibromatosis 1 – a consensus overview. *Hum Pathol* 2017;**67**:1–10. https://doi.org/10.1016/j.humpath.2017.05.010.

Moimas S, Novati F, Ronchi G, et al. Effect of vascular endothelial growth factor gene therapy on post-traumatic peripheral nerve regeneration and denervation-related muscle atrophy. *Gene Ther* 2013;**20**(10):1014–21. https://doi.org/10.1038/gt.2013.26.

Molliver DC, Wright DE, Leitner ML, et al. IB4-binding DRG neurons switch from NGF to GDNF dependence in early postnatal life. *Neuron* 1997;**19**(4):849–61. https://doi.org/10.1016/s0896-6273(00)80966-6.

Nodari A, Previtali SC, Dati G, et al. Alpha6beta4 integrin and dystroglycan cooperate to stabilize the myelin sheath. *J Neurosci* 2008;**28**(26):6714–9. https://doi.org/10.1523/JNEUROSCI.0326-08.2008.

O'Brien JP, Mackinnon SE, MacLean AR, Hudson AR, Dellon AL, Hunter DA. A model of chronic nerve compression in the rat. *Ann Plast Surg* 1987;**19**(5):430–5. https://doi.org/10.1097/00000637-198711000-00008.

Ochoa J, Fowler TJ, Gilliatt RW. Anatomical changes in peripheral nerves compressed by a pneumatic tourniquet. *J Anat* 1972;**113**(Pt 3):433–55.

Papalia I, Tos P, Stagno d'Alcontres F, Battiston B, Geuna S. On the use of the grasping test in the rat median nerve model: a re-appraisal of its efficacy for quantitative assessment of motor function recovery. *J Neurosci Methods* 2003;**127**(1):43–7. https://doi.org/10.1016/s0165-0270(03)00098-0.

Pasmant E, Sabbagh A, Spurlock G, et al. NF1 microdeletions in neurofibromatosis type 1: from genotype to phenotype. *Hum Mutat* 2010;**31**(6):E1506–18. https://doi.org/10.1002/humu.21271.

Penas C, Navarro X. Epigenetic modifications associated to neuroinflammation and neuropathic pain after neural trauma. *Front Cell Neurosci* 2018;**12**:158. https://doi.org/10.3389/fncel.2018.00158.

Pham K, Gupta R. Understanding the mechanisms of entrapment neuropathies. *Neurosurg Focus* 2009;**26**(2):E7. https://doi.org/10.3171/FOC.2009.26.2.E7.

Poppler LH, Parikh RP, Bichanich MJ, et al. Surgical interventions for the treatment of painful neuroma: a comparative meta-analysis. *Pain* 2018;**159**(2):214–23. https://doi.org/10.1097/j.pain.0000000000001101.

Previtali SC, Feltri ML, Archelos JJ, Quattrini A, Wrabetz L, Hartung H. Role of integrins in the peripheral nervous system. *Prog Neurobiol* 2001;**64**(1):35–49. https://doi.org/10.1016/s0301-0082(00)00045-9.

Prudner BC, Ball T, Rathore R, Hirbe AC. Diagnosis and management of malignant peripheral nerve sheath tumors: current practice and future perspectives. *Neurooncol Adv* 2020;**2**(Suppl 1):i40–i49. https://doi.org/10.1093/noajnl/vdz047.

Que J, Cao Q, Sui T, Du S, Kong D, Cao X. Effect of FK506 in reducing scar formation by inducing fibroblast apoptosis after sciatic nerve injury in rats. *Cell Death Dis* 2013;**4**:e526. https://doi.org/10.1038/cddis.2013.56.

Ray WZ, Mahan MA, Guo D, Guo D, Kliot M. An update on addressing important peripheral nerve problems: challenges and potential solutions. *Acta Neurochir (Wien)* 2017;**159**(9):1765–73. https://doi.org/10.1007/s00701-017-3203-3.

Reid AJ, de Luca AC, Faroni A, et al. Long term peripheral nerve regeneration using a novel PCL nerve conduit. *Neurosci Lett* 2013;**544**:125–30. https://doi.org/10.1016/j.neulet.2013.04.001.

Rosen HR, Ammer K, Mohr W, Bock P, Kornek GV, Firbas W. Chemically-induced chronic nerve compression in rabbits – a new experimental model for the carpal tunnel syndrome.

Langenbecks Arch Chir 1992;**377**(4):216–21. https://doi.org/10.1007/BF00210276.

Rydevik B, Lundborg G. Permeability of intraneural microvessels and perineurium following acute, graded experimental nerve compression. *Scand J Plast Reconstr Surg* 1977;**11**(3):179–87. https://doi.org/10.3109/02844317709025516.

Rydevik B, Lundborg G, Bagge U. Effects of graded compression on intraneural blood blow. An in vivo study on rabbit tibial nerve. *J Hand Surg Am* 1981;**6**(1):3–12. https://doi.org/10.1016/s0363-5023(81)80003-2.

Salzer JL, Bunge RP. Studies of Schwann cell proliferation. I. An analysis in tissue culture of proliferation during development, Wallerian degeneration, and direct injury. *J Cell Biol* 1980;**84**(3):739–52. https://doi.org/10.1083/jcb.84.3.739.

Savastano LE, Laurito SR, Fitt MR, Rasmussen JA, Gonzalez Polo V, Patterson SI. Sciatic nerve injury: a simple and subtle model for investigating many aspects of nervous system damage and recovery. *J Neurosci Methods* 2014;**227**:166–80. https://doi.org/10.1016/j.jneumeth.2014.01.020.

Scholz J, Finnerup NB, Attal N, et al. The IASP classification of chronic pain for ICD-11: chronic neuropathic pain. *Pain* 2019;**160**(1):53–9. https://doi.org/10.1097/j.pain.0000000000001365.

Schwartz MA, DeSimone DW. Cell adhesion receptors in mechanotransduction. *Curr Opin Cell Biol* 2008;**20**(5):551–6. https://doi.org/10.1016/j.ceb.2008.05.005.

Sdrulla AD, Guan Y, Raja SN. Spinal cord stimulation: clinical efficacy and potential mechanisms. *Pain Pract* 2018;**18**(8):1048–67. https://doi.org/10.1111/papr.12692.

Siemionow M, Brzezicki G. Chapter 8: Current techniques and concepts in peripheral nerve repair. *Int Rev Neurobiol* 2009;**87**:141–72. https://doi.org/10.1016/S0074-7742(09)87008-6.

Sommer C, Leinders M, Uceyler N. Inflammation in the pathophysiology of neuropathic pain. *Pain* 2018;**159**(3):595–602. https://doi.org/10.1097/j.pain.0000000000001122.

Sommerich CM, Lavender SA, Buford JA, Banks JJ, Korkmaz SV, Pease WS. Towards development of a nonhuman primate model of carpal tunnel syndrome: performance of a voluntary, repetitive pinching task induces median mononeuropathy in *Macaca fascicularis*. *J Orthop Res* 2007;**25**(6):713–24. https://doi.org/10.1002/jor.20363.

Spinner RJ, Kline DG. Surgery for peripheral nerve and brachial plexus injuries or other nerve lesions. *Muscle Nerve* 2000;**23**(5):680–95. https://doi.org/10.1002/(sici)1097-4598(200005)23:5<680::aid-mus4>3.0.co;2-h.

Staedtke V, Bai RY, Blakeley JO. Cancer of the peripheral nerve in neurofibromatosis type 1. *Neurotherapeutics* 2017;**14**(2):298–306. https://doi.org/10.1007/s13311-017-0518-y.

Stone JJ, Spinner RJ. Go for the gold: a "plane" and simple technique for resecting benign peripheral nerve sheath tumors.

Oper Neurosurg (Hagerstown) 2020;**18**(1):60–8. https://doi.org/10.1093/ons/opz034.

Stossel M, Wildhagen VM, Helmecke O, et al. Comparative evaluation of chitosan nerve guides with regular or increased bendability for acute and delayed peripheral nerve repair: a comprehensive comparison with autologous nerve grafts and muscle-in-vein grafts. *Anat Rec (Hoboken)* 2018;**301**(10):1697–713. https://doi.org/10.1002/ar.23847.

Swieboda P, Filip R, Prystupa A, Drozd M. Assessment of pain: types, mechanism and treatment. *Ann Agric Environ Med* 2013; Spec no. **1**:2–7.

Szabo RM, Sharkey NA. Response of peripheral nerve to cyclic compression in a laboratory rat model. *J Orthop Res* 1993;**11**(6):828–33. https://doi.org/10.1002/jor.1100110608.

Taskinen HS, Roytta M. The dynamics of macrophage recruitment after nerve transection. *Acta Neuropathol* 1997;**93**(3):252–9. https://doi.org/10.1007/s004010050611.

Teixeira MJ, da Paz MG, Bina MT, et al. Neuropathic pain after brachial plexus avulsion–central and peripheral mechanisms. *BMC Neurol* 2015;**15**:73. https://doi.org/10.1186/s12883-015-0329-x.

Tibbs GR, Posson DJ, Goldstein PA. Voltage-gated ion channels in the PNS: novel therapies for neuropathic pain? *Trends Pharmacol Sci* 2016;**37**(7):522–42. https://doi.org/10.1016/j.tips.2016.05.002.

Tos P, Battiston B, Ciclamini D, Geuna S, Artiaco S. Primary repair of crush nerve injuries by means of biological tubulization with muscle-vein-combined grafts. *Microsurgery* 2012;**32**(5):358–63. https://doi.org/10.1002/micr.21957.

Tos P, Ronchi G, Nicolino S, et al. Employment of the mouse median nerve model for the experimental assessment of peripheral nerve regeneration. *J Neurosci Methods* 2008;**169**(1):119–27. https://doi.org/10.1016/j.jneumeth.2007.11.030.

Tricaud N, Perrin-Tricaud C, Bruses JL, Rutishauser U. Adherens junctions in myelinating Schwann cells stabilize Schmidt–Lanterman incisures via recruitment of p120 catenin to E-cadherin. *J Neurosci* 2005;**25**(13):3259–69. https://doi.org/10.1523/JNEUROSCI.5168-04.2005.

Tsuda M. Microglia in the spinal cord and neuropathic pain. *J Diabetes Investig* 2016;**7**(1):17–26. https://doi.org/10.1111/jdi.12379.

Varejao AS, Melo-Pinto P, Meek MF, Filipe VM, Bulas-Cruz J. Methods for the experimental functional assessment of rat sciatic nerve regeneration. *Neurol Res* 2004;**26**(2):186–94. https://doi.org/10.1179/016164104225013833.

Vuka I, Vucic K, Repic T, Ferhatovic Hamzic L, Sapunar D, Puljak L. Electrical stimulation of dorsal root ganglion in the context of pain: a systematic review of in vitro and in vivo animal model studies. *Neuromodulation* 2018;**21**(3):213–24. https://doi.org/10.1111/ner.12722.

Wall EJ, Massie JB, Kwan MK, Rydevik BL, Myers RR, Garfin SR. Experimental stretch neuropathy. Changes in nerve conduction under tension. *J Bone Joint Surg Br* 1992;**74**(1):126–9.

Watanabe M, Yamaga M, Kato T, Ide J, Kitamura T, Takagi K. The implication of repeated versus continuous strain on nerve function in a rat forelimb model. *J Hand Surg Am* 2001;**26**(4):663–9. https://doi.org/10.1053/jhsu.2001.24142.

Whitlock EL, Tuffaha SH, Luciano JP, et al. Processed allografts and type I collagen conduits for repair of peripheral nerve gaps. *Muscle Nerve* 2009;**39**(6):787–99. https://doi.org/10.1002/mus.21220.

Yamaguchi T, Osamura N, Zhao C, Zobitz ME, An KN, Amadio PC. The mechanical properties of the rabbit carpal tunnel subsynovial connective tissue. *J Biomech* 2008;**41**(16):3519–22. https://doi.org/10.1016/j.jbiomech.2007.06.004.

28 The Neuroscience of Functional Neurosurgery

Joseph S. Bell, T. J. Florence, Maya Harary, Maxwell D. Melin, Hiro Sparks, and Nader Pouratian

28.1 Introduction to the Neuroscience of Functional Neurosurgery

Functional neurosurgery is the branch of neurosurgery that seeks to restore or improve neurologic function by manipulation of neural activity. Of course, no branch of neurosurgery is agnostic to the function of the brain, but since Jean Talairach popularized the term it has nevertheless come to encompass a group of techniques treating movement disorders, pain, epilepsy, and psychiatric disease in which the neurosurgical intervention is designed to alter function. The history of functional neurosurgery is tightly linked to the development of stereotaxy, and many functional techniques rely on the use of stereotactic localization. They may involve both ablative procedures and the implantation of devices for chronic stimulation. The increasing power of cross-sectional imaging, rapid miniaturization of implantable electronics, and exponential increase in neural recording density has permitted an explosion of development in functional neurosurgery. It is one of the most exciting fields in neurosurgery, and one where the emerging discoveries of basic neuroscience are being rapidly and continually applied to the design of new therapies. Here we present a brief review of the pathobiology functional neurosurgery seeks to address, with the aim of providing an accessible introduction to neurosurgeons and others who may wish to further its progress.

28.2 Parkinson's Disease

28.2.1 Introduction

Parkinson's disease (PD) is the second most common neurodegenerative disease, with an overall prevalence of 300 per 100,000, which increases greatly with age (de Lau and Breteler, 2006). It is characterized by a classic triad of bradykinesia, rigidity, and resting tremor. Additional non-motor symptoms can also be present, including psychiatric disturbances, cognitive impairment, sleep disturbances, pain, and autonomic dysfunction (Magrinelli et al., 2016). Symptoms of PD severely impact quality of life and the lack of disease-modifying therapies has led to treatments that are targeted toward symptom reduction and quality of life improvement. Neurosurgical treatment of PD primarily consists of deep brain stimulation (DBS) of the basal ganglia, which provides similar therapeutic effects to dopamine replacement medication, with reduced side effects.

28.2.2 Pathobiology of Parkinson's Disease

Although advancing age is the primary risk factor for developing PD, genetics and environmental factors are thought to determine disease risk and severity (Blauwendraat et al., 2020). Parkinson's disease is predominantly a sporadic condition, with over 90% of cases appearing in the absence of any family history. These cases are thought to result from a complex interplay of genetic and environmental factors. To date, roughly 90 risk-modifying loci have been identified, demonstrating the role of many low-penetrance genes in contributing to PD risk. As few as 10% of cases are familial with incompletely identified monogenetic causes. In such cases, PD tends to manifest at an earlier age and with atypical clinical features.

Parkinson's disease is defined by a specific set of histologic criteria: the loss of dopaminergic cells in the substantia nigra pars compacta (SNpc). The presence of intraneuronal Lewy bodies (LBs), eosinophilic protein aggregates containing high levels of α-synuclein, is also often associated with PD. Although neuronal loss is most apparent in the SNpc, LBs can be found throughout the brain of PD patients. However familial PD patients with mutations in the *Parkin* gene usually do not present with LBs.

Although PD cytopathology is very well characterized, less is known about the molecular events that lead to the hallmark neurodegeneration. For the better part of the twentieth century, the neurotoxic/environmental hypothesis of PD was of prime interest to those who studied the disease, largely due to work with neurotoxic 1-methyl-4-phenyl-1,2,3,6-tetrahydropyridine (MPTP) animal models (Meredith and Rademacher, 2011). Oxidative stress, mitochondrial dysfunction, and abnormal protein aggregation are all being explored as potential drivers of PD neurodegeneration, with the interest in protein aggregation being driven primarily by the more recent discovery of PD genes. The known and well-studied Parkinson's genes, including α-synuclein, parkin, and ubiquitin C-terminal hydrolase L1 (*UCHL-1*), are all thought to participate in the ubiquitin proteasome pathway – compelling findings in light of PD's hallmark LB pathology (Dauer and Przedborski, 2003). Uncovering the molecular mechanisms behind PD neurodegeneration will present major opportunities to advance therapy for the disease.

At the circuit level, PD motor dysfunction is thought to arise primarily from severe (>70%) loss of SNpc dopamine neurons (Galvan and Wichmann, 2008). Loss of these neurons leads to dopamine hypoactivity in the striatum, a region critically involved in action selection and movement initiation. This dopamine depletion in the striatum has different but likely additive consequences in the direct and indirect pathways of the basal ganglia (BG), both key pathways in the selection and suppression of motor programs. Preferential expression of excitatory D_1 receptors in the direct pathway neurons leads to hypoactivity of this pathway when dopamine release is restricted, while preferential expression of the inhibitory D_2 receptor in the

indirect pathway leads to its hyperactivity (Figure 28.1). The imbalance of these pathways is thought to inhibit motor output via their increased inhibition of thalamocortical and brainstem motor systems. Conversely, high dopamine states (such as levodopa administration) can reverse this phenomenon and give rise to dyskinesias.

While this two-pathway BG model may explain bradykinesias and dyskinesias in corresponding low and high dopamine states, there are many motor and non-motor aspects of PD that are still not fully explained. In particular, this model does not adequately explain the emergence of rigidity and tremor, which may be explained by different circuits entirely. Neurosurgical treatment is also at odds with this model of the BG, as pallidotomy, or globus pallidus interna (GPi) DBS tend to paradoxically reduce hyperkinesia, although this model would predict the opposite (Brown and Eusebio, 2008). Of particular interest to the neurosurgical therapeutics is the emerging appreciation of the hyperdirect pathway (Gradinaru et al., 2009). In addition to a richer expansion of the BG two-pathway model, further exploration is needed to clarify the role of different circuits in contributing to the full range of PD symptoms, as there is evidence to suggest that multiple circuits and neurotransmitters are involved.

28.2.3 Animal Models of Parkinson's Disease

Several PD animal models are available to researchers and are generally derived from neurotoxic chemicals or genetic modification. Of the neurotoxic models, MPTP,

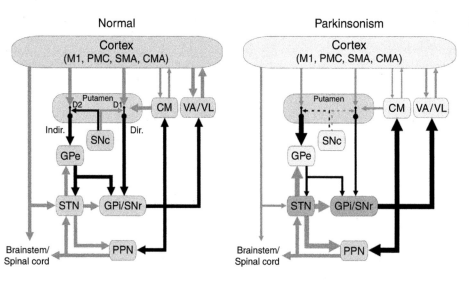

Figure 28.1 The basal ganglia circuit.

6-hydroxydopamine (6-OHDA), paraquate, and rotenone have been most widely used. These neurotoxins are thought to promote neurodegeneration through reactive oxygen species (ROS) formation (Dauer and Przedborski, 2003). Of these neurotoxins, MPTP is the most widely used because it has been shown to induce parkinsonism in humans, and symptoms respond to levodopa treatment in a nearly identical fashion to PD patients. MPTP-treated non-human primates also show similar patterns of neurodegeneration to PD patients. They respond to subthalamic nucleus (STN) DBS and thus offer a means to study the mechanisms underlying DBS therapy. Rodents are not as sensitive to MPTP toxicity as primates, but still provide an adequate model. There are two points where this model diverges from PD patients: neurons are not always lost in other monoaminergic nuclei, and the appearance of classical LBs has not yet been shown convincingly (Forno et al., 1993). Despite these shortcomings, MPTP has still been widely used for studying PD in a variety of animal models.

The advent of newer genetic murine and fly models of PD may offer another window to study the disorder, although these models have not been studied as extensively as some neurotoxic models. Based on the known monogenic causes of PD, multiple genetic mouse and fly models – including α-synuclein, leucine-rich repeat kinase 2 (*LRKK2*), PTEN Induced Kinase 1 (*PINK1*), Parkin, Protein deglycase (*DJ1*), and ATPase Cation Transporting 13A2 (*ATP13A2*) mutants- have been created with varying success at replicating PD movement abnormalities. Transgenic mice generally show increased sensitivity to neurotoxic chemicals such as MPTP and are found to model α-synuclein aggregation and nigrostriatal dopamine loss by some authors. However, the extent of SNpc dopamine cell loss in certain genetic approaches has been questioned, as several authors have failed to find degeneration in some of these models. It remains to be seen why some genetic models do not show the pronounced SNpc dopamine loss characteristic of PD, but stronger compensatory mechanisms remains one possibility. While the neurotoxic models have historically been a better system to study the effects of SNpc degeneration, genetic models offer an excellent window into the cell biology and biochemistry of PD and LB formation that may occur through similar pathways in sporadic patients.

28.3 Essential Tremor

28.3.1 Introduction

Essential tremor (ET) is the most common adult movement disorder, with a prevalence of 1%. Essential tremor is characterized by a progressively worsening postural and/or kinetic tremor that classically affects the hands and arms in a bilateral, slightly asymmetric fashion (Deuschl et al., 2011). Although this is the most common presentation of ET, tremor can also manifest in the head, voice, face, or trunk. In addition to action tremor, the defining feature of this disorder is a lack of any other neurological symptoms, although this notion of tremor as the isolated sign or symptom is evolving (Louis et al., 2020). Neurosurgical treatment of ET principally consists of thalamotomy or DBS.

28.3.2 Pathobiology of Essential Tremor

Despite the widespread prevalence of ET, little is known about the pathogenesis of this disorder. Evidence from genome-wide association studies (GWAS) and familial genotyping have identified substantial genetic heterogeneity, with some forms of ET inherited in an autosomal dominant fashion with incomplete penetrance, while others appear to be sporadic and result from a combination of genetic and environmental susceptibilities (Clark and Louis, 2015). Study of ET has been challenged by the absence of definitive biomarkers; clinical history and physical examination remain the only tools to diagnose ET.

Although the pathological processes leading to ET are still debated, more is known about the circuit level changes that occur with the disorder. Essential tremor symptoms very likely arise due to rhythmic activity in the cortico-ponto-cerebello-thalamo-cortical loop. Patients show elevated cerebellar metabolism at rest and with movement. Furthermore, burst activity in the ventral intermediate thalamus (VIM, which receives significant input from the cerebellum) has been shown to strongly correlate with tremor activity (Hua and Lenz, 2005). Animal models of ET also show increased rhythmic activity in the inferior olive. Together, this evidence likely indicates the role of faulty movement execution circuits in ET pathogenesis.

Several lines of evidence indicate cerebellar dysfunction may be responsible for ET. Magnetic resonance spectroscopy has revealed decreased levels of *N*-acetylaspartate in the cerebellum of ET patients, which is thought to be a marker of neuronal loss or dysfunction. Additional imaging studies have found cerebellar γ-aminobutyric acid (GABA) hypoactivity, as well as decreased $GABA_A$ and $GABA_B$ expression in the dentate nucleus, lending credence to the "GABA hypothesis" of ET. Pathological studies have pointed to Purkinje cell degeneration, climbing fiber pathology, and the emergence of axonal torpedoes in the cerebellum, although these findings are controversial. Additional studies have argued for the heterogeneity of ET pathology findings, citing the variable presence of cerebellar changes and brainstem LBs in post-mortem samples (Louis et al., 2006).

28.3.3 Animal Models of Essential Tremor

Despite the wide number of tremor animal models available, there are few validated models that capture ET's presentation (Pan et al., 2018). The classic model of ET is the harmaline-induced model. Harmaline is a $GABA_A$ inverse agonist that induces transient postural and kinetic tremor. This compound induces rhythmic burst firing in the inferior olivary nuclei (ION) that is transmitted via climbing fibers to Purkinje cells and other downstream regions (Handforth, 2012). Given this compound's primary action in the ION, authors have begun to question its validity in light of pathological findings in ET patients (Louis and Lenka, 2017). Despite concern about the underlying mechanism, the harmaline model has shown reasonable face and predictive validity when ET pharmacotherapy is administered. One drawback of the model is the acute nature of tremor, usually not lasting more than several hours. The model also does not capture the progressively worsening nature of ET. About half of the drugs reported to suppress harmaline tremor suppress ET in clinical trials (Handforth, 2012).

The $GABA_{A1}$ knockout mouse is the next widely used model of ET. Mice lacking the α1 subunit of the $GABA_A$ receptor display a postural and kinetic tremor, as well as motor incoordination that is characteristic of ET patients (Kralic et al., 2005). There is a greater than 50% reduction of $GABA_{A1}$ expression in the cerebellum, although this is mitigated by increased tonic conductance in the mutant channels. This model has also been shown to respond to propranolol, primidone, and ethanol, all known to alleviate tremor in human patients. While other animal models exist, models must be selected carefully in order to closely recapitulate ET symptoms. Many models of tremor exhibit overlapping tremor subtypes and additional movement problems such as ataxia or dystonia, casting doubt on their ability to model the "essential" nature of ET.

28.4 Dystonia

28.4.1 Introduction

Dystonia is a movement disorder in which muscle contractions, often of opponent muscle groups, cause abnormal postures and twisting movements (Breakefield et al., 2008). Dystonia is heterogeneous, and arises from many distinct genetic and anatomic causes. Primary dystonias are disorders in which the dystonia is the principal clinical feature, and occur in the absence of macroscopically obvious brain pathology, whereas secondary dystonias accompany other neurodegenerative and movement disorders or arise from a traumatic, infectious, or vascular brain injury. Neurosurgical treatments for dystonia historically have included thalamotomy and pallidotomy, although in the modern era these lesion-based treatments have been largely replaced by DBS (Kupsch et al., 2003).

28.4.2 Pathobiology of Dystonia

Primary dystonias are frequently stratified by age of onset, and causal genetic lesions have been characterized for a variety of primary dystonias, particularly those emerging in childhood. Most commonly, these are inherited in an autosomal dominant fashion, and influence a variety of cell biological processes (Tanabe et al., 2009). However, the mechanisms that result in dystonic movements remain mostly unclear. For example, early onset torsion dystonia (DYT1) is a severe form of childhood-onset generalized dystonia. DYT1 is caused by mutations of torsinA, an ATPase localized to the nuclear envelope and endoplasmic reticulum associated with processing of synaptic vesicles. Although torsinA may be relatively enriched in the basal ganglia, it is ubiquitously expressed in neurons throughout the cortex, hippocampus, and cerebellum. Rodents expressing mutant torsinA demonstrate subtle motor deficits, but not overt dystonia. Consequently, while these animals have been important for understanding the underlying cell biology of torsinA, they have not explained the emergence of the clinical phenotype (Oleas et al., 2013).

Other primary dystonias also result from mutations that have the potential to impair neurons, but have not yet revealed a mechanism for the resulting circuit pathology. DYT6 generalized dystonia is caused by mutations in *THAP1*, a DNA binding protein which may co-localize with torsinA, but whose function remains unexplained. DYT11 myoclonus dystonia is caused by a mutation in *SGCE*, a transmembrane sarcoglycan which localizes to both muscles and inhibitory postsynaptic sites. DYT12, the rapid-onset dystonia–parkinonism syndrome, is caused by mutations in the α3 subunit of the Na^+–K^+-ATPase (*ATP1A3*). This lesion has the potential to impair the ability of neurons to maintain rapid firing rates and recycle synaptic vesicles, but it is unclear why patients function normally before the onset of symptoms and subsequently experience rapid decompensation. DYT5 dopa-responsive dystonia is notable for its response to dopamine replacement, and can result from mutations in both *GCH1* and tyrosine hydroxylase. Both of these mutations result in deficient dopamine biosynthesis, and suggest the clearest links between mutations and circuit pathology because of their known effects on the dopaminergic circuit.

Several lines of evidence suggest that abnormalities in synaptic plasticity, and specifically GABAergic inhibition, contribute to dystonia. GABA agonists, including benzodiazepines and baclofen, are modestly helpful for dystonic patients. Patients undergoing cortical transcranial magnetic stimulation exhibit reduced inhibition of muscle activation to the second of two closely spaced stimulating pulses. Patients also exhibit impaired temporal discrimination thresholds. Interestingly, even *DYT1* carriers without dystonic movements exhibit these abnormalities, but it is not known whether they cause dystonia, are an effect of abnormal movements, or an additional endophenotype of a shared causal lesion. However, the fact that patients with dystonia can often relieve episodes of posturing by touching a nearby body part argues that sensory circuits can modify the disease process.

28.4.3   Animal Models of Dystonia

Mutations recapitulating the genetics of the human dystonias DYT1, DYT11, and DYT12 have been generated in worms, fruit flies, and mice (Oleas et al., 2013). Although these models exhibit biochemical and electrophysiological abnormalities reminiscent of human disease, none of them results in overt dystonia. For example, a knock-in mouse generated with the most common symptomatic human mutation in the *torsinA* gene showed a subtle increase in slips in a beam walking test, reduced striatal dopamine release, and impaired neurotransmission in cultured neurons, but not abnormal posturing.

Separate phenotypic models of dystonia with behavioral features reminiscent of human symptoms map to distinct loci (Wilson and Hess, 2013). The *tottering* mouse exhibits episodic dystonic movements caused by mutations in the voltage-gated calcium channel $Ca_V2.1$. Importantly, mutation of this channel in only cerebellar Purkinje neurons is sufficient to reproduce the dystonic phenotype, and cerebellar resection or silencing Purkinje neurons abolishes it. Similar cerebellar dysfunction and rescue has been observed in *dt* rats, which derive from a different mutation in the protein caytaxin.

Phenotypic models have also been produced using pharmacologic lesions (Wilson and Hess, 2013). Dystonia may accompany both MPTP-induced Parkinsonism (discussed above), as well as chronic L-DOPA administration. Anatomic models have been generated by microinjection of the GABA antagonist bicuculline, the AMPA agonist kainic acid, into the globus pallidus, substantia nigra, and thalamus in both rodents and non-human primates. These models support the evolving consensus that dystonia can arise from dysfunction at many nodes in motor circuits involving the basal ganglia, cortex, cerebellum, and dopaminergic system, and that pro-dystonic lesions in one part of the motor circuit may potentiate the effects of lesions in other parts.

28.5   Epilepsy

28.5.1   Introduction

Epilepsy is a brain disease characterized by an enduring propensity for epileptic seizures, which are transient episodes of neurologic signs or symptoms that arise from abnormal excessive or synchronous brain activity. Epilepsy is heterogeneous, and may arise due to genetic, developmental, infectious, vascular, traumatic, metabolic, or neoplastic causes. Appropriate therapy is determined both by the etiology and the neuroanatomy of the brain areas they arise from. Neurosurgical involvement in epilepsy includes both diagnostic and therapeutic procedures that allow intracranial neurophysiologic recordings, therapeutic electrical stimulation, and disconnection or resection of structures that permit the generation or propagation of seizure activity.

28.5.2   Pathobiology of Epilepsy

Seizures are induced by increases in excitation or reductions in inhibition that lead to recurrent and self-sustaining activity. Accordingly, early genetic studies identified mutations in ion channels and neurotransmitter receptors. Although it is tempting to describe epilepsy as an imbalance between excitation and inhibition, this description is incomplete. If excitation and inhibition are unbalanced, why does the epileptic brain seize for brief episodes and not constantly? One explanation is that a particular level of activity or network state is required to trigger a seizure. Forms of epilepsy in which seizures occur only during particular stages of sleep support this idea. The characteristic timescale of seizures – intermittent, brief, and usually self-terminating events – suggests that mechanisms underlying synaptic plasticity and homeostasis may contribute. Consistently, both presynaptic and postsynaptic mechanisms have been implicated (Casillas-Espinosa et al., 2012). Mechanisms regulating synaptic transmission are also important targets for pharmacologic treatment. For example, the commonly used drug levetiracetam was initially identified during a drug screen in epileptic mice. The subsequent discovery that it targeted the synaptic vesicle protein SV2A enabled the development of a more potent analog, brivaracetam.

Although initial targeted genetic studies focused on ion channels and the regulation of cell excitability, subsequent unbiased screens have identified genes with diverse effects on neuronal cell biology, physiology, and development (Epi4K Consortium et al., 2013). Abnormal network connectivity can occur as the result of alterations in neuronal proliferation, differentiation, migration, synapse formation, cell death, and survival, and all of these developmental processes have been implicated in the creation of epileptogenic networks. For example, sequencing of human brain tissue samples from subjects with epilepsy and focal cortical dysplasia type II demonstrated somatic mutations in the kinase *mTOR*, which led to altered neuronal migration and seizures in mouse models.

The use of brain stimulation to treat epilepsy has highlighted the complex anatomy underlying seizure generation, and DBS for refractory epilepsy has been attempted targeting the thalamus, subthalamic nucleus, caudate, hippocampus, and cerebellum (Li and Cook, 2018). The best studied of these targets is the anterior nucleus of the thalamus (ANT), which was subjected to a randomized sham-controlled clinical trial, resulting in FDA approval in 2018. Interest in this site was motivated by its location in the circuit of Papez, a recurrent circuit linking the hippocampus and mesial temporal structures often involved in epilepsy with the cingulate and thalamus (Oikawa et al., 2001; Figure 28.2).

The mechanism by which DBS works at target tissues is unclear. Neural recordings near DBS sites in the GPi conducted for PD suggest that cell bodies near the stimulating electrodes are inhibited. This could be due to depolarization block or activation of presynaptic inhibition (Herrington et al., 2016). However, it is also possible that stimulation exerts its greatest effect on passing axons that arise from cells distant to the stimulating electrode. No similar data exist to describe the direct effect of stimulation on the ANT. Interestingly, while studies have shown DBS for PD to be most effective at high frequencies, ANT data in rats describe similar seizure control at both low and high frequencies, suggesting that the underlying mechanism could be different.

Epilepsy has also been surgically treated by vagus nerve stimulation (VNS). The mechanism by which VNS reduces seizures is unclear. The vagus nerve projects

Figure 28.2 The circuit of Papez.

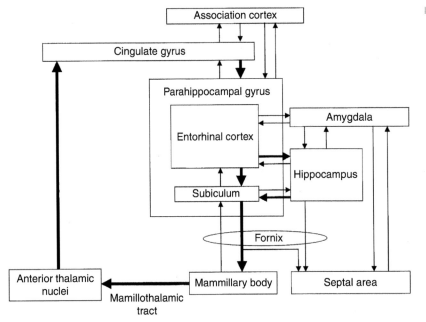

predominantly to the nucleus of the solitary tract (NTS), which in turn sends projections throughout the brainstem, including the monoaminergic nuclei. Noradrenergic and serotonergic neurons from these nuclei are activated by VNS and project widely throughout the brain, and are the most likely substrate for the VNS effect (Krahl and Clark, 2012). However, NTS neurons also project widely into the hypothalamus and thalamus and it is possible these projections contribute.

28.5.3 Animal Models of Epilepsy

Experimental animal models of both congenital and acquired forms of epilepsy have been used since at least the nineteenth century, beginning with studies of epileptic dogs, and induction of seizures in cats, rabbits, and guinea pigs (Grone and Baraban, 2015). Modern epilepsy research continues to benefit from a comparative approach, although rodents are widely used. Many techniques have been used to model acquired epilepsies, including electric shock, proconvulsive drugs, hypoxia, hyperthermia, viral infection, tumor transplantation, and trauma (Becker, 2018). For example, administration of the glutamate analog kainic acid causes acute seizures, and also causes the induction of recurrent spontaneous seizures, or *kindling*, even after the drug has been removed.

Genetic model organisms including mice, zebrafish, and fruit flies have allowed for forward genetic screens to identify new genes that cause phenotypes resembling human epilepsies, as well as targeted gene disruptions that model known human mutations (Wong and Roper, 2016). Epileptogenic alleles often result in model organisms with phenotypes that differ from their human counterparts. For example, tuberous sclerosis complex (TSC) is caused by autosomal dominant mutations in the *Tsc1* and *Tsc2* genes (regulators of *mTOR*, described above) that result in cortical dysplasia, the formation of cortical tubers, and epilepsy. Numerous rodent models of TSC have been generated by both germline- and tissue-specific knockout of the *Tsc1* and *Tsc2* genes, resulting in a variety of phenotypes which incompletely reproduce features of the human disease. *Tsc2* mutant heterozygote rats develop rare cortical tubers, but not epilepsy. *Tsc1* and *Tsc2* heterozygote mice demonstrate learning deficits, but no pathologic abnormalities of the brain or seizures.

Even without complete phenotypic correspondence, animal models of epilepsy have proved useful. For example, analysis of the *Drosophila* mutant Shaker, which exhibits leg shaking during ether anesthesia, ultimately led to the cloning of the first voltage-gated potassium channel and identification of human mutations associated with episodic ataxia and seizures. Dravet syndrome, a pediatric epilepsy syndrome associated with intellectual disability and drug-resistant seizures, is caused by mutations in the voltage-gated sodium channel *Scn1A*. Zebrafish generated with similar mutations were subsequently used to screen a large drug library to identify a new treatment.

28.6 Chronic Pain

28.6.1 Introduction

Pain that persists beyond normal healing and lacks the warning function of nociception can be referred to as chronic pain (CP). Human neuroimaging and electrophysiological evidence suggests that chronic pain arises from centrally mediated changes in neuronal plasticity, regardless of the inciting etiology. Thus, some authors assume that treatment-refractory CP is mostly neuropathic central pain. However, CP from different sources responds differently to neuromodulation. For example, long-term success of periventricular gray matter (PVG) or ventral posterior thalamus (VP) stimulation has been reported to be 70–73% for failed back surgery syndrome and as low as 14% for post-stroke pain (Rasche et al., 2006). This uncertainty is exacerbated by a variability of results of neuromodulation efficacy, reflecting the limitations of pain assessment tools and study design.

28.6.2 Pathobiology of Chronic Pain

Pain perception arises from a network that includes the spinal cord, internal capsule, posterior hypothalamus, amygdala, striatum, and cortex. Accumulating evidence suggests that pain perception likely involves both top-down and bottom-up systems. Human electrophysiological studies of neuronal coherence and causality modeling suggest that PVG/periaqueductal gray (PAG) exerts ascending modulation upon VP in a bottom-up circuit. Meanwhile, ablation of the anterior cingulate cortex (ACC) appears to act top-down to diminish the emotional saliency of pain perception while leaving nociception unaltered.

Many nodes within the putative pain network have been subject to attempts at lesioning and stimulation. DBS was first applied to treat cancer CP over six decades ago following reports of analgesia in patients receiving septal DBS for psychiatric disorders. In the modern era the PVG and VP are targeted most commonly. The anterior cingulate cortex, ventral striatum, internal capsule, and centromedian thalamic nuclei also remain promising targets (Frizon et al., 2020).

The mechanisms by which DBS influences the pain network are not clearly delineated. Early reports that PVG/PAG DBS increases cerebrospinal endorphins could not be replicated. More recently, reports of association between CP and increased thalamic firing suggest that altered rhythmic activity within the VP plays a central role. The clinical observation that DBS is analgesic at lower frequencies (50 Hz) and hyperalgesic at higher frequencies (>70 Hz) implies DBS may disrupt pathological high-frequency oscillations or augment diminished low-frequency oscillations, especially in thalamofugal projections. Conversely, multiple time-frequency analyses have identified increased alpha oscillatory power in the PVG/PAG and anterior cingulate, and greater alpha coherence within affective networks is correlated with increased attention toward pain. Disruption of alpha synchrony within these networks represents an additional possible mechanism by which stimulation modulates pain perception (Green et al., 2009).

28.6.3 Animal Models of Chronic Pain

There are two primary considerations for the selection of nociceptive animal models: the method of insult and the consequent end-point measurement. The most useful models recapitulate the nociceptive mechanisms of a specific clinical condition (Gregory et al., 2013). As pain is a multidimensional experience, measures of nociception should be assessed in conjunction with more complicated behaviors like place aversion and socialization that may capture the affective component of pain. Murine and rat models are among the most frequently used mammalian models for nociception studies, and specific models have been developed based on injection of irritants, surgical incisions, direct nerve injury, and tumor transfection (Mogil, 2009).

28.6.4 Challenges in Chronic Pain

Challenges associated with the quantification and standardization of pain perception among humans also extend to animal models of CP. Several human studies have noted that reduction of pain intensity is not always associated with overall benefits in quality of life. The possibility that addressing nociception alone is inadequate has prompted the search for new targets, such as the ventral striatum, which could better modulate the cognitive and affective aspects of pain. Durability is also a challenge; up to one half of patients who derive

benefit during trials of neuromodulation do not experience long-term relief. Failed attempts to recover early pain relief have included increasing amplitude or insertion of a second electrode (Kumar et al., 1997). Modifications to stimulation parameters, including closed-loop and intermittent stimulation, have shown benefits. Still, further investigation is required to better understand predictors of long-term efficacy and mechanisms by which tolerance to stimulation develops.

28.7 Psychiatric Disease

28.7.1 Introduction

Psychosurgery has been a central part of modern functional neurosurgery since its inception. Prior to the development of neuroleptic medication in the mid-twentieth century, psychiatric disease was a particularly significant source of morbidity, relegating patients to life in psychiatric asylums; this need drew many neurosurgeons to the budding field of psychosurgery. Mostly notably, the prefrontal leucotomy was developed by Egas Moniz and later popularized by Walter Freeman to treat a range of psychiatric conditions, at times with loose clinical indication. Ethical backlash, alongside the significant positive impact of new neuroleptic medications, stunted work in this field until the late twentieth century at all but a handful of centers. Despite advances in treatment, a considerable portion of patients remain refractory, and psychiatric disease remains a significant source of morbidity and mortality. The continuous developments in neuromodulation, increased understanding of the neurobiology of psychiatric disease, and rigorous ethical regulatory review, have made psychosurgery once again an active area of inquiry.

28.7.2 Obsessive Compulsive Disorder

Obsessive compulsive disorder (OCD) is a relatively common psychiatric disorder with a prevalence of 2%, and is characterized by distressing repetitive thoughts which trigger compulsive behaviors. Similar to PD, the neural substrate of OCD has been localized to the cortico-striato-thalamo-cortical circuitry. Whereas PD localizes to the more posterior motor circuit, OCD is associated with dysregulation of the anterior circuit involving the orbito-frontal cortex, ventral striatum (VS), and ACC, which is involved with executive functioning and emotional regulation. Anterior capsulotomy and anterior cingulotomy have both shown good efficacy in the treatment of OCD (Pepper et al., 2019). Treatment-refractory

OCD is the only FDA-approved indication for DBS psychosurgery, based on studies demonstrating significant symptom improvement with ventral capsule (VC)/VS and STN DBS.

28.7.3 Depression

Major depressive disorder (MDD) is a particularly common and insidious disorder, contributing to significant worldwide morbidity and mortality. Like other psychiatric diseases, depression is understood as a dysregulation of functional neural networks as opposed to the dysfunction of a single network node. The brain areas that have been implicated in depression include the anterior capsule, the ACC, the subgenual cingulate (SGC), and the ventro-medial prefrontal cortex (Abosch and Cosgrove, 2008). While murine models of depression do exist – namely, the tail suspension, forced swim, and sucrose preference tests – these are predominantly used for pharmaceutical research and lack applicability to psychosurgery (Nestler and Hyman, 2010). Prior to the age of DBS, surgical treatment of intractable MDD was lesion-based – anterior capsulotomy, anterior cingulotomy, and subcaudate tractotomy. These procedures have a response rate reported in the 40–70% range in small open-label patient series. DBS has been used for MDD with mixed results. Two recent randomized controlled trials (RCTs), RECLAIM trial targeting VC/VS and BROADEN trial targeting the SGC, were terminated early due to failure to meet expected response at interim analysis. Other studies, targeting the ventral portion of the anterior limb of the internal capsule and SGC, have shown positive outcomes.

28.7.4 Addiction

Addiction is a complex psychiatric disorder with significant morbidity, mortality, and economic impact (Bari et al., 2018). Addiction is particularly difficult to study given multiple dimensions of disease heterogeneity. Patients can have an addiction to a range of stimuli, such as drugs of abuse, food, and sex. Much of our understanding of the pathobiology of addiction comes from animal studies of classical and associative learning and reward processing using the operant conditioning chamber. Addictive substances co-opt the physiologic reward circuitry of the limbic cortico-striatal–thalamo-cortical (CSTC) – specifically the dopaminergic signalling of ventral tegmental area (VTA) onto the nucleus accumbens (NAc) (Nestler, 2005). Supraphysiologic dopamine release, signal duration, and altered dopamine responsiveness leading to limbic dysregulation are central to the pathophysiology of addiction (Figure 28.3). Although neuroimaging and animal studies have consistently implicated a number of limbic structures (Wang et al., 2018), these may be more or less involved in different stages of the addictive cycle of intoxication, tolerance, withdrawal, and craving. Furthermore, the longer-term progression of the disease is impacted by a patient's psychosocial circumstances. While animal models of addiction continue to be

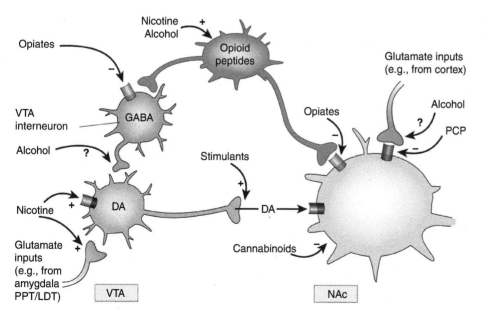

Figure 28.3 Mechanisms of drugs of abuse.

fundamental to our understanding of addiction patho-physiology, they are fraught with inherent translational limitations due to the inability to capture these heterogeneities. Human studies have primarily focused on STN and NAc stimulation, which have shown promising outcomes in small numbers of patients with a range of substance addictions including alcohol, heroin, and cocaine.

28.7.5 Challenges in Psychosurgery

There are several persistent challenges in the study of neurosurgery for psychiatric disease. First is the difficulty in objectively classifying disease phenotypes. For example, MDD is diagnosed by the presence of at least five of nine symptoms according to the *Diagnostic and Statistical Manual of Mental Disorders, 5th Edition*; this means that two MDD patients may only overlap in one disease symptom. Due to this heterogeneity, treatment may be effective in one MDD phenotype but not in another. There is an effort to address this issue through the development of Research Domain Criteria (RDoC), which aim to integrate nuanced assessment of psycho-cognitive behaviors, functional neuroimaging, and electrophysiology in defining disease phenotypes. The linking of RDoC phenotypic axes to in-vivo recordings may help generate electrophysiologic biomarkers for psychiatric disease that could be used to modulate stimulation parameters in a closed-loop DBS system, akin to the responsive neurostimulation (RNS) model in epilepsy surgery (Bari et al., 2018).

28.8 Emerging Applications and Challenges in Functional Neurosurgery

28.8.1 Introduction

Here we highlight promising technological developments in active transition from fundamental laboratory neuroscience to operative technique. This list is not meant to be comprehensive; further, with the pace of development in the field, it will become rapidly outdated. The work below shares the exciting potential to expand what we think of as "neurosurgical" problems.

28.8.2 Central Thalamic Stimulation for Disorders of Consciousness

While a comprehensive definition of consciousness has escaped philosophers and neuroscientists alike, brain injury leading to impaired states of consciousness is a common neurosurgical problem. In support of

a working clinical definition, Plumb and Posner noted that to be conscious, a patient must be both awake and aware (Posner et al., 2007). This concept informs much of our current clinical thinking with respect to disorders of consciousness (DOC). Outside of brain death, DOCs encompass three states: coma, vegetative state, and minimally conscious state. As alertness and sensory awareness are actively regulated processes, each state corresponds to damage to distinct brain regions. Coma patients suffer from damage to the reticular system and its thalamic projections resulting in a closed-eye state lacking sleep–wake cycles and do not respond meaningfully to external stimuli. Damage to thalamocortical connections that spare the brainstem lead either to vegetative state (VS), characterized by evident sleep–wake cycles but lacking responses to external stimuli, or minimally conscious state (MCS), in which a patient displays variable but discernible responses. Vegetative state and MCS may represent a spectrum of extent of thalamocortical damage.

Incomplete damage represents an opportunity for augmentation by DBS. The central thalamic nucleus directs broad connections throughout the striatum and cortex and appears to play a significant role in the regulation of alertness and arousal. A small but growing cohort of patients has undergone implantation of DBS electrodes into the bilateral central thalamus with the goal of addressing DOCs (Shah and Schiff, 2010). In the most dramatic example, a traumatic brain injury patient who had been in a minimally conscious state for 6 years regained intelligible speech and sustained attention after CT-DBS. Significant work remains to demonstrate the generalizability of this result and to understand its mechanism.

28.8.3 Limbic Stimulation for Disorders of Memory

Wilder Penfield's compelling descriptions of evoking experiential memory with brain stimulation raised the possibility that neural memory systems can be controlled (Penfield and Perot, 1963). With more than 130 million adults projected to be living with Alzheimer's disease (AD) by 2050, definitive neurosurgical treatment of memory disorders would be of great benefit to humanity. As such, there has been significant recent effort in evaluating DBS targets throughout the limbic system. Results to date have been mixed, likely reflecting that what we experience as a memory reflects a range of processes including encoding, consolidation, and retrieval over multiple timescales, each with a partially overlapping substrate.

This may partially explain the surprising observation that extra-hippocampal stimulation has shown more promise than direct hippocampal stimulation. Such sites include the fornices, which have led to subjective reports of intense deja vu in patients and, together with the nucleus basalis of Meynert, may have some effect in slowing progression of AD symptoms. Meanwhile, stimulation of the entorhinal cortex tends to improve memory performance on derived experimental tasks, but primarily when used during memory encoding. In sum, these results suggest that DBS strategies for supporting memory must rely on a nuanced understanding and recapitulation of native brain memory processes (Mankin and Fried, 2020).

28.8.4 Neural Prostheses: Reading and Writing Data Via Brain–Computer Interfaces

Excitingly, brain–computer interface (BCI) technology is beginning to reach maturity. Ongoing developments in systems neurobiology, parallel computing, and semiconductor manufacturing bring tantalizingly close the widespread ability to directly read from, and write to, the neural data stream. Leaders in this space include the Brain Gate consortium (Hochberg et al., 2012), which by 2012 published results in which two tetraplegic patients with 96-probe cortical recording arrays controlled a robotic arm to feed themselves. More recently, a multidisciplinary group demonstrated direct decoding of speech from surface electrode recording of dominant frontal cortex.

Some of the most significant developments in enabling BCI have been in data stream analysis. Broadly, there are two significant problems – spike sorting and dimensionality. Spike sorting refers to identifying the action potentials of individual neurons from recorded voltage deflections. In crowded cortex, this is akin to identifying the shouts of individual fans on a multi-track recording of a rock concert. Achieving rapid spike sorting has been aided by work in parallel and distributed computing, with origins in machine learning and database infrastructure required for large-scale data projects like Google Maps.

The dimensionality problem is similarly significant. The spike rate of a single neuron can be represented on a one-dimensional line like ticker tape, but the instantaneous firing rates of three neurons recorded simultaneously trace a trajectory through a three-dimensional space like a fly buzzing around a fruit bowl. The instantaneous activity of the firing rates of 100 simultaneously recorded neurons can be thought of as representing a point in a 100-dimensional "activity space," a daunting construct to understand. However, connected neurons are likely to have correlated activity, and thus neural activity occupies a lower-dimensional region, or manifold, within the higher-dimensional space. But finding such a pattern within high-dimensional data is difficult. One approach is dimensionality reduction, in which some aspect of data structure is preserved as the data are projected on, or embedded in, some lower-dimensional space (Pang et al., 2016). Dimensionality reduction applied to large-scale neural recordings has demonstrated that population activity traces characteristic, elegantly circular trajectories during tasks like reaching for objects or walking (Shenoy et al., 2013).

Writing data directly to the nervous system allows clinicians to bypass dysfunctional sensory systems, output systems, or even to replace the processing function of damaged brain centers themselves. Input neuroprostheses are not new. The cochlear implant, which has existed since the late 1970s, exemplifies how development of such devices relies on clever engineering combined with a functional understanding of underlying neurophysiology and anatomy. Recent promising examples include the restoration of walking muscle recruitment in paraplegic spinal cord injury patients via patterned stimulation of spinal motor pools. A similar strategy, taking advantage of patterned stimulation of visual cortex, has been able to restore rudimentary vision in a select group of patients with acquired blindness. In each case, significant hurdles remain toward restoring useful function, but these developments represent significant promise.

28.8.5 Future Techniques for Fine-Scale Manipulation of Neural Activity

Genetic engineering presents significant promise for the field of functional neurosurgery because it will allow for the manipulation of neural activity in defined cell types with spatial and temporal precision. Such precise manipulation is now routinely accomplished in the laboratory using optogenetics, the strategy of expressing light-gated ion channels in neurons to directly control activity with flashes of light (Deisseroth, 2011). Control can be genetically refined: by making the expression of an opsin dependent on specific gene promoters, expression of these channels can be programmed to occur only within specific cell types. Thus, light-controlled inhibition can be obtained by directing expression to GABAergic neurons; conversely, an area can be excited by expression in glutaminergic neurons. Spatial refinement can also be achieved via selective activation of specific nerve terminals: in a theoretical example, to activate only dopaminergic neurons within the subthalamic nucleus, one could express an optogenetic transgene within all dopaminergic neurons, then implant an optical fiber to activate only those terminals within the STn. A related strategy, termed chemogenetics, makes use of genetically encoded receptors for novel drug ligands to manipulate activity. Most excitingly, with the implantation of dopaminergic neurons derived from autologous induced pluripotent stem cells, the era of transgenics in functional neurosurgery has already begun (Schweitzer et al., 2020).

Figure acknowledgements

The following image is reprinted from Galvan and Wichmann (2008), with permission: Figure 28.1

The following image is reprinted from Oikawa et al., 2001, with permission: Figure 28.2

The following image is reprinted from Nestler, 2005, with permission: Figure 28.3

References

Abosch A, Cosgrove GR. Biological basis for the surgical treatment of depression. *Neurosurg Focus* 2008;**25**(1):E2. https://doi.org/10.3171/FOC/2008/25/7/E2.

Bari A, DiCesare J, Babayan D, Runcie M, Sparks H, Wilson B. Neuromodulation for substance addiction in human subjects: a review. *Neurosci Biobehav Rev* 2018;**95**:33–43.

Becker AJ. Review: Animal models of acquired epilepsy: insights into mechanisms of human epileptogenesis. *Neuropathol Appl Neurobiol* 2018;**44**(1):112–29. https://doi.org/10.1111/nan.12451.

Blauwendraat C, Nalls MA, Singleton AB. The genetic architecture of Parkinson's disease. *Lancet Neurol* 2020;**19**(2):170–8.

Breakefield XO, Blood AJ, Li Y, Hallett M, Hanson PI, Standaert DG. The pathophysiological basis of dystonias. *Nat Rev Neurosci* 2008;**9**(3):222–34.

Brown P, Eusebio A. Paradoxes of functional neurosurgery: clues from basal ganglia recordings. *Mov Disord* 2008;**23** (1):12–20; quiz 158.

Casillas-Espinosa PM, Powell KL, O'Brien TJ. Regulators of synaptic transmission: roles in the pathogenesis and treatment of epilepsy. *Epilepsia* 2012;**53**(Suppl 9):41–58.

Clark LN, Louis ED. Challenges in essential tremor genetics. *Rev Neurol* 2015;**171**(6–7):466–74. https://doi.org/10.1016/j.neurol.2015.02.015.

Dauer W, Przedborski S. Parkinson's disease: mechanisms and models. *Neuron* 2003;**39**(6):889–909. https://doi.org/10.1016/s0896-6273(03)00568-3.

de Lau LML, Breteler MMB. Epidemiology of Parkinson's disease. *Lancet Neurol* 2006;**5**(6):525–35. https://doi.org/10.1016/S1474-4422(06)70471-9.

Deisseroth K. Optogenetics. *Nat Methods* 2011;**8**(1):26–9. https://doi.org/10.1038/nmeth.f.324.

Deuschl G, Raethjen J, Hellriegel H, Elble R. Treatment of patients with essential tremor. *Lancet Neurol* 2011;**10** (2):148–61. https://doi.org/10.1016/S1474-4422(10)70322-7.

Epi4K Consortium, Epilepsy Phenome/Genome Project, Allen AS, et al. De novo mutations in epileptic encephalopathies. *Nature* 2013;**501**(7466):217–21. https://doi.org/10.1038/nature12439

Forno LS, DeLanney LE, Irwin I, Langston JW. Similarities and differences between MPTP-induced parkinsonsim and Parkinson's disease. Neuropathologic considerations. *Adv Neurol* 1993;**60**:600–08.

Frizon LA, Yamamoto EA, Nagel SJ, Simonson MT, Hogue O, Machado AG. Deep brain stimulation for pain in the modern era: a systematic review. *Neurosurgery* 2020;**86**(2):191–202. https://doi.org/10.1093/neuros/nyy552.

Galvan A, Wichmann T. Pathophysiology of parkinsonism. *Clin Neurophysiol* 2008;**119**(7):1459–74. https://doi.org/10.1016/j.clinph.2008.03.017.

Gradinaru V, Mogri M, Thompson KR, Henderson JM, Deisseroth K. Optical deconstruction of parkinsonian neural circuitry. *Science* 2009;**324**(5925):354–9. https://doi.org/10.1126/science.1167093.

Green AL, Wang S, Stein JF, et al. Neural signatures in patients with neuropathic pain. *Neurology* 2009;**72**(6):569–71. https://doi.org/10.1212/01.wnl.0000342122.25498.8b.

Gregory NS, Harris AL, Robinson CR, Dougherty PM, Fuchs PN, Sluka KA. An overview of animal models of pain: disease models and outcome measures. *J Pain* 2013;**14** (11):1255–69. https://doi.org/10.1016/j.jpain.2013.06.008.

Grone BP, Baraban SC. Animal models in epilepsy research: legacies and new directions. *Nat Neurosci* 2015;**18**(3):339–43. https://doi.org/10.1038/nn.3934.

Handforth A. Harmaline tremor: underlying mechanisms in a potential animal model of essential tremor. *Tremor Other Hyperkinet Mov* 2012;**2**:02-92-769-1. https://doi.org/10.7916/D8TD9W2P.

Herrington TM, Cheng JJ, Eskandar EN. Mechanisms of deep brain stimulation. *J Neurophysiol* 2016;**115**(1):19–38. https://doi.org/10.1152/jn.00281.2015.

Hochberg LR, Bacher D, Jarosiewicz B, et al. Reach and grasp by people with tetraplegia using a neurally controlled robotic arm. *Nature* 2012;**485**(7398):372–5. https//doi.org/10.1038/nature11076.

Hua SE, Lenz FA. Posture-related oscillations in human cerebellar thalamus in essential tremor are enabled by voluntary motor circuits. *J Neurophysiol* 2005;**93**(1):117–27. https://doi .org/10.1152/jn.00527.2004.

Krahl SE, Clark KB. Vagus nerve stimulation for epilepsy: a review of central mechanisms. *Surg Neurol Int* 2012;**3**(Suppl 4):S255–9. https://doi.org/10.4103/2152-7806.103015.

Kralic JE, Criswell HE, Osterman JL, et al. Genetic essential tremor in γ-aminobutyric acidA receptor α1 subunit knockout mice. *J Clin Invest* 2005;**115**(3):774–9. https://doi.org/10.1172 /JCI23625.

Kumar K, Toth C, Nath RK. Deep brain stimulation for intractable pain: a 15-year experience. *Neurosurgery* 1997;**40** (4):736–46; discussion 746–7. https://doi.org/10.1097/0000612 3-199704000-00015.

Kupsch A, Kuehn A, Klaffke S, et al. Deep brain stimulation in dystonia. *J Neurol* 2003;**250**(Suppl 1):I47–52. https://doi.org/10 .1007/s00415-003-1110-2.

Li MCH, Cook MJ. Deep brain stimulation for drug-resistant epilepsy. *Epilepsia* 2018;**59**(2):273–90. https://doi.org/10.1111/ epi.13964.

Louis ED, Bares M, Benito-Leon J, et al. Essential tremor-plus: a controversial new concept. *Lancet Neurol* 2020;**19**(3):266–70. https://doi.org/10.1016/S1474-4422(19)30398-9.

Louis ED, Lenka A. The olivary hypothesis of essential tremor: time to lay this model to rest? *Tremor Other Hyperkinet Mov* 2017;**7**:473. https://doi.org/10.7916/D8FF40RX.

Louis ED, Vonsattel JPG, Honig LS, Ross GW, Lyons KE, Pahwa R. Neuropathologic findings in essential tremor. *Neurology* 2006;**66**(11):1756–9. https://doi.org/10.1212/01 .wnl.0000218162.80315.b9.

Magrinelli F, Picelli A, Tocco P, et al. Pathophysiology of motor dysfunction in parkinson's disease as the rationale for drug treatment and rehabilitation. *Parkinsons Dis* 2016;**2016**:9832839. https://doi.org/10.1155/2016/9832839.

Mankin EA, Fried I. Modulation of human memory by deep brain stimulation of the entorhinal–hippocampal circuitry. *Neuron* 2020;**106**(2):218–35. https://doi.org/10.1016/j .neuron.2020.02.024.

Meredith GE, Rademacher DJ. MPTP mouse models of Parkinson's disease: an update. *J Parkinsons Dis* 2011;**1** (1):19–33. https://doi.org/10.3233/JPD-2011-11023.

Mogil JS. Animal models of pain: progress and challenges. *Nat Rev Neurosci* 2009;**10**(4):283–94. https://doi.org/10.1038/nrn2606.

Nestler EJ. Is there a common molecular pathway for addiction? *Nat Neurosci* 2005;**8**(11):1445–9. https://doi.org/10.1038/nn1578.

Nestler EJ, Hyman SE. Animal models of neuropsychiatric disorders. *Nat Neurosci* 2010;**13**(10):1161–9. https://doi.org/10 .1038/nn.2647.

Oikawa H, Sasaki M, Tamakawa Y, Kamei A. The circuit of Papez in mesial temporal sclerosis: MRI. *Neuroradiology* 2001;**43**(3):205–10. https://doi.org/10.1038/nn.2647.

Oleas J, Yokoi F, DeAndrade MP, Pisani A, Li Y. Engineering animal models of dystonia. *Mov Disord* 2013;**28**(7):990–1000. https://doi.org/10.1002/mds.25583.

Pan M-K, Ni C-L, Wu Y-C, Li Y-S, Kuo S-H. Animal models of tremor: relevance to human tremor disorders. *Tremor Other Hyperkinet Mov* 2018;**8**:587. https://doi.org/10.7916 /D89S37MV.

Pang R, Lansdell BJ, Fairhall AL. Dimensionality reduction in neuroscience. *Curr Biol* 2016;**26**(14):R656–60. https://doi.org/ 10.1016/j.cub.2016.05.029.

Penfield W, Perot P. The brain's record of auditory and visual experience. A final summary and discussion. *Brain* 1963;**86**:595–696. https://dooi.org/10.1093/brain/86.4.595.

Pepper J, Zrinzo L, Hariz M. Anterior capsulotomy for obsessive-compulsive disorder: a review of old and new literature. *J Neurosurg* 2019;1–10. Online ahead of print. https:// doi.org/10.3171/2019.4.JNS19275

Posner JB, Saper CB, Schiff N, Plum F. *Plum and Posner's Diagnosis of Stupor and Coma*, 4th ed. Oxford University Press, 2007.

Rasche D, Rinaldi PC, Young RF, Tronnier VM. Deep brain stimulation for the treatment of various chronic pain syndromes. *Neurosurg Focus* 2006;**21**(6):E8. https://doi.org/10 .3171/foc.2006.21.6.10.

Schweitzer JS, Song B, Herrington TM, et al. Personalized iPSC-derived dopamine progenitor cells for Parkinson's disease. *N Engl J Med* 2020;**382**(20):1926–32. https://doi.org/10.1056 /NEJMoa1915872.

Shah SA, Schiff ND. Central thalamic deep brain stimulation for cognitive neuromodulation – a review of proposed mechanisms and investigational studies. *Eur J Neurosci* 2010;**32**(7):1135–44. https://doi.org/10.1111/j.1460-9568 .2010.07420.x.

Shenoy KV, Sahani M, Churchland MM. Cortical control of arm movements: a dynamical systems perspective. *Annu Rev Neurosci* 2013;**36**:337–59. https://doi.org/10.1146/annurev-neuro-062111-150509.

Tanabe LM, Kim CE, Alagem N, Dauer WT. Primary dystonia: molecules and mechanisms. *Nat Rev Neurol* 2009;**5** (11):598–609. https://doi.org/10.1038/nrneurol.2009.160.

Wang TR, Moosa S, Dallapiazza RF, Elias WJ, Lynch WJ. Deep brain stimulation for the treatment of drug addiction. *Neurosurg Focus* 2018;**45**(2):E11. https://doi.org/10.3171/2018 .5.FOCUS18163.

Wilson BK, Hess EJ. Animal models for dystonia. *Mov Disord* 2013;**28**(7):982–9. https://doi.org/10.1002/mds.25526.

Wong M, Roper SN. Genetic animal models of malformations of cortical development and epilepsy. *J Neurosci Methods* 2016;**260**:73–82. https://doi.org/10.1016/j .jneumeth.2015.04.007.

Neuroradiology: Focused Ultrasound in Neurosurgery

Massimiliano Del Bene, Roberto Eleopra, Francesco Prada, and Francesco DiMeco

29.1 Historical Perspective

Ultrasound (US) is a longitudinal mechanical wave characterized by a frequency higher than 20,000 Hz. Technically, US generation is possible because of the outbreaking discovery of the piezoelectric effect by the Curie brothers in 1880 and of the inverse effect by Gabriel Lippmann one year later (O'Brien, 2017). The first concrete application for piezoelectric technology was during World War I, when, in 1917, Paul Langevin developed an ultrasonic submarine detector (Katzir, 2012). The subsequent progress has led to the introduction of the piezoelectric technology in all sectors. Concerning medical applications, the most significant is represented by US-based imaging and treatment. The first study on therapeutic applications of US was from Raimar Pohlman in 1938. At that time, it was thought that US treatment would have cured all kinds of illness such as arthritis, gastric ulcers, eczema, asthma, hemorrhoids, urinary incontinence, elephantiasis, and angina pectoris (Gersten and Kawashoma, 1955; James et al., 1960; Smith et al., 1966). In 1942, William Fry, a physicist of naval sonar research, and his brother, Francis Fry, began research at the Bioacoustic Research Laboratory. They finally developed a focused US device able to align four US transducers to produce a punctiform lesion with no damage to the neighboring tissue. The first study on brain applications was in 1942 by Lynn and Putnam, who treated 37 animals (dogs, cats, and monkeys) with high-frequency focused US waves. They were able to create focal damage in the targeted cortical and subcortical territories with only minor effects on the surrounding areas (Lynn et al., 1942). The first therapeutic use to treat a brain pathology, in a patient, was in 1950, by Lars Leksell. For this application, he designed a specific frame and US transducer and used it to treat psychiatric disorders. He subsequently renounced to the method because of lack of imaging feedback and the need for craniotomies. In 1955, William and Francis Fry performed the first partial basal ganglia ablation through a craniotomy (Fry et al., 1955). This subsequently led to Russell Meyers and William Fry treating numerous patients affected from various brain pathologies, in particular Parkinson's disease (Fry and Meyers, 1962). Over the years, several reports have described different brain applications. In 1968 Dr. Robert Heimburger exploited, for the first time, a focused US device to treat brain cancer, under US guidance (Heimburger, 1985). In the 1970s, a computer-controlled focused US system guided by a US scanner was specifically developed to treat brain tumor patients (Heimburger, 1985). In 1993, Hynynen and colleagues reported the first combination with magnetic resonance imaging (MRI) to guide and monitor tissue damage. The term MRI-guided focused ultrasound (MRgFUS) was coined (Hynynen et al., 1993). In 1998, Hynynen and Jolesz demonstrated the feasibility of using a large phased-array transducer for transcranial focusing and ablation. They also predicted the benefits of cavitation for transcranial treatments (Hynynen and Jolesz, 1998). In 1999, the Moonen group, introduced real-time temperature feedback for the first time in preclinical, studies demonstrating the feasibility of fully automatic FUS control based on MRI thermometry (Vimeaux et al., 1999). Relying on these experiences and advances, focused US applications in the brain have demonstrated an impressive growth that continues to the present day.

29.2 Mechanisms of Action

29.2.1 Thermal Effect

Heat generation is caused by the transfer of US energy to the tissue. This is mainly based on three mechanisms. When a mechanical wave such as US propagates in a tissue, this determines the succession of compressions and rarefactions, which determines micrometric tissue shearing and therefore heat (Nyborg, 2001). The second mechanism is based on non-linear wave generation that occurs when the wave propagates in a heterogeneous medium, which can determine the formation of waves with supra-harmonic frequencies from the fundamental frequency. These can be absorbed by the tissue, thus inducing heat generation (Hynynen, 1987; Khokhlova et al., 2006; Medel et al., 2012). The third mechanism is cavitation through (i) the absorption of the energy generated by cavitation, and (ii) scattering and superior absorption of US in the region of cavitation (Medel et al., 2012). The principle of FUS relies on focusing multiple US transducers on a small volume to concentrate the desired amount of energy to obtain the heating (Figure 29.1). This allows limitation of the therapeutic effect at the region of interest. The limit of this approach is represented by the dimension of the focal volume, which is millimetric and can be extended only by moving the focus to the surrounding areas. As an alternative, pulsed ultrasound with short duty cycles (5–10%) minimizes the temporal average US intensity, thus leading to minimal heat generation and allowing for the non-thermal mechanical effects to take place

(Frenkel et al., 2006; O'Neill et al., 2009). Cerebral ablative procedures are carried out fixing the patient's head in a stereotactic frame for safe and secure placement within the FUS transducer. Targeting and procedure monitoring are performed under image guidance: this allows fusion of accurate preoperative images (CT and MRI) to intraoperative MRI coupled with the FUS transducer for planning, while exploiting quasi real-time MR thermometry to monitor location and temperatures at the focal spot. Several techniques are used to assess lesioning outcome (Allen et al., 2021; Franzini et al., 2020; Wang et al., 2018).

29.2.2 Mechanical Effects

As stated above, US is a longitudinal mechanical wave whose cycle is based on alternating negative (rarefactive) and positive (compressive) phases. This physical principle explains the two mechanical effects of focused US: (i) acoustic cavitation and (ii) radiation forces/acoustic streaming.

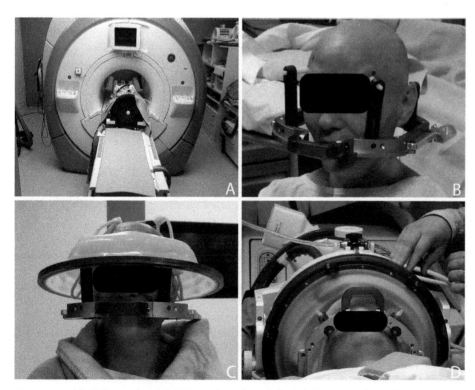

Figure 29.1 MRgFUS procedure. MRgFUS is performed in a dedicated MRI suite, exploiting the hardware from Insightech. It consists of a specific MRI-compatible helmet equipped with 1024 US transducers (A). The patient's head is shaved to improve US transmission and immobilized by a stereotactic head frame (B). A silicone barrier is positioned on the head to fill the helmet with cooled degassed water in order to maximize acoustic coupling and to prevent scalp heating (C, D). The procedure is performed under real-time MRI thermometry and passive cavitation detectors feedback to prevent excessive heating or cavitation (D).

29.2.2.1 Acoustic Cavitation

Acoustic cavitation describes the US-induced oscillations in size of gas-filled bubbles within a liquid medium (Dalecki, 2004; Hersh et al., 2016; Medel et al., 2012). When a US wave hits a gas-filled bubble, this is subjected to rarefactions and compressions, thus determining repetitive changes in size. When the pressure wave amplitude is low, the phenomenon is stable, alternating bubble expansions and reduction, and is called non-inertial cavitation. Otherwise, when the pressure wave amplitude increases, this can determine a bubble collapse, which produces violent shock waves and high-velocity jets, with potentially harmful effects on the adjacent tissues. This manifestation is defined inertial cavitation (Krasovitski et al., 2011). Notably, acoustic cavitation may rely on US-induced nucleation of gas bubbles within the tissue or on synthetic microbubbles that are administered as a US imaging contrast agent. In this latter case, a lower power of US can determine similar cavitation effects, thus reducing the risks for inertial cavitation (Medel et al., 2012; Sokka et al., 2003; Tran et al., 2005; Figure 29.1). Acoustic cavitation can exert a mechanical effect on surrounding structures (in particular interfaces) or can induce cell death if the oscillating bubble damages the cell membrane. With these premises, the cavitation damage is less predictable than thermal damage. In general, it depends on microbubbles (MBs) and US-related factors: MBs composition, concentration, and distribution as well as US frequency and amplitude are to be taken into account (Allen et al., 2021; Franzini et al., 2020; Wang et al., 2018). In particular, the higher the frequency, the higher the amplitude needed to obtain the cavitation. This is why, for therapeutic purposes, high frequencies are usually avoided when dealing with cavitation (Jagannathan et al., 2009).

29.2.2.2 Radiation Forces/Acoustic Streaming

When a FUS beam hits a tissue, it exerts a force alongside the direction of the beam. This force is defined radiation force. If sufficient, the force may induce a selective displacement in the focus excepting the surrounding tissues and thus producing a strain in the tissue (Hancock et al., 2009). Similarly, when the US wave produces a radiation force in a fluid medium this may lead to a circulation of the liquid that can augment convection and produce shear forces that ultimately can determine tissue changes and damage. This phenomenon is known as acoustic streaming (Frenkel et al., 2000, 2001).

29.3 Clinical Applications

Focused ultrasound is on the verge of shifting from bench to bedside thanks to many therapeutic modalities already approved by regulatory bodies for clinical application. The main clinically approved FUS application regards the use of thermal lesioning for movement disorders, but other targets such as the hippocampus for epilepsy or the anterior limb of the internal capsule for psychiatric disorders are being investigated under clinical trials (Franzini et al., 2019). Furthermore, other FUS modalities are under investigation such as BBB opening, neuromodulation, or sonodynamic therapy. In the following paragraphs, the principal clinical applications of FUS in neurosurgery will be revised also providing an overview of the future advances (Figure 29.1).

29.3.1 Functional Neurosurgery

29.3.1.1 Essential Tremor

Essential tremor (ET) represents the most frequent movement disorder, affecting an estimated 2.2% of the population (Louis and Ottman, 2014). Essential tremor is a debilitating condition that can prejudice patients' ability to write, eat, shave, perform everyday activities, and work a job. The treatment is based on medical therapy involving beta blockers or barbiturates even though 30% of patients are refractory to therapy finally requiring a functional neurosurgical approach (Louis, 2016). The first-line surgical treatment is represented by deep brain stimulation (DBS) to target the ventral intermediate nucleus (VIM) of the thalamus (Weintraub and Elias, 2017). Relying on the observation's derived from DBS, MRgFUS has been proposed as treatment for ET. Several pilot studies reported the thermal ablation of the VIM to achieve tremor improvements ranging from 75% to 81% with only marginal complications (Elias et al., 2013; Gallay et al., 2016; Lipsman et al., 2013; Weintraub and Elias, 2017). In 2016, Elias et al. published the results from a randomized controlled trial which compared unilateral MRgFUS thalamotomy to a sham procedure (Elias et al., 2016). They observed that the hand-tremor scores improved much more with thalamotomy (from 18.1 points at baseline to 9.6 at 3 months) than with the sham procedure (from 16.0 to 15.8 points). Notably, the improvement in the MRgFUS harm was maintained at 12 months. Adverse events included gait disturbance in 36% of patients and paresthesias or numbness in 38% with some degree of recovery at one year (Elias et al., 2016).

These results led Kim and colleagues to compare MRgFUS, radiofrequency, and DBS. They did not observe any difference in outcome but rather a lower incidence of complications for the MRgFUS group (Kim et al., 2017). In 2017, a further validation of the efficacy of MRgFUS came from a multicenter randomized trial that confirmed the stability of tremor suppression after MRgFUS thalamotomy at 2 years without delayed complications (Chang et al., 2018). Relying on these studies, the FDA approved the MRgFUS treatment for ET in 2016. Giordano and colleagues recently published a systematic review and meta-analysis comparing unilateral MRgFUS to unilateral and bilateral DBS (Giordano et al., 2020). Bilateral DBS appeared significantly superior to MRgFUS and unilateral DBS ($p < 0.001$), but no difference was observed between MRgFUS and unilateral DBS ($p < 0.198$), while postoperative quality of life improvement was better with MRgFUS thalamotomy than DBS ($p < 0.001$) (Giordano et al., 2020). Therefore, a long-term follow-up (5 years) of 44 ET patients which underwent to unilateral MRgFUS revealed that this treatment is an effective and safe procedure with a significant relief and improvement of tremor (Sinai et al., 2019). In the last two years, several studies have addressed multiple aspects of MRgFUS treatment of ET encompassing technical improvements, treatment modalities, indications, imaging interpretation and clinical outcome (Chapman et al., 2020; D'Souza et al., 2019; Ito et al., 2020; Jones et al., 2019; Kapadia et al., 2020; Keil et al., 2020; Lehman et al., 2020; McDannold et al., 2020b; Paff et al., 2020; Ranjan et al., 2019b; Su et al., 2020; Weidman et al., 2019). These reports globally sustain the efficacy and potentiality of this application fostering the research in this field.

The treatment is currently approved also in Europe, Korea, Canada, Japan, Russia, Taiwan, and the Middle East. Different clinical trials are ongoing in USA and Europe to validate staged bilateral treatments.

29.3.1.2 Chronic Neuropathic Pain

Chronic neuropathic pain is a common condition, affecting 7–10% of the general population. The etiology and pathophysiology are not well-defined (Attal, 2000; Colloca et al., 2017). The International Association for Study of Pain (IASP) has recently published a new definition of neuropathic pain according to which neuropathic pain is defined as "pain caused by a lesion or disease of the somatosensory system" (www.iasp-pain.org/resources/painDefinition). Treatment is based on a variety of medical therapies, including non-steroidal anti-inflammatory drugs (NSAIDs), antiepileptic drugs, sodium-channel blockers, antidepressants,

local anesthetics, opioids, capsaicin, and N-methyl-D-aspartate antagonists. Notably, these therapies are not universally effective because only half of patients experience a 30 50% relief with the current therapeutic approaches (Attal, 2000; Colloca et al., 2017; Jung and Chang, 2018). Functional neurosurgery, by targeting the contralateral thalamus through DBS or ablation (e.g., radiofrequency), may play a role, especially in those cases of pain refractory to medical treatments. In this frame, MRgFUS perfectly fits as a non-invasive way to obtain a thermal ablation of the contralateral thalamus. Martin and coworkers reported nine cases of patients affected by different forms of chronic neuropathic pain who were treated by contralateral thalamotomies exploiting MRgFUS. Interestingly, all patients described an instantaneous relief during sonication followed by a mean of 68% reduction 2 days after treatment and a mean of 57% relief at 1 year (Martin et al., 2009). These positive results were confirmed by Jeanmonod and coworkers (Gallay et al., 2018; Jeanmonod et al., 2012). Notably, they reported one case of bleeding in the target with ischemia in the motor thalamus. This led them to introduce a cavitation detector to exclude potential cavitation and to maintain the sonication temperature below 60° C (Jeanmonod et al., 2012). Even being small reports, these studies provide the proof of concept and preliminary evidence of safety and feasibility of MRgFUS treatment for chronic pain neuropathy. Regulatory approvals for the treatment of neuropathic pain have been achieved in Europe, Korea, the Middle East, and Russia and clinical trials are ongoing in the United States (Jung and Chang, 2018).

29.3.1.3 Parkinson's Disease

Parkinson's disease (PD) is a degenerative condition affecting 1.5% of people over the age of 70 and 0.15% of the general population (Dobrakowski et al., 2014). The progressive loss of function of dopaminergic neurons in the basal ganglia leads to akinesia/bradykinesia, resting tremors, and muscular rigidity. Surgical treatment is based on DBS and ablation using as targets the subthalamic nucleus, the globus pallidus pars interna (GPi), and the VIM, among others (Delong and Wichmann, 2015; Katz et al., 2015; Metman and Slavin, 2015). These areas have also been proposed as target for MRgFUS. Magara and colleagues reported the initial experience with MRgFUS pallidothalamic tractotomy (PTT) (Magara et al., 2014). The study demonstrated the safety, feasibility, accuracy, and durability of the MRgFUS PTT. They exploited repetitive sonications (repetition of the final temperatures 4–5 times) to achieve an effective lesioning.

They finally obtained a reduction of 60.9% in Unified Parkinson Disease Rating Scale (UPDRS) score and 56.7% improvement in global symptoms relief at the 3 months follow-up (Magara et al., 2014). Differently, MRgFUS thalamotomy is particularly indicated for tremor-dominant PD. Bond et al. designed a double-blinded randomized controlled trial demonstrating the effectiveness of unilateral MRgFUS thalamotomy in tremor-dominant PD. They observed a mean of 50% improvement in hand tremor at 3 months compared with a 22% improvement of the sham procedures. The 1-year tremor scores showed a reduction of 40.6% (Bond et al., 2017). Moreover, an open-label pilot study demonstrated the feasibility and efficacy of MRgFUS unilateral subthalamotomy. The procedure resulted in a mean improvement of the MDS-UPDRS III scores of 53% in the off-medication state and of 47% in the on-medication state at 6 months (Martínez-Fernández et al., 2018). The other relevant target for surgical treatment of PD, in particular for dyskinesia, is the GPi. In 2018, the results of a phase II clinical trial on unilateral MRgFUS pallidotomy were published (Jung et al., 2018). Patients' outcomes showed several significant improvements: (i) 32.2% in the "medication-off" UPDRS part III score and (ii) 52.7% in UDysRS at the 6-month follow-up; (iii) 39.1% and (iv) 42.7% at the 1-year follow-up; and in (v) quality of life (QoL). Recently, Yangyang Xu and colleagues demonstrated the efficacy and safety profile of MRgFUS in 80 parkinsonian patients through a systematic review of the related literature (Xu et al., 2021). Similarly to ET, in the last two years, a number of reports have presented technical improvements, new indications, innovative treatment modalities, imaging interpretation, and clinical outcome in PD treatment (Boutet et al., 2019; Dang et al., 2019; Ebani et al., 2020; Foffani et al., 2019; Fusco et al., 2019; Gagliardo et al., 2020; Gallay et al., 2019a, 2019b, 2019c; Keil et al., 2020; Martínez-Fernández and Pineda-Pardo, 2019; McDannold et al., 2020a, 2020b; Meng et al., 2020; Miller et al., 2020; Moosa et al., 2019; Rodriguez-Rojas et al., 2020; Shah et al., 2020; Sharma et al., 2020; Walters and Shah, 2019). At present, the use of MRgFUS to treat medication-refractory PD is approved in Israel, Europe, Korea, Russia, and – for tremor-dominant PD only – also in the USA. Numerous ongoing trials are underway to demonstrate the feasibility of treating the different aspects of PD also considering bilateral ablation through staged treatments. Furthermore, even if experimental, the possibility of opening the blood–brain barrier (BBB) with MRgFUS is under study in an effort to enhance the delivery of neurotherapeutics; among the

others: genes, growth factors, stem cells, neuroprotective and/or neurorestorative drugs, and anti-alpha synuclein antibodies (Fan et al., 2017; Jung and Chang, 2018; Lin et al., 2016; Long et al., 2017).

29.3.1.4 Obsessive-Compulsive Disorder and Major Depressive Disorder

Obsessive compulsive disorder (OCD) and major depressive disorder (MDD) are highly prevalent conditions, affecting 2% and 11% of the population, respectively. Current treatments include medications, ablative surgery, DBS, and stereotactic radiosurgery. Notably, up to 30% of cases are "treatment-resistant" (Davidson et al., 2020). Surgical targets are usually part of the limbic system and include the anterior limb of the internal capsule (ALIC), subgenual cingulate cortex, anterior cingulate cortex, and ventral striatum (Jung and Chang, 2018). The first experience in MRgFUS application for OCD was in 2015 by Jung et al. In this study, medically refractory OCD patients underwent bilateral ablation of ALIC. The MRgFUS led to an improvement in Yale–Brown Obsessive Compulsive Scale (Y-BOCS) scores (mean 33%), along with higher improvements in Hamilton Anxiety Rating Scale (HAM-A) (mean 69.4%) and Hamilton Depression Rating Scale (HAM-D) (mean 61.1%) scores, without causing neuropsychological or neurological complications at 6 months follow-up. Notably, the greater result was for the MDD component (Jung et al., 2015a, 2015b; Jung and Chang, 2018). Symptom improvement was stable for both OCD and MDD at 2 years following MRgFUS (Jung et al., 2015a, 2015b; Jung and Chang, 2018; Kim et al., 2018). Recently, the safety and efficacy of MRgFUS capsulotomy in OCD and MDD patients have been confirmed by a report on two phase I trials (Davidson et al., 2020). Recently, a clinical trial has begun to treat OCD patients in Canada. MRI-guided focused ultrasound for OCD or MDD is not approved by any regulatory bodies worldwide.

29.3.1.5 Emerging Applications in Functional Neurosurgery

29.3.1.5.1 Neuromodulation

Focused ultrasound can influence (stimulate or suppress) neuronal activity. Neuromodulation can be achieved with high or low frequencies exploiting mainly the mechanical effect of US through several mechanisms including cavitation, direct effects on neural ion channels, and plasma membrane deformation (Deffieux et al., 2013; Fiani et al., 2020; Fomenko et al., 2018;

Tyler et al., 2008; Wahab et al., 2012; Younan et al., 2013). Different low-frequency sonication parameters have been demonstrated to enhance neural firing, suppress cortical (and epileptic) discharges, and modify behavior when directed to cortical and subcortical brain regions (Fomenko et al., 2018). High frequency may exert similar neuromodulatory activity as demonstrated by target verification prior to definitive ablation during procedures for tremor (Elias et al., 2013). Examples of neuromodulation include inducing activity in hippocampal regions, stimulating motor responses, altering frontal eye field responses, inducing sensory responses, and treatment of refractory epilepsy (Fiani et al., 2020; Fomenko et al., 2018). Several trials on human application of low-intensity FUS for treatment of Alzheimer's disease, epilepsy, disorders of consciousness, and Parkinson's disease have begun (Darrow, 2019; Fiani et al., 2020; Fomenko et al., 2018; Ranjan et al., 2019a). Future applications may encompass, among the others, human brain mapping, and nonsurgical treatments for functional neurological disorders.

29.3.1.5.2 Ablative Approaches

Ablation may represent the ideal treatment for focal lesion causing functional disturbances such as hypothalamic hamartomas, tuberous sclerosis, and temporal lobe epilepsy (Jung and Chang, 2018).

29.3.1.5.3 Blood–Brain Barrier Permeabilization

The BBB represents one of the main obstacles to medical treatments in neurological diseases. Through its mechanical effect, MRgFUS can produce a temporary BBB disruption so as to allow an enhanced accumulation of drugs or compounds in the brain. This mechanism is under study for several conditions, for instance Parkinson's disease and Alzheimer's disease (Fan et al., 2017; Fiani et al., 2020; Jung and Chang, 2018; Lin et al., 2016; Long et al., 2017).

29.3.2 Neuro-Oncology

29.3.2.1 Thermal Ablation

Depending on US parameters and sonication time, thermal effect can finally result in hyperthermia (42–45°C) and then in ablation (>50°C). The latter consists of a thermocoagulative necrosis related to denaturation of proteins, while hyperthermia can result in cell death depending on the exposure–time relationship (Lepock,

2005). Several reports have described this approach, starting as preliminary experiences, in the 1980s, with CT or US guidance and the need for a craniectomy (Guthkelch et al., 1991; Heimburger, 1985; Park et al., 2006). The results were encouraging (Park et al., 2006; Ram et al., 2006), thus sustaining the research which finally led Coluccia and colleagues. to report the first case of a recurrent glioblastoma patient successfully treated with MRgFUS without the need for a craniectomy (Coluccia et al., 2014). Notably, during the initial experiences, several complications were described, mainly related to bleeding or the formation of secondary lesions in the insonation path (Hynynen and Clement, 2007; McDannold et al., 2010; Ram et al., 2006). Thermal ablation presents also several limitations: (i) the focus volume is limited, thus requiring repeated sonication at multiple adjacent points to cover the entire tumor; (ii) the bone shield limits the indications, with it still being impossible to treat superficial or skull base tumors. Currently, three trials are ongoing (NCT00147056, NCT01473485, and NCT03028246) addressing the safety and feasibility of thermal ablation in gliomas, brain metastases, and benign tumors in adult and pediatric patients. One trial has concluded (NCT01698437), although results are still not available. Some preclinical studies have proposed the combination of US contrast agents and MRgFUS to enhance tissue damage thanks to mechanical effects, thus reducing the time-averaged acoustic power, the heating, and the potential damage to healthy surrounding structures (McDannold et al., 2006; Yu et al., 2004). Another interesting approach, even if mainly preclinical, is interstitial FUS. It relies on a US transducer enveloped in a cooling catheter to produce precise thermal ablation even in the case of large tumors in a way similar to radiofrequency or laser ablation (Canney et al., 2013; Christian et al., 2014; N'Djin et al., 2014).

29.3.2.2 Blood–Brain Barrier Disruption

The BBB is crucial to protect the central nervous system, but on the other hand, it also protects tumors from treatment. Focused US allows a precise, repeatable, safe BBB opening (Bunevicius et al., 2020; K.-T. Chen et al., 2019; Deng et al., 2012; Idbaih et al., 2019; Lamsam et al., 2018; Mainprize et al., 2019; Meng et al., 2018; Park et al., 2020; Sheikov et al., 2004; Sheybani and Price, 2019; Zaki Ghali et al., 2019). The mechanism is based on low-frequency US to induce a mechanical stimulation (stable cavitation) of the endothelial cells, and in general of the BBB so as to induce a time-limited permeability due to (i) disruption of the tight junction, (ii) induced transcytosis, (iii) increased caveolins; and (iv) decreased P-glycoprotein (P-gp; Deng et al., 2012; Lionetti et al., 2009; Sheikov et al., 2004, 2008). To maximize the effect while reducing the insonation power, exogenous microbubbles, US contrast agents can be exploited (Bunevicius et al., 2020; K.-T. Chen et al., 2019; Idbaih et al., 2019; Lamsam et al., 2018; Mainprize et al., 2019; Park et al., 2020; Zaki Ghali et al., 2019). The enhanced permeability has immediate onset and lasts up to 8 h (Idbaih et al., 2019; Lamsam et al., 2018; Mainprize et al., 2019; Zaki Ghali et al., 2019). The BBB disruption is evaluated with gadolinium enhancement in MRI (Idbaih et al., 2019; Mainprize et al., 2019; Park et al., 2020; Zaki Ghali et al., 2019). In preclinical models, BBB disruption has allowed the enhanced delivery of trastuzumab, doxorubicin, temozolomide, methotrexate, viruses, and cells (Bunevicius et al., 2020; K.-T. Chen et al., 2019; Lamsam et al., 2018; Mainprize et al., 2019; Zaki Ghali et al., 2019). Recently, a growing body of literature has been published reporting the results of the first patient applications. A single-center trial (NCT02253212) demonstrated the safety and efficacy of an implantable, pulsed (low-intensity) US device (SonoCloud-1; CarThera, Paris, France) with microbubble injection to disrupt the BBB in association with carboplatin administration in 21 patients with recurrent GBM (Idbaih et al., 2019). In 2018, Mainprize and colleagues demonstrated the safety and feasibility of BBB opening with an instantaneous 15–50% increased gadolinium enhancement on T_1-weighted MRI, and resolution nearly 20 h after (Mainprize et al., 2019). In 2020, Park and colleagues demonstrated the safety and feasibility of repetitive MRgFUS BBB opening in the same targets in association with a standard chemotherapy protocol in glioblastoma patients (Park et al., 2020). On the basis of these results, several trials have been started aiming at confirming the safety, demonstrating the efficacy, and identifying the ideal compounds and US parameters: NCT02343991, NCT03551249, NCT03616860, NCT04063 514, NCT04446416, NCT04440358, NCT04417088, NCT03712293, NCT03626896, NCT03714243, NCT03744 026. In addition, even if still preclinical, several research lines are trying to develop experimental approaches to obtain the maximum effectiveness with FUS. Among others, gene therapy, cell therapy, viral therapy, liposome encapsulation, nanoparticle conjugation, immunotherapy, and modified microbubbles are the most promising (Bunevicius et al., 2020; K.-T. Chen et al., 2019; Lamsam et al., 2018; Sheybani and Price, 2019; Zaki Ghali et al., 2019).

29.3.2.3 Emerging Applications in Neuro-Oncology

29.3.2.3.1 Focused Ultrasound-Enhanced Liquid Biopsy

Liquid biopsy represents one of the most relevant unmet clinical needs in neuro-oncology. Several approaches have been proposed and are under study, ranging from cell-free nucleic acids to proteins and extracellular vesicles. All these entities are extremely rare in peripheral blood, thus requiring cumbersome methodologies to enrich and characterize the biomarkers (D'Soouza et al., 2009; Pacia et al., 2020; Zhu et al., 2020). Low-frequency FUS may induce, through a mechanical effect, the permeabilization of BBB and the release of molecules from tumor cells. In the preclinical setting, this possibility has already been demonstrated in two reports from the Hong Chen Group in 2020. They were able to (i) statistically increase the blood concentrations of glial fibrillary acidic protein (GFAP) and myelin basic protein (MBP) by sonicating a normal brain tissue of a porcine model, and (ii) increase the plasma concentration of mRNA from glioblastoma (GBM) in a murine model (Pacia et al., 2020; Zhu et al., 2020). Notably, they did not observe any adverse effect.

29.3.2.3.2 Immunomodulation

Focused US can induce a complex immunomodulation relying on both thermal and mechanical effects. Heating leads to overexpression of heat shock proteins, which can stimulate immune response (Hu et al., 2005). Permeabilization of the BBB determines an increase of bidirectional flow, across the BBB, of antigens, immune cells, and proinflammatory molecules/chemokines. Tumor cells sonoporation or mechanical disruption produces a great amount of tumor-derived debris and new antigens able to stimulate dendritic cells (Chen et al., 2015b; Hu et al., 2007). In addition, FUS can influence tumor-related immunosuppression, augment tumor-infiltrating lymphocytes population, and induce sterile inflammation in healthy brain (Cohen-Inbar et al., 2016; Hu et al., 2007; Kovacs et al., 2017; Lu et al., 2009; Mauri et al., 2018). Most of the aforementioned considerations have been derived from systemic tumors and provide the basis for a translation of FUS immunomodulation in brain tumor patients, especially in combination with immunotherapeutic approaches (Chen et al., 2015a; Curley et al., 2017; Sheybani and Price, 2019).

29.3.2.3.3 Sensitization to Chemotherapy and Radiotherapy

As stated above, FUS can induce BBB disruption, thus opening the door to new chemotherapeutic approaches but also enhancing the bioavailability and efficacy of the already available. Hyperthermia can influence the tumor microenvironment, determining an increase in blood flow which leads to higher concentration of drugs, oxygen, and metabolites. This pro-trophic setting stimulates tumor metabolism but also tumor exposition to chemotherapeutic compounds, finally enhancing tumor sensitivity to chemotherapy and radiotherapy (Finley et al., 2011; Kampinga, 2006; Song et al., 2005; Yu et al., 2006). In addition, during the cell cycle, cells are more sensitive to hyperthermia in S phase, which is also the phase of relative resistance to radiotherapy (Guthkelch et al., 1991). Prior exposition to radiation therapy can determine a higher efficacy of FUS in inducing BBB disruption (White et al., 2020). Relying on these aspects, FUS with chemotherapy and radiotherapy may have a synergistic and additive effect in tumor treatment in a final effort to maximize the efficacy while reducing the side effects.

29.3.2.3.4 Sonodynamic Therapy

Sonodynamic therapy (SDT) is an extremely promising technique based on the combination of a sonosensitizer compound such as 5-aminolevulinic acid (5-ALA) and FUS to generate ROS able to damage tumor cell DNA, thus inducing apoptosis (Bilmin et al., 2019). Sonodynamic therapy represents the ideal solution to achieve a high specificity of damage in a non-invasive fashion. Indeed, FUS can reach tumors located deep in the brain, non-invasively and with high accuracy. On the other hand, depending on the features of the sonosensitizer, it is possible to increment the specificity of damage. For instance, 5-ALA is metabolized specifically by glioma cells and not by the neighbor healthy parenchyma, while sodium fluorescein is able to accumulate where the BBB is disrupted by the tumor. In both cases, the final tumoricidal effect will be reached only in the tumor. Recently, growing interest is fostering research in SDT exploiting 5-ALA or fluorescein in preclinical models, and is obtaining encouraging results (Bilmin et al., 2019; Prada et al., 2020b; Sheehan et al., 2020; Suehiro et al., 2018; Wu et al., 2019). A phase 0, first in human, open-label study of intravenous aminolevulinic acid hydrochloride (ALA) and an MR-guided FUS device in patients with recurrent high-grade glioma will be completed in 2024 (NCT04559685).

29.3.3 Neurovascular

29.3.3.1 Ischemic Stroke

Stroke is one of the most common reasons for permanent deficits and death in most developed countries. In particular, arterial ischemic stroke (AIS) represents 70–80% of all types of stroke (Donnan et al., 2008). So far, treatment has been based on mechanical thrombolysis and intravenous thrombolysis to obtain the recanalization and to finally improve outcome (Z. Chen et al., 2019). Sonothrombolysis through transcranial Doppler (TCD) or transcranial color-coded sonography (TCCS) with or without t-PA is a promising alternative for the treatment of AIS (Z. Chen et al., 2019; Ricci et al., 2012). The mechanism is based on the mechanical effect of US on the blood flow surrounding the thrombus. This stimulation may also induce better distribution of t-PA at the level of the obstruction (Alexandrov et al., 2004a; Skoloudik et al., 2006; Tsivgoulis and Alexandrov, 2007). The addition of US contrast agents can be exploited to obtain cavitation and microbubbles blast to better dissolve the thrombus (Auboire et al., 2018; Prada et al., 2019; Rubiera et al., 2008). Several trials have addressed the efficacy of sonothrombolysis in AIS (Dwedar et al., 2014; Eggers et al., 2005, 2008). Eggers et al. (2005, 2008) and Dwedar et al. (2014) have proved that sonothrombolysis can increase the recanalization rate and improve the outcomes of acute middle cerebral artery occlusion. Differently, CLOTBUST (Alexandrov et al., 2004a)and Molina et al. (2006) demonstrated that continuous TCD can enhance t-PA based recanalization in AIS even if does not influence patients outcomes (Alexandrov et al., 2004b). The TUCSON trial (Molina et al., 2009) found that the combination of US, microbubbles, and t-PA leads to a better recanalization rate and to a better outcome. In contrasr, Differently, the NOR-SASS trial (Nacu et al., 2017) did not observe any clinical effect in unselected AIS patients. In 2019, Zhouqing Chen performed a meta-analysis of the existing randomized controlled trials. They concluded that "t-PA," "NIHSS > 15," "Treatment time ≤ 150 min," and "Age ≤ 65 years" are potential favorable factors for efficacy outcomes of sonothombolysis. Sonothrombolysis can increase the rate of recanalization in AIS although without significant improvement in neurological outcome (Z. Chen et al., 2019). The same year, Alexandrov et al. published the results from CLOTBUST-ER, a multi-center, double-blind, phase 3, randomized controlled trial. The aim of the trial was to dissect whether an operator-independent transcranial (low-power, high-frequency) US device could improve outcome in combination with t-PA after AIS. The trial was stopped after the second interim analysis because of futility (Alexandrov et al., 2019). AIS application still needs to be better addressed and dissected even considering the application of MRgFUS techinques (Ilyas et al., 2018; Zafar et al., 2019). Furthermore, the endovascular sonolysis approach, even in combination with microbubbles, has to be mentioned, which is achieving promising results (Dixon et al., 2019; Kuliha et al., 2013).

29.3.3.2 Hemorrhagic Stroke

Intracerebral hemorrhage (ICH) is the second big chapter of the cerebrovascular accidents, behind AIS. Treatment is based on surgery, which carries significant risks. Several studies have demonstrated, in a preclinical setting, the safety and feasibility of inducing a lysis of the hematoma exploiting FUS to liquefy the clot to be finally aspirated through a burr hole. This may be performed also under MR guidance in a highly accurate and non-invasive fashion (Harnof et al., 2014; Ilyas et al., 2018; Monteith et al., 2013a, 2013b; Zafar et al., 2019). Interestingly, FUS can also determine an effect named histotripsy, which exploits the mechanical cavitation to disrupt a tissue. Histotripsy has been applied in a porcine model of ICH with promising results in terms of safety and feasibility (Gerhardson et al., 2017, 2020).

29.4 Conclusions

Focused ultrasound is an extremely promising technique that is still in its infancy, in particular for neurological applications. Several technical advances (e.g., microbubbles, sonosensitizers, low- and high-frequency helmets, skull compensation, MRI guidance, real-time thermometry) have fostered the research, thus leading to an impressive number of preclinical studies. While the mainstay to treat brain diseases is currently MR-guided FUS, many other devices are currently being used for clinical application to treat brain diseases and others are under development, ranging from single-element navigated devices to implantable devices (Idbaih et al., 2019; Pouliopoulos et al., 2020; Prada et al., 2020a). This leads us to believe that in the near future several diseases will be treated in a completely different way thanks to innovative and non-invasive approaches provided by FUS.

Figure acknowledgements

The following image obtained with consent is credited to the authors of this chapter: Figure 29.1

References

Alexandrov AV, Demchuk AM, Burgin WS, Robinson DJ, Grotta JC. Ultrasound-enhanced thrombolysis for acute ischemic stroke: phase I. Findings of the CLOTBUST trial. *J Neuroimaging* 2004a;**14**:113–17.

Alexandrov AV, Köhrmann M, Soinne L, et al. Safety and efficacy of sonothrombolysis for acute ischaemic stroke: a multicentre, double-blind, phase 3, randomised controlled trial. *Lancet Neurol* 2019;**18**:338–47. www.sciencedirect.com/science/article/pii/S1474442219300262.

Alexandrov AV, Molina CA, Grotta JC, et al. Ultrasound-enhanced systemic thrombolysis for acute ischemic stroke. *N Engl J Med* 2004b;**351**:2170–8.

Allen SP, Prada F, Xu Z, et al. A preclinical study of diffusion-weighted MRI contrast as an early indicator of thermal ablation. *Magn Reson Med* 2021;**85**(4):2145–59. https://doi.org/10.1002/mrm.28537.

Attal N. Chronic neuropathic pain: mechanisms and treatment. *Clin J Pain* 2000;**16**:S118–30.

Auboire L, Sennoga CA, Hyvelin J-M, et al. Microbubbles combined with ultrasound therapy in ischemic stroke: a systematic review of in-vivo preclinical studies. *PLoS One* 2018;**13**:e0191788.

Bilmin K, Kujawska T, Grieb P. Sonodynamic therapy for gliomas. perspectives and prospects of selective sonosensitization of glioma cells. *Cells* 2019;**8**(11):1428. https://doi.org/10.3390/cells8111428.

Bond AE, Shah BB, Huss DS, et al. Safety and efficacy of focused ultrasound thalamotomy for patients with medication-refractory, tremor-dominant Parkinson disease: a randomized clinical trial. *JAMA Neurol* 2017;**74**:1412–8. https://doi.org/10.1001/jamaneurol.2017.3098.

Boutet A, Gwun D, Gramer R, et al. The relevance of skull density ratio in selecting candidates for transcranial MR-guided focused ultrasound. *J Neurosurg* 2019;**132**(6):1785–91. https://doi.org/10.3171/2019.2.JNS182571.

Bunevicius A, McDannold NJ, Golby AJ: Focused ultrasound strategies for brain tumor therapy. *Oper Neurosurg* 2020;**19**:9–18. https://doi.org/10.1093/ons/opz374.

Canney MS, Chavrier F, Tsysar S, Chapelon J-Y, Lafon C, Carpentier A. A multi-element interstitial ultrasound applicator for the thermal therapy of brain tumors. *J Acoust Soc Am* 2013;**134**:1647–55.

Chang JW, Park CK, Lipsman N, et al. A prospective trial of magnetic resonance-guided focused ultrasound thalamotomy for essential tremor: results at the 2-year follow-up. *Ann Neurol* 2018;**83**:107–14.

Chapman M, Park A, Schwartz M, Tarshis J. Anesthesia considerations of magnetic resonance imaging-guided focused ultrasound thalamotomy for essential tremor: a case series. *Can J Anaesth* 2020;**67**:877–84.

Chen K-T, Wei K-C, Liu H-L. Theranostic strategy of focused ultrasound induced blood–brain barrier opening for CNS disease treatment. *Front Pharmacol* 2019;**10**:86. https://doi.org/10.3389/fphar.2019.00086.

Chen P-Y, Hsieh H-Y, Huang C-Y, Lin C-Y, Wei K-C, Liu H-L. Focused ultrasound-induced blood–brain barrier opening to enhance interleukin-12 delivery for brain tumor immunotherapy: a preclinical feasibility study. *J Transl Med* 2015a;**13**:93.

Chen P-Y, Wei K-C, Liu H-L. Neural immune modulation and immunotherapy assisted by focused ultrasound induced blood–brain barrier opening. *Hum Vaccin Immunother* 2015b;**11**:2682–7.

Chen Z, Xue T, Huang H, et al. Efficacy and safety of sonothombolysis versus non-sonothombolysis in patients with acute ischemic stroke: a meta-analysis of randomized controlled trials. *PLoS One* 2019;**14**:e0210516. https://doi.org/10.1371/journal.pone.0210516.

Christian E, Yu C, Apuzzo MLJ. Focused ultrasound: relevant history and prospects for the addition of mechanical energy to the neurosurgical armamentarium. *World Neurosurg* 2014;**82**:354–65.

Cohen-Inbar O, Xu Z, Sheehan JP. Focused ultrasound-aided immunomodulation in glioblastoma multiforme: a therapeutic concept. *J Ther Ultrasound* 2016;**4**:2.

Colloca L, Ludman T, Bouhassira D, et al. Neuropathic pain. *Nat Rev Dis Prim* 2017;**3**:17002.

Coluccia D, Fandino J, Schwyzer L, et al. First noninvasive thermal ablation of a brain tumor with MR-guided focused ultrasound. *J Ther Ultrasound* 2014;**2**:17. https://doi.org/10.1186/2050-5736-2-17.

Curley CT, Sheybani ND, Bullock TN, Price RJ. Focused ultrasound immunotherapy for central nervous system pathologies: challenges and opportunities. *Theranostics* 2017;**7**:3608–23. www.thno.org/v07p3608.htm.

D'Souza AL, Tseng JR, Pauly KB, et al. A strategy for blood biomarker amplification and localization using ultrasound. *Proc Natl Acad Sci U S A* 2009;**106**:17152–7.

D'Souza M, Chen KS, Rosenberg J, et al. Impact of skull density ratio on efficacy and safety of magnetic resonance-guided focused ultrasound treatment of essential tremor. *J Neurosurg* 2019;**132** (5):1392–7. https://doi.org/10.3171/2019.2.JNS183517.

Dalecki D. Mechanical bioeffects of ultrasound. *Annu Rev Biomed Eng* 2004;**6**:229–48.

Dang TTH, Rowell D, Connelly LB/ Cost-effectiveness of deep brain stimulation with movement disorders: a systematic review. *Mov Disord Clin Pract* 2019;**6**:348–58.

Darrow DP. Focused ultrasound for neuromodulation. *Neurotherapeutics* 2019;**16**:88–99.

Davidson B, Hamani C, Rabin JS, et al. Magnetic resonance-guided focused ultrasound capsulotomy for refractory obsessive compulsive disorder and major depressive disorder: clinical and imaging results from two phase I trials. *Mol Psychiatry* 2020;**25**:1946–57. https://doi.org/10.1038/s41380-020-0737-1.

Deffieux T, Younan Y, Wattiez N, Tanter M, Pouget P, Aubry J-F. Low-intensity focused ultrasound modulates monkey visuomotor behavior. *Curr Biol* 2013;**23**:2430–3. https://doi.org/10.1016/j.cub.2013.10.029.

DeLong MR, Wichmann T. Basal ganglia circuits as targets for neuromodulation in Parkinson disease. *JAMA Neurol* 2015;**72**:1354–60.

Deng J, Huang Q, Wang F, et al. The role of caveolin-1 in blood–brain barrier disruption induced by focused ultrasound combined with microbubbles. *J Mol Neurosci* 2012;**46**:677–87. https://doi.org/10.1007/s12031-011-9629-9.

Dixon AJ, Li J, Rickel J-MR, Klibanov AL, Zuo Z, Hossack JA. Efficacy of sonothrombolysis using microbubbles produced by a catheter-based microfluidic device in a rat model of ischemic stroke. *Ann Biomed Eng* 2019;**47**:1012–22.

Dobrakowski PP, Machowska-Majchrzak AK, Labuz-Roszak B, Majchrzak KG, Kluczewska E, Pierzchała KB. MR-guided focused ultrasound: a new generation treatment of Parkinson's disease, essential tremor and neuropathic pain. *Interv Neuroradiol* 2014;**20**:275–82. https://doi.org/10.15274/INR-2014-10033.

Donnan GA, Fisher M, Macleod M, Davis SM. Stroke. *Lancet* 2008;**371**:1612–23.

Dwedar AZ, Ashour S, Haroun M, et al. Sonothrombolysis in acute middle cerebral artery stroke. *Neurol India* 2014;**62**:62–5. https://doi.org/10.4103/0028-3886.128308.

Ebani EJ, Kaplitt MG, Wang Y, Nguyen TD, Askin G, Chazen JL. Improved targeting of the globus pallidus interna using quantitative susceptibility mapping prior to MR-guided focused ultrasound ablation in Parkinson's disease. *Clin Imaging* 2020;**68**:94–8.

Eggers J, König IR, Koch B, Händler G, Seidel G. Sonothrombolysis with transcranial color-coded sonography and recombinant tissue-type plasminogen activator in acute middle cerebral artery main stem occlusion: results from a randomized study. *Stroke* 2008;**39**:1470–5.

Eggers J, Seidel G, Koch B, König IR. Sonothrombolysis in acute ischemic stroke for patients ineligible for rt-PA. *Neurology* 2005;**64**:1052–4.

Elias WJ, Huss D, Voss T, et al. A pilot study of focused ultrasound thalamotomy for essential tremor. *N Engl J Med* 2013;**369**:640–8.

Elias WJ, Lipsman N, Ondo WG, et al. A randomized trial of focused ultrasound thalamotomy for essential tremor. *N Engl J Med* 2016;**375**:730–9. https://doi.org/10.1056/NEJMoa1600159.

Fan C-H, Lin C-Y, Liu H-L, Yeh C-K. Ultrasound targeted CNS gene delivery for Parkinson's disease treatment. *J Control Release* 2017;**261**:246–62.

Fiani B, Lissak IA, Soula M, et al. The emerging role of magnetic resonance imaging-guided focused ultrasound in functional neurosurgery. *Cureus* 2020;**12**:e9820. https://doi.org/10.7759/cureus.9820.

Finley DS, Pouliot F, Shuch B, et al. Ultrasound-based combination therapy: potential in urologic cancer. *Expert Rev Anticancer Ther* 2011;**11**:107–13.

Foffani G, Trigo-Damas I, Pineda-Pardo JA, et al. Focused ultrasound in Parkinson's disease: a twofold path toward disease modification. *Mov Disord* 2019;**34**:1262–73.

Fomenko A, Neudorfer C, Dallapiazza RF, Kalia SK, Lozano AM. Low-intensity ultrasound neuromodulation: an overview of mechanisms and emerging human applications. *Brain Stimul* 2018;**11**:1209–17. www.sciencedirect.com/science/article/pii/S1935861X18302961.

Franzini A, Moosa S, Prada F, Elias WJ. Ultrasound ablation in neurosurgery: current clinical applications and future perspectives. *Neurosurgery* 2020;**87**:1–10.

Franzini A, Moosa S, Servello D, et al. Ablative brain surgery: an overview. *Int J Hyperthermia* 2019;**36**:64–80. www.ncbi.nlm.nih.gov/pubmed/31537157.

Frenkel V, Kimmel E, Iger Y. Ultrasound-facilitated transport of silver chloride (AgCl) particles in fish skin. *J Control Release* 2000;**68**:251–61.

Frenkel V, Etherington A, Greene M, et al. Delivery of liposomal doxorubicin (Doxil) in a breast cancer tumor model: investigation of potential enhancement by pulsed-high intensity focused ultrasound exposure. *Acad Radiol* 2006;**13**:469–79. https://doi.org/10.1016/j.acra.2005.08.024.

Frenkel V, Gurka R, Liberzon A, Shavit U, Kimmel E. Preliminary investigations of ultrasound induced acoustic streaming using particle image velocimetry. *Ultrasonics* 2001;**39**:153–6. https://doi.org/10.1016/s0041-624x(00)00064-0.

Fry WJ, Barnard JW, Fry EJ, Krumins RF, Brennan JF. Ultrasonic lesions in the mammalian central nervous system. *Science* 1955;**122**:517–8.

Fry WJ, Meyers R. Ultrasonic method of modifying brain structures. *Confin Neurol* 1962;**22**:315–27.

Fusco P, De Sanctis F, Di Carlo S, et al. Dexmedetomidine sedation in magnetic resonance-guided focused ultrasound thalamotomy: a case series of 3 patients. *A&A Pract* 2019;**12**:406–08.

Gagliardo C, Cannella R, Quarrella C, et al. Intraoperative imaging findings in transcranial MR imaging-guided focused ultrasound treatment at 1.5T may accurately detect typical lesional findings correlated with sonication parameters. *Eur Radiol* 2020;**30**:5059–70.

Gallay MN, Moser D, Federau C, Jeanmonod D. Anatomical and technical reappraisal of the pallidothalamic tractotomy with the incisionless transcranial MR-guided focused ultrasound. A technical note. *Front Surg* 2019a;**6**:2.

Gallay MN, Moser D, Federau C, Jeanmonod D. Radiological and thermal dose correlations in pallidothalamic tractotomy with MRgFUS. *Front Surg* 2019b;**6**:28.

Gallay MN, Moser D, Jeanmonod D. Safety and accuracy of incisionless transcranial MR-guided focused ultrasound functional neurosurgery: single-center experience with 253 targets in 180 treatments. *J Neurosurg* 2018;1–10. Online ahead of publication. https://thejns.org/view/journals/j-neurosurg/aop/article-10.3171-2017.12.JNS172054.xml.

Gallay MN, Moser D, Rossi F, et al. Incisionless transcranial MR-guided focused ultrasound in essential tremor: cerebellothalamic tractotomy. *J Ther Ultrasound* 2016;**4**:5.

Gallay MN, Moser D, Rossi F, et al. MRgFUS Pallidothalamic tractotomy for chronic therapy-resistant Parkinson's disease in 51 consecutive patients: single center experience. *Front Surg* 2019c;**6**:76.

Gerhardson T, Sukovich JR, Chaudhary N, et al. Histotripsy clot liquefaction in a porcine intracerebral hemorrhage model. *Neurosurgery* 2020;**86**:429–36. https://doi.org/10.1093/neuros/nyz089.

Gerhardson T, Sukovich JR, Pandey AS, Hall TL, Cain CA, Xu Z. Effect of frequency and focal spacing on transcranial histotripsy clot liquefaction, using electronic focal steering. *Ultrasound Med Biol* 2017;**43**:2302–17.

Gersten JW, Kawashima E. Recent advances in fundamental aspects of ultrasound and muscle. *Br J Phys Med* 1955;**18**:106–09.

Giordano M, Caccavella VM, Zaed I, et al. Comparison between deep brain stimulation and magnetic resonance-guided focused ultrasound in the treatment of essential tremor: a systematic review and pooled analysis of functional outcomes. *J Neurol Neurosurg Psychiatry* 2020;**91**(12):1270–8. https://doi.org/10.1136/jnnp-2020-323216.

Guthkelch AN, Carter LP, Cassady JR, et al. Treatment of malignant brain tumors with focused ultrasound hyperthermia and radiation: results of a phase I trial. *J Neurooncol* 1991;**10**:271–84.

Hancock HA, Smith LH, Cuesta J, et al. Investigations into pulsed high-intensity focused ultrasound-enhanced delivery: preliminary evidence for a novel mechanism. *Ultrasound Med Biol* 2009;**35**:1722–36.

Harnof S, Zibly Z, Hananel A, et al. Potential of magnetic resonance-guided focused ultrasound for intracranial hemorrhage: an in vivo feasibility study. *J Stroke Cerebrovasc Dis* 2014;**23**:1585–91. www.sciencedirect.com/science/article/pii/S1052305713005612.

Heimburger RF. Ultrasound augmentation of central nervous system tumor therapy. *Indiana Med* 1985;**78**:469–76.

Hersh DS, Kim AJ, Winkles JA, Eisenberg HM, Woodworth GF, Frenkel V. Emerging applications of therapeutic ultrasound in neuro-oncology: moving beyond tumor ablation. *Neurosurgery* 2016;**79**:643–54. https://doi.org/10.1227/NEU.0000000000001399.

Hu Z, Yang XY, Liu Y, et al. Release of endogenous danger signals from HIFU-treated tumor cells and their stimulatory effects on

APCs. *Biochem Biophys Res Commun* 2005;**335**:124–31. https://doi.org/10.1016/j.bbrc.2005.07.071.

Hu Z, Yang XY, Liu Y, et al. Investigation of HIFU-induced anti-tumor immunity in a murine tumor model. *J Transl Med* 2007;**5**:34. https://doi.org/10.1186/1479-5876-5-34.

Hynynen K. Demonstration of enhanced temperature elevation due to nonlinear propagation of focussed ultrasound in dog's thigh in vivo. *Ultrasound Med Biol* 1987;**13**:85–91. https://doi.org/10.1016/0301-5629(87)90078-0.

Hynynen K, Clement G. Clinical applications of focused ultrasound – the brain. *Int J Hyperthermia* 2007;**23**:193–202. https://doi.org/10.1080/02656730701200094.

Hynynen K, Darkazanli A, Unger E, Schenck JF. MRI-guided noninvasive ultrasound surgery. *Med Phys* 1993;**20**:107–15. https://doi.org/10.1118/1.597093.

Hynynen K, Jolesz FA. Demonstration of potential noninvasive ultrasound brain therapy through an intact skull. *Ultrasound Med Biol* 1998;**24**:275–83. https://doi.org/10.1016/s0301-5629(97)00269-x.

Idbaih A, Canney M, Belin L, et al. Safety and feasibility of repeated and transient blood–brain barrier disruption by pulsed ultrasound in patients with recurrent glioblastoma. *Clin Cancer Res* 2019;**25**:3793–801. https://doi.org/10.1158/1078-0432.CCR-18-3643.

Ilyas A, Chen C-J, Ding D, et al. Magnetic resonance-guided, high-intensity focused ultrasound sonolysis: potential applications for stroke. *Neurosurg Focus* 2018;**44**:E12.

Ito H, Yamamoto K, Fukutake S, Odo T, Kamei T. Two-year follow-up results of magnetic resonance imaging-guided focused ultrasound unilateral thalamotomy for medication-refractory essential tremor. *Intern Med* 2020;**59**:2481–3.

Jagannathan J, Sanghvi NT, Crum LA, et al. High-intensity focused ultrasound surgery of the brain: part 1 – a historical perspective with modern applications. *Neurosurgery* 2009;**64**:201.

James JA, Dalton GA, Bullen MA, Freundlich HF, Hopkins JC. The ultrasonic treatment of Meniere's disease. *J Laryngol Otol* 1960;**74**:730–57.

Jeanmonod D, Werner B, Morel A, et al. Transcranial magnetic resonance imaging–guided focused ultrasound: noninvasive central lateral thalamotomy for chronic neuropathic pain. *Neurosurg Focus* 2012;**32**(1):E1. https://doi.org/10.3171/2011.10.FOCUS11248.

Jones RM, Kamps S, Huang Y, et al. Accumulated thermal dose in MRI-guided focused ultrasound for essential tremor: repeated sonications with low focal temperatures. *J Neurosurg* 2019;**132**(6):1802–9. https://doi.org/10.3171/2019.2.JNS182995.

Jung HH, Chang WS, Rachmilevitch I, Tlusty T, Zadicario E, Chang JW. Different magnetic resonance imaging patterns after transcranial magnetic resonance-guided focused ultrasound of the ventral intermediate nucleus of the thalamus and anterior limb of the internal capsule in patients with essential tremor or obsessive-com. *J Neurosurg* 2015b;**122**:162–8. https://doi.org/10.3171/2014.8.JNS132603.

Jung HH, Kim SJ, Roh D, et al. Bilateral thermal capsulotomy with MR-guided focused ultrasound for patients with treatment-refractory obsessive-compulsive disorder: a proof-of-concept study. *Mol Psychiatry* 2015a;**20**:1205–11. https://doi.org/10.1038/mp.2014.154.

Jung NY, Chang JW. Magnetic resonance-guided focused ultrasound in neurosurgery: taking lessons from the past to inform the future. *J Korean Med Sci* 2018;**33**:e279. https://doi.org/10.3346/jkms.2018.33.e279.

Jung NY, Park CK, Kim M, Lee PH, Sohn YH, Chang JW. The efficacy and limits of magnetic resonance-guided focused ultrasound pallidotomy for Parkinson's disease: a Phase I clinical trial. *J Neurosurg* 2018; https://doi.org/10.3171/2018.2.JNS172514. Online ahead of print.

Kampinga HH. Cell biological effects of hyperthermia alone or combined with radiation or drugs: a short introduction to newcomers in the field. *Int J Hyperthermia* 2006;**22**:191–6. https://doi.org/10.1080/02656730500532028.

Kapadia AN, Elias GJB, Boutet A, et al. Multimodal MRI for MRgFUS in essential tremor: post-treatment radiological markers of clinical outcome. *J Neurol Neurosurg Psychiatry* 2020;**91**:921–7. https://doi.org/10.1136/jnnp-2020-322745.

Katz M, Luciano MS, Carlson K, et al. Differential effects of deep brain stimulation target on motor subtypes in Parkinson's disease. *Ann Neurol* 2015;**77**:710–9. https://doi.org/10.1002/ana.24374.

Katzir S. Who knew piezoelectricity? Rutherford and Langevin on submarine detection and the invention of sonar. *Notes Rec R Soc* 2012;**66**:141–57. https://doi.org/10.1098/rsnr.2011.0049.

Keil VC, Borger V, Purrer V, et al. MRI follow-up after magnetic resonance-guided focused ultrasound for non-invasive thalamotomy: the neuroradiologist's perspective. *Neuroradiology* 2020;**62**:1111–22. https://doi.org/10.1007/s00234-020-02433-9.

Khokhlova VA, Bailey MR, Reed JA, Cunitz BW, Kaczkowski PJ, Crum LA. Effects of nonlinear propagation, cavitation, and boiling in lesion formation by high intensity focused ultrasound in a gel phantom. *J Acoust Soc Am* 2006;**119**:1834–48. https://doi.org/10.1121/1.2161440.

Kim M, Jung NY, Park CK, Chang WS, Jung HH, Chang JW. Comparative evaluation of magnetic resonance-guided focused ultrasound surgery for essential tremor. *Stereotact Funct Neurosurg* 2017;**95**:279–86. https://doi.org/10.1159/000478866.

Kim SJ, Roh D, Jung HH, Chang WS, Kim C-H, Chang JW. A study of novel bilateral thermal capsulotomy with focused ultrasound for treatment-refractory obsessive-compulsive disorder: 2-year follow-up. *J Psychiatry Neurosci* 2018;**43**:170188. https://doi.org/10.1503/jpn.170188.

Kovacs ZI, Kim S, Jikaria N, et al. Disrupting the blood–brain barrier by focused ultrasound induces sterile inflammation. *Proc Natl Acad Sci U S A*, 2017;**114**:E75–84.

Krasovitski B, Frenkel V, Shoham S, Kimmel E. Intramembrane cavitation as a unifying mechanism for ultrasound-induced bioeffects. *Proc Natl Acad Sci U S A* 2011;**108**:3258–63.

Kuliha M, Roubec M, Jonszta T, et al. Safety and efficacy of endovascular sonolysis using the EkoSonic endovascular system in patients with acute stroke. *Am J Neuroradiol* 2013;**34**:1401–06. www.ajnr.org/content/34/7/1401.abstract.

Lamsam L, Johnson E, Connolly ID, Wintermark M, Hayden Gephart M. A review of potential applications of MR-guided focused ultrasound for targeting brain tumor therapy. *Neurosurg Focus* 2018;**44**:E10.

Lehman VT, Lee KH, Klassen BT, et al. MRI and tractography techniques to localize the ventral intermediate nucleus and dentatorubrothalamic tract for deep brain stimulation and MR-guided focused ultrasound: a narrative review and update. *Neurosurg Focus* 2020;**49**:E8.

Lepock JR. Measurement of protein stability and protein denaturation in cells using differential scanning calorimetry. *Methods* 2005;**35**:117–25.

Lin C-Y, Hsieh H-Y, Chen C-M, et al. Non-invasive, neuron-specific gene therapy by focused ultrasound-induced blood–brain barrier opening in Parkinson's disease mouse model. *J Control Release* 2016;**235**:72–81. https://doi.org/10.1016/j.jconrel.2016.05.052.

Lionetti V, Fittipaldi A, Agostini S, Giacca M, Recchia FA, Picano E. Enhanced caveolae-mediated endocytosis by diagnostic ultrasound in vitro. *Ultrasound Med Biol* 2009;**35**:136–43. https://doi.org/10.1016/j.ultrasmedbio.2008.07.011.

Lipsman N, Schwartz ML, Huang Y, et al. MR-guided focused ultrasound thalamotomy for essential tremor: a proof-of-concept study. *Lancet Neurol* 2013;**12**:462–8.

Long L, Cai X, Guo R, et al. Treatment of Parkinson's disease in rats by Nrf2 transfection using MRI-guided focused ultrasound delivery of nanomicrobubbles. *Biochem Biophys Res Commun* 2017;**482**:75–80.

Louis ED. Treatment of medically refractory essential tremor. *N Engl J Med* 2016;**375**:792–3. https://doi.org/10.1056/NEJMe1606517.

Louis ED, Ottman R. How many people in the USA have essential tremor? Deriving a population estimate based on epidemiological data. *Tremor Other Hyperkinet Mov (N Y)* 2014;**4**:259.

Lu P, Zhu X-Q, Xu Z-L, Zhou Q, Zhang J, Wu F. Increased infiltration of activated tumor-infiltrating lymphocytes after high intensity focused ultrasound ablation of human breast cancer. *Surgery* 2009;**145**:286–93.

Lynn JG, Zwemer RL, Chick AJ, Miller AE. A new method for the generation and use of focused ultrasound in experimental biology. *J Gen Physiol* 1942;**26**:179–93. https://doi.org/10.1085/jgp.26.2.179.

Magara A, Bühler R, Moser D, Kowalski M, Pourtehrani P, Jeanmonod D. First experience with MR-guided focused ultrasound in the treatment of Parkinson's disease. *J Ther Ultrasound* 2014;**2**:11.

Mainprize T, Lipsman N, Huang Y, et al. Blood–brain barrier opening in primary brain tumors with non-invasive MR-guided focused ultrasound: a clinical safety and feasibility study. *Sci Rep* 2019;**9**:321. https://doi.org/10.1038/s41598-018-36340-0.

Martin E, Jeanmonod D, Morel A, Zadicario E, Werner B. High-intensity focused ultrasound for noninvasive functional neurosurgery. *Ann Neurol* 2009;**66**:858–61.

Martínez-Fernández R, Pineda-Pardo JA. Magnetic resonance-guided focused ultrasound for movement disorders: clinical and neuroimaging advances. *Curr Opin Neurol* 2020;**33**:488–97.

Martínez-Fernández R, Rodríguez-Rojas R, Del Álamo M, et al. Focused ultrasound subthalamotomy in patients with asymmetric Parkinson's disease: a pilot study. *Lancet Neurol* 2018;**17**:54–63.

Mauri G, Nicosia L, Xu Z, et al. Focused ultrasound: tumour ablation and its potential to enhance immunological therapy to cancer. *Br J Radiol* 2018;**91**:20170641.

McDannold N, Clement GT, Black P, Jolesz F, Hynynen K. Transcranial magnetic resonance imaging- guided focused ultrasound surgery of brain tumors: initial findings in 3 patients. *Neurosurgery* 2010;**66**:323–32; discussion 332. https://doi.org/10.1227/01.NEU.0000360379.95800.2F.

McDannold NJ, Vykhodtseva NI, Hynynen K. Microbubble contrast agent with focused ultrasound to create brain lesions at low power levels: MR imaging and histologic study in rabbits. *Radiology* 2006;**241**:95–106.

McDannold NJ, White PJ, Cosgrove GR. MRI-based thermal dosimetry based on single-slice imaging during focused ultrasound thalamotomy. *Phys Med Biol*: 2020a;**65**(23):235018. https://doi.org/10.1088/1361-6560/abb7c4.

McDannold N, White PJ, Cosgrove GR. Using phase data from MR temperature imaging to visualize anatomy during MRI guided focused ultrasound neurosurgery. *IEEE Trans Med Imaging* 2020b;**39**(12):3821–30. https://doi.org/10.1109/TMI.2020.3005631.

Medel R, Monteith SJ, Elias WJ, et al. Magnetic resonance-guided focused ultrasound surgery: Part 2: a review of current and future applications. *Neurosurgery* 2012;**71**:755–63.

Meng Y, Pople CB, Kalia SK, et al. Cost-effectiveness analysis of MR-guided focused ultrasound thalamotomy for tremor-dominant Parkinson's disease. *J Neurosurg* 2020. https://doi.org/10.3171/2020.5.JNS20692. Online ahead of print.

Meng Y, Suppiah S, Surendrakumar S, Bigioni L, Lipsman N. Low-intensity MR-guided focused ultrasound mediated disruption of the blood–brain barrier for intracranial metastatic diseases. *Front Oncol* 2018;8:338. www.frontiersin.org/article/10.3389/fonc.2018.00338.

Metman LV, Slavin KV. Advances in functional neurosurgery for Parkinson's disease. *Mov Disord* 2015;30:1461–70.

Miller TR, Guo S, Melhem ER, et al. Predicting final lesion characteristics during MR-guided focused ultrasound pallidotomy for treatment of Parkinson's disease. *J Neurosurg* 2020;134(3):1083–90. https://doi.org/10.3171/2020.2.JNS192590.

Molina CA, Barreto AD, Tsivgoulis G, et al. Transcranial ultrasound in clinical sonothrombolysis (TUCSON) trial. *Ann Neurol* 2009;66:28–38.

Molina CA, Ribo M, Rubiera M, et al. Microbubble administration accelerates clot lysis during continuous 2-MHz ultrasound monitoring in stroke patients treated with intravenous tissue plasminogen activator. *Stroke* 2006;37:425–9.

Monteith SJ, Harnof S, Medel R, et al. Minimally invasive treatment of intracerebral hemorrhage with magnetic resonance-guided focused ultrasound. *J Neurosurg* 2013a;118:1035–45.

Monteith SJ, Kassell NF, Goren O, Harnof S. Transcranial MR-guided focused ultrasound sonothrombolysis in the treatment of intracerebral hemorrhage. *Neurosurg Focus* 2013b;34:E14.

Moosa S, Martínez-Fernández R, Elias WJ, Del Alamo M, Eisenberg HM, Fishman PS. The role of high-intensity focused ultrasound as a symptomatic treatment for Parkinson's disease. *Mov Disord* 2019;34:1243–51. https://doi.org/10.1002/mds.27779.

N'Djin WA, Burtnyk M, Lipsman N, et al. Active MR-temperature feedback control of dynamic interstitial ultrasound therapy in brain: in vivo experiments and modeling in native and coagulated tissues. *Med Phys* 2014;41:93301.

Nacu A, Kvistad CE, Naess H, et al. NOR-SASS (Norwegian Sonothrombolysis in Acute Stroke Study): randomized controlled contrast-enhanced sonothrombolysis in an unselected acute ischemic stroke population. *Stroke* 2017;48:335–41.

Nyborg WL: Biological effects of ultrasound: development of safety guidelines. Part II: general review. *Ultrasound Med Biol* 2001;27:301–33.

O'Brien Jr WD. Ultrasound – biophysics mechanisms. *Prog Biophys Mol Biol* 2007;93:212–55. https://pubmed.ncbi.nlm.nih.gov/16934858.

O'Neill BE, Vo H, Angstadt M, Li KPC, Quinn T, Frenkel V. Pulsed high intensity focused ultrasound mediated nanoparticle delivery: mechanisms and efficacy in murine muscle. *Ultrasound Med Biol* 2009;35:416–24.

Pacia CP, Zhu L, Yang Y, et al. Feasibility and safety of focused ultrasound-enabled liquid biopsy in the brain of a porcine model. *Sci Rep* 2020;10:7449. https://doi.org/10.1038/s41598-020-64440-3.

Paff M, Boutet A, Neudorfer C, et al. Magnetic resonance-guided focused ultrasound thalamotomy to treat essential tremor in nonagenarians. *Stereotact Funct Neurosurg* 2020;98:182–6. https://doi.org/10.1159/000506817.

Park J, Jung S, Jung T, Lee M. Focused ultrasound surgery for the treatment of recurrent anaplastic astrocytoma: a preliminary report. *AIP Conf Proc* 2006;829:238–40. https://aip.scitation.org/doi/abs/10.1063/1.2205473.

Park SH, Kim MJ, Jung HH, et al. Safety and feasibility of multiple blood–brain barrier disruptions for the treatment of glioblastoma in patients undergoing standard adjuvant chemotherapy. *J Neurosurg* 2020. https://thejns.org/view/journals/j-neurosurg/aop/article-10.3171-2019.10.JNS192206/article-10.3171-2019.10.JNS192206.xml. Online ahead of print.

Pouliopoulos AN, Wu S-Y, Burgess MT, Karakatsani ME, Kamimura HAS, Konofagou EE. A clinical system for non-invasive blood–brain barrier opening using a neuronavigation-guided single-element focused ultrasound transducer. *Ultrasound Med Biol* 2020;46:73–89.

Prada F, Franzini A, Moosa S, et al. In vitro and in vivo characterization of a cranial window prosthesis for diagnostic and therapeutic cerebral ultrasound. *J Neurosurg* 2020a. https://doi.org/10.3171/2019.10.JNS191674. Online ahead of print.

Prada F, Kalani MYS, Yagmurlu K, et al. Applications of focused ultrasound in cerebrovascular diseases and brain tumors. *Neurotherapeutics* 2019;16:67–87. https://doi.org/10.1007/s13311-018-00683-3.

Prada F, Sheybani N, Franzini A, et al. Fluorescein-mediated sonodynamic therapy in a rat glioma model. *J Neurooncol* 2020b;148:445–54. https://doi.org/10.1007/s11060-020-03536-2.

Ram Z, Cohen ZR, Harnof S, et al. Magnetic resonance imaging-guided, high-intensity focused ultrasound for brain tumor therapy. *Neurosurgery* 2006;59:946–9.

Ranjan M, Boutet A, Bhatia S, et al. Neuromodulation beyond neurostimulation for epilepsy: scope for focused ultrasound. *Expert Rev Neurother* 2019a;19:937–43.

Ranjan M, Elias GJB, Boutet A, et al. Tractography-based targeting of the ventral intermediate nucleus: accuracy and clinical utility in MRgFUS thalamotomy. *J Neurosurg* 2019b. https//doi.org/10.3171/2019.6.JNS19612. Online ahead of print.

Ricci S, Dinia L, Del Sette M, et al. Sonothrombolysis for acute ischaemic stroke. *Cochrane Database Syst Rev* 2012;10:CD008348.

Rodriguez-Rojas R, Pineda-Pardo JA, Martinez-Fernandez R, et al. Functional impact of subthalamotomy by magnetic resonance-guided focused ultrasound in Parkinson's disease: a hybrid PET/MR study of resting-state brain metabolism. *Eur J Nucl Med Mol Imaging* 2020;47:425–36. https://doi.org/10.1007/s00259-019-04497-z.

Rubiera M, Ribo M, Delgado-Mederos R, et al. Do bubble characteristics affect recanalization in stroke patients treated with microbubble-enhanced sonothrombolysis? *Ultrasound Med Biol* 2008;**34**:1573–77.

Shah BR, Lehman VT, Kaufmann TJ, et al. Advanced MRI techniques for transcranial high intensity focused ultrasound targeting. *Brain* 2020;**143**:2664–72.

Sharma VD, Patel M, Miocinovic S. Surgical treatment of Parkinson's disease: devices and lesion approaches. *Neurotherapeutics* 2020;**17**(4):1525–38. https://doi.org/10.1007/s13311-020-00939-x.

Sheehan K, Sheehan D, Sulaiman M, et al. Investigation of the tumoricidal effects of sonodynamic therapy in malignant glioblastoma brain tumors. *J Neurooncol* 2020;**148**:9–16.

Sheikov N, McDannold N, Sharma S, Hynynen K. Effect of focused ultrasound applied with an ultrasound contrast agent on the tight junctional integrity of the brain microvascular endothelium. *Ultrasound Med Biol* 2008;**34**:1093–104. https://doi.org/10.1016/j.ultrasmedbio.2007.12.015.

Sheikov N, McDannold N, Vykhodtseva N, Jolesz F, Hynynen K. Cellular mechanisms of the blood–brain barrier opening induced by ultrasound in presence of microbubbles. *Ultrasound Med Biol* 2004;**30**:979–89. https://doi.org/10.1016/j.ultrasmedbio.2004.04.010.

Sheybani ND, Price RJ. Perspectives on recent progress in focused ultrasound immunotherapy. *Theranostics* 2019;**9**:7749–58. https://doi.org/10.7150/thno.37131.

Sinai A, Nassar M, Eran A, et al. Magnetic resonance-guided focused ultrasound thalamotomy for essential tremor: a 5-year single-center experience. *J Neurosurg* 2019. https://doi.org/10.3171/2019.3.JNS19466. Online ahead of print.

Skoloudik D, Bar M, Skoda O, et al. Efficacy of sonothrombotripsy versus sonothrombolysis in recanalization of intracranial arteries. *Eur J Neurol* 2006;**13**:180.

Smith AN, Fisher GW, Macleod IB, Preshaw RM, Stavney LS, Gordon D. The effect of ultrasound on the gastric mucosa and its secretion of acid. *Br J Surg* 1966;**53**:720–5.

Sokka SD, King R, Hynynen K. MRI-guided gas bubble enhanced ultrasound heating in in vivo rabbit thigh. *Phys Med Biol* 2003;**48**:223–41.

Song CW, Park HJ, Lee CK, Griffin R. Implications of increased tumor blood flow and oxygenation caused by mild temperature hyperthermia in tumor treatment. *Int J Hyperthermia* 2005;**21**:761–7.

Su JH, Choi EY, Tourdias T, et al. Improved VIM targeting for focused ultrasound ablation treatment of essential tremor: a probabilistic and patient-specific approach. *Hum Brain Mapp* 2020;**41**:4769–88.

Suehiro S, Ohnishi T, Yamashita D, et al. Enhancement of antitumor activity by using 5-ALA-mediated sonodynamic therapy to induce apoptosis in malignant gliomas: significance of high-intensity focused ultrasound on 5-ALA-SDT in a mouse glioma model. *J Neurosurg* 2018;**129**:1416–28. https://doi.org/10.3171/2017.6.JNS162398.

Tran BC, Jongbum Seo, Hall TL, Fowlkes JB, Cain CA. Effects of contrast agent infusion rates on thresholds for tissue damage produced by single exposures of high-intensity ultrasound. *IEEE Trans Ultrason Ferroelectr Freq Control* 2005;**52**:1121–30. https://doi.org/10.1109/tuffc.2005.1503998.

Tsivgoulis G, Alexandrov AV. Ultrasound-enhanced thrombolysis in acute ischemic stroke: potential, failures, and safety. *Neurotherapeutics* 2007;**4**:420–7. https://doi.org/0.1016/j.nurt.2007.05.012.

Tyler WJ, Tufail Y, Finsterwald M, Tauchmann ML, Olson EJ, Majestic C. Remote excitation of neuronal circuits using low-intensity, low-frequency ultrasound. *PLoS One* 2008;**3**:e3511. https://doi.org/10.1371/journal.pone.0003511.

Vimeux FC, De Zwart JA, Palussiére J, et al. Real-time control of focused ultrasound heating based on rapid MR thermometry. *Invest Radiol* 1999;**34**:190–3. https://doi.org/10.1097/00004424-199903000-00006.

Wahab RA, Choi M, Liu Y, Krauthamer V, Zderic V, Myers MR. Mechanical bioeffects of pulsed high intensity focused ultrasound on a simple neural model. *Med Phys* 2012;**39**:4274–83. https://doi.org/10.1118/1.4729712.

Walters H, Shah BB. Focused ultrasound and other lesioning therapies in movement disorders. *Curr Neurol Neurosci Rep* 2019;**19**:66. https://doi.org/10.1007/s11910-019-0975-2.

Wang TR, Bond AE, Dallapiazza RF, et al. Transcranial magnetic resonance imaging-guided focused ultrasound thalamotomy for tremor: technical note. *Neurosurg Focus* 2018;**44**:E3.

Weidman EK, Kaplitt MG, Strybing K, Chazen JL. Repeat magnetic resonance imaging-guided focused ultrasound thalamotomy for recurrent essential tremor: case report and review of MRI findings. *J Neurosurg* 2019. https://doi.org/10.3171/2018.10.JNS181721. Online ahead of print.

Weintraub D, Elias WJ: The emerging role of transcranial magnetic resonance imaging-guided focused ultrasound in functional neurosurgery. *Mov Disord* 2017;**32**:20–7.

White PJ, Zhang Y-Z, Power C, Vykhodtseva N, McDannold N. Observed effects of whole-brain radiation therapy on focused ultrasound blood–brain barrier disruption. *Ultrasound Med Biol* 2020;**46**:1998–2006. www.sciencedirect.com/science/article/pii/S030156292030185X.

Wu S-K, Santos MA, Marcus SL, Hynynen K. MR-guided focused ultrasound facilitates sonodynamic therapy with 5-aminolevulinic acid in a rat glioma model. *Sci Rep* 2019;**9**:10465. https://doi.org/10.1038/s41598-019-46832-2.

Xu Y, He Q, Wang M, et al. Safety and efficacy of magnetic resonance imaging-guided focused ultrasound neurosurgery for Parkinson's disease: a systematic review. *Neurosurg Rev* 20219;**44**(1):115–27. https://doi.org/10.1007/s10143-019-01216-y.

Younan Y, Deffieux T, Larrat B, Fink M, Tanter M, Aubry J-F. Influence of the pressure field distribution in transcranial ultrasonic neurostimulation. *Med Phys* 2013;40:82902.

Yu T, Li SL, Zhao JZ, Mason TJ. Ultrasound: a chemotherapy sensitizer. *Technol Cancer Res Treat* 2006;5:51–60.

Yu T, Wang G, Hu K, Ma P, Bai J, Wang Z. A microbubble agent improves the therapeutic efficiency of high intensity focused ultrasound: a rabbit kidney study. *Urol Res* 2004;32:14–9.

Zafar A, Quadri SA, Farooqui M, et al. MRI-guided high-intensity focused ultrasound as an emerging therapy for stroke: a review. *J Neuroimaging* 2019;29:5–13. https://doi.org/10.1111/jon.12568.

Zaki Ghali MG, Srinivasan VM, Kan P. Focused ultrasonography-mediated blood–brain barrier disruption in the enhancement of delivery of brain tumor therapies. *World Neurosurg* 2019;131:65–75. https://doi.org/10.1016/j.wneu.2019.07.096.

Zhu L, Nazeri A, Pacia CP, Yue Y, Chen H. Focused ultrasound for safe and effective release of brain tumor biomarkers into the peripheral circulation. *PLoS One* 2020;15:e0234182. https://doi.org/10.1371/journal.pone.0234182.

Chapter 30

Magnetic Resonance Imaging in Neurosurgery

David J. Segar, Jasmine A. Thum, Dhiego Bastos, and Alexandra J. Golby

30.1 Introduction

The adoption of magnetic resonance imaging (MRI) into clinical practice brought about a revolution in the diagnosis and treatment of neurological illness, and has dramatically advanced the study of brain anatomy. Early MRI resolved structures in the brain with comparatively poor resolution on the order of 2.5 mm, with limited methods of amplifying contrast between different tissues (Duyn and Korestsky, 2011). Advances in imaging sequences and analytical methods, combined with improvements in spatial resolution and contrast modalities, have dramatically increased the diagnostic and treatment utility of MRI in neurosurgery. Over time, MRI has been used to study and diagnose nervous system diseases of all kinds, from brain tumors, to stroke, to multiple sclerosis. Today, MRI techniques enable the in-vivo study of brain microstructure, connectivity, functional activity, tissue composition, and blood flow; supports surgical planning; and provides critical feedback during selected neurosurgical interventions.

The use of MRI in neurosurgery and neuroscientific research is broad; this chapter will focus on a subset of MRI modalities used in neurosurgical research and clinical treatment, and their relevance to neurosurgical disease. This will hopefully lay the groundwork for readers who are interested in conducting further research in this field. For more detailed fundamentals on MRI physics, we direct readers to *MRI Physics for Radiologists: A Visual Approach* by Alfred L. Horowitz (1994), or 'Understanding MRI: basic MR physics for physicians', a review article by Currie et al. (2013). Throughout this chapter we will refer readers to additional resources for more in-depth review of specific subject matter.

30.2 Magnetic Resonance Imaging Basics

Four main components are necessary to create and measure an MR signal. The main magnet coil, usually superconducting metal cooled to near absolute zero with liquid helium to lower electrical resistance, creates a constant magnetic field (B_0), measured in tesla (T). When an object is placed in this field, it can reduce field homogeneity. Shim coils can be added to either actively or passively improve the magnetic field homogeneity.

Three sets of gradient coils positioned along x-, y-, and z-axes are used for localization and generate electric fields in the same direction as B_0, but with variable field strengths along the length of the coils (Figure 30.1).

Radiofrequency (RF) coils transmit high-frequency electromagnetic energy to, and receive RF signal from, the imaged tissue. For cranial imaging, an additional RF coil is usually positioned around the head to maximize receipt of the emitted RF signal from the spherical surface. The field produced by the RF coils, also known as B_1, interacts with B_0 to produce an output signal that is ultimately reconstructed into an image. The variation in RF pulse enables different sequence acquisitions (i.e., T_1, T_2).

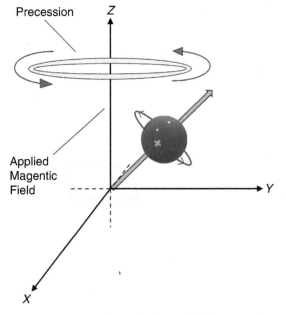

Figure 30.1 Image of x, y, and z planes of hydrogen ion relaxation fields.

MRI creates images by perturbing the individual magnetic fields of hydrogen ions, and measures how they return to their randomly oriented magnetic moment. When placed within a strong magnetic field, protons within the imaged tissue become aligned with the external field. An RF pulse disturbs the alignment of these protons, causing magnetization in a direction offset from the primary B_0 magnetic field. After the pulse ends, molecules relax back to their original alignment. The T_1 signal defines what is referred to as the longitudinal relaxation rate, along the z-axis, whereas the T_2 signal defines the transverse relaxation rate, as protons fall out of phase along the x–y plane.

The variation in relaxation efficiency between molecules of different types leads to variation in signal, which translates into characteristic imaging features for different types of tissues. For example, free water and lipid membranes are inefficient at the energy exchange required to return to their polarized states, and therefore have long T_1 relaxation times. In contrast, the short T_1 value seen in fat corresponds to a more efficient rate of energy transfer, allowing faster return to a longitudinally magnetized state.

The ability to differentiate tissue types with MRI has tremendous clinical utility in neurosurgery. Vasogenic edema leads to increased T_2 signal due to increased interstitial water content, while cytotoxic edema and ischemia can more effectively be detected using diffusion-weighted imaging, which has revolutionized imaging in ischemic stroke. The addition of contrast agents, usually chelates of gadolinium, results in T_1 shortening, or an increase in T_1 signal (with a minimal effect on T_2 sequences). The addition of contrast agents may be particularly useful for identification of tumors or inflammation, where disruption of the blood–brain barrier permits extravasation of the contrast into surrounding tissue.

Spin echo (SE) and gradient echo (GRE) sequences are based around measurements of repetition time (TR) and echo time (TE) of the hydrogen ions. For additional detail on these sequences, we recommend review articles by Jung and Weigel (2013) and Markl and Leupold (2012).

30.3 Physiologic Magnetic Resonance Imaging

30.3.1 Diffusion Magnetic Resonance Imaging

Diffusion-weighted MRI sequences measure the local diffusion of water molecules. Diffusion-weighted imaging (DWI), which is commonly used clinically for early detection of ischemia, measures diffusion in three dimensions, and after subtraction of T_2 components, an apparent diffusion coefficient (ADC) maps overall diffusivity in the brain. Multiple factors, including cell density and tissue microstructure contribute to the degree and direction of water molecule motion (Le Bihan, 2003).

While conventional MRI sequences effectively visualize delayed vasogenic edema several hours after infarct (Allen et al., 2012; Hjort et al., 2005; Madai et al., 2014; Nagaraja et al., 2020; Siemonsen et al., 2009), DWI can be used to visualize early signs of brain ischemia within several minutes after an occlusion of a major cerebral artery (Hjort et al., 2005). The ability to detect early ischemic change has helped revolutionize the treatment of ischemic stroke, providing essential information for treatments that rely on early detection, such as endovascular thrombectomy.

Diffusion tensor imaging (DTI) was developed to map the direction of fiber orientation by quantification of fractional anisotropy, or the tendency for water to diffuse selectively in one direction more than another (Le Bihan, 2003). By calculating the net directional movement of water molecules, DTI sequences capture the anisotropy present in different tissue types, and, with additional processing, can be used to highlight the directionality of coherent white matter fibers in a given voxel. In white matter containing tightly packed myelinated axons, the diffusion of water is greatest parallel to the fibers allowing inferences about the presence and orientation of white matter tracts. The data are then analyzed in a process called tractography using a variety of models to output processed images which display the trajectory of white matter tracts. Diffusion MRI-based white matter tracking techniques are now commonly used in preoperative planning for brain tumor surgeries (Figure 30.2), and are gaining traction as a supplementary method when targeting input and output pathways associated with deep brain nuclei. Numerous diffusion techniques have been developed, with newer methods often demonstrating higher directional or structural resolution.

The ability to non-invasively map the three-dimensional structure of white matter tracts provides valuable information for presurgical planning in multiple settings. White matter tracts can be visualized adjacent to a tumor or vascular malformation to guide extent of resection, assist with risk stratification and inform patient counseling. Alternatively, tractography may guide optimal placement of a deep brain electrode or a focused ultrasound lesion. However, the reliability and validity of DTI methods, and

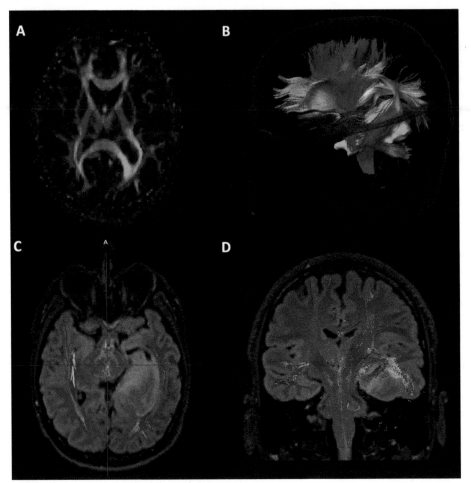

Figure 30.2 Diffusion map and fiber tracking on patient with a left mesial temporal infiltrative glioma. (A) Directionally-color encoded diffusion tensor imaging map; (B) Tractography reconstruction of the language and motor fiber tracts; (C) Midaxial T2-weighted FLAIR image showing the aforementioned fiber tracts in relation to the tumor; (D) Midcoronal T2-weighted FLAIR image showing fiber tracts.

the significant variability between different techniques has slowed the widespread adoption of tractography in surgical planning (Essayed et al., 2017).

Differences in diffusion MRI (dMRI) tracking algorithms and thresholds have a substantial impact on the resulting tracts, which presents an ongoing challenge when using tractography for targeting in cases requiring high levels of accuracy, such as in DBS. The more common deterministic diffusion tensor algorithms calculate fiber orientations, and will generate the same tract patterns with repeated use of the algorithm. Probabilistic algorithms, on the other hand, generate a probabilistically determined distribution of tract locations – these methods are computationally intense, and create additional complexity and sources of variation (Calabrese et al., 2014). In neurosurgical preoperative planning, deterministic tractography allows for more rapid calculation, as well as more

straightforward visualization of tracts in 3D space (Calabrese et al., 2014; Essayed et al., 2017). However, when evaluating the location of a DBS electrode contact, probabilistic tracts can provide a particular advantage, allowing assignment of a probability of contact between the electrode and tract (Pouratian et al., 2011), rather than an all or none calculation created with deterministic methods (Calabrese et al., 2014).

Conventional, single-tensor, deterministic DTI is unable to map multiple directions of fiber orientation within a single voxel, which limits the accurate visualization of heterogeneous or crossing tracts. Advanced techniques, including several high-angular resolution diffusion imaging (HARDI) methods have surpassed conventional DTI when resolving crossing fibers. These include diffusion spectrum imaging (DSI) and q-ball imaging (QBI; Kuo et al., 2008), developed to overcome this challenge, enabling accurate visualization of structures with dense crossing fibers such as the optic chiasm, centrum semiovale, or brainstem (Kuo et al., 2008; Wedeen et al., 2008). Other methods including deterministic two-tensor tractography have also been developed to better resolve crossing fibers. These advanced DTI methods promise to be valuable for the study of detailed structural connectomic studies of the human brain, and are critical components of large-scale studies of neural connectivity such as the Human Connectome Project, which aim to map functional neural connectivity in vivo and distribute these data and tools for research (Hagmann et al., 2007; Human Connectome Project, n.d.; Wedeen et al., 2008). In addition, these sequences will continue to have direct implications for neurosurgical planning (Becker et al., 2020; Calabrese et al., 2014; Essayed et al., 2017).

Diffusion MRI has broad utility as both a clinical and a research tool, and an array of adaptations in hardware and analysis have further improved the quality of information that can be gleaned from collected data. In order to obtain the highest-fidelity diffusion imaging, recent research suggests that the highest possible gradient strengths should be used. Huang and colleagues describe more robust resolution of axon diameters with increasing gradient field strengths, suggesting that this will likely lead to higher gradient strengths being developed for use in medical applications (Huang et al., 2015).

Furthermore, diffusion imaging provides limited structural information when voxels contain substantial free water, such as in the presence of vasogenic edema (Bergmann et al., 2020; Pasternak et al., 2009). Several groups have begun to explore free water modeling methods to account for signal occurring secondary to extracellular fluid. By creating distinct compartments, with one tensor representing free water, and another representing tissue, free water techniques may be able to provide more robust representation of the underlying tissue structure especially in regions affected by vasogenic edema such as around tumors (Bergmann et al., 2020; Pasternak et al., 2009).

Conventional tractography is also limited spatially by the size of the imaging voxel, which limits investigation of tissue microstructure. While high field and ultra-high-field MRI may address some of these difficulties by increasing the signal to noise ratio and creating smaller voxels, other methods such as track density imaging (TDI) increase spatial resolution using post-processing, by incorporating information from outside the voxel of interest (Calamante et al., 2010). Methods which allow for improved definition of tissue microstructure may be of significant research and clinical value. Thalamic nuclei, for example, have proven difficult to resolve using conventional techniques and may be better segmented using high resolution TDI, which better differentiates small white matter tracts within a structure. Clinical targeting of thalamic nuclei (e.g., ventralis intermedius) for procedures such as DBS or focused ultrasound (FUS) thalamotomy relies on indirect targeting, and the further development of imaging techniques able to resolve thalamic nuclei may enable direct targeting of traditionally obscured structures (Su et al., 2020). For a review of direct thalamic targeting methods, both dMRI and other advanced techniques, we recommend the comprehensive reviews by Shah et al. (2020) and Gravbrot et al. (2020).

Thalamic segmentation is one example of tractography based atlasing. White matter atlases using DTI may be used to provide powerful representation of deep white matter tracts, which can be used to examine both healthy and pathological brain anatomy in individual living subjects, rather than extrapolating from existing cadaveric atlases. As with other techniques, different atlasing techniques will lead to variation in results, and these limitations must be considered if using an atlas technique for clinical or research purposes (de Haan and Karnath, 2017). For additional detailed discussion of tractography based atlases, including their use in neurosurgical patients, limitations, and future developments, we refer the reader to several articles by Mori et al. (2009), O'Donnell et al. (2016), Figley et al. (2017), and Zhang et al. (2020).

30.3.2 Functional Magnetic Resonance Imaging

Functional MRI (fMRI) is an extension of MRI, often using naturally occurring contrast agents based on biologic metabolic processes, which provides additional information on biologic function. Specifically, fMRI is an indirect measure of neuronal activity which can be related to local blood flow, oxidative glucose metabolism, glycolysis, or other metabolic processes. Therefore, depending on the clinical or research application, it is important to understand the biological basis of the measured signals so that measurements and results can be properly interpreted. A summary of the biologic underpinnings of fMRI can be found in Raichle's "Behind the scenes of functional brain imaging: a historical and physiological perspective" (Raichle, 1998).

One common endogenous contrast agent used for fMRI is paramagnetic deoxyhemoglobin in venous blood. Using

GRE imaging techniques, blood oxygenation level-dependent (BOLD) contrast can act as a proxy for changes in blood flow or brain metabolism, which varies with changes in neural activity. The biophysiologic underpinnings are described further by Hillman (2014).

Functional MRI has become an effective tool for pre-surgical planning, often used in challenging epilepsy and tumor surgeries for lesions near critical language, motor, or other eloquent cortex (Figure 30.3; Petrella et al., 2006; Rosen and Savoy, 2012; Silva et al., 2017). As changes from baseline BOLD signal may be small, fMRI results are limited by signal to-noise-ratio, as well as the ability of the patient to effectively perform a desired task. Furthermore, perilesional BOLD changes, due for example to edema, hemosiderin, or neurovascular decoupling, may obscure interpretation of fMRI. More advanced methods may reduce signal artifact and increase spatial resolution and signal to noise ratio, improving sensitivity of signal detection. Additional challenges as well as techniques in presurgical fMRI are reviewed in detail by Silva et al. (2017).

Several newer methods have expanded the role of fMRI in brain science and neurosurgery. Resting-state fMRI was developed as a method to evaluate functional connectivity by comparing patterns of activation across distributed regions during continuous fMRI acquisition obtained at rest. Resting-state oscillations are often confounded by non-neural oscillations including cardiac and respiratory patterns, but an increasing body of literature supports the finding that resting-state BOLD changes likely reflect neuronal activity (Birn et al., 2006, 2008; Chang et al., 2009; Damoiseaux et al., 2006; Nir et al., 2008; Shmuel et al., 2002; van den Heuvel and Hulshoff Pol, 2010). The nuances of resting-state fMRI and its role in functional connectivity are described in detail in a 2010 review by van den Heuvel and Hulshoff Pol. Resting-state methods have been studied as a potential non-invasive biomarker for quantifying pathologic changes associated with disease, and may prove useful for the non-invasive mapping of cognitive and emotional networks, regions which are not traditionally defined as eloquent, but may still have significant implications on patient outcome if affected by pathology or surgical resection (Catalino et al., 2020). Resting-state fMRI may augment decision making in epilepsy and tumor surgery, by improving identification of an epileptic zone and by better defining critical cognitive networks to enable more complete and safer resections (Boerwinkle et al. 2017; Böttger et al., 2011; Catalino et al., 2020; Lee et al., 2013; Leuthardt et al., 2018; Roland et al., 2017; Shimony et al., 2009).

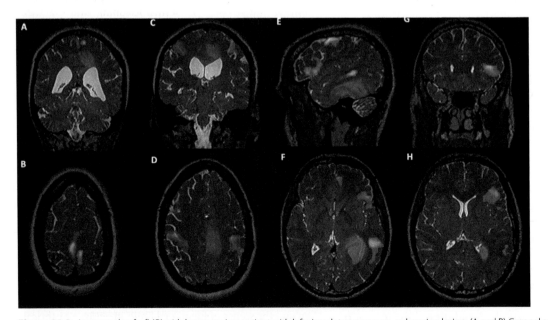

Figure 30.3 An example of a fMRI with language in a patient with left cingulate gyrus non- enhancing lesion. (A and B) Coronal and axial T2-weighted image showing BOLD activation during bilateral toe wiggle task; (C and D) Coronal and axial T2-weighted image showing BOLD activation during bilateral hand clench task; (E and F) Coronal and axial T2-weighted image showing BOLD activation during auditory naming; (G and H) Coronal and axial T2- weighted image showing BOLD activation during sentence completion.

All conventional fMRI methods are limited by their temporal resolution, often on the order of seconds, which limits their ability to evaluate the myriad neural processes operating at higher frequencies. A novel proposed method for functional mapping is based on MR elastography (MRE), which quantifies tissue biomechanical properties by imaging an externally induced mechanical soundwave, compared in some cases to the imaging counterpart to palpation, commonly used by physicians for diagnostic purposes (Mariappan et al., 2010). A pad placed under the patient generates shear waves using mechanical energy; the propagation of those waves through tissue allows for quantitative mapping of tissue stiffness using MRI (Mariappan et al., 2010; Muthupillai and Ehman, 1996). While the mechanism is different than in diffusion fMRI, preliminary exploration of functional MRE (fMRE) similarly relies on detecting cellular mechanical changes with comparatively high temporal resolutions on the order of 100 ms (Muthupillai and Ehman, 1996; Patz et al., 2019). An aspirational gold standard in functional imaging would combine high spatial resolution of ultra-high-field MRI with the temporal resolution of electrical or optical techniques, fMRE, and other techniques may offer an exciting window into whole-brain in-vivo physiology, allowing for exploration of more complex and temporally dynamic physiology (Patz et al., 2019).

30.3.3 Perfusion and Cerebral Blood Flow

Perfusion imaging has been developed with the goal of quantifying tissue perfusion, typically defied as the delivery of blood at the capillary level, which significantly impacts oxygen and nutrient delivery to tissue (Jahng et al., 2014). Dynamic susceptibility contrast (DSC) and dynamic contrast-enhanced MRI both rely on the delivery of a contrast bolus. Dynamic susceptibility contrast methods are used extensively in the clinical setting for measurement of cerebral ischemia and brain tumor perfusion via repeated measurements of T_2 signal loss over time. Dynamic constrast enhanced (DCE) MRI also relies on a contrast bolus and serial image acquisition, using T_1-weighted images and tracer pharmacokinetic modeling to infer physiologic differences in tissue. Dynamic constrast-enhanced methods have been applied extensively to other organ systems, but are increasingly applied to intracranial applications. Dynamic constrast-enhanced MRI may help measure both perfusion and vascular permeability. Together, these metrics are under investigation as adjunct methods of differentiating tumor grade and differentiating tumor recurrence from radiation necrosis, both of critical importance in neuro-oncology treatment planning (Law et al., 2004; Morabito et al., 2019).

30.4 Intraoperative Magnetic Resonance Imaging

Magnetic resonance imaging has been used successfully in neurosurgical operating rooms since the 1990s, and was developed to address several intraoperative challenges, including the identification of residual tumor during resection, reduction of navigation accuracy secondary to brain shift, and monitoring of thermal lesioning with MR thermometry (Figure 30.4; Jolesz, 2011). Identification of residual tumor is a natural use of the technology, provided that the tumor is visible on MRI, and a radiologist experienced in interpreting intraoperative MRI (iMRI) is available to review the images. Intraoperative MRI remains the most reliable tool for assessing extent of resection during surgery. As additional sequences become available, iMRI may be

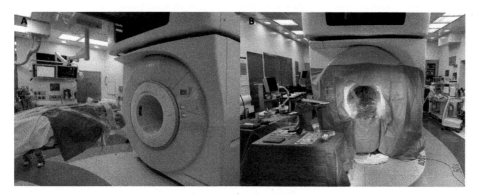

Figure 30.4 The intraoperative MRI in the Advanced Multimodality Image Guided Operating (AMIGO) suite at Brigham and Women's Hospital, Harvard Medical School. (A) Patient being prepared for an intraoperative MRI during tumor resection; here the MRI moves to scan a patient in the OR during a craniotomy (B) Patient undergoing Laser Interstitial Thermal Therapy for mesial temporal lobe epilepsy; here the machine is draped for an in-bore procedure.

able to provide more information about surrounding tissue, better delineating tumor margins, and assessing the integrity of any nearby tissue for infiltration or normal function with evaluation of multiple sequences. These advantages have led to increasing use in tumor surgery, and have also had particularly wide adoption in pediatric neurosurgery (Levy et al., 2009).

After a craniotomy, entrance of air, egress of cerebrospinal fluid (CSF) and tissue resection and retraction cause brain shift which may render standard intraoperative navigation techniques increasingly inaccurate vas the surgery progresses. While an ultimate goal remains to monitor brain shift continuously during surgery, utilizing iMRI allows for updated registration and can improve understanding of intraoperative anatomy (Gering et al., 2001). Furthermore, some procedures, including DBS and stereotactic drug injection, may be performed inside an intraoperative magnet, allowing for adjustments in targeting of deep brain structures and confirmatory imaging during the procedure. These methods provide improved accuracy when compared to frame-based stereotaxy with preoperative imaging alone (Larson et al., 2012; Starr et al., 2010).

The development of MR thermometry has enabled significant advancement in thermal lesioning methods. Temperature-sensitive MR images are based on the calculated change in the temperature-dependent shift in proton resonant frequency, which is acquired using a fast spoiled gradient echo (FSPGR) sequence (Hynynen and McDannold, 2004). In both laser interstitial thermal therapy (LITT; Figure 30.5), and MR-guided FUS ablation, MR thermometry plays a key role in defining tissue temperature changes, which allow for minimally invasive thermal lesions to be created safely with assessment of temperature change in near real time. Certain limitations do exist – for example, gas in the field (created by tissue cavitation or surgically introduced during a biopsy, for example) distorts local magnetic fields, and may lead to areas of signal drop out. Experts in the field predict that with improved rapid temperature monitoring, closed-loop systems may provide increased safety and efficacy, enabling control mechanisms based directly on MR temperature readings (Salomir et al., 2000). Additional novel uses of MR thermometry may further improve therapeutic targeting. McDannold and colleagues have demonstrated that phase data obtained during MR thermometry for focused ultrasound allows for visualization of the internal capsule and potentially other structures that could be used to refine procedural targeting (McDannold et al., 2020).

30.5 Ultra-High-Field Magnetic Resonance Imaging

While clinical MRI scanners primarily use field strengths from 1.5 to 3T, modern, high-field MR machines may reach field strengths of up to 10.5T for infrequent human imaging, and 11.7T, primarily for research purposes. Scanners in the 7T range were approved for clinical use in 2017, and scanners at or above the 7T field strength are considered ultra-high-field imaging modalities. Higher field strengths enable increased signal to noise, allowing for higher spatial resolution when examining structural features (Duyn, 2012; Ladd et al., 2018). However, the higher field strengths also present challenges, including greater susceptibility artifacts, worsening of movement artifact, and more frequent presence of side effects such as transient dizziness, nausea or metallic taste (van Osch and Webb, 2014). For an in-depth review of the physics and human applications of ultra-high-field MRI, fMRI and MRS, we direct the readers to the insightful review by Ladd and colleagues (2018).

Several applications highlight the benefit of high-field MRI in clinical neurosurgery. When exploring medically refractory epilepsy, non-lesional pathology presents a challenge for surgical management, as the optimal target may be difficult or impossible to identify. A number of sites now incorporate 7T MRI in such cases, with the goal of identifying lesions that were too subtle to resolve on a 1.5 or 3T scanner – if a lesion is identified, such cases may become substantially more amenable to surgical intervention. In a 2016 study of 21 patients with refractory, focal epilepsy and unremarkable conventional brain MRIs, 7T FLAIR and GRE imaging identified six lesions that had not been visible at 3T. After the identification of these subtle lesions that correlated with epileptic onset, four of these patients underwent epilepsy surgery with focal cortical dysplasia identified on tissue examination. All four patients had seizure reduction after surgery (Ciantis et al., 2016).

Potential applications for ultra-high-field MRI are broad and could include evaluation of any aspect of the brain where current resolution or signal to noise is inadequate. Uses include study of disease progression in multiple sclerosis (Zurawski et al., 2020), evaluation of cortical layers and substructure demonstrated by Duyn et al. (2007) with 7T phase-contrast imaging, and improved resolution of cerebral vasculature with ultra-high field MR angiography (MRA) (Heverhagen et al., 2008; Park et al., 2018). Studies with 7T MRA are able to image vasculature with a resolution of 0.2–0.3 mm,

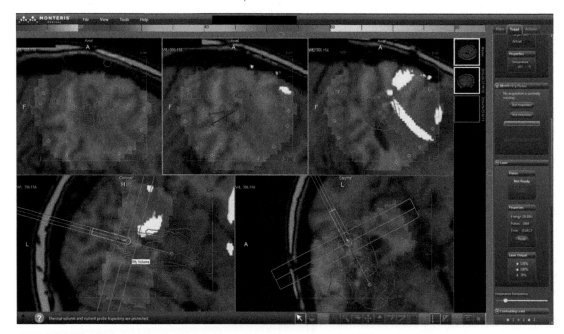

Figure 30.5 Laser Interstitial Thermal Therapy NeuroBlate (Monteris Medical, MN, USA) software display. The targeted lesion can be contoured slice-by-slice to guide the ablation. The software executes the treatment allowing the user to monitor real-time thermal imaging. Adjustments can be made during treatment. Here, a blue contour line demonstrates a predicted zone of ablation. The three parallel red lines traversing the ablation zone each correspond to the axial imaging planes show in the top 3 panels.

allowing reliable imaging of lenticulostriate or basilar perforating vessels, which are not reliably demonstrated on lower field strength imaging, and can typically only be visualized on invasive, digital subtraction angiography (Heverhagen et al., 2008; Kang et al., 2009, 2010). This improved microvascular resolution could have substantial implications for diagnosis of cerebrovascular disease, arteriovenous malformations (AVMs), and intracranial stenosis, and may also prove a valuable tool during preoperative planning for aneurysm and AVM surgeries (Park et al., 2018).

Similar principles allow for more detailed connectomic and functional imaging when using ultra-high-field fMRI. Increased field strength enables exploration of the relationship between structure and function with higher spatial resolution, such as the detailed examination of the function of ocular dominance columns by Yacoub et al. (2008). High-resolution fMRI also allows for functional imaging of human cortical layers, allowing for the measurement of layer-specific responses with substantial research applications in cognitive neuroscience (Lawrence et al., 2019).

Additional MR methods such as MR spectroscopy (MRS) also benefit from the increased signal to noise offered by ultra-high-field strengths. Conventional proton MRS allows non-invasive detection of several metabolites, and has been used to explore a variety of pathological conditions, including brain tumor classification and evaluation of dementia (Howe and Opstad, 2003; Kantarci et al., 2004). By increasing the signal to noise ratio using high MR field strengths, more robust quantification of brain neurochemical composition is possible, including distinct separation of glutamate from glutamine, which was not previously well differentiated by lower-resolution imaging (Godlewska et al., 2017; Ladd et al., 2018). In glioma, prognostically valuable IDH mutations are associated with the accumulation of 2-hydroxyglutarate (2-HG). While monitoring 2-HG levels has been proposed as a method of tracking disease progression, standard MRS techniques have failed to provide adequate signal detection. The increased signal to noise in ultra-high-field MRS has enabled quantification of 2-HG, among other metabolites, and such methods may prove valuable in monitoring post-surgical recurrence and response to therapy (Emir et al., 2016).

30.6 Conclusion

MRI is a uniquely powerful and versatile tool for tissue characterization relative to other common clinical imaging modalities such as computed tomography or x-ray. The wide range of imaging parameters associated with MRI acquisition allow for a broad array of current clinical applications and potential research findings, which may be translated to clinical use. A fundamental understanding of underlying physics and relationship to tissue composition is necessary to identify opportunities for novel imaging sequences and clinical applications in this field. MRI techniques are currently being applied to translational efforts to improve care in presurgical mapping, increased specificity for DBS/anatomic targeting, diagnosing structuring lesions (i.e., epileptogenic regions), quantifying brain perfusion, and improving non-invasive diagnostics (i.e., identifying inflammation, tumor, stroke, demyelination, etc.) and monitoring therapeutics. Substantial strides continue to improve understanding of brain organization through tractography and functional imaging as a counterpart to invasive neurophysiology. Newer sequences, including advanced tractography, will hopefully help further spatially define deep brain structures such as ventral intermediate thalamus (VIM), which are currently difficult to visualize with conventional techniques. Such techniques could have significant implications for future surgical treatment. Further advances in MR technology, including hardware, acquisition sequences and processing are likely to have a substantial impact on understanding of brain function and disease, and will contribute to improved tools for combating these diseases.

Figure acknowledgements

The following image is credited to the authors of this chapter: Figure 30.1
The following images obtained with consent are credited to the authors of this chapter: Figures 30.2–30.5

References

Allen LM, Hasso AN, Handwerker J, Farid H. Sequence-specific MR imaging findings that are useful in dating ischemic stroke. *Radiographics* 2012;**32**(5):1285–97; discussion 1297–9. https://doi.org/10.1148/rg.325115760.

Becker D, Scherer M, Neher P, et al. Going beyond diffusion tensor imaging tractography in eloquent glioma surgery – high-resolution fiber tractography: Q-ball or constrained spherical deconvolution? *World Neurosurg* 2020;**134**:e596–609. https://doi.org/10.1016/j.wneu.2019.10.138.

Bergmann Ø, Henriques R, Westin C-F, Pasternak O. Fast and accurate initialization of the free-water imaging model parameters from multi-shell diffusion MRI. *NMR Biomed* 2020;**33**(3):e4219. https://doi.org/10.1002/nbm.4219.

Birn RM, Diamond JB, Smith MA, Bandettini PA. Separating respiratory-variation-related fluctuations from neuronal-activity-related fluctuations in fMRI. *Neuroimage* 2006;**31**(4):1536–48. https://doi.org/10.1016/j.neuroimage.2006.02.048.

Birn RM, Smith MA, Jones TB, Bandettini PA. The respiration response function: the temporal dynamics of fMRI signal fluctuations related to changes in respiration. *Neuroimage* 2008;**40**(2):644–54. https://doi.org/10.1016/j.neuroimage.2007.11.059.

Boerwinkle VL, Mohanty D, Foldes ST, et al. Correlating resting-state functional magnetic resonance imaging connectivity by independent component analysis-based epileptogenic zones with intracranial electroencephalogram localized seizure onset zones and surgical outcomes in prospective pediatric intractable epilepsy study. *Brain Connect* 2017;**7**(7):424–42. https://doi.org/10.1089/brain.2016.0479.

Böttger J, Margulies DS, Horn P, et al. A software tool for interactive exploration of intrinsic functional connectivity opens new perspectives for brain surgery. *Acta Neurochir (Wien)* 2011;**153**(8):1561–72. https://doi.org/10.1007/s00701-011-0985-6.

Calabrese E, Badea A, Coe CL, Lubach GR, Styner MA, Johnson GA. Investigating the tradeoffs between spatial resolution and diffusion sampling for brain mapping with diffusion tractography: time well spent? *Hum Brain Mapp* 2014;**35**(11):5667–85. https://doi.org/10.1002/hbm.22578.

Calamante F, Tournier J-D, Jackson GD, Connelly A. Track-density imaging (TDI): super-resolution white matter imaging using whole-brain track-density mapping. *Neuroimage* 2010;**53**(4):1233–43. https://doi.org/10.1016/j.neuroimage.2010.07.024.

Catalino MP, Yao S, Green DL, Laws ER, Golby AJ, Tie Y. Mapping cognitive and emotional networks in neurosurgical patients using resting-state functional magnetic resonance imaging. *Neurosurg Focus* 2020;**48**(2):E9. https://doi.org/10.3171/2019.11.FOCUS19773.

Chang C, Cunningham JP, Glover GH. Influence of heart rate on the BOLD signal: the cardiac response function. *Neuroimage* 2009;**44**(3):857–69. https://doi.org/10.1016/j.neuroimage.2008.09.029.

Ciantis AD, Barba C, Tassi L, et al. 7T MRI in focal epilepsy with unrevealing conventional field strength imaging. *Epilepsia* 2016;**57**(3):445–54. https://doi.org/10.1111/epi.13313.

Currie S, Hoggard N, Craven IJ, Hadjivassiliou M, Wilkinson ID. Understanding MRI: basic MR physics for physicians. *Postgrad Med J* 2013;**89**(1050):209–23. https://doi.org/10.1136/postgradmedj-2012-131342.

Damoiseaux JS, Rombouts S a. RB, Barkhof F, et al. Consistent resting-state networks across healthy subjects. *Proc Natl Acad Sci U S A* 2006;**103**(37):13848–53. https://doi.org/10.1073/pnas.0601417103.

de Haan B, Karnath H-O. 'Whose atlas I use, his song I sing?' – The impact of anatomical atlases on fiber tract contributions to cognitive deficits after stroke. *Neuroimage* 2017;**163**:301–09. https://doi.org/10.1016/j.neuroimage.2017.09.051.

Duyn JH. The future of ultra-high field MRI and fMRI for study of the human brain. *Neuroimage* 2012;**62**(2):1241–8. https://doi.org/10.1016/j.neuroimage.2011.10.065.

Duyn JH, Koretsky AP. Novel frontiers in MRI of the brain. *Curr Opin Neurol* 2011;**24**(4):386–93. https://doi.org/10.1097/WCO.0b013e328348972a.

Duyn JH, van Gelderen P, Li T-Q, de Zwart JA, Koretsky AP, Fukunaga M. High-field MRI of brain cortical substructure based on signal phase. *Proc Natl Acad Sci U S A* 2007;**104**(28):11796–801. https://doi.org/10.1073/pnas.0610821104.

Emir UE, Larkin SJ, Pennington N de, et al. Noninvasive quantification of 2-hydroxyglutarate in human gliomas with *IDH1* and *IDH2* mutations. *Cancer Res* 2016;**76**(1):43–9. https://doi.org/10.1158/0008-5472.CAN-15-0934.

Essayed WI, Zhang F, Unadkat P, Cosgrove GR, Golby AJ, O'Donnell LJ. White matter tractography for neurosurgical planning: a topography-based review of the current state of the art. *Neuroimage Clin* 2017;**15**:659–72. https://doi.org/10.1016/j.nicl.2017.06.011.

Figley TD, Mortazavi Moghadam B, Bhullar N, Kornelsen J, Courtney SM, Figley CR. Probabilistic white matter atlases of human auditory, basal ganglia, language, precuneus, sensorimotor, visual and visuospatial networks. *Front Hum Neurosci* 2017;**11**. https://doi.org/10.3389/fnhum.2017.00306.

Gering DT, Nabavi A, Kikinis R, et al. An integrated visualization system for surgical planning and guidance using image fusion and an open MR. *J Magn Reson Imaging* 2001;**13**(6):967–75. https://doi.org/10.1002/jmri.1139.

Godlewska BR, Clare S, Cowen PJ, Emir UE. Ultra-high-field magnetic resonance spectroscopy in psychiatry. *Front Psychiatry*. 2017;**8**:123. https://doi.org/10.3389/fpsyt.2017.00123.

Gravbrot N, Saranathan M, Pouratian N, Kasoff WS. Advanced imaging and direct targeting of the motor thalamus and dentato-rubro-thalamic tract for tremor: a systematic review. *Stereotact Funct Neurosurg* 2020;**98**(4):220–40. https://doi.org/10.1159/000507030.

Hagmann P, Kurant M, Gigandet X, et al. Mapping human whole-brain structural networks with diffusion MRI. *PLoS One* 2007;**2**(7):e597. https://doi.org/10.1371/journal.pone.0000597.

Heverhagen JT, Bourekas E, Sammet S, Knopp MV, Schmalbrock P. Time-of-flight magnetic resonance angiography at 7 Tesla. *Invest Radiol* 2008;**43**(8):568–73. https://doi.org/10.1097/RLI.0b013e31817e9b2c.

Hillman EMC. Coupling mechanism and significance of the BOLD signal: a status report. *Annu Rev Neurosci* 2014;**37**:161–81. https://doi.org/10.1146/annurev-neuro-071013-014111.

Hjort N, Christensen S, Sølling C, et al. Ischemic injury detected by diffusion imaging 11 minutes after stroke. *Ann Neurol* 2005;**58**(3):462–5. https://doi.org/10.1002/ana.20595.

Horowitz AL. *MRI Physics for Radiologists – A Visual Approach.* Springer, 1994. www.springer.com/gp/book/9780387943725.

Howe FA, Opstad KS. 1H MR spectroscopy of brain tumours and masses. *NMR Biomed* 2003;**16**(3):123–31. https://doi.org/10.1002/nbm.822.

Huang SY, Nummenmaa A, Witzel T, et al. The impact of gradient strength on in vivo diffusion MRI estimates of axon diameter. *Neuroimage*. 2015;**106**:464–72. https://doi.org/10.1016/j.neuroimage.2014.12.008.

Human Connectome Project. 2020. www.humanconnectomeproject.org/about/

Hynynen K, McDannold N. MRI guided and monitored focused ultrasound thermal ablation methods: a review of progress. *Int J Hyperthermia* 2004;**20**(7):725–37. https://doi.org/10.1080/02656730410001716597.

Jahng G-H, Li K-L, Ostergaard L, Calamante F. Perfusion magnetic resonance imaging: a comprehensive update on principles and techniques. *Korean J Radiol* 2014;**15**(5):554–77. https://doi.org/10.3348/kjr.2014.15.5.554.

Jolesz FA. Intraoperative imaging in neurosurgery: where will the future take us? *Acta Neurochir Suppl* 2011;**109**:21–5. https://doi.org/10.1007/978-3-211-99651-5_4.

Jung BA, Weigel M. Spin echo magnetic resonance imaging. *J Magn Reson Imaging* 2013;**37**(4):805–17. https://doi.org/10.1002/jmri.24068.

Kang C-K, Park C-A, Kim K-N, et al. Non-invasive visualization of basilar artery perforators with 7T MR angiography. *J Magn Reson Imaging* 2010;**32**(3):544–50. https://doi.org/10.1002/jmri.22250.

Kang C-K, Park C-A, Lee H, et al. Hypertension correlates with lenticulostriate arteries visualized by 7T magnetic resonance angiography. *Hypertension* 2009;**54**(5):1050–6. https://doi.org/10.1161/HYPERTENSIONAHA.109.140350.

Kantarci K, Petersen RC, Boeve BF, et al. [1]H MR spectroscopy in common dementias. *Neurology* 2004;**63**(8):1393–8. https://doi.org/10.1212/01.wnl.0000141849.21256.ac.

Kuo L-W, Chen J-H, Wedeen VJ, Tseng W-YI. Optimization of diffusion spectrum imaging and q-ball imaging on clinical MRI system. *Neuroimage*. 2008;**41**(1):7–18. https://doi.org/10.1016/j.neuroimage.2008.02.016.

Ladd ME, Bachert P, Meyerspeer M, et al. Pros and cons of ultra-high-field MRI/MRS for human application. *Prog Nucl Magn Reson Spectrosc* 2018;**109**:1–50. https://doi.org/10.1016/j.pnmrs.2018.06.001.

Larson PS, Starr PA, Bates G, Tansey L, Richardson RM, Martin AJ. An optimized system for interventional MRI guided stereotactic surgery: preliminary evaluation of targeting accuracy. *Neurosurgery.* 2012;**70**(OPERATIVE):ons95–ons103. https://doi.org/10.1227/NEU.0b013e31822f4a91.

Law M, Yang S, Babb JS, et al. Comparison of cerebral blood volume and vascular permeability from dynamic susceptibility contrast-enhanced perfusion MR imaging with glioma grade. *Am J Neuroradiol* 2004;**25**(5):746–55.

Lawrence SJD, Formisano E, Muckli L, de Lange FP. Laminar fMRI: applications for cognitive neuroscience. *Neuroimage.* 2019;**197**:785–91. https://doi.org/10.1016/j.neuroimage.2017.07.004

Le Bihan D. Looking into the functional architecture of the brain with diffusion MRI. *Nat Rev Neurosci* 2003;**4**(6):469–80. https://doi.org/10.1038/nrn1119.

Lee MH, Smyser CD, Shimony JS. Resting-state fMRI: a review of methods and clinical applications. *Am J Neuroradiol* 2013;**34**(10):1866–72. https://doi.org/10.3174/ajnr.A3263.

Leuthardt EC, Guzman G, Bandt SK, et al. Integration of resting state functional MRI into clinical practice – a large single institution experience. *PLoS One* 2018;**13**(6):e0198349. https://doi.org/10.1371/journal.pone.0198349.

Levy R, Cox RG, Hader WJ, Myles T, Sutherland GR, Hamilton MG. Application of intraoperative high-field magnetic resonance imaging in pediatric neurosurgery. *J Neurosurg Pediatr* 2009;**4**(5):467–74. https://doi.org/10.3171/2009.4.PEDS08464.

Madai VI, Galinovic I, Grittner U, et al. DWI intensity values predict FLAIR lesions in acute ischemic stroke. *PLoS One.* 2014;**9**(3):e92295. https://doi.org/10.1371/journal.pone.0092295.

Mariappan YK, Glaser KJ, Ehman RL. Magnetic resonance elastography: a review. *Clin Anat* 2010;**23**(5):497–511. https://doi.org/10.1002/ca.21006.

Markl M, Leupold J. Gradient echo imaging. *J Magn Reson Imaging* 2012;**35**(6):1274–89. https://doi.org/10.1002/jmri.23638.

McDannold N, White PJ, Cosgrove GR. Using phase data from MR temperature imaging to visualize anatomy during MRI guided focused ultrasound neurosurgery. *IEEE Trans Med Imaging* 2020;**39**(12):3821–30. https://doi.org/10.1109/TMI.2020.3005631

Morabito R, Alafaci C, Pergolizzi S, et al. DCE and DSC perfusion MRI diagnostic accuracy in the follow-up of primary and metastatic intra-axial brain tumors treated by radiosurgery with cyberknife. *Radiat Oncol* 2019;**14**(1):65. https://doi.org/10.1186/s13014-019-1271-7.

Mori S, Oishi K, Faria AV. White matter atlases based on diffusion tensor imaging. *Curr Opin Neurol* 2009;**22**(4):362–9. https://doi.org/10.1097/WCO.0b013e32832d954b.

Muthupillai R, Ehman RL. Magnetic resonance elastography. *Nat Med* 1996;**2**(5):601–03. https://doi.org/10.1038/nm0596-601.

Nagaraja N, Forder JR, Warach S, Merino JG. Reversible diffusion-weighted imaging lesions in acute ischemic stroke: a systematic review. *Neurology* 2020;**94**(13):571–87. https://doi.org/10.1212/WNL.0000000000009173.

Nir Y, Mukamel R, Dinstein I, et al. Interhemispheric correlations of slow spontaneous neuronal fluctuations revealed in human sensory cortex. *Nat Neurosci* 2008;**11**(9):1100–08. https://doi.org/10.1038/nn.2177.

O'Donnell LJ, Suter Y, Rigolo L, et al. Automated white matter fiber tract identification in patients with brain tumors. *Neuroimage Clin* 2016;**13**:138–53. https://doi.org/10.1016/j.nicl.2016.11.023.

Park C-A, Kang C-K, Kim Y-B, Cho Z-H. Advances in MR angiography with 7T MRI: from microvascular imaging to functional angiography. *NeuroImage.* 2018;**168**:269–78. https://doi.org/10.1016/j.neuroimage.2017.01.019.

Pasternak O, Sochen N, Gur Y, Intrator N, Assaf Y. Free water elimination and mapping from diffusion MRI. *Magn Reson Med* 2009;**62**(3):717–30. https://doi.org/10.1002/mrm.22055.

Patz S, Fovargue D, Schregel K, et al. Imaging localized neuronal activity at fast time scales through biomechanics. *Sci Adv* 2019;**5**(4):eaav3816. https://doi.org/10.1126/sciadv.aav3816.

Petrella JR, Shah LM, Harris KM, et al. Preoperative functional MR imaging localization of language and motor areas: effect on therapeutic decision making in patients with potentially resectable brain tumors. *Radiology* 2006;**240**(3):793–802. https://doi.org/10.1148/radiol.2403051153.

Pouratian N, Zheng Z, Bari AA, Behnke E, Elias WJ, DeSalles AAF. Multi-institutional evaluation of deep brain stimulation targeting using probabilistic connectivity-based thalamic segmentation. *J Neurosurg* 2011;**115**(5):995–1004. https://doi.org/10.3171/2011.7.JNS11250.

Raichle ME. Behind the scenes of functional brain imaging: a historical and physiological perspective. *Proc Natl Acad Sci* 1998;**95**(3):765–72. https://doi.org/10.1073/pnas.95.3.765.

Roland JL, Griffin N, Hacker CD, et al. Resting-state functional magnetic resonance imaging for surgical planning in pediatric patients: a preliminary experience. *J Neurosurg Pediatr* 2017;**20**(6):583–90. https://doi.org/10.3171/2017.6.PEDS1711.

Rosen BR, Savoy RL. fMRI at 20: has it changed the world? *Neuroimage.* 2012;**62**(2):1316–24. https://doi.org/10.1016/j.neuroimage.2012.03.004.

Salomir R, Vimeux FC, de Zwart JA, Grenier N, Moonen CT. Hyperthermia by MR-guided focused ultrasound: accurate temperature control based on fast MRI and a physical model of local energy deposition and heat conduction. *Magn Reson Med*

2000;43(3):342–7. https://doi.org/10.1002/(sici)1522-2594(200003)43:3<342::aid-mrm4>3.0.co;2-6.

Shah BR, Lehman VT, Kaufmann TJ, et al. Advanced MRI techniques for transcranial high intensity focused ultrasound targeting. *Brain* 2020;143(9).2664–72. https://doi.org/10.1093/brain/awaa107.

Shimony JS, Zhang D, Johnston JM, Fox MD, Roy A, Leuthardt EC. Resting-state spontaneous fluctuations in brain activity: a new paradigm for presurgical planning using fMRI. *Acad Radiol* 2009;16(5):578–83. https://doi.org/10.1016/j.acra.2009.02.001.

Shmuel A, Yacoub E, Pfeuffer J, et al. Sustained negative BOLD, blood flow and oxygen consumption response and its coupling to the positive response in the human brain. *Neuron* 2002;36(6):1195–210. https://doi.org/10.1016/s0896-6273(02)01061-9.

Siemonsen S, Mouridsen K, Holst B, et al. Quantitative T2 values predict time from symptom onset in acute stroke patients. *Stroke* 2009;40(5):1612–6. https://doi.org/10.1161/STROKEAHA.108.542548.

Silva MA, See AP, Essayed WI, Golby AJ, Tie Y. Challenges and techniques for presurgical brain mapping with functional MRI. *Neuroimage Clin* 2017;17:794–803. https://doi.org/10.1016/j.nicl.2017.12.008.

Starr PA, Martin AJ, Ostrem JL, Talke P, Levesque N, Larson PS. Subthalamic nucleus deep brain stimulator placement using high-field interventional magnetic resonance imaging and a skull-mounted aiming device: technique and application accuracy. *J Neurosurg* 2010;112(3):479–90. https://doi.org/10.3171/2009.6.JNS081161.

Su JH, Choi EY, Tourdias T, et al. Improved Vim targeting for focused ultrasound ablation treatment of essential tremor: a probabilistic and patient-specific approach. *Hum Brain Mapp.* 2020;41(17):4769–88. https://doi.org/10.1002/hbm.25157.

van den Heuvel MP, Hulshoff Pol HE. Exploring the brain network: a review on resting-state fMRI functional connectivity. *Eur Neuropsychopharmacol* 2010;20(8):519–34. https://doi.org/10.1016/j.euroneuro.2010.03.008.

van Osch MJP, Webb AG. Safety of ultra-high field MRI: what are the specific risks? *Curr Radiol Rep* 2014;2(8):61. https://doi.org/10.1007/s40134-014-0061-0.

Wedeen VJ, Wang RP, Schmahmann JD, et al. Diffusion spectrum magnetic resonance imaging (DSI) tractography of crossing fibers. *Neuroimage* 2008;41(4):1267–77. https://doi.org/10.1016/j.neuroimage.2008.03.036.

Yacoub E, Harel N, Uğurbil K. High-field fMRI unveils orientation columns in humans. *Proc Natl Acad Sci* 2008;105(30):10607–12. https://doi.org/10.1073/pnas.0804110105.

Zhang F, Xie G, Leung L, et al. Creation of a novel trigeminal tractography atlas for automated trigeminal nerve identification. *Neuroimage* 2020;220:117063. https://doi.org/10.1016/j.neuroimage.2020.117063.

Zurawski J, Tauhid S, Chu R, et al. 7T MRI cerebral leptomeningeal enhancement is common in relapsing-remitting multiple sclerosis and is associated with cortical and thalamic lesions. *Mult Scler* 2020;26(2):177–87. https://doi.org/10.1177/1352458519885106.

Chapter 31

Brain Mapping

Anthony T. Lee, Cecilia Dalle Ore, and Shawn L. Hervey-Jumper

31.1 Introduction

Maximizing the extent of resection is fundamental in both glioma and epilepsy surgery. Careful consideration is necessary when lesions are within or neighbor eloquent cortex in order to minimize permanent postoperative neurological deficits, which themselves are associated with worse overall survival and lower quality of life (Duffau et al., 2003; Han et al., 2018; Keles et al., 2004; Rahman et al., 2017). A wide array of intraoperative and extraoperative techniques have been established to guide surgical planning, including direct electrical stimulation (DES) for sensorimotor and language mapping, as well as multimodal adjuncts including functional and resting-state magnetic resonance imaging (fMRI and rs-fMRI), diffusion tensor imaging (DTI), magnetoencephalography (MEG), and intraoperative imaging (IOI).

In this chapter, we review the principles of DES for sensorimotor and language mapping, with a particular focus on the advances in cognitive and systems neuroscience that underlie the language circuits probed by the most common intraoperative tasks. We then highlight the efforts to expand the use of non-invasive imaging modalities for neurosurgical planning.

31.2 Sensorimotor Mapping

Monitoring motor-evoked potentials (MEPs) of direct cortical or subcortical DES has become the mainstay of identifying the motor cortex and its descending motor fibers (De Witt Hamer et al., 2012). There are two general methods for stimulating cortical and subcortical fibers: (1) monopolar stimulation, which uses short trains of high frequency (250–500 Hz) square wave monophasic pulses delivered via a single-tipped probe; and (2) bipolar stimulation, which uses low frequency (60 Hz) to deliver long biphasic pulses via a 5-mm spaced stimulator probe (Bello et al., 2014; Szelényi et al., 2011). Due to the configuration of the stimulators and differences in current spread, these two methods vary in their sensitivity

and specificity for evoking MEPs. Because the current spread is confined to the 5-mm space on the stimulator tip, bipolar stimulation is targeted with high specificity for identifying cortical and subcortical motor pathways. Detection of a motor response subcortically with bipolar stimulation indicates that the motor tract is nearby (within 5 mm). Because the monopolar acts as a point source, the current spread is larger (at roughly 20 mm), which significantly increases its sensitivity in eliciting MEPs. A comparison of the two techniques found that bipolar stimulation detected subcortical pathways in only 20% of cases, whereas monopolar stimulation identified descending motor pathways in 100% of the same cases (Gogos et al., 2020). Furthermore, the shape of the current spread from monopolar stimulation falls linearly with every 1 mm of distance. Therefore, monopolar stimulation is useful for estimating the proximity of the probe to the white matter tract, with a linear relationship of 1 mA of current for every 1 mm of (up to 25 mA) (Bello et al., 2014; Plans et al., 2017; Prabhu et al., 2011). Thus, monopolar and bipolar stimulation appear to be complementary tools, and when combined with continuous MEP monitoring during resection, outperforms the use of each technique in its isolation in detecting corticospinal tracts and avoiding postoperative morbidity (Gogos et al., 2020).

With regard to awake versus asleep motor mapping, there are few advantageous for performing motor mapping awake. Outcomes between awake and asleep motor mapping are comparably excellent in extent of resection and functional outcomes (Han et al., 2018; Magill et al., 2018). While awake mapping affords the theoretical advantage of having the patient voluntarily move the affect muscle group to confirm motor function following changes in MEPs, awake motor mapping may have increased risk of seizures (Gonen et al., 2014; Nossek et al., 2013). Transcranial MEPs are also often painful and poorly tolerated, and DES involving supplementary motor areas may affect regions involved in movement planning and initiation causing apraxia, which can mimic stimulation of the motor pathway and cause tumor resection to stop prematurely despite the functional recovery that occurs following supplementary motor area resections (Fernández Coello et al., 2013; Young et al., 2020).

31.3 Language Mapping

Identification of language sites with DES can be performed using low-frequency bipolar stimulation (60 Hz, 1.0 ms biphasic square wave) with concurrent electrocorticography using a 16-channel electrode and holder assembly (Grass Model CE1, Natus Medical Inc.). Stimulation begins at 2 mA and then increases until positive sites are identified, after-discharge potentials occur, or a maximum current of 5 mA is reached (Roux et al., 2017). A positive stimulation site is preserved after repeat testing results in >50% error rate. Intraoperative testing can test multiple domains of language, including picture naming, repetition, reading, writing, syntax, and comprehension. Because each of these domains is driven by overlapping, yet distinct language processing networks, intraoperative testing requires balancing comprehensiveness with efficiency to minimize permanent postoperative language deficits. Initial theoretical language models posited a dual-stream framework, whereby the 'dorsal stream' engages sensorimotor processing to produce the phonology of speech, whereas the 'ventral stream' captures the semantic meaning of language. As described below, advances in cognitive and linguistic neuroscience have begun to describe distinctly more complex language processing networks for each language task.

31.3.1 Picture and Auditory Naming

Pioneered by Penfield and later popularized by Ojemann, picture naming (PN) of line drawings is the most common task in intraoperative language mapping (Ojemann et al., 1989; Ojemann and Mateer, 1978; Penfield and Roberts, 1959; Snodgrass and Vanderwart, 1980). In one study, 58% of glioma patients had at least one cortical site with stimulation-induced PN deficit (Sanai et al., 2008), and subsequent studies have mapped naming errors to specific cortical areas and language processing systems.

Picture naming errors can be categorized into six subtypes: semantic paraphasias (dog → "cat"), circumlocutions (tree→ "plant with leaves"), phonological paraphasias (deletions or substitutions of syllables), neologisms (made-up words), performance errors (slurred or stuttered responses), and no response errors (Corina et al.,

2010). Direct electrical stimulation of the posterior middle temporal gyrus (pMTG) and anterior supramarginal gyrus (SMG) (both regions of the ventral lexical-semantic stream) can result in in semantic paraphasias, while DES of the posterior superior temporal sulcus (STS; a region in the dorsal phonological stream) results in phonological paraphasias, neologisms, and circumlocutions. DES of the posterior supramarginal gyrus (pSMG), a region that is also within the dorsal production stream, evoked significantly more performance errors.

Naming in response to auditory stimuli in the absence of visual cues can also be used in intraoperative language testing. In auditory naming (AN), participants name an object upon hearing a description: e.g. "An animal with feathers that flies." "Bird". Interestingly, DES experiments have supported differential localization of AN and PN, in particular an anterior–posterior gradient for AN within the dominant temporal lobe. Stimulation of the anterior temporal lobe resulted in preferential deficits in AN, whereas stimulation of the posterior temporal region resulted in equal AN and PN deficits (Hamberger et al., 2001). Importantly, removal of AN sites resulted in both AN and PN deficits despite preservation of PN sites in all patients, which may infer that processing of AN occurs upstream to PN (Hamberger et al., 2005).

Within the ventral semantic stream, studies have attempted to determine whether naming retrieval in the temporal lobe occurs in a modality-independent (heteromodal) or -dependent (unimodal) manner. Using electrocorticography (ECoG) in the left anterior temporal lobe (ATL) of temporal lobe epilepsy (TLE) patients, Abel et al. (2015) found that cortical responses were near-identical for responses to picture and auditory stimuli of famous US politicians during a naming task, arguing for a heteromodal processing for proper naming. In a large cohort of patients undergoing parallel ECoG and functional MRI, Forseth and colleagues showed participants PN and AN trials, together with non-semantic control conditions using scrambled pictures and reversed speech, to identify heteromodal responses in middle fusiform gyrus, intraparietal sulcus, and inferior frontal gyrus (IFG). Importantly, the activity from these regions preceded articulation and were absent in control conditions. Intraoperative DES confirmed the middle fusiform gyrus to disrupt performance in PN and AN while having limited effects on sentence repetition, convincingly demonstrating the middle fusiform gyrus as a key lexical semantic hub for heteromodal naming (Forseth et al., 2018).

Subcortical stimulation mapping of white matter (WM) tracts has also identified several language tracts critical in naming, again in a manner consistent with the dual-stream model of language processing. The dorsal stream is served by the superior longitudinal fasciculus (SLF)/arcuate fasciculus (AF), while the ventral stream has two separate pathways: (1) the direct ventral pathway, which is comprised of the interior fronto-occipital fascicle (IFOF) that connects the occipital lobe, parietal lobe, and the posterotemporal cortex with the frontal lobe, and (2) the indirect ventral pathway, which is comprised of the inferior longitudinal fascicle (ILF; running below the IFOF) that connects the posterior occipitotemporal region and the temporal pole (Duffau et al., 2013). Stimulation of the AF near the superior insular sulcus has resulted in phonemic paraphasia, while stimulation of the IFOF within the roof of the temporal horn and extreme capsule has elicited semantic paraphasia (Benzagmout et al., 2007; Duffau, 2005, 2008; Duffau et al., 2014; Plaza et al., 2007). Stimulation of ILF has also been shown to cause semantic paraphasias (Bello et al., 2007).

31.3.2 Repetition

Conduction aphasia, first described in 1874 by Wernicke, is a syndrome characterized by phonological paraphasia and impairment in repetition with otherwise fluent speech production and perception (Buchsbaum et al., 2011; Damasio and Damasio, 1980; Goodglass, 1992; Leonard et al., 2019). The classical Wernicke–Geschwind model of language posits damage to the WM tracts of the dorsal stream as the primary driver in conduction aphasia (Geschwind, 1965).

The specific WM tracts that subserve the dorsal pathway are the three bundles of the SLF (Catani et al., 2005; Saur et al., 2008): the most medial direct pathway corresponding to the AF, which connects the middle and inferior temporal gyri with the precentral and inferior frontal gyri, and two more lateral indirect pathways – an anterior portion (SLFIII) connecting the ventral premotor cortex with the supramarginal gyrus, and the posterior portion (SLFII) connecting the angular gyrus with the posterior temporal area. Imaging studies show that the AF and SLFIII are recruited in connecting the cortical regions in word repetition (WR) (Fridriksson et al., 2010; Makris et al., 2005; Martino et al. 2013). Consistent with subcortical stimulation for naming, subcortical stimulation of the AF can induce phonological and articulatory disorders during word repetition. Direct electric stimulation of

IFOF either caused no deficits or produced semantic paraphasias (Moritz-Gasser and Duffau, 2013).

Evidence from recent voxel-based lesion mapping (VBLM) studies have begun to expand conduction aphasia beyond WM tracts to also encompass cortical regions, particularly in the posterior planum temporum of the left Sylvian parietal–temporal region (Spt), an area encompassing the supramarginal and angular gyri and posterior superior temporal cortex (Baldo et al., 2012; Buchsbaum et al., 2011; Dell et al., 2013; Fridriksson et al., 2010). As is the case in speech production, the role of Spt in repetition is believed to involve auditory guidance for providing real-time sensory feedback as the motor speech unit reaches its auditory target (Hickok and Poeppel, 2000, 2004; Hickok et al., 2003), and damage to the AF and/or Spt disrupts this sensory–motor integration (Buchsbaum et al., 2011; Parker et al., 2014; Rogalsky et al., 2015). Direct electrical stimulation studies have implicated cortical regions, whereby stimulation of the posterior superior temporal gyrus (pSTG) and supramaginal gyrus resulted in patients with decreased repetition of words and intact semantic knowledge (Anderson et al., 1999; Quigg and Fountain, 1999; Quigg et al., 2006). The use of pseudo-words may be a confounding factor to these experiments, as repetition of known words may theoretically be compensated by lexical retrieval pathways in the ventral stream, raising the possibility that non-word repetition (NWR) tasks may be more sensitive to identifying effective AF function. Indeed, significantly more repetition errors were identified when using NWR than WR tasks intr-operatively (Sierpowska et al., 2017).

Extending even further beyond serial, feedforward models of processing between nodes in the dorsal stream, recent ECoG studies have begun to illustrate a more distributed, parallel language processing network that incorporates recurrent processing nodes throughout the peri-Sylvian territory. By combining ECoG and DES, a large peri-Sylvian network was activated throughout all stages of a word repetition task, including dorsal stream nodes in the posterior temporal region that were immune to DES stimulation for speech production during word repetition (Leonard et al., 2019).

31.3.3 Reading

Whether the brain contains a region for "word images" or a visual word form area (VWFA) that contains visual representation of words specifically dedicated to reading dates back to Charcot, Dejerine, and Wernicke in the late nineteenth century. First established primarily from brain-damaged patients with acquired dyslexia (either lexical or phonological dyslexia), contemporary dual-stream models separate reading into two pathways: (1) the lexical–semantic pathway for orthographically irregular (i.e., irregularly spelled) words, whereby words are directly recognized as lexicon members and mapped onto verbal semantic representations; and (2) the phonological pathway for unknown or pseudo-words, whereby words are read using grapheme to phoneme rules (i.e., spelling–sound correspondences). Thus, patients with phonological dyslexia can read irregular words but not pseudo-words, whereas those with lexical dyslexia have difficulty reading irregular words but not pseudo-words (Beauvois and Dérouesné, 1979; Coltheart et al., 2001; Damasio and Damasio, 1983; Funnell, 1983; Warrington and Shallice, 1980).

Voxel-based lesion mapping studies have begun to identify differing neural substrates associated with these disassociated processes. Damage to the left inferior–parietal and left inferofrontal regions was linked to phonological dyslexia (Fiez et al., 2006; Rapcsak et al., 2009), while neuroimaging studies supported localization of the phonological pathway to the supramarginal gyrus, left posterior superior temporal gyrus, and the pars opercularis of the inferior frontal gyrus (Graves et al., 2008; Paulesu et al., 1993). For the lexical–semantic pathway, neuroimaging studies highlighted activation of the left basal temporal language area, the posterior part of the middle temporal gyrus, and the pars triangularis of the inferior frontal gyrus (Jobard et al., 2003).

In his monogram, Ojemann (1998) found reading sites that were distinct from naming in temporal–parietal and frontal areas. In awake language experiments using PN and reading tasks, Roux et al. (2004) also found reading sites that were both distinct and more numerous than naming sites in the dominant supramarginal, angular, posterior superior temporal gyrus (STG), dominant middle temporal gyrus (MTG), and dominant IFG and middle frontal gyrus (MFG). Naming interference sites were categorized as articulatory sites (evoking a visible orofacial contraction), anomia sites (unable to name the image during stimulation, but successful naming upon cessation of stimulation), and speech arrest (inability to say anything with stimulation, without visible orofacial contraction). Reading interference sites were similarly categorized into articulatory sites, pure reading arrest sites (patient stops reading and resumes upon cessation of stimulation, without obvious orofacial contraction), paraphasia sites (fluent speech with incomprehensible word choices), and sites that elicited ocular movements.

Overall, significantly more reading interference sites were mapped compared to PN interference sites, with the majority (~70%) of reading sites occurring adjacent to naming sites. Of speech arrest sites, 95% were commonly shared between PN and reading tasks, while only 65% of anomia sites during naming tasks resulted in reading deficits. This French-based study also investigated PN and reading sites in a subset of bilingual patients. They found that although the overall distribution of naming and reading sites for bilingual patients were no different than monolingual patients, language- and reading-specific sites were distributed across temporoparietal and frontal regions, suggesting a separate anatomic network for processing aspects of a second language (Roux et al., 2004).

To find evidence of cortical sites subserving dorsal phonological and ventral lexical-semantic reading streams, Roux and colleagues then asked patients to read frequent, but irregular French words along with pronounceable pseudowords. Irregular words were defined as words that contained at least one irregular/inconsistent segment whose pronunciation could not be obtained by letter–phoneme correspondence (i.e., monseir, oignon). Pseudowords were letters that could be pronounced in French without close orthographic neighbors. Thus, reading irregular words accessed phonological output lexicon and assembled phonological representations within the ventral stream, whereas pseudoword reading required sublexical orthography-to-phonology processing (Roux et al., 2012). Using this approach, the authors found that stimulation of anterior/inferior portion of left supramarginal gyrus resulted in pseudoword deficits, whereas stimulation of the left STG resulted in word deficits, highlighting that lexical and sublexical processes could be anatomically disassociated in "dual-stream" manner (Roux et al., 2012).

Direct electrical stimulation of the left basal posterotemporal cortex (BPTC), which includes the left middle and posterior fusiform gyrus and the posterior third of the inferior temporal gyrus, has also uncovered disassociations between naming and reading (Cohen et al., 2000; Dehaene et al., 2002; Dehaene and Cohen, 2011). Gil-Robles et al. (2013) found that stimulation of the BPTC resulted in deficits of reading short sentences but not articulatory or naming difficulties. During DES, patients reported difficulties with reading words and had to resort to "letter-by-letter" reading. The left middle fusiform gyrus (lmFG) has also been implicated in a series of patients undergoing DES and ECoG for epilepsy surgery (Hirshorn et al., 2016). With electrodes in the lmFG, patients were shown words, bodies, or scrambled objects, with words eliciting the strongest responses in the lmFG. Intraoperative stimulation of the lmFG was performed during language testing with orthographic stimuli (words and letters) and non-orthographic objects (faces and pictures). Supportive of a role for the lmFG in visual word form processing, stimulation of the lmFG specifically increased errors and response times to letter and word naming compared to non-orthographic stimuli. Furthermore, postoperative language assessment of one patient who underwent surgical resection of the left BPTC showed acquired alexia and its characteristic letter-by-letter reading (Hirshorn et al., 2016).

31.4 Adjunctive Multimodal Intraoperative Technologies

31.4.1 Task-Based and Resting-State Functional MRI

Functional MRI (fMRI) measures the oxy/deoxyhemoglobin ratio, sampled sequentially over time, to produce the blood oxygen level-dependent (BOLD) signal. fMRI can be used in a task-based or resting-state paradigm, with a temporal resolution of 3–5 s and spatial resolution of 1–1.5 mm (Volkow et al., 1997). In a task-based paradigm, motor or language responses are averaged to produce activation maps (Håberg et al., 2004; Khanna et al., 2015), and at some centers, Wada testing for language localization has been replaced by language-based fMRI (Wagner et al., 2012). However, task-based fMRI by definition is limited to brain functions that are represented by tasks, and certain patient factors such as baseline neurological deficits, age, cognitive impairment, or poor cooperation may preclude patient participation. The accuracy of fMRI varies widely when compared to the gold standard DES, with reported sensitivities and specificities of 5% to 100% and 0% to 98%, respectively, for language mapping. Much of the variation is from studies that have used arbitrary distance thresholds to determine accuracy (Ellis et al., 2020).

Resting-state fMRI (rs-fMRI) mitigates many of the limitations of task-based fMRI. Instead of actively participating in a task, data for rs-fMRI are acquired in a 10–15-min recording session with the patient lying still. Resting-state fMRI analyzes the correlations of very low-frequency (<0.1 Hz) BOLD signals across the brain, with the presumption that functionally connected brain regions demonstrate baseline synchronous activity when the brain is not engaged in any task (Biswal et al., 1995; Fox and Snyder, 2005). Validation of rs-fMRI in recapitulating task-based fMRI has been seen across many behavioral task-based paradigms, specifically those in motor, language, and visual tasks (Cordes et al., 2000; Smith et al., 2009). Resting-state fMRI possesses distinct advantages: multiple brain function networks can be extracted from the same imaging data set and acquisition can occur under sedation.

Resting-state fMRI has typically corresponded well when compared to task-based fMRI and DES. In general, rs-fMRI captures a broader activation of sensorimotor cortex, whereas task-based fMRI shows more focal responses, as driven by the specific task such as finger tapping (Dierker et al., 2017). Furthermore, rs-fMRI often includes cortical regions upstream of node of activity such that rs-fMRI often includes supplementary motor regions whereas DES primarily detects precentral gyrus activation. Resting-state fMRI has good sensitivity, but relatively less specificity, when compared to DES, with receiver-operative characteristic curves of 0.89 and 0.76 (AUC, areas under curve), for motor and language, respectively in adults (Mitchell et al., 2013), and an AUC of 0.77 for sensorimotor mapping in the pediatric population (Roland et al., 2019). The implication of rs-fMRI for language mapping is less clear. Resting-state fMRI operationally captures a far more distributed language network than DES, but whether each region is an active (as opposed to parallel or compensatory) pathway in language processing requires intraoperative DES, which itself may not be sensitive enough to detect language deficits beyond obvious speech arrest.

The main limitations of rs-fMRI remain the lack of direct neuronal activity and the selection of the resting state networks (RSNs). Seed-based connectivity requires individualized seed placement that often is precluded by mass effect from tumors, whereas RSNs from independent component analysis (ICA) are not standardized across patients and dependent on specific ICA settings to prevent "overmodeling" and split networks. Advances in supervised machine learning have the potential to address these issues, but are limited by the data used to train neural networks.

31.4.2 Diffusion Tensor Imaging

Diffusion tensor imaging images WM tracts by leveraging the diffusion properties of water molecules in neural tissue. In gray matter and CSF, water molecules diffuse randomly in Brownian motion (i.e., isotropically), whereas in WM, diffusion of water molecules is linearly bounded by the parallel axonal membranes traversing through the tissue (i.e., anisotropically). This anisotropy is mathematically represented by a 3D ellipsoid, termed the diffusion tensor, and then projected back onto the MRI (Beaulieu, 2002; Pierpaoli et al., 1996). Thus, DTI lacks any functional information but captures structural details about connectivity, with a spatial resolution of 2–2.5 mm (Zeineh et al., 2012). Tracts that are routinely imaged by DTI include corticospinal tracts, optic radiation (e.g., Meyer's loop), and language pathways, such as the arcuate fasiculus, superior longitudinal fasiculus, inferior longitudinal fasculus, and inferior frontal-occipital fasciculus.

The performance and clinical utility of DTI is constrained by its significant limitations. Compared to post-mortem dissections, Meyer's loop had a spatial precision of 1 mm (Sherbondy et al., 2008). Patients with loss of arcuate fasciculate fibers were twice as likely to suffer from postoperative aphasia (Negwer et al., 2018). Compared to DES, stimulation within 6 mm of a language fiber tract resulted in intraoperative dysphasia in 16 of 21 DES-positive language sites (Leclercq et al., 2010). Diffusion tensor imaging can also be used for surgical planning of intramedullary spinal cord tumors (Choudhri et al., 2014) and to differentiate glioblastoma from abscesses and metastases (Toh et al., 2011).

Because DTI is constructed indirectly by measurements of water molecule diffusion, lesions such as brain tumors or stroke can dramatically influence the diffusion properties, and hence distort the anatomy of the calculated fiber tracts (Duffau, 2014). Studies have shown significant differences in projected DTI tracts among software vendors (Feigl et al., 2014), and accurately located DTI tracts do not always result in clinically reliable fiber diameters (Kinoshita et al., 2005). Even the seed region of interest (ROI) is reliant on physician placement, although theoretically one could functionally combine ROIs as assessed by fMRI to more holistically ground DTI projections (Kleiser et al., 2010; Schonberg et al., 2006).

31.4.3 Magentoencephalography

Unlike DTI and fMRI, MEG directly measures neuronal activity by capturing the minuscule change in magnetic field generated by postsynaptic currents of neocortical pyramidal neurons (Hari et al., 2000). With sensitive magnetic field detectors, called superconductor quantum interference devices (SQUIDs), capable of detecting 10–100 femtotesla (10 billion times weaker than the Earth's magnetic field), MEG captures a spatial resolution of 2–3 mm and matches EEG in temporal resolution (<1 mm) (Tovar-Spinoza et al., 2008). It achieves such high fidelity because magnetic signals are unaffected by intervening tissues between the probe and neuron, and because the probe is not in physical contact with the scalp, it is less immune to muscle artifacts (Baillet, 2017). Indeed, the millisecond temporal resolution at millimeter resolution across the entire brain, achieved entirely non-invasively, is a hallmark of MEG compared to other functional mapping techniques.

Used primarily for preoperative localization of epileptogenic foci (Englot et al., 2015; Hamandi et al., 2016; Tovar-Spinoza et al., 2008), MEG has also been shown to have high concordance with WADA for hemispheric dominance (Doss et al., 2009; Papanicolaou et al., 2004). More recent work has leveraged resting-state MEG functional connectivity as a means for preoperative tumor evaluation (Guggisberg et al., 2008). Patients with intrinsic brain tumors display disrupted functional connectivity, which also correlate with global neurocognitive dysfunction (Bartolomei et al., 2006a, 2006b; Bosma et al., 2008a, 2008b). Specifically, functional brain mapping of low functional connectivity (LFC) sites were found to have a 100% negative predictive value for presence of eloquent cortex during DES (Martino et al., 2011), while motor-evoked MEG signals were within 1-cm margins of DES-positive motor sites (Tarapore et al., 2012b). Furthermore, tumor patients with resection of LFC tissue had 0% rate of new neurological deficit at 6-month follow-up (Tarapore et al., 2012a). Interestingly, the degree of resected high-functional connectivity (but DES-negative) tissue correlated with auditory naming or language syntactic deficits, suggesting that MEG may be more sensitive than DES in detecting higher-order language processing (Lee et al., 2020).

Limitations of MEG center primarily upon the capital expenditure necessary to house the SQUID and shield it from surrounding magnetic interference. Given that MEG is still in its infancy in terms of clinical application, institutions typically fund MEG as a strategic research investment without the ability to recover appreciable clinical revenue. Another limitation lies in the rich and complex nature of MEG signals, which require sophisticated post-acquisition processing pipelines to isolate and interpret biological signals from MEG source data (Baillet, 2017).

31.4.4 Intraoperative Imaging

A primary limitation to preoperative functional neuro-imaging is the brain shift that results following craniotomy and tumor debulking. Studies have estimated upwards of 5 mm of target registration errors may occur (Stieglitz et al., 2013). Intraoperative imaging aims to address these drawbacks. Using charge-coupled device cameras that capture the emission spectrum during metabolic changes in cerebral blood volume and oxygenation that occurs with neuronal activity, IOI is able to directly project functional maps onto the views from intraoperative microscopes while patients undergo awake craniotomy and functional testing.

Although IOI generally has shown good concordance to DES, few studies have rigorously assessed intermodality accuracy (Cannestra et al., 2000, 2004; Pouratian et al., 2000). A recent study by Oelschlagel et al. (2020) showed "high agreement" between IOI-generated functional maps and DES-positive motor sites in 2/2 patients, while only 1/8 patients had high concordance between IOI and DES for language tasks. These authors concluded that the use of IOI for motor site identification seemed to be beneficial given its highly resolved intraoperative spatial maps, while the technique proved too unspecific for language localization.

31.5 Conclusion

Intraoperative and extraoperative brain mapping strategies are commonly applied to maximize the extent of lesion resection while minimizing morbidity. All available surgical tools and techniques rely on the principles of cognitive neuroscience. The gold standard for intraoperative identification of cortical and subcortical functional regions is DES; however, functional imaging using magnetoencephalography, diffusion tensor imaging MRI, and resting-state functional MRI may aid surgical planning and intraoperative decision making.

References

Abel TJ, Rhone AE, Nourski KV, et al. Direct physiologic evidence of a heteromodal convergence region for proper naming in human left anterior temporal lobe. *J Neurosci* 2015;**35**:1513–20. https://doi.org/10.1523/JNEUROSCI.3387-14.2015.

Anderson JM, Gilmore R, Roper S, et al. Conduction aphasia and the arcuate fasciculus: a reexamination of the Wernicke–Geschwind model. *Brain Lang* 1999;**70**:1–12. https://doi.org/10.1006/brln.1999.2135.

Baillet S. Magnetoencephalography for brain electrophysiology and imaging. *Nat Neurosci* 2017;**20**:327–39. https://doi.org/10.1038/nn.4504.

Baldo JV, Katseff S, Dronkers NF. Brain regions underlying repetition and auditory-verbal short-term memory deficits in aphasia: evidence from voxel-based lesion symptom mapping. *Aphasiology* 2012;**26**:338–54. https://doi.org/10.1080/02687038.2011.602391.

Bartolomei F, Bosma I, Klein M, et al. How do brain tumors alter functional connectivity? A magnetoencephalography study. *Ann Neurol* 2006a;**59**:128–38. https://doi.org/10.1002/ana.20710.

Bartolomei F, Bosma I, Klein M, et al. Disturbed functional connectivity in brain tumour patients: evaluation by graph analysis of synchronization matrices. *Clin Neurophysiol* 2006b;**117**:2039–49. https://doi.org/10.1016/j.clinph.2006.05.018.

Beaulieu C. The basis of anisotropic water diffusion in the nervous system – a technical review. *NMR Biomed* 2002;**15**:435–55. https://doi.org/10.1002/nbm.782.

Beauvois MF, Dérouesné J. Phonological alexia: three dissociations. *J Neurol Neurosurg Psychiatry* 1979;**42**:1115–24. https://doi.org/10.1136/jnnp.42.12.1115.

Bello L, Gallucci M, Fava M, et al. Intraoperative subcortical language tract mapping guides surgical removal of gliomas involving speech areas. *Neurosurgery* 2007;**60**:67–80; discussion 80. https://doi.org/10.1227/01.NEU.0000249206.58601.DE.

Bello L, Riva M, Fava E, et al. Tailoring neurophysiological strategies with clinical context enhances resection and safety and expands indications in gliomas involving motor pathways. *Neuro Oncol* 2014;**16**:1110–28. https://doi.org/10.1093/neuonc/not327

Benzagmout M, Gatignol P, Duffau H. Resection of World Health Organization Grade II gliomas involving Broca's area: methodological and functional considerations. *Neurosurgery* 2007;**61**:741–52; discussion 752. https://doi.org/10.1227/01.NEU.0000298902.69473.77.

Biswal B, Zerrin Yetkin F, Haughton VM, Hyde JS. Functional connectivity in the motor cortex of resting human brain using echo-planar MRI. *Magn Reson Med* 1995;**34**:537–41. https://doi.org/10.1002/mrm.1910340409.

Bosma I, Douw L, Bartolomei F, et al. Synchronized brain activity and neurocognitive function in patients with low-grade glioma: a magnetoencephalography study. *Neuro Oncol* 2008a;**10**:734–44. https://doi.org/10.1215/15228517-2008-034

Bosma I, Stam CJ, Douw L, et al. The influence of low-grade glioma on resting state oscillatory brain activity: a magnetoencephalography study. *J Neurooncol* 2008b;**88**:77–85. https://doi.org/10.1007/s11060-008-9535-3.

Buchsbaum BR, Baldo J, Okada K, et al. Conduction aphasia, sensory-motor integration, and phonological short-term memory – an aggregate analysis of lesion and fMRI data. *Brain*

Lang 2011;**119**:119–28. https://doi.org/10.1016/j
.bandl.2010.12.001.

Cannestra AF, Bookheimer SY, Pouratian N, et al. Temporal
and topographical characterization of language cortices using
intraoperative optical intrinsic signals. *Neuroimage*
2000;**12**:41–54. https://doi.org/10.1006/nimg.2000.0597.

Cannestra AF, Pouratian N, Forage J, Bookheimer SY,
Martin NA, Toga AW. Functional magnetic resonance imaging
and optical imaging for dominant-hemisphere perisylvian
arteriovenous malformations. *Neurosurgery* 2004;**55**:804–12;
discussion 812. https://doi.org/10.1227/01
.neu.0000137654.27826.71.

Catani M, Jones DK, ffytche DH. Perisylvian language networks
of the human brain. *Ann Neurol* 2005;**57**:8–16. https://doi.org
/10.1002/ana.20319.

Choudhri AF, Whitehead MT, Klimo P, Montgomery BK,
Boop FA. Diffusion tensor imaging to guide surgical planning in
intramedullary spinal cord tumors in children. *Neuroradiology*
2014;**56**:169–74. https://doi.org/10.1007/s00234-013-1316-9.

Cohen L, Dehaene S, Naccache L, et al. The visual word form area:
spatial and temporal characterization of an initial stage of reading
in normal subjects and posterior split-brain patients. *Brain*
2000;**123**:291–307. https://doi.org/10.1093/brain/123.2.291.

Coltheart M, Rastle K, Perry C, Langdon R, Ziegler J. DRC:
a dual route cascaded model of visual word recognition and
reading aloud. *Psychol Rev* 2001;**108**:204–56. https://doi.org/10
.1037/0033-295x.108.1.204.

Cordes D, Haughton VM, Arfanakis K, et al. Mapping
functionally related regions of brain with functional
connectivity MR imaging. *Am J Neuroradiol* 2000;**21**:1636–44.

Corina DP, Loudermilk BC, Detwiler L, Martin RF, Brinkley JF,
Ojemann G. Analysis of naming errors during cortical
stimulation mapping: implications for models of language
representation. *Brain Lang* 2010;**115**:101–12. https://doi.org/10
.1016/j.bandl.2010.04.001.

Damasio AR, Damasio H. The anatomic basis of pure alexia.
Neurology 1983;**33**:1573. https://doi.org/10.1212/wnl.33.12
.1573.

Damasio H, Damasio AR. The anatomical basis of conduction
aphasia. *Brain* 1980;**103**:337–50. https://doi.org/10.1093/brain/
103.2.337.

De Witt Hamer PC, Robles SG, Zwinderman AH, Duffau H,
Berger MS. Impact of intraoperative stimulation brain mapping
on glioma surgery outcome: a meta-analysis. *J Clin Oncol*
2012;**30**:2559–65. https://doi.org/10.1200/JCO.2011.38.4818.

Dehaene S, Cohen L. The unique role of the visual word form
area in reading. *Trends Cogn Sci* 2011;**15**:254–62. https://doi.org
/10.1016/j.tics.2011.04.003.

Dehaene S, Le Clec'H G, Poline JB, Le Bihan D, Cohen L. The
visual word form area: a prelexical representation of visual words
in the fusiform gyrus. *Neuroreport* 2002;**13**:321–5. https://doi.org
/10.1097/00001756-200203040-00015.

Dell GS, Schwartz MF, Nozari N, Faseyitan O, Branch Coslett H.
Voxel-based lesion-parameter mapping: identifying the neural
correlates of a computational model of word production.
Cognition 2013;**128**:380–96. https://doi.org/10.1016/j
.cognition.2013.05.007.

Dierker D, Roland JL, Kamran M, et al. Resting-state functional
magnetic resonance imaging in presurgical functional mapping:
sensorimotor localization. *Neuroimaging Clin N Am*
2017;**27**:621–33. https://doi.org/10.1016/j.nic.2017.06.011.

Doss RC, Zhang W, Risse GL, Dickens DL. Lateralizing
language with magnetic source imaging: validation based on the
Wada test. *Epilepsia* 2009;**50**:2242–8. https://doi.org/10.1111/j
.1528-1167.2009.02242.x.

Duffau H. Lessons from brain mapping in surgery for low-grade
glioma: insights into associations between tumour and brain
plasticity. *Lancet Neurol* 2005;**4**:476–86. https://doi.org/10.1016
/S1474-4422(05)70140-X.

Duffau H. The anatomo-functional connectivity of language
revisited: new insights provided by electrostimulation and
tractography. *Neuropsychologia* 2008;**46**:927–34. https://doi.org
/10.1016/j.neuropsychologia.2007.10.025.

Duffau H. The dangers of magnetic resonance imaging
diffusion tensor tractography in brain surgery. *World
Neurosurg* 2014;**81**:56–8. https://doi.org/10.1016/j
.wneu.2013.01.116.

Duffau H, Capelle L, Denvil D, et al. Usefulness of
intraoperative electrical subcortical mapping during surgery for
low-grade gliomas located within eloquent brain regions:
functional results in a consecutive series of 103 patients.
J Neurosurg 2003;**98**:764–78. https://doi.org/10.3171/jns
.2003.98.4.0764.

Duffau H, Herbet G, Moritz-Gasser S. Toward a
pluri-component, multimodal, and dynamic organization of the
ventral semantic stream in humans: lessons from stimulation
mapping in awake patients. *Front Syst Neurosci* 2013;**7**:44. https://
doi.org/10.3389/fnsys.2013.00044

Duffau H, Moritz-Gasser S, Mandonnet E. A re-examination
of neural basis of language processing: proposal of a dynamic
hodotopical model from data provided by brain stimulation
mapping during picture naming. *Brain Lang* 2014;**131**:1–10.
https://doi.org/10.1016/j.bandl.2013.05.011.

Ellis DG, White ML, Hayasaka S, Warren DE, Wilson TW,
Aizenberg MR. Accuracy analysis of fMRI and MEG activations
determined by intraoperative mapping. *Neurosurg Focus*
2020;**48**:E13. https://doi.org/10.3171/2019.11.FOCUS19784.

Englot DJ, Nagarajan SS, Imber BS, et al. Epileptogenic zone
localization using magnetoencephalography predicts seizure
freedom in epilepsy surgery. *Epilepsia* 2015;**56**:949–58. https://
doi.org/10.1111/epi.13002.

Feigl GC, Hiergeist W, Fellner C, et al. Magnetic resonance
imaging diffusion tensor tractography: evaluation of anatomic
accuracy of different fiber tracking software packages. *World*

Neurosurg 2014;**81**:144–50. https://doi.org/10.1016/j .wneu.2013.01.004.

Fernández Coello A, Moritz-Gasser S, Martino J, Martinoni M, Matsuda R, Duffau H. Selection of intraoperative tasks for awake mapping based on relationships between tumor location and functional networks. *J Neurosurg* 2013;**119**:1380–94. https://doi .org/10.3171/2013.6.JNS122470.

Fiez JA, Tranel D, Seager-Frerichs D, Damasio H. Specific reading and phonological processing deficits are associated with damage to the left frontal operculum. *Cortex* 2006;**42**:624–43. https://doi.org/10.1016/s0010-9452(08)70399-x.

Forseth KJ, Kadipasaoglu CM, Conner CR, Hickok G, Knight RT, Tandon N. A lexical semantic hub for heteromodal naming in middle fusiform gyrus. *Brain* 2018;**141**:2112–26. https://doi.org/10.1093/brain/awy120.

Fox MD, Snyder AZ, Vincent JL, Corbetta M, Van Essen DC, Raichle ME. The human brain is intrinsically organized into dynamic, anticorrelated functional networks. *Proc Natl Acad Sci U S A* 2005;**102**(27):9673–8. https://doi.org/10.1073/pnas .0504136102.

Fridriksson J, Kjartansson O, Morgan PS, et al. Impaired speech repetition and left parietal lobe damage. *J Neurosci* 2010;**30**:11057–61. https://doi.org/10.1523/JNEUROSCI.1120- 10.2010.

Funnell E. Phonological processes in reading: new evidence from acquired dyslexia. *Br J Psychol* 1983;**74**:159–80. https://doi .org/10.1111/j.2044-8295.1983.tb01851.x.

Geschwind N. Disconnexion syndromes in animals and man. I.*Brain* 1965;**88**:237–94. https://doi.org/10.1093/brain/88 .2.237.

Gil-Robles S, Carvallo A, Jimenez MM, et al. Double dissociation between visual recognition and picture naming: a study of the visual language connectivity using tractography and brain stimulation. *Neurosurgery* 2013;**72**:678–86. https:// doi.org/10.1227/NEU.0b013e318282a361.

Gogos AJ, Young JS, Morshed RA, et al. Triple motor mapping: transcranial, bipolar, and monopolar mapping for supratentorial glioma resection adjacent to motor pathways. *J Neurosurg* 2020;**134**(6):172837. https://doi.org/10.3171/2020.3 .JNS193434.

Gonen T, Grossman R, Sitt R, et al. Tumor location and IDH1 mutation may predict intraoperative seizures during awake craniotomy. *J Neurosurg* 2014;**121**:1133–8. https://doi.org/10 .3171/2014.7.JNS132657.

Goodglass H. Diagnosis of conduction aphasia. In Kohn SE (Ed.), *Conduction Aphasia*. New York: Psychology Press, 1992, pp. 49–60.

Graves WW, Grabowski TJ, Mehta S, Gupta P. The left posterior superior temporal gyrus participates specifically in accessing lexical phonology. *J Cogn Neurosci* 2008;**20**:1698–710. https:// doi.org/10.1162/jocn.2008.20113.

Guggisberg AG, Honma SM, Findlay AM, et al. Mapping functional connectivity in patients with brain lesions. *Ann Neurol* 2008;**63**:193–203. https://doi.org/10.1002/ana.21224.

Håberg A, Kvistad KA, Unsgård G, Haraldseth O. Preoperative blood oxygen level-dependent functional magnetic resonance imaging in patients with primary brain tumors: clinical application and outcome. *Neurosurgery* 2004;**54**:902–15. https:// doi.org/10.1227/01.neu.0000114510.05922.f8.

Hamandi K, Routley BC, Koelewijn L, Singh KD. Non-invasive brain mapping in epilepsy: applications from magnetoencephalography. *J Neurosci Methods* 2016;**260**: 283–91. https://doi.org/10.1016/j.jneumeth.2015.11.012.

Hamberger MJ, Goodman RR, Perrine K, Tamny T. Anatomic dissociation of auditory and visual naming in the lateral temporal cortex. *Neurology* 2001;**56**:56–61. https://doi.org/10 .1212/wnl.56.1.56.

Hamberger MJ, Seidel WT, Mckhann GM, Perrine K, Goodman RR. Brain stimulation reveals critical auditory naming cortex. *Brain* 2005;**128**:2742–9. https://doi.org/10.1093 /brain/awh621

Han SJ, Morshed RA, Troncon I, et al. Subcortical stimulation mapping of descending motor pathways for perirolandic gliomas: assessment of morbidity and functional outcome in 702 cases. *J Neurosurg* 2018;**131**:201–08. https://doi.org/10.3171 /2018.3.JNS172494.

Hari R, Levänen S, Raij T. Timing of human cortical functions during cognition: role of MEG. *Trends Cogn Sci* 2000;**4**:455–62. https://doi.org/10.1016/s1364-6613(00)01549-7.

Hickok G, Buchsbaum B, Humphries C, Muftuler T. Auditory- motor interaction revealed by fMRI: speech, music, and working memory in area Spt. *J Cogn Neurosci* 2003;**15**:673–82. https://doi.org/10.1162/089892903322307393.

Hickok G, Poeppel D. Towards a functional neuroanatomy of speech perception. *Trends Cogn Sci* 2000;**4**:131–8. https://doi .org/ 10.1016/s1364-6613(00)01463-7.

Hickok G, Poeppel D. Dorsal and ventral streams: a framework for understanding aspects of the functional anatomy of language. *Cognition* 2004;**92**:67–99. https://doi.org/10.1016/j .cognition.2003.10.011.

Hirshorn EA, Li Y, Ward MJ, Richardson RM, Fiez JA, Ghuman AS. Decoding and disrupting left midfusiform gyrus activity during word reading. *Proc Natl Acad Sci U S A* 2016;**113**:8162–7. https://doi.org/10.1073/pnas.1604126113.

Jobard G, Crivello F, Tzourio-Mazoyer N. Evaluation of the dual route theory of reading: a metanalysis of 35 neuroimaging studies. *Neuroimage* 2003;**20**:693–712. https://doi.org/10.1016/ S1053-8119(03)00343-4.

Keles GE, Lundin DA, Lamborn KR, Chang EF, Ojemann G, Berger MS. Intraoperative subcortical stimulation mapping for hemispherical perirolandic gliomas located within or adjacent to the descending motor pathways: evaluation of morbidity and assessment of functional outcome in 294 patients. *J Neurosurg* 2004;**100**:369–75. https://doi.org/10.3171/jns.2004.100.3.0369.

Khanna N, Altmeyer W, Zhuo J, Steven A. Functional neuroimaging: fundamental principles and clinical applications. *Neuroradiol J* 2015;**28**:87 96. https://doi.org/10.1177 /1971400915576311.

Kinoshita M, Yamada K, Hashimoto N, et al. Fiber-tracking does not accurately estimate size of fiber bundle in pathological condition: initial neurosurgical experience using neuronavigation and subcortical white matter stimulation. *Neuroimage* 2005;**25**:424–9. https://doi.org/10.1016/j .neuroimage.2004.07.076.

Kleiser R, Staempfli P, Valavanis A, Boesiger P, Kollias S. Impact of fMRI-guided advanced DTI fiber tracking techniques on their clinical applications in patients with brain tumors. *Neuroradiology* 2010;**52**:37–46. https://doi.org/10.1007/s00234-009-0539-2.

Leclercq D, Duffau H, Delmaire C, et al. Comparison of diffusion tensor imaging tractography of language tracts and intraoperative subcortical stimulations. *J Neurosurg* 2010;**112**:503–11. https://doi.org/10.3171/2009.8.JNS09558.

Lee AT, Faltermeier C, Morshed RA, et al. The impact of high functional connectivity network hub resection on language task performance in adult low- and high-grade glioma. *J Neurosurg* 2020;**134**(3):1102–112. https://doi.org/10.3171/2020 .1.JNS192267.

Leonard MK, Cai R, Babiak MC, Ren A, Chang EF. The peri-Sylvian cortical network underlying single word repetition revealed by electrocortical stimulation and direct neural recordings. *Brain Lang* 2019;**193**:58–72. https://doi.org/10.1016 /j.bandl.2016.06.001.

Magill ST, Han SJ, Li J, Berger MS. Resection of primary motor cortex tumors: feasibility and surgical outcomes. *J Neurosurg* 2018;**129**:961–72. https://doi.org/10.3171/2017 .5.JNS163045.

Makris N, Kennedy DN, McInerney S, et al. Segmentation of subcomponents within the superior longitudinal fascicle in humans: a quantitative, in vivo, DT-MRI study. *Cereb Cortex* 2005;**15**:854–69. https://doi.org/10.1093/cercor/bhh186

Martino J, De Witt Hamer PC, Berger MS, et al. Analysis of the subcomponents and cortical terminations of the perisylvian superior longitudinal fasciculus: a fiber dissection and DTI tractography study. *Brain Struct Funct* 2013;**218**:105–21. https:// doi.org/10.1007/s00429-012-0386-5.

Martino J, Honma SM, Findlay AM, et al. Resting functional connectivity in patients with brain tumors in eloquent areas. *Ann Neurol* 2011;**69**:521–32. https://doi.org/10.1002/ana.22167.

Mitchell TJ, Hacker CD, Breshears JD, et al. A novel data-driven approach to preoperative mapping of functional cortex using resting-state functional magnetic resonance imaging. *Neurosurgery* 2013;**73**:969–83. https://doi.org/10.1227/NEU .0000000000000141.

Moritz-Gasser S, Duffau H. The anatomo-functional connectivity of word repetition: insights provided by awake brain tumor surgery. *Front Hum Neurosci* 2013;**7**:405. https:// doi.org/10.3389/fnhum.2013.00405.

Negwer C, Beurskens E, Sollmann N, et al. Loss of subcortical language pathways correlates with surgery-related aphasia in patients with brain tumor: an investigation via repetitive navigated transcranial magnetic stimulation-based diffusion tensor imaging fiber tracking. *World Neurosurg* 2018;**111**: e806–18. https://doi.org/10.1016/j.wneu.2017.12.163.

Nossek E, Matot I, Shahar T, et al. Intraoperative seizures during awake craniotomy: incidence and consequences: analysis of 477 patients. *Neurosurgery* 2013;**73**:135–40; discussion 140. https://doi.org/10.1227/01.neu.0000429847.91707.97.

Oelschlägel M, Meyer T, Morgenstern U, et al. Mapping of language and motor function during awake neurosurgery with intraoperative optical imaging. *Neurosurg Focus* 2020;**48**:E3. https://doi.org/10.3171/2019.11.FOCUS19759.

Ojemann G. Intraoperative investigations of the neurobiology of reading. In Euler CV, Lundberg I, Llinás RR (Eds.), *Basic Mechanisms in Cognition and Language with Special Reference to Phonological Problems in Dyslexia.* Elsevier, 1998: p. 288.

Ojemann G, Mateer C. Human language cortex: localization of memory, syntax, and sequential motor-phoneme identification systems. *Science* 1979;**205**:1401–03. https://doi.org/10.1126/sci ence.472757.

Ojemann G, Ojemann J, Lettich E, Berger M. Cortical language localization in left, dominant hemisphere. An electrical stimulation mapping investigation in 117 patients. *J Neurosurg* 1989;**71**:316–26. https://doi.org/10.3171/jns.1989.71.3.0316.

Papanicolaou AC, Simos PG, Castillo EM, et al. Magnetocephalography: a noninvasive alternative to the Wada procedure. *J Neurosurg* 2004;**100**:867–76. https://doi.org/10 .3171/jns.2004.100.5.0867.

Parker J, Prejawa S, Hope TM et al. Sensory-to-motor integration during auditory repetition: a combined fMRI and lesion study. *Front Hum Neurosci* 2014;**8**:24. https://doi.org/10 .3389/fnhum.2014.00024.

Paulesu E, Frith CD, Frackowiak RS. The neural correlates of the verbal component of working memory. *Nature* 1993;**362**:342–5. https://doi.org/10.1038/362342a0.

Penfield W, Roberts L. *Speech and Brain Mechanisms.* Princeton: Princeton University Press, 1959.

Pierpaoli C, Jezzard P, Basser PJ, Barnett A, Di Chiro G. Diffusion tensor MR imaging of the human brain. *Radiology* 1996;**201**:637–48. https://doi.org/10.1148/radiology .201.3.8939209.

Plans G, Fernández-Conejero I, Rifà-Ros X, Fernández-Coello A, Rosselló A, Gabarrós A. Evaluation of the high-frequency monopolar stimulation technique for mapping and monitoring the corticospinal tract in patients with supratentorial gliomas. A proposal for intraoperative management based on neurophysiological data analysis in a series of 92 patients. *Neurosurgery* 2017;**81**:585–94. https://doi.org/10.1093/neuros/nyw087.

Plaza M, Gatignol P, Cohen H, Berger B, Duffau H. A Discrete area within the left dorsolateral prefrontal cortex involved in visual–verbal incongruence judgment. *Cerebr Cortex* 2007;**18**:1253–9. https://doi.org/10.1093/cercor/bhm169.

Pouratian N, Bookheimer SY, O'Farrell AM, et al. Optical imaging of bilingual cortical representations. Case report. *J Neurosurg* 2000;**93**:676–81. https://doi.org/10.3171/jns.2000.93.4.0676.

Prabhu SS, Gasco J, Tummala S, Weinberg JS, Rao G. Intraoperative magnetic resonance imaging-guided tractography with integrated monopolar subcortical functional mapping for resection of brain tumors. Clinical article. *J Neurosurg* 2011;**114**:719–26. https://doi.org/10.3171/2010.9.JNS10481.

Quigg M, Fountain NB. Conduction aphasia elicited by stimulation of the left posterior superior temporal gyrus. *J Neurol Neurosurg Psychiatry* 1999;**66**:393–6. https://doi.org/10.1136/jnnp.66.3.393.

Quigg M, Geldmacher DS, Elias WJ. Conduction aphasia as a function of the dominant posterior perisylvian cortex. Report of two cases. *J Neurosurg* 2006;**104**:845–8. https://doi.org/10.3171/jns.2006.104.5.845.

Rahman M, Abbatematteo J, De Leo EK, et al. The effects of new or worsened postoperative neurological deficits on survival of patients with glioblastoma. *J Neurosurg* 2017;**127**:123–31. https://doi.org/10.3171/2016.7.JNS16396.

Rapcsak SZ, Beeson PM, Henry ML, et al. Phonological dyslexia and dysgraphia: cognitive mechanisms and neural substrates. *Cortex* 2009;**45**:575–91. https://doi.org/10.1016/j.cortex.2008.04.006.

Rogalsky C, Poppa T, Chen KH, et al. Speech repetition as a window on the neurobiology of auditory-motor integration for speech: a voxel-based lesion symptom mapping study. *Neuropsychologia* 2015;**71**:18–27. https://doi.org/10.1016/j.neuropsychologia.2015.03.012.

Roland JL, Hacker CD, Snyder AZ, et al. A comparison of resting state functional magnetic resonance imaging to invasive electrocortical stimulation for sensorimotor mapping in pediatric patients. *NeuroImage Clin* 2019;**23**:101850. https://doi.org/10.1016/j.nicl.2019.101850.

Roux FE, Durand JB, Djidjeli I, Moyse E, Giussani C. Variability of intraoperative electrostimulation parameters in conscious individuals: language cortex. *J Neurosurg* 2017;**126**:1641–52. https://doi.org/10.3171/2016.4.JNS152434.

Roux FE, Durand JB, Jucla M, Réhault E, Reddy M, Démonet JF. Segregation of lexical and sub-lexical reading processes in the left perisylvian cortex. *PLoS One* 2012;**7**:e50665. https://doi.org/10.1371/journal.pone.0050665.

Roux FE, Lubrano V, Lauwers-Cances V, Trémoulet M, Mascott CR, Démonet JF. Intra-operative mapping of cortical areas involved in reading in mono- and bilingual patients. *Brain* 2004;**127**:1796–810. https://doi.org/10.1093/brain/awh204.

Sanai N, Mirzadeh Z, Berger MS. Functional outcome after language mapping for glioma resection. *N Engl J Med* 2008;**358**:18–27. https://doi.org/10.1056/NEJMoa067819.

Saur D, Kreher BW, Schnell S, et al. Ventral and dorsal pathways for language. *Proc Natl Acad Sci U S A* 2008;**105**:18035–40. https://doi.org/10.1073/pnas.0805234105.

Schonberg T, Pianka P, Hendler T, Pasternak O, Assaf Y. Characterization of displaced white matter by brain tumors using combined DTI and fMRI. *Neuroimage* 2006;**30**:1100–11. https://doi.org/10.1016/j.neuroimage.2005.11.015.

Sherbondy AJ, Dougherty RF, Napel S, Wandell BA. Identifying the human optic radiation using diffusion imaging and fiber tractography. *J Vis* 2008;**8**:12.1–1211. https://doi.org/10.1167/8.10.12.

Sierpowska J, Gabarrós A, Fernandez-Coello A, et al. Words are not enough: nonword repetition as an indicator of arcuate fasciculus integrity during brain tumor resection. *J Neurosurg* 2017;**126**:435–45.

Smith SM, Fox PT, Miller KL, et al. Correspondence of the brain's functional architecture during activation and rest. *Proc Natl Acad Sci* 2009;**106**:13040–5. https://doi.org/10.1073/pnas.0905267106.

Snodgrass JG, Vanderwart M. A standardized set of 260 pictures: norms for name agreement, image agreement, familiarity, and visual complexity. *J Exp Psychol Hum Learn* 1980;**6**:174–215. https://doi.org/10.1037//0278-7393.6.2.174.

Stieglitz LH, Fichtner J, Andres R, et al. The silent loss of neuronavigation accuracy: a systematic retrospective analysis of factors influencing the mismatch of frameless stereotactic systems in cranial neurosurgery. *Neurosurgery* 2013;**72**:796–807. https://doi.org/10.1227/NEU.0b013e318287072d.

Szelényi A, Senft C, Jardan M, et al. Intra-operative subcortical electrical stimulation: a comparison of two methods. *Clin Neurophysiol* 2011;**122**:1470–5. https://doi.org/10.1016/j.clinph.2010.12.055.

Tarapore PE, Martino J, Guggisberg AG, et al. Magnetoencephalographic imaging of resting-state functional connectivity predicts postsurgical neurological outcome in brain gliomas. *Neurosurgery* 2012a;**71**:1012–22. https://doi.org/10.1227/NEU.0b013e31826d2b78.

Tarapore PE, Tate MC, Findlay AM et al. Preoperative multimodal motor mapping: a comparison of magnetoencephalography imaging, navigated transcranial magnetic stimulation, and direct cortical stimulation. *J Neurosurg* 2012b;**117**:354–62. https://doi.org/10.3171/2012.5.JNS112124.

Toh CH, Wei KC, Ng SH, Wan YL, Lin CP, Castillo M. Differentiation of brain abscesses from necrotic glioblastomas and cystic metastatic brain tumors with diffusion tensor imaging. *Am J Neuroradiol* 2011;**32**:1646–51. https://doi.org/10.3174/ajnr.A2581.

Tovar-Spinoza ZS, Ochi A, Rutka JT, Go C, Otsubo H. The role of magnetoencephalography in epilepsy surgery. *Neurosurg Focus* 2008;**25**:E16. https://doi.org/10.3171/FOC/2008/25/9/E16.

Volkow ND, Rosen B, Farde L. Imaging the living human brain: magnetic resonance imaging and positron emission tomography. *Proc Natl Acad Sci U S A* 1997;**94**:2787–8. https://doi.org/10.1073/pnas.94.7.2787.

Wagner K, Hader C, Metternich B, Buschmann F, Schwarzwald R, Schulze-Bonhage A. Who needs a Wada test? Present clinical indications for amobarbital procedures. *J Neurol Neurosurg Psychiatry* 2012;**83**:503–09. https://doi.org/10.1136/jnnp-2011-300417.

Warrington EK, Shallice T. Word-form dyslexia. *Brain* 1980;**103**:99–112. https://doi.org/10.1093/brain/103.1.99.

Young JS, Morshed RA, Mansoori Z, Cha S, Berger MS. Disruption of frontal aslant tract is not associated with long-term postoperative language deficits. *World Neurosurg* 2020;**133**:192–5. https://doi.org/10.1016/j.wneu.2019.09.128.

Zeineh MM, Holdsworth S, Skare S, Atlas SW, Bammer R. Ultra-high resolution diffusion tensor imaging of the microscopic pathways of the medial temporal lobe. *Neuroimage* 2012;**62**:2065–82. https://doi.org/10.1016/j.neuroimage.2012.05.065.

Index